Comments about *Everlasting Health*

and *The Truth About Children's Health*   by Robert Bernardini, M.S.

"This book is a masterpiece! A brilliant combination of modern science and innate wisdom, *Everlasting Health* is a compendium of invaluable information, resources, and references. Bernardini unravels the complexities, misunderstandings, and deceptions in our modern health-care system, and serves up a compelling, original, and workable recipe for health. This book will save you money and can save your life and preserve life for our future generations."

Dale Paula T⌐⌐"

R⌐⌐   ert

"This is the best health book I've ever   ɔrdered
to friends and family – that's how impo

Do

"This is a vitally important book. The autʰ   ⌐ᵤₑ ɲis research and has discovered the probable causes for most illnesses and diseases. He then shows the courage to confront big business, the government, and the medical establishment, and reveals the misinformation that is propagated due to greed and power. He exposes the numerous dangers in our food supply and environment and then explains in clear and understandable English how to live to achieve optimal health. He especially emphasizes how crucial a nutritious diet and clean environment are for the proper growth and development of infants and children. The fundamental theme throughout the book: We must live by the laws of nature in order to stay or become healthy. I think Robert's books are excellent!"

Tracy Cousins, M.D., Pathologist

"I used to spend about $200 a month on supplements. Since reading your book, last month I spent $0 and I feel better than ever!"

Stan J, Maryland

"I thought your book was magnificent! It should be required reading in every school!"   W.E. Rose, California

" You are to be commended for all the years you have worked so hard to improve the health of mankind."   A.W. Thompson, Kentucky

"Robert's new book, *Everlasting Health*, is astonishingly comprehensive and really an encyclopedia of how to attain good health. I recommend you read it cover-to-cover with a highlighter and note pad handy. Do you need information about heart disease, arthritis, cancer, diabetes, autism, asthma, ADHD, or memory problems? This book has all of these and a great deal more. It concentrates on helping you address these problems in a supportive, holistic way, while at the same time shedding light on the oftentimes damaging effects of mainstream medical practices and drugs. Robert references an amazingly wide range of scientific research for validation which will allow the reader to prove to his or her physician, or any other

non-believer, that what's in this book is not hocus-pocus, but is indeed based on valid science. The most damaging thing you could do to your health might very well be to not read this book!"   David Getoff, CCN, CTN, CNC, FAAIM
Vice president of the non-profit Price-
Pottenger Nutrition Foundation

"Positively one of the best books of the millennium. This may look like an ordinary book, but it is really a health encyclopedia with important information worth reading and re-reading. As a parent, guardian, or practitioner, you can make you child's future brighter and healthier. Free from physical, mental, and emotional disease that have threatened our children for years. As a holistic dentist for the past 32 years I have been treating children nutritionally not only for their dental needs but as a whole person, head, mind, and body. Important concepts are highlighted in my favorite sections called Food for Thought. Robert has put more information in one book than you could possibly ask for."
Steven N. Green, DDS

"The author fearlessly addresses an array of controversial topics including birth defects, infertility, soy, vaccines, and SIDS. He gives extensive advice on what to avoid but also has plenty of support and resources on ways to deal with any problem. I particularly enjoyed his Food for Thought sections where he dares to tell you the politics behind many of our government policies and how they are harmful."   Janice M. Curtin
Weston A Price Foundation

"Absolutely one of the most important books of our time. Not just for children, but for adults, our society, and our very survival."
Gregory Pouls, D.C.
Maile Pouls, Ph.D.

"This is one of the finest resources on the market. . .I recommend each and every one of my patients have one and get one for someone they love. It is not just informative, but it could save your and your child's life."
Chadwick Hawk, D.C.

"Well researched and offers great advancement toward a better life for not only adults, but children as well."   Aajonus Vonderplanitz, Ph.D.

"Bravo! Every Parent in America should have this book!"
Cheryl Peterson, massage therapist

"I read your book and tried some of your suggestions...the improvements I saw with my 13-year-old son include more consistent schoolwork – his reading went from a D to an A. He is less hyper and he gets far fewer ear infections. My husband and I have both noticed an increase in energy and an overall feeling of well-being. A book I wouldn't be without."
Samantha Ayers, parent

Everlasting Health

Humanity's Guide to Understanding, Avoiding, and Reversing Disease

"We can't solve problems by using the same
kind of thinking we used when we created them."
—Albert Einstein

"Any intelligent fool can make things bigger, more complex, and more violent.
It takes a touch of genius – and a lot of courage – to move in the opposite
direction."
—Albert Einstein

"Even if you are a minority of one, the truth is still the truth."
— Gandhi

"Genius is the ability to recognize the truth."
—Bernardini

"Take no part in the unfruitful works of darkness, but instead expose them."
—Eph 5:11

by Robert Bernardini, M.S.

This publication is designed to provide accurate and authoritative information in regard to the subject matter covered. It is sold with the understanding that the publisher is not engaged in rendering medical, legal or other professional services. If such advice or other expert assistance is required, the services of a competent professional person should be sought. The ideas and suggestions contained in this book are not intended as a substitute for the appropriate care of a licensed health care practitioner. Qualified medical assistance should always be sought before beginning any treatments. The following is intended for educational purposes only. Suggestions are not made to treat a specific condition.

Thanks to Ashland University, Ashland Ohio, for use of lab facilities for cover photo. Cover photo by Finlay & Finlay Photography, Ashland ,Ohio, March 12, 2009.

Publisher's Cataloging-in-Publication
(Provided by Quality Books, Inc.)

Bernardini, Robert.
    Everlasting health: humanity's guide to
    understanding, avoiding and reversing disease / by
    Robert Bernardini.
p.cm.
Includes bibliographical references and index.
LCCN 2008942652
ISBN-13: 978-0-9703269-9-7
ISBN-10: 0-9703269-9-8

1. Health –Popular works. 2. Medicine, Preventive—
Popular works.   I.Title.

RA776.B47 2009   613
                        QBI08-600353

Table of Contents

Forward

"The most damaging thing you could do to your health might very well be to not read this book!" *David J. Getoff, CCN, CTN, CNC, FAAIM*

I became acquainted with author Robert Bernardini several years ago when he sent a copy of his first health book *The Truth About Children's Health* to the Price-Pottenger Nutrition Foundation for possible inclusion in their catalog. Although many board members (I am on this non-profit's board) read prospective books, fate set it up that I was to read and comment on his. I took the book with me on a flight to one of the many nutritional medicine conferences I attend or present at each year and I couldn't put it down! I remember being upset that the flight was too short to finish it. I was amazed that this author, who has since become a friend, had been able to put so much factual valid information into a book on children's health. I liked the book so much that I bought 100 copies and gave them out free to any of my patients who were new or expecting parents

Robert's new book, *Everlasting Health*, is just as good if not better than his first one. It's astonishingly comprehensive and is really an encyclopedia of how to attain and keep good health. I recommend you read it cover-to-cover with a highlighter and a note pad handy. Now I'll be giving it to my patients who promise me they'll read it.

Health is an extremely complex topic and most people have more misinformation than facts. It would even be safe to say that the "facts" that are generally believed by both the medical profession and the public are actually more wrong than right. This abundant and pervasive quantity of misinformation serves to do two things extremely well: It continues to make the medical pharmaceutical industry billions of dollars a year; and it continues to hold the public at a far lower level of health then they deserve and could easily attain.

Everlasting Health gives people a phenomenal amount of pertinent information that allows them to whittle away at virtually any health problem easily and without great expense or risk. Do you need information about heart disease, cancer, diabetes, autism, asthma, ADHD, or memory problems? This book has all of these and a great deal more. Most importantly, it concentrates on helping you address these problems in a supportive, holistic way, while at the same time shedding light on the oftentimes damaging effects of mainstream medical practices and drugs.

Many authors go about writing their books to cover only a small area or single topic of health or disease. Others are more comprehensive but go into very little depth on each subject. A third group tries to be both broad and thorough, but never takes the time to put in important reference citations from scientific books or journals to validate what they are writing about. This is often because no such documentation exists to back up their beliefs.

Robert obviously decided to write the best, most comprehensive, thoroughly scientific book on improving health that he possibly could. In order to make certain that "all bases were covered" and that he was not simply going with accepted but often wrong medical beliefs, he accessed and referenced an amazingly wide range of scientific research for validation. This allows the reader to prove to his or her physician, or any other non-believer, that what was learned from this book is not hocus-pocus, but is indeed based on valid science.

Today, science is often used to mislead. The pharmaceutical industry often conducts five to ten studies before finally managing to have one or two that show their drug works better than a placebo or has side effects acceptable to the FDA to be granted approval. When a study result looks like it is going to be against what the manufacture was hoping for, the study is stopped, never published, never given to the FDA, and a new study is begun. Oftentimes studies that are in the minority of research and not valid scientifically are quoted in order to make a point that is not even true. Since research showing that using foods or supplements to treat disease will not make any money for the drug companies, we have a very important bias problem.

The result is that you may often read a news report bashing alternative methods of regaining health or supplementation of certain nutrients, when in reality, the nutritional scientist such as myself or Robert (but not your physician) would know that possibly hundreds of other research studies clearly show these alternative methods to be enormously beneficial. News and good quality science rarely have much to do with one another and sadly, due to money, power, and politics, medicine, and medical education is biased towards pharmaceutical drugs and is often not very scientific at all.

Robert has done an exceptional job of teaching us what his exhaustive research has shown to be the most valid scientific data available to date. If you care about your health and the health of your family, I highly recommend that you take this information to heart and learn from it. It's presented in an easy-to-understand and entertaining way, rare for a book of such depth and insight. I suggest you decide right now that the best thing for your and your family's health is to learn what Robert's new book has to teach you. Keep the entire family healthy, pain-free, and energetic all the way into old age!

The most damaging thing you could do to your health might very well be to not read this book. Thank you, Robert, for your efforts and desire to help the public. It is sorely needed.

David J. Getoff, *CCN, CTN, CNC, FAAIM*
> Elected Member: American College of Nutrition & International
> College of Integrative Medicine
> Fellow: American Association of Integrative Medicine
> Board certified clinical nutritionist
> Board certified traditional naturopath

Introduction

Imagine you're driving in your car on a stormy night, and you hear a strange knocking from under the hood. Immediately, you start worrying the car may stall or even catch on fire. As your imagination runs wild, your heart races, your hands get sweaty, and a knot forms in your stomach. You pull over to check it out and notice the only thing wrong is that the hood latch is loose. "What a relief," you think. Your heart rate returns to normal, your hands stop sweating, and the knot in your stomach relaxes.

Stress is a major cause of illness, and a major cause of stress is doubt. If an experienced mechanic heard the same noise while driving, he or she would probably shrug it off and never worry about it. However, someone who doesn't know enough could get so flustered they might end up driving into a ditch.

If you have a health challenge, wouldn't you be less stressed if you knew exactly what the problem really is? Unlike a car mechanic who can most often find the exact cause of an automobile's malfunction, medical doctors usually cannot. They still don't know what causes the common cold, let alone cancer. Their technologies, drugs, and advice don't seem to be fixing us that well either. Why are Alzheimer's, diabetes, prostate cancer, breast cancer, ADHD, depression, AIDS, SIDS, birth defects all at or nearing epidemic levels?

There are reasons for disease that either the doctors don't know or are not telling you. However, realize that everything, disease included, has cause. What most people don't realize is that the causes of disease are not as difficult to understand or esoteric as the scientists and medical profession makes them sound. In fact, the causes are (they have to be) based on fundamental laws of nature and matter – laws that anyone can comprehend. For example, although a physicist might develop a fancy mathematical formula to show how an apple falls to the ground, anyone can understand that the apple does, in fact, fall.

Pulitzer Prize winning novelist and world famous agriculturist Louis Bromfield, wrote,

> Man is never able to impose his own law upon Nature nor to alter her laws, but he can, by working with her, accomplish much, whether it is in dynamos or the airplane or the earth or the body of man himself. The man who loves Nature comes nearer to an understanding of God. . .and the good earth and true faith have never been removed from one another. They are as near today as they were ten thousand years ago.(1)

This book unravels the complexities, misunderstandings, deceptions, and outright lies that have, as part of the modern health-care system, kept virtually everyone slaves to that system. Once you understand why a disease occurs, you can take steps to avoid it, stop it from getting worse, or even reverse it. That, my friend, is the last thing the health-care system wants. So it hides behind technical jargon, advanced degrees, exclusive organizations, and fancy technology to keep us begging for mercy. Once you read this book, you'll be able to give yourself and your loved ones that mercy.

You'll learn that any disease starts because of conditions that are usually easy to control. You may simply need to avoid the toxin(s) that causes it or supply a key nutrient that's lacking. The hard part is finding those things out. I've done that for you, and you hold these findings in your hands. Now all you need to do is follow directions.

Another major benefit from reading this book is that it details how you can save money in not just one, but four different ways on your health expenses. First: You'll no longer spend money on the everyday products and foods that cause or add to your sickness. Second: You'll no longer spend money on drugs and treatments that are either worthless or cause disease. Third: You will no longer spend money on many vitamins, herbs, supplements, and other so-called "natural" ways to prevent or treat disease, most of which are harmful or worthless. Fourth: You'll learn what the most nutritious and disease-fighting foods, supplements, and treatments are that give you the most for your money.

While doing the experiments and research for this book, I made some startling discoveries. One is that most adult diseases actually get started due to conditions the person experienced earlier in his or her life – not just earlier as an adult, but as far back as childhood, infancy, while in the womb, and even before conception. Cancer, heart disease, diabetes, arthritis, depression, and other maladies just don't appear out of nowhere. Nearly all diseases, even the common cold, result from conditions building up in an individual over time. Eventually, the bad overtakes the good, and the disease manifests.

In order to fully understand disease, why it happens, and how you can avoid it, it's best to understand it from the very beginning. Once you know how and why it starts, you can take the necessary steps for healing or avoidance. All with a clear conscience and certainty that you are doing the right things – the things that will stop your pain and keep you healthy for the rest of your life.

You're going to learn why, unfortunately, it's getting harder to get and stay healthy. You'll discover how following mainstream medical advice will make you more susceptible to heart failure, memory loss, and impotence. You're going to understand why adults and especially children are becoming sick or impaired earlier and earlier in life, and what the ramifications of this trend are for the human race as a whole.

You'll notice that I devote a lot of time and space to the health of children. This is not just a preference on my part, but a necessity if we are to fully understand disease and how it manifests. Yes, children are our future, but just as importantly, they are our barometer. Like the canary in the coal mine, children are extremely sensitive. If there's something wrong in our environment children will most likely be the one's to suffer first. (For an even more in-depth review of children's health, see my book *The Truth About Children's Health*.)

Besides, who doesn't have a child in his or her life? If you are a parent and your children are grown, they may be thinking of starting a family. You may have grandchildren. Think of your siblings' children, and your friends'. Wouldn't it be nice for you to be able to help them get and stay healthy too? Think of the pain, suffering, and expense you'll be saving them.

If you're an adult reading this who is older than about 45 years of age, I'd like you to think back to your childhood. How many adults did you know had diabetes, heart disease, or cancer? More poignantly, how many children did you know had leukemia, brain cancer, diabetes, attention deficit-hyperactivity disorder (ADHD), arthritis, multiple sclerosis, asthma, cancer, autism, or were obese? Chances are you knew a few. Perhaps the kid down the street had asthma. Maybe a neighbor's friend was a little chubby.

Now children and adolescents are getting these diseases in epidemic numbers. There are whole hospitals devoted to children's cancer alone. Along with physical sicknesses, emotional and behavioral problems are increasing and becoming more severe. When as a child growing up did you ever, ever hear of another child or adolescent shooting, stabbing, or killing someone else? Now shooting sprees in schools happen with agonizing frequency. Harold E. Buttram, M.D., sums up this disturbing trend:

> American children today may be confronted with the greatest difficulty and danger that can be placed on any generation, that of a subtle deterioration in health, largely the result of an increasingly hostile and toxic environment. Considering the circumstances, the marvel is that many do turn out well…Children are much more vulnerable to toxic exposures than adults…In the present case, the ultimate cure must rest with the children…Increasing health problems in children today largely involve two closely related and interacting systems of the body, the immune system and the brain and nervous system. Health problems involving these systems express themselves as various manifestations of crippled immune systems, delayed development, and "minimal brain dysfunction." …Allergic disorders such as asthma are rapidly increasing, both in frequency and severity. Although more difficult to quantify statistically, susceptibility to common viral infections and their complications appears to have increased on a scale largely unknown in earlier generations, as indicated by the increasing numbers of children who are becoming dependent on frequent or prolonged courses of antibiotics…Corresponding increases have taken place in behavioral disorders, attention deficit hyperactive disorder (ADHD), and learning disabilities. ADHD, with its long-term

consequences in terms of impaired learning capacity and social adjustment difficulties that commonly ensue in later adolescence, is arguably one of the foremost health problems of our times. Although statistics confirm the increasing prevalence of ADHD and related problems among children, statistics alone do not tell the entire story. Many factors involved are subtle and intangible and are difficult to measure statistically.

Perhaps the best way to gain insight into the pervasiveness of the problem is to talk with veteran teachers with a perspective of 20 or 30 years teaching experience. In our office we have asked a number of these teachers, inquiring if they have observed a change in children during their teaching careers. Without exception, they have replied there has been a dramatic change, most notably since the 1970s. Steadily increasing numbers of children, they report, are restless, impulsive, less focused, less able to maintain sustained concentration, and therefore, less able to learn...

We believe that meaningful progress will best come about through public education. Large portions of the public are already seeking sound guidance in this area. Above all, there should be freedom of choice in matters pertaining to health. Those seeking health for themselves and their families must return to more natural patterns of living. This requires effort and, very often, the braving of public opinion. This cannot come about in a society where basic freedoms in the health field are denied. (2)

Statistics from a variety of sources and over long periods of time have been used to identify the deteriorating health trends in ourselves and our children. The prudent thing to do is to recognize these trends and attempt to figure out why they are occurring. We must not ignore these warning signs with denial or a Pollyanna attitude. If we do, we might witness in the not too distant future many diverse and widespread tragedies affecting ourselves, our children, and our society.

However, as useful and helpful as statistics are, we must not allow them to usurp our own common sense. We must evaluate everything with our own keen eye and judgment and use scientific information as a guideline, but not a rule. Always ask yourself these two questions when given information: "Does this make sense using nature as the standard?" and, "What have I seen or experienced in my own world?" Don't necessarily believe somebody just because he or she is on the nightly news, has a stethoscope around his or her neck, is in the papers or is a so-called "expert." Make yourself the expert. Learn to seek answers, not just accept what is foisted upon you: The truth is often quiet and the truth is often hidden. Truth doesn't advertise and it's not in it for the money. It just is.

You must scrutinize closely the information you receive from the government and the mass media. Policy decisions, guidelines, and laws are oftentimes made not so much for the preservation of our health, but for the preservation of profits. Big money can do big things, including influencing our government. A study showed that almost half of the leading officials at the Food and Drug Administration (FDA) had at one time worked for organizations the agency is mandated to regulate.(3) Similarly, many FDA officials quit to go to work for a company in the field they were once regulating. The battle lines between the regulated and the regulator are not as clear as one is led to believe.

The findings I present in this book are mostly not mine but are from other researchers, doctors, medical journals and textbooks, newspapers, health professionals, and government reports. I document and reference everything of importance so you can see that I'm not exaggerating or making anything up. You may not believe something in this book because I say it, but you may believe it when you realize it's what others believe based on their own research.

This book is not just a summary of research, but also a compilation of my own discoveries in my quest for better health. Starting in infancy, I have had a number of health problems, some quite serious. My parents told me of the time when I was just a baby, and they had to slap me to keep me from plunging into unconsciousness. I got the measles, mumps, had ear infections, headaches, allergies, sinusitis, and poison ivy so bad my eyes swelled shut and I couldn't go to school. When I was 13, I fell on my head and cracked it open, almost bleeding to death waiting for the ambulance. That was the end of my football career, and instead, my neck vertebrae got messed up and arthritic. As recently as just a few years ago, when I would run, I would hear a clicking in my head near where my skull had cracked. I had tendon problems, vision problems, blood sugar problems, thyroid problems, a circulatory issue that doctors couldn't help me with. My digestion was so bad, at one point, I weighed just 95 pounds.

After spending my childhood, adolescence, and early adulthood in one kind of misery or another, I finally started using my education in biology, chemistry, physics, and engineering to figure out why I was suffering and how to alleviate it. After years of study, research, and experimentation, I rooted out not only the things that are truly health promoting, but learned why they are so on the most fundamental scientific levels. Knowing this takes away the doubt and guesswork and helps keep you committed to a healthier lifestyle. Most, if not all, of the recommendations I give you I have done myself. I believe they are the reason I'm not just still alive and able to write this book, but perform and feel better than I ever have. There may be other ways to get healthy, but I know for sure, the ways I detail in this book, work.

There are a few health concepts I present in this book that are quite revolutionary. You'll know them when you read them. When you do, you may say, "That's nuts! That's exactly the opposite of what I've heard all my life!" Believe me, when I first heard them, I was skeptical too. However, after more research and experimenting, I discovered these seemingly heretical theories are absolutely correct. If you don't believe these concepts straight away, that's understandable. Maybe I'm just planting a seed, and as you go on with your life, you'll gradually realize the old accepted theories just don't make sense anymore. Maybe you'll courageously experiment on your own to test their validity. But please, do me a favor and don't discount them just because "everybody knows" or "all the experts say" they aren't true. Most great advances of civilization occurred when a common belief was turned on its head.

For example, did you know that immediately after Orville Wright flew for the first time in a heavier that air flying machine, several newspapers refused to print the story insisting that "everyone knows" man can't fly! If the Wright brothers believed what "everybody knows," we might still be taking trains. By the way, this historic flight was made on December 17, 1903 at Kitty Hawk, North Carolina, and it lasted 12 seconds.

Or that in 1630, Galileo published his *Dialogue on the Two Chief Systems of the World*, which contradicted the accepted theory that the earth is fixed and is the center of the universe. He proved that Copernicus was right – that the earth revolves around the sun and is not the center of the universe. Nonetheless, he was threatened with jail and forced to recant his theories before the Inquisition at Rome in 1633. Popular opinion may be popular, but that doesn't mean it's correct.

Please keep in mind that everything I present here is designed to give you the power over your health and well-being. Not a doctor, government agency, high-tech machine, or germ. I want to empower you so you can be free of sickness, free of pain, free of misery. You'll see that attaining good health for the rest of your life is not as complicated as you've been led to believe. So buckle up, try to keep an open mind, and enjoy the ride. I'm going to show you that there's nothing wrong under the hood that you and nature can't fix.

Special Notice

The content of this book is presented in a sequential order that builds as it goes, so I suggest you read it as you would read a novel. Skipping around will not allow you to fully understand and appreciate not just the technical information, but the theoretical concepts. There's also some overlap in the information. For example, heart disease is discussed at length in the chapter on cardiovascular diseases, but some important information is also revealed in the chapter on asthma, obesity, and others. If you must skip around, please eventually read the whole book, since that's the only way you'll be able to learn all the secrets, suppressed information, and methods, that can help you understand, avoid, and reverse just about any disease.

CHAPTER I

People of the U.S.A.

This book in large part addresses health problems in the United States, which are then used to understand health issues for humanity as a whole. Therefore, to understand the scope of our subject, let's first consider who we are, how we live, and how we are changing.

- Currently (November, 2009) there were 307,950,412 people in the U.S. (The world population is 6,797,479,914) There's one birth every 8 seconds, one death every 13 seconds, one new immigrant every 26 seconds, and a net gain of one person every 12 seconds. By the year 2050, there will be approximately 419.9 million people in the U.S.
- Roughly 51 percent are women and 49 percent men – that equates to about 5.2 million more women than men.
- There were 35.9 million people 65 years of age or older in 2003. That's 12.3 percent of the total population. By the year 2030 there'll be about 71.5 million older persons (twice the number in 2000) and will comprise 20 percent of the population by 2030.
- The average family size is 3.14 people, 80 percent of Americans adults have graduated high school, and 24 percent have a college education.
- There's an estimated 2-3 million Americans that experience homelessness over the course of a given year. For most, it is a short, one-time event, but for some it lasts for long periods. Those who experience chronic homelessness are most often single, poor adults with prevalent disabilities. It's estimated that the number of elderly persons who are homeless will grow substantially as the baby boom generation ages. Roughly 9.2 percent of families live below the poverty level and 12.4 percent of individuals live below the poverty level (close to 34 million people).
- In 2000, non-Hispanic whites comprised 75.1 percent of the population. By 2050, they will comprise only 50.1 percent.
- In 2000, Hispanics comprised 12.5 percent of the population. By 2050 they are expected to comprise 24.4 percent.
- In 2000, Asians comprised 0.38 percent of the population. By 2050 they are expected to comprise 8.0 percent.
- In 2000, Blacks comprised 12.3 percent of the population. By 2050 they are expected to comprise 14.6 percent.
- The United States ranks 49th in the world in life expectancy at 77.43 years. Andorra is first at 83.50 years, and Botswana is last at 34.19 year.

- The top five leading causes of death are heart disease, cancer, accidents, stroke, and diabetes, in that order. [1,2]

Food for Thought

The United States has the fastest growing population of all developing countries. We grow by about 2.5 million people a year. That's like adding a city the size of San Diego every year. The first U.S. Census was conducted in 1790 by U.S Marshals who weren't even given paper to use to complete their task. They came up with a total count of 3.9 million. Conducting a census isn't cheap. In 1990 it cost $2.6 billion.

Concerning the leading causes of death in the U.S., here's an interesting note: A report was published in the *Journal of the American Medical Association (JAMA) – the m*ost widely circulated medical journal in the world – that estimates there are approximately 250,000 deaths per year in the U.S. due to physician errors. That means that doctors are the third leading cause of death behind cancer and heart disease.[3] Some of the medical errors that cause death include surgical errors, drug interactions, and misdiagnoses. Other errors that occur that are not deadly include things like amputating the wrong limb or sending a child home with the wrong family.

Consumer Reports magazine reported that one in six Americans who have ever taken a prescription drug experienced a side effect that was serious enough to send them to the hospital.[4] Since over 50 percent of Americans are on some form of daily prescription medication, there are a lot of people going to the hospital because of negative reactions to their drugs. The disclaimers on the drug ads make it sound like side effects hardly ever happen (based on clinical trials), but when you look at the actual numbers of real people having real problems, it is definitely significant.

The Most Sensitive

Our health is in large part affected if not determined by the conditions we are subject to as children. However, children are not just "little adults." Their exploratory behavior, increased biological sensitivity, and different diet make them more vulnerable and susceptible to environmental contaminants. Keep in mind that most if not all studies of exposures to and possible health effects of environmental toxins have used adults. The same exposure to children would magnify their health risks. The National Research Council states:

> The data strongly suggest that exposure to neurotoxic compounds at levels believed to be safe for adults could result in permanent loss of brain function if it occurred during the prenatal or early childhood period of brain development. This information is particularly relevant to dietary exposure to pesticides, since

policies that established safe levels of exposure to neurotoxic pesticides for adults could not be assumed to adequately protect a child less than four years of age.(5)

The National Academy of Sciences says that infants are likely to be 10 times more sensitive to any single pesticide than an adult. Furthermore, the additive effects of pesticides consumed in combination are not considered when regulating pesticides; nor are multiple routes of exposure (food, water, household use). There are 275 pesticides allowed on food and 102 of these were detected by the FDA from 1990 through 1992 on just 22 different fruits and vegetables.(6) So the additive effect of simultaneous exposure to multiple pesticides presents a real-world risk to infants and children.

Yet, there are no standards to protect infants, children, or anyone else from the effects of multiple pesticides on food, around the house or from any other source, for that matter. Indeed, the EPA has just begun to consider the combined effects of certain groups of pesticides, but once again, the studies focus on adults, not children. The likely effect of multiple pesticide exposure is probably synergetic (similar to adding 2 plus 2 and getting 5), and may even be exponential (similar to adding 2 plus 2 and getting 20). There are so many chemicals in our environment these days there is no way studies could be performed to determine the health risks of every combination. What's more, different people may have different levels of sensitivity to various chemicals or combinations of chemicals "generally considered safe," and these may not apply to you or your child. The only way to eliminate the risks is to eliminate the chemicals.

Children are more sensitive and more easily harmed, placing them at special risk for adverse effects from toxic exposure. Their metabolic mechanisms for processing and excreting toxic substances are not fully developed. Children are especially sensitive because of their different pathways of absorption, tissue distribution, ability to biotransform and eliminate chemicals, and the manners in which they respond to chemicals and radiation.

Children go through various stages of development – fetal, newborn, an infant, school age, adolescent – and each stage may be particularly vulnerable to specific toxins. For example, infants are more vulnerable to the effects of secondhand smoke because their lung capacity is still increasing. Toddlers' respiratory rates are more rapid, so they are more vulnerable to air pollutants than an adult might be. Several organ systems, including the nervous, immune, reproductive, and endocrine systems, which are not fully developed at birth, may "demonstrate particular sensitivity during the postnatal [newborn] period."(7)

The reproductive system is also vulnerable to the toxic effects of chemical pollutants and pesticides – whether exposure occurs in the womb or in early childhood. This can interfere with normal sexual development. This exposure may also be contributing to declining male reproductive health in general in the industrialized world.(8,9)

In many cases infants and children suffer far more serious damage than adults do. Aspirin, for example, can cause Reye's syndrome (a condition that kills 80 percent of its victims) in children and teenagers, but it does not cause this condition in adults. Lead causes permanent loss of mental capacity when infants and children are exposed at levels of little consequence to adults. Phenobarbital, a sedative in adults, produces hyperactivity in most children. Ritalin produces hyperactivity in most adults but is a sedative in children. Infants under six months of age suffer methemoglobinemia, or "blue baby syndrome," from nitrate exposure at levels that are safe for older children and adults. Radiation treatment for brain cancer in children under four can cause major cognitive problems later in life, but appear not to cause cognitive problems if performed after age eight.(10)

Therefore, children can be viewed as our weakest link. They are the "canary in the coal mine," and manifestations of diseases in children warn us that something is wrong in our environment and we as adults should do something about it. Protecting ourselves necessitates protecting our children.

A study in the journal *Cancer Research* reported a sevenfold increase in cancer rates when animals were exposed to carcinogens starting in infancy, as compared with exposure only during adulthood.(11) A review of the scientific literature in 1992 (we've known for that long) found that exposure to chemicals early in life (dosing animals in utero, in infancy, and in adulthood), increases the rate of cancer in the exposed population and that these cancers generally occur earlier in life.(12)

This is an important point. Exposure to toxins (and other stressors such as deficient diet, emotional stress, and physical inactivity) is taking its toll on people earlier and earlier in life. Once, only older people got cancer – and few of them at that. Then, middle-aged people started getting it. Now, our children are getting it and dying from it. Cancer is just one manifestation of ill health. There are many others such as ADHD, autism, childhood diabetes, asthma, and so on. Some of those conditions were not even defined in the scientific and medical literature until recently since they were either so rare, or they simply did not exist. People are getting sicker younger and younger – physically, mentally, and emotionally. It's not by chance – it's because our bodies are not being treated and cared for the way nature intended.

Not only can children suffer devastating effects from environmental toxins that go unnoticed or are relatively harmless for adults, they may also respond more acutely to these toxins at much smaller exposures simply because their bodies are smaller and not fully developed. That sensitivity is present even before a baby is born. Many environmental toxins can cross the placenta, thus exposing the fetus. Air pollutants and toxins from secondhand smoke, or if the mother smokes herself, can impact the fetus. A pregnant mother who had been overexposed to lead would have stored it in her bones, from which it could escape and be potentially harmful to the fetus as well.

The risk of exposure more than multiplies after birth. Infants spend much time exploring their world through touch, taste, and movement. Their curiosity puts them at greater risk to exposure from environmental hazards. They put their fingers and objects they find in their mouths and spend their time crawling on the floor, where household chemicals, pesticides, and other environmental toxins accumulate. Since they spend more time outdoors, have an increased respiratory rate, and high levels of activity, they have increased exposure to air pollution. (Yet keeping them in deprives them of sunlight – important, as we shall see.) Safe levels of pesticides and food additives are calculated for lifetime exposure to adults. Those may be grossly underestimated or even just erroneous for a child, however.

A child's rapid growth during the first years of life requires proportionally more food and liquid consumption than an adult needs. Furthermore, their bodies naturally absorb more of what they eat and drink. Therefore, any pesticides or chemicals in their food will be taken in more fully and at higher levels and do more harm faster and more permanently.

A growing child will typically eat more of certain foods such as apples and bananas per unit body weight than adults. But produce (if not organically grown) may be more highly contaminated than the foods adults typically eat. Children also drink more water, thus increasing their potential exposure to any toxins in it – including those such as chlorine added to sanitize it or fluoride.

A faster and more responsive metabolism and rapid growth and development are the basic reasons for an infant's increased vulnerability to any toxic substance. After birth the most pronounced period of growth is the first year of life, during which the human infant triples in weight. Different organs grow at different rates as the infant matures, creating a roulette of infant organ susceptibility. For instance, the brain of a newborn child grows rapidly and is particularly sensitive to toxic substances. Not only that, but where an infant's brain weighs about 33 percent what an adult brain weighs, the infant body weighs about 4 percent of an adult body. That relatively large brain grows rapidly in the newborn child, achieving 50 percent of its adult weight by six months of age. Seventy-five percent of all brain cells are present by age two.[13,14] In contrast, children do not attain even 50 percent of adult weight in the liver, heart, and kidneys until age nine.[15]

During puberty, there are rapid metabolic and physiological changes that increase the impact of environmental toxins. As adolescents enter the work force through summer jobs or jobs after school, or start smoking, drinking, or experimenting with drugs, any harmful effects of exposures are magnified.

In general, rapid growth increases the risk of cancer from toxic exposure. The NAS Committee on Pesticides in the Diets of Infants and Children concluded that in the absence of other factors, "Direct carcinogens are more potent in rapidly growing animals," adding that "infants and children are subject to rapid tissue growth and development, which will have an impact on cancer risk."[16] Does this have an effect on their health? It appears so. The incidence of childhood brain cancer and childhood leukemia has increased 33 percent since 1973.(17) Cancer now kills more children under age 14 than any other disease.

Hazardous substances such as lead, Polychlorinated Biphenyls (PCBs), asbestos, radon, solvents, pesticides, food additives, and air pollution have found their way into the schools, homes, food, and playgrounds. Resultant exposures to these toxins can have significant impacts on children's health, putting them at risk of developing learning disabilities, chronic and acute respiratory diseases, neurological problems, asthma, bronchitis, and cancer. Consider this: Dr. Roger D. Masters says that children absorb up to 50 percent of the lead they ingest, compared with only 8 percent for adults. Even low exposures to toxins in early childhood and even in the womb can have permanent effects on intelligence and behavior.(18)

Our children are under protected. There are very few data banks that have information on children's exposures, and again, risk assessments do not routinely differentiate between adults and children. However, the Federal government has officially recognized the vulnerability of children. On April 21, 1999 an Executive Order was issued by the White House titled *Protection of Children From Environmental Health Risks and Safety Risks*. Part of this order is quoted below:

> A growing body of scientific knowledge demonstrates that children may suffer disproportionately from environmental health risks and safety risks. These risks arise because: children's neurological, immunological, digestive, and other bodily systems are still developing; children eat more food, drink more fluids, and breathe more air in proportion to their body weight than adults; children's size and weight may diminish their protection from standard safety features; and children's behavior patterns may make them more susceptible to accidents because they are less able to protect themselves. Therefore, to the extent permitted by law and appropriate, and consistent with the agency's mission, each Federal agency:
>
> (a) shall make it a high priority to identify and assess environmental health risks and safety risks that may disproportionately affect children; and
>
> (b) shall ensure that its policies, programs, activities, and standards address disproportionate risks to children that result from environmental health risks or safety risks.(19)

In the words of Dr. Lynn Goldman, Assistant Administrator for the EPA: "We can no longer behave as though all environments were created equal. Children especially bear the brunt of environmental pollution in our most polluted environments, and they must be protected."(20)

CHAPTER II

Overweight & Obesity

Nearly seven of every 10 U.S. adults are overweight, and about three of every 10 are obese. Since 1991, the prevalence of obesity has increased 75 percent (Obesity is defined as being more than 30 percent above ideal body weight.) The younger you are the more chance you have of becoming fat. For example, people born in 1964 become obese about 27 percent faster than people born in 1957.[1,2]

The Centers for Disease Control's (CDC) 2000 report on Nutrition and Physical Activity found that the percentage of children and adolescents who are overweight has more than doubled in the past 30 years. Most of the increase has occurred since the late 1970s. Nearly 30 percent of U.S. children are considered overweight or obese, and the U.S. has the highest rates of obesity among teenagers than other industrialized countries.[3,4,5]

In December 2008, the National Center for Health Statistics reported that more Americans are obese (34 percent) than overweight (32.7 percent), and six out of every hundred Americans (6 percent) are extremely obese. Estimates are that by the year 2030, 86 percent of American adults will be overweight and 51 percent obese. Thirty-two percent of children are by definition overweight, 16 percent obese, and 11 percent extremely obese.[6] If all the dietary advice you hear from mainstream media, nutritionists, and doctors were correct, would this be happening?

Obesity has increased in every state, in both sexes and across all age groups, all races, all educational levels, and among smokers and non-smokers alike. By region, the largest increases were seen in the South, with a 67 percent increase in the number of obese people. Georgia had the largest increase: 101 percent.

The CDC estimates that 300,000 deaths a year are caused by obesity and it's considered the second most preventable cause of death in the U.S. behind smoking. It's estimated that if this trend continues, it could lower the average life expectancy of 77.6 years in the U.S. by as much as five years.[7]

Being overweight and obese isn't cheap. The amount of money spent on illnesses associated with obesity has increased more than tenfold between 1987 and 2002: In 1987, $3.6 billion was spent compared to $36.5 billion in 2002.[8] Restaurants are even installing bigger furniture to accommodate larger people.

Why So Heavy?

Why are so many people overweight? Two reasons: Improper nutrition and lack of exercise. We'll look at exercise first.

As the weight of adults and children alike has increased, physical activity has gone down. About 17 percent of adults ages 45-64 and 23 percent of adults aged 65-74 are physically inactive. Forty percent of adults engage in no leisure-time physical activity at all. Nearly half of young people ages 12 to 21 are not vigorously active on a regular basis. Participation in all types of physical activity declines as children and adolescents get older. The percentage of high school students who participate in daily physical education classes has declined in recent years from 42 percent in 1991 to 25 percent in 1995. Forty percent of high school students are not enrolled in any type of physical education class. Even toddlers are not getting enough exercise with an average of only 20 minutes a day compared to the recommended one hour per day.[9,10] The ever-present television and the explosion of the Internet have not helped matters when it comes to exercise. We and our children are much more likely to sit in front of a screen than go out and play.

It's obvious that we're simply not getting enough exercise. Remember the old saying "a sound body, a sound mind?" Science bears that out. One of the recommendations for people with clinical depression is physical exercise. It's a stress reliever and a self-esteem builder. It causes the release of endorphins, the body's natural "feel-good" chemicals. Exercise simply makes you feel better. Physical activity often reduces the symptoms of depression and has been found to be just as effective as medication in reducing these symptoms. It also improves the quality of sleep and even helps older adults reduce the amount of cognitive decline they experience as they age.

The benefits of physical activity are everywhere. Regular walking helps reduce pain and improves the function of joints for people with arthritis. There was a 58 percent decrease in falls among older women who exercise regularly. Life expectancy increases almost 6 years if a person exercises regularly, and medical costs go down (especially for women) when one exercises.[11]

CDC Director Jeffrey P. Koplan says that the American lifestyle of convenience and inactivity has had a devastating toll on every segment of society, particularly on children. Research shows that 60 percent of overweight five- to 10-year-old children already have at least one risk factor for heart disease, including hyperlipidemia (increased levels of fat in the blood) and elevated blood pressure or insulin levels. Koplan says, "Overweight and physical inactivity account for more than 300,000 premature deaths each year in the U.S., second only to tobacco-related deaths. Obesity is an epidemic and should be taken as seriously as any infectious disease epidemic. Obesity and overweight are linked to the nation's number one killer – heart disease – as well as diabetes and other chronic conditions."[12]

Obese children and adolescents are more likely to become obese adults. This extra weight carries with it increased risks for heart disease, high blood pressure, stroke, diabetes, some types of cancer, gallbladder disease, and osteoporosis. Even the health of the parents has a tremendous effect on whether a child will be obese or not: Children with two obese parents stand an 80 percent chance of being obese themselves and a 40 percent chance if one parent is obese. Sadly, "once you're fat, you're fat:" Eighty percent of obese teenagers will become obese adults.(13)

The damage of obesity in young people is real. Using ultrasound- imaging techniques, doctors saw that the blood vessels of some overweight 10-year-old children were as thick as those of heavy adult smokers. These children risk having a heart attack or stroke decades sooner than normal weight children (14)

Nutrient Poor/Nutrient Dense:
Your Key to Real and Lasting Weight Loss

As important as exercise is for staying trim, improper nutrition is the major force behind obesity and being overweight. It's not the quantity of food we eat as much as the quality of it that determines if we are overweight or not. If your food doesn't have enough (and the right kinds of) vitamins, minerals, essential fatty acids, trace minerals, and so on for your body to function properly, the *appastat* (the part of the brain that tells you you're hungry) continues to sense hunger and you continue to want to eat. (The appastat is the part of the brain in the *arcuate nucleus* in the *hypothalamus*, an endocrine gland just below the pituitary gland which is pretty much right in the middle of your brain.) If, on the other hand, the foods we eat are nutrient dense, the body will sense that it has everything it needs to function, the appastat will be turned off and you will sense fullness and no longer feel the need to eat. There's no will power involved here – it's all automatic.

Consider that most of today's food are woefully lacking in nutrients. Just since 1975, the amount of vitamins and minerals in many foods has plummeted. For example, apples have 41 percent less vitamin A, broccoli has 50 percent less vitamin A and calcium, sweet peppers have 31 percent less vitamin C, collard greens have 45 percent less vitamin A 60 percent less potassium and 85 percent less magnesium. I go into much more detail on the inadequacy of our food supply and soils in a later chapter, but suffice it here to say that the food you find in a typical grocery store is not as nutrient dense as it once was, and not nutrient dense enough to nourish you adequately and turn off the appastat and your hunger.(15) Therefore, you never feel satisfied, and continue to want to eat.

All this talk about "lite" foods is really misguided. First, these foods are usually lower in fat content. But, fat is not the demon it's made out to be, and in fact, the right kind of fats are absolutely necessary not just for good health, but for weight control too. Second, these lite foods have usually been stripped of the nutrients the appastat and body needs to sense fullness. Again, if the nutrients aren't in the food, you continue to feel hungry, you continue to eat food with calories, and you continue to gain weight. You can and will lose weight if you eat the right foods that are dense in nutrition, not "lite." To be nourished adequately so you lose weight, you need to replace the nutrient poor foods with nutrient dense foods. I call this the Nutrient Dense Diet, or NDD for short.

What kinds of foods are nutrient poor? Consider that cooking destroys many vitamins, fats, and enzymes and degrades carbohydrates and proteins. Second, food grown by conventional methods lack many important minerals. Third, over-processed foods are nutrient deficient foods: every step of a processing method robs the food of nutrition. So raw, untampered with foods that are organically grown are nutritionally superior foods. (I discuss organic food in more detail later, but for now, just understand that it *is* important.)

Food for Thought

"Heat is one of the most damaging elements in the food preparation process. Vitamin C and the B-complex vitamins are particularly vulnerable to heat. Carotenoids and retinoids are also heat-sensitive. In addition, exposure to water during cooking can leach out the vitamins, minerals, and flavonoids from the food," so states nutritionist Jerry Ryan, Ph.D.[16] Canning causes about twice the loss of nutrients than freezing does, and refining food is very destructive. When wheat is made into white bread, the flour loses 70 percent of its vitamins, minerals, and fiber, 25 percent of its protein, and 80 percent of its magnesium, copper, and potassium. It's been shown that if orange juice is stored in plastic, it loses almost all its vitamin C, but if it's stored in glass, it retains much of it. There's even more vitamin C in orange juice you squeeze yourself and drink right away. Just cut an organic orange in half and squeeze each half into a glass or bowl. It only takes a half a minute and will not only get you the most nutritious juice, but improve your grip and hand strength too.

The food that is very nutrient poor and largely to blame for the tendency to overeat is refined carbohydrates, commonly called starches. You find it in cookies, bagels, chips, pasta, pizza, hamburger buns, bread, cereals, and so on. The flour used to make these products is over processed and stripped of valuable vitamins and minerals that we need in order to feel satisfied. Even the Centers for Disease Control (CDC) admits that carbohydrates are the main reason Americans are gaining weight.[17] The liver takes these refined flours and carbohydrates and converts them into triglycerides (blood fat). When there's too much fat in the blood, it gets deposited in tissues as fat.

High-fructose corn sweeteners (HFCS) are also nutrient poor and are having a major impact on the obesity rate. These sweeteners are now used in place of sucrose (table sugar) to sweeten soft drinks, fruit juices, and just about everything else that needs sweetening simply because they are less expensive than sugar. They're made from refined corn and are devoid of vitamins, minerals, and enzymes.

HFCS are worse than sugar because fructose is converted into fat and raises triglycerides more than any other sugar. Whereas sucrose breaks down into glucose molecules the body can use as fuel, fructose is oftentimes converted by the liver into fat and cholesterol. Fructose also does not stimulate insulin secretion and has been shown to cause insulin resistance. Since insulin tends to turn off your hunger, this won't happen when you consume these sweeteners.

Considering that soft drinks are now made with HFCS and that the consumption of soft drinks has soared in recent years, hand-in-hand with obesity. It's easy to see that soft drink consumption is a major reason people are gaining weight. A simple way to lose weight is to cut out all products that contain high-fructose corn sweeteners. Even if you consume similar products that use sucrose (no aspartame or *Splenda*, please), you'll be better off.

One more food that is surprisingly contributing to Americans being overweight is pasteurized, low-fat milk. In a recent study involving 12,000 children, weight gain was observed in children consuming low-fat milk, but not those who drank full-fat milk. The more reduced-fat milk they drank, the more, and faster they gained weight.[18] I will discuss milk and the importance of fat more in depth as we go, but know that pasteurized milk and low-fat milk are not the great things the media make them out to be. This is another example of a food that is not nutrient dense causing weight gain.

What foods are nutrient dense? Ideally, the food should be uncooked, unprocessed, and from fertile, clean soil. These foods include some vegetables and vegetable juices, eggs, dairy, and meat. Other items such as whole grains can be included, but sparingly so. I discuss the kinds of foods that nourish you throughout this book that are part of the NDD (Nutrient Dense Diet), and you'll see that getting properly nourished is not complicated. There's no need to take a lot of supplements either – almost all of them are contaminated, over-processed, and made from inferior materials.

Food for Thought

"Sometimes the most toxic thing in a person's diet is the herbal products they are using," says Dr. Richard Schulze, a world-renowned natural health practitioner.[19] Most herbs on the market today are grown using pesticides. Ninety-nine percent of the herbs sold in the U.S. are grown in countries that have no regulations on pesticides – they're grown in third world countries where they can use things like DDT and organophosphates, which have been banned in the U.S. To make matters worse, many herbs are subjected to intense fumigation and irradiation when they get to U.S. docks.

Does this matter? The National Academy of Sciences stated that "the potential risks posed by cancer-causing pesticides. . .are over one million additional cancer cases in the U.S. population over our lifetimes."[20] Researchers at the University of Southern California showed that children living in homes where household and garden pesticides were used had as much as a sevenfold greater chance of developing childhood leukemia.[21] Even if the herbs have been grown organically, they are oftentimes fumigated with toxic sprays to kill pests on dried herbs. Ethylene oxide (linked to birth defects, spontaneous abortions, and cancer) is one such fumigant. Manufacturers claim that the gas residues are long gone before the herbs reach the consumer, but are they're not. The half-life of these poisons is longer than the shelf life of the supplement.

Many herbal products are extracts of the herbs, but extracts use solvents to extract the active ingredient. One of the solvents typically used is hexane, which is a known carcinogen. Manufacturers claim all of it is removed before the product is sold, but there is always some residue left behind in the final product. Hexane is not only carcinogenic; it may also cause central nervous system toxicity if consumed over a long period of time (as herbal supplements often are).

Besides pesticides, additives and encapsulating materials can be harmful too. Magnesium stearate, or stearic acid, is added to over 90 percent of the vitamin and mineral products on the market as a flowing agent (so the powders don't get gooey and foul up the machines). Problem is, stearic acid has been shown to inhibit certain immune system cells (T-cells). In an article published in the journal *Immunology*, the authors noted, "Stearic acid inhibits T-cell dependent immune responses. Plasma membrane integrity is significantly impaired, leading to a loss of membrane potential and ultimately cell function and viability."[22] Other researchers at East Carolina University School of Medicine said, "When cells were exposed to stearic acids and palmitic acids, there was a dramatic loss of cell viability after 24 hours. Cell death was induced by stearic and palmitic acid."[23] An article in the *American Journal of Medical Science* said, "Palmitates and stearates caused cardiac and other types of cells to undergo programmed cell death."[24] Manufactureres and sellers of supplements will typically say that the amount of magnesium stearate (or other additives) are insignificant and won't do any harm. Well, if they're insignificant, why use them? Because they ARE significant and DO have effects on your body.

Sodium benzoate (benzoate of soda) and potassium sorbate are preservatives used in most liquid vitamin and mineral products. They are added to prevent the growth of mold or insects (by killing them and anything else that's alive in the product) simply to increase shelf life (these products would go bad after just a few days without the preservatives making them nearly impossible to market effectively).

Over the past decade or so, there have been many products made from fruits and berries, or mineral mixtures that claim to heal everything from arthritis to heart disease. But all of these products have preservatives, and these preservatives kill. In fact, Dr. Harvey W. Wiley, the man instrumental in getting the Pure Food and Drug Act passed in 1906, wanted sodium benzoate outlawed as a preservative. But of course, big business prevailed, and all Dr. Wiley could do was admonish consumers to read labels and not buy anything with sodium benzoate in it (such as white flour products, which it's still in).

Even the Material Safety Data Sheet (a sheet from the government telling the hazards of each chemical) for sodium benzoate says that if it's swallowed, to ". . .call a physician immediately; Induce vomiting. Give oxygen or artificial respiration as needed." The Chemical Analysis Data Sheet on sodium benzoate says to "Store away from food and beverages." And yet, it's put in everything from vitamin drinks to sodas.

Other ingredients in pills and capsules include binders, lubricants, sweeteners, dispensing agents, film formers, coatings and glaze (shellac), disintegrants, artificial coloring and flavorings, silicon dioxide, talc. You may think that these are in such low quantities that they would be insignificant. But consider that by taking just 3 pills or capsules a day, over the course of a year you'll consume nearly 1,100 of them. That's enough to fill a shoe box. Do you really subject yourself to all those impurities every day?

In addition, the vitamins or minerals themselves can be toxic. More than half of people in the U.S take a multivitamin everyday. In 2007, people in the U.S. spent about $23 billion dollars on dietary supplements that include more than one vitamin or mineral. As many as one in ten consumers of multivitamins are overdosing on certain nutrients, and over the past eight years, some 30,000 reports of adverse events (liver damage, drug interactions) associated with vitamin use have been reported through the federal government's monitoring system.(25)

Over the past several years, there's been an explosion in what are now being called *functional foods* – foods with added vitamins and minerals – with the thought of improving them (putting back in what processing took out). Some cereals have a dizzying array of added nutrients as do orange juice, sports drinks, and vitamin waters. But consuming these products can lead to overdosing on many of these nutrients, not just because the consumer is getting too much of them, but because these added ingredients are mostly unnatural and over-processed vitamins and minerals anyway.

The mere drying of herbs (usually with high heat which is essentially cooking them) causes changes to their chemical and electrical properties rendering them much less effective and even harmful. Herbs are only truly effective when used fresh soon after harvesting. Isolated vitamins and minerals, as most supplements are, lack the cofactors the body needs to process and use them correctly. When consumed, the body tries to compensate for the lack of balancing nutrients, and leaches them out of tissues, which causes deficiencies. You may increase your level of vitamin C, but cause a deficiency of fatty acids, for example, somewhere else. There are only a very few supplements I recommend taking since they are of such fundamental importance and the underpinning of so many biochemical reactions that I believe supplying them even in less than ideal forms (from food) is better than not getting them at all.

Why do some people seem to get results from taking herbs or vitamins? Some of their symptoms may have been alleviated, but consider that when the body is exposed to toxic substances (these products and drugs included), it reacts by increasing hormone levels, adrenaline being one of them. This "rush," (similar to a rush from caffeine), may in fact cause a cessation of symptoms for a time. But true healing has not occurred, and symptoms will return in one form or another later on. Therefore, it's best to get your vitamins, minerals, and everything else from food. A great vitamin/mineral supplement is freshly made vegetable juice.

If you are overweight or suffering from any kind of ailment, the food you have been eating is probably far from ideal. Not only is it not clean and nutrient dense, but it is downright addictive. In this regard, it will take some will power – sometimes a lot of will power – to stay away from the ice cream, chips, donuts and so on. In fact, Dr. John Hoebel at Princeton University in New Jersey showed that test animals fed a diet containing 25 percent sugar were thrown into a state of anxiety when the sugar was removed and showed symptoms similar to those when people come off morphine and nicotine. (This is a testament to the fact that sugar is in fact a drug, as we'll later see.) Dr. Ann Kelley at the University of Wisconsin Medical School identified changes in test animals' brain chemistry after eating a diet full of junky foods similar to changes caused by the extended use of morphine or heroin.[26] That's the bad news.

The good news is, "right is might" and "like attracts like," meaning, the more good food you eat, the healthier your cells become and the more they want more good food. Feeling healthy is addictive too – you just need a nudge in the right direction. Now that you're going to know what that is, it won't be that hard. Knowledge brings conviction.

To start things off, I'd like to introduce you to your new, nutrient dense, multi-vitamin/mineral. Eating this once or twice a day will go far in getting every cell in your body nourished and satisfied. This food has been shown to help curb your appetite and supply just about every nutrient you need. It's raw, unprocessed, and relatively inexpensive too. This food is bee pollen, and it's one of the best, most complete foods you can eat.

It has: vitamins C (ascorbic acid), D, E, K, B_1(thiamine), B_2 (riboflavin), B_3 (niacin), B_5,(pantothenic acid), B_6 (pyridoxine), B_{12} (methylcobalamin), biotin, folic acid, provitamin A, pantothenic acid, calcium, phosphorus, iron, copper, potassium, magnesium, manganese, silica, sulphur, sodium, zinc, iodine, chlorine, boron, molybdenum, selenium, essential fatty acids, enzymes, beta carotene, amino acids, proteins, peptones, rutin, DNA, RNA, and more.

If you were to see all these ingredients listed on a vitamin bottle, you'd think it was the best multi-vitamin/mineral ever. It's the only food on earth that contains 185 known nutritional ingredients including 22 amino acids (all 8 essential ones) needed by the human body for complete health. Bee pollen contains an average of 20 percent protein, so you may be able to get your full-day's complement of protein (45-60 grams of pure protein) by consuming seven ounces of fresh (not dried) bee pollen.

Warning: Do Not feed bee pollen, honey, or other hive products to infants under a year and a half old. There may be a small amount of mold and spores in these products that the babies undeveloped system cannot handle.

Writings over 2000 years old reveal that Egyptian physicians called honey with pollen the "universal healer." Writings from ancient Greece and Rome, Russia and the Orient all praise the nutritious and healing products of the bee hive.(27,28) It's been called "the greatest body builder on earth" by some with no negative side effects. Bee pollen has reportedly helped scores of different health conditions – not surprising since it's such a complete, natural and raw food. A study published in the *Journal of the National Cancer Institute* showed that tumors in mice were substantially delayed if they were fed bee pollen and that "seven mice in this series were still tumor-free at 56 to 62 weeks of age, when the tests were terminated."(29)

Bee pollen was shown to significantly lower serum lipid levels. An article published in the journal *Atherosclerosis* says, "The most pronounced reduction in lipid metabolism and in the severity of plaque formation occurred after the pollen extract had been applied. The total cholesterol content in serum and liver homogenate was depressed by 67% and 45%, respectively. . .Atherosclerotic plaque intensity at 12 weeks. . .averaged 85.5% in HFD-fed animals [high-fat diet] vs. 33.7% in pollen extract-treated rabbits."(30)

Bee pollen has been shown to reduce or eliminate cravings for heavy protein food and aids in the digestion of other foods. One study showed that the average daily food consumption of test subjects was 15 percent to 20 percent less than those not taking the bee pollen.(31) This is because the dense nutrition of the bee pollen is being sensed by the hypothalamus, shutting off the appastat and the feelings of hunger. Bee pollen contains phenylalanine, a natural amino acid that works on the appestat too. Bee pollen also contains lecithin, a substance that helps dissolve and flush fat from the body.

Ironically, bee pollen has been shown to help those recovering from chronic illnesses and those who need to gain weight. To me, that's the measure of a truly a good food: no matter what the condition, it brings the body back to normal (homeostasis). Bee pollen is also reported to help reduce cravings from addictions – so eliminating those junky foods from your diet will be easier. It's also reported to have helped overcome retardation and other developmental problems in children, and it seems to have anti-cancer properties as well.(32)

Unfortunately, I can't get into all the wonderful things bee pollen (your new multi-vitamin/mineral) can do – it would take a whole book to do so. But here's a partial list of problems it has reportedly helped: allergies, tumor formation, hypoglycemia, diabetes, snoring, weight loss, depression, acne, atherosclerosis, stroke, headaches, backaches, fatigue, insomnia, menstruation problems, arthritis, psoriasis, senility, hair growing, gray hair turning back to color, eczema, helps dogs with arthritis, leg pains, colds and flu, emphysema, ADHD, hay fever, headaches, Parkinson's disease, impotence, constipation, sinusitis, fatigue, bronchitis.

When taking bee pollen to help lose weight, it's best to consume it an hour or so before meals. If your weight is normal, you can take it with or after meals. But I must warn you to start any supplementation program under the supervision of a qualified health care professional. Bee pollen has rarely been known to trigger allergic reactions in some people, and should be started at very low quantities, even as little as a few pollen granules per day. Go slow, be careful, and read and follow label directions. Never heat bee pollen since that destroys most of its nutritive value. Bee pollen is a food, not a drug, and its effects may take a while to manifest. Don't expect improvement overnight, although it may happen. Take if for at least three months and then evaluate if you feel a difference.

Here are a few stories of the power of bee pollen I can't help but share with you (these are just testimonials, mind you, and not scientific studies, but they are impressive none the less):

> Seventy year old Noel Johnson, based on exercise, diet and bee pollen, was able to reverse a long-standing heart condition, going from bed-ridden to champion long-distance runner, boxer and as he describes it, stud at 80. Also healed arthritis, gout, and bursitis.

> A doctor wrote about a five year old child: "This is a severely developmentally delayed floppy child whose differential includes a structural abnormality in the brain or a genetic abnormality, some of which may be diagnosed by chromosome analysis or genetic screen." Parent's tried every possible approach with no improvement. The Easter Seals Rehab Center listed the child as "1. Severe receptive and expressive speech language delay; 2. Immature neuromotor functioning; 3. Delay in development of play/cognitive skills; 4. Questionable hearing acuity/perception; 5. Severe delays in all areas of development; 6. Severe hypotonia." Her mother began to give [bee pollen], and slow progress began: lost rag-doll floppiness, clung to mother when held. Later noted that her eyes fixed on colorful objects with interest; able to scoot body forward while sitting on couch; rolled over for the first time; reached with operational arm for articles; skin color better; able to drink from cup. Improvement continued onward: Colleen is alert and interested in things around her – this fact alone is 'medically impossible' – and is beginning to speak. She smiles, laughs, loves, hugs and kisses."

Woman, late twenties, suffered numerous health problems: had stopped menstruating, lost hair, frequent headaches and backaches, fatigued, and sensitivity to cosmetics. On taking bee pollen had more relaxed feeling in her body, and in just days was sleeping better. After eight months on pollen began having regular menstrual periods for the first time in seven years. Had increased strength, sounder sleep more cheerful disposition, thicker and healthier hair, no more problems with chills. Another woman, after giving birth to her last child, was depressed and hormones messed up, with irregular periods. Within three months of taking bee pollen, started having normal periods and moods leveled off. Nails started growing strong and long, and no longer split and chipped off.(33)

Not all bee pollen is created equal. You need to get it from areas of low pollution and it can't be heated or stored too long before sale. If it's improperly stored or handled, it will lose up to 75 percent of its nutritive value within twelve months. The only way to preserve live bee pollen is by keeping it cold, so never buy pollen that isn't refrigerated. (Short periods of non-refrigeration like that experienced for shipping do no great harm.) It should taste sweet and fresh and feel spongy and soft – any hard and crunchy granules have lost nutritive value. See Resource Guide for good brands.

How much bee pollen should you take? Start slowly with just a few granules a day, and slowly work up to a tablespoon twice a day. I repeat, some people are allergic to bee pollen, so check with your doctor and start slowly. If you're active, you can take more – I take three full tablespoons a day. Taking bee pollen, along with getting off sugar, may make a startling difference in your health and your weight.

Sweet & Sour

Another effective way to lose weight is by taking the edge off your appetite a few minutes before you eat by drinking a special beverage I call the Total Health Drink (THD). It not only supplies many vitamins and minerals in an easy-to-absorb form, but prepares your stomach so it can digest the food you eat more efficiently. You make it at home from fresh and natural ingredients, it tastes great, and costs very little. Although you can find the ingredients at any grocery store, these won't work. That's because the kind they sell at regular grocery stores are processed and heat-treated, which ruins the nutritive value. You must use the exact kinds I recommend that are available at health food stores, catalogs, or on-line stores, to get the maximum effectiveness.

Here's the recipe: Two teaspoons unheated, raw honey and 2 teaspoons to 2 tablespoons raw apple cider vinegar in an 8 ounce glass of spring or filtered water. (See the Resource Guide for brands.) Mix, stir, and drink ten minutes before mealtime. Do this before lunch and dinner, and you will not only eat less, but have better digestion (say goodbye to antacids) and more energy throughout the day.

You can mix several days worth at once and store it in a glass bottle in the refrigerator. The vinegar must be raw and it must be apple cider vinegar. White vinegar or other kinds do not work and are even harmful. Start with the lower amount of vinegar – 2 teaspoons and see how it goes. If you feel you need more, go up to the 2 tablespoons. After drinking it, rinse your mouth out with water, since the acid in the vinegar may not be good for tooth enamel. But don't worry, you won't be dissolving your teeth, it's just a precaution. Don't use metal when handling vinegar, but stainless steel is OK.

How effective is this drink? Dr. Carol Johnston, professor of nutrition at Arizona State University has done numerous studies on the benefits of vinegar. She reported that those who took the two tablespoons before meals lost an average of two pounds over four weeks. The people who didn't take it didn't lose any weight and some actually increased weight over the study period. That may not sound like a big weight loss, but it's something, and just one of the ways your body is going to come to its normal, correct weight when you eat better. Dr. Johnston also said the vinegar helped with blood-glucose levels in diabetes, and I explore this in more depth in the diabetes chapter.(34)

If you're worried about the honey in the recipe, don't be. Since it has not been heated, it still contains all the vitamins, minerals, and most importantly, the enzymes that help digest itself and other foods. It reacts totally differently in the body than the other heat-treated honey that will rot your teeth and cause diabetes. Unheated honey on the other hand, is good for diabetics since its active enzymes actually replace the insulin that's lacking and helps blood sugar. In fact, the honey you will be using is known to improve many other health problems too, similar to what you read about concerning bee pollen.

Food for Thought

Can you really get noticeable results from such simple things as honey and vinegar? After all, you've eaten honey and vinegar many times in the past without seeing any effects.

Please consider that you've probably been consuming second-rate, processed, and life-*less* forms that actually cause the body to work harder. Now, you will be consuming vibrant, life-*giving* forms that supply energy and help your body function the way it's supposed to. The difference is like night and day. Over time, it adds up to be very, very significant. Although nature is often simple, never underestimate its powers – especially its powers to heal.

The Total Health Drink has been shown to help a wide variety of health problems besides excess weight. The health benefits that vinegar may help include: acid reflux, acid indigestion, blood sugar/diabetes control, arthritis, blood pressure, colds, constipation, diarrhea, indigestion, increasing metabolism, fatigue, fibromyalgia, headaches, kidney and liver problems, skin problems and others. Since apple cider vinegar helps cut mucus and phlegm, it also helps with asthma.

Science is beginning to recognize the benefits of apple cider vinegar. A study in Japan showed that those taking vinegar had "enhanced glycogen repletion in liver and skeletal muscle," meaning they recovered from fatigue faster. Vinegar has been clinically shown to help in calcium absorption, kidney function, hypertension, ear infections, and cancer. As I said, many studies have shown vinegar helps with blood-sugar control.[35,36,37,38,39,40]

Apple cider vinegar contains 19 of the 22 minerals essential for human health and is rich in amino acids, vitamins, enzymes, pectin, and some valuable fruit acids such as acetic and malic acids.

Malic acid is known to help soften and dissolve gall and kidney stones and is important in energy production (it's needed by enzymes in ATP synthesis). Malic acid is believed to be the most potent aluminum detoxifier and may help Alzheimer's disease, since aluminum may be a major contributor to impaired brain function.

Another benefit of malic acid may be for pain relief, especially in cases of fibromyalgia (FM). It's believed that malic acid can reverse low oxygen levels in muscle tissue, and along with magnesium, can bring significant pain relief experienced from fibromyalgia. In one study reported in the *Journal of Nutritional Medicine*, "All patients reported significant subjective improvement of pain within 48 hours of starting [magnesium and malic acid supplementation]. . .This appears to be a very promising approach to the management of FM."[41] I discuss magnesium in greater detain throughout the book (telling you the best way to supplement it), but understand here that most if not all cases of FM exhibit a magnesium deficiency, so getting magnesium levels back up is imperative for recovery (all drugs and soft drinks deplete magnesium).

Another thing that would probably help fibromyalgia significantly, since it appears it is due in part to low oxygen levels in the tissues, is the breathing technique I detail in the chapter on asthma. So those three things: apple cider vinegar, magnesium, and the special breathing technique (not deep breathing) will go far in alleviating the pain of FM.

Apple cider vinegar is also believed to thin the blood and prevent blood clots. It's rich in potassium (about 15 mg per tablespoon), which is known to lower blood pressure and relax blood vessels. Potassium is believed to be one of the most important minerals for good health since it is so necessary for the proper functioning of the heart and muscles. D.C. Jarvis, M.D., said that potassium is found in just the right amounts in natural apple cider vinegar and "is so essential to the life of every living thing that without it there would be no life."[42] Potassium's main function is to promote cell, tissue and organism growth and is necessary to replace dead cells and tissues. Good sources of potassium besides apple cider vinegar are root vegetables including potatoes, beets, parsnips, turnips, raw, unsalted nuts, melons, peaches, avocados, tomatoes, and bananas.

Humans are not the only ones who benefit from apple cider vinegar. The *Encyclopedia of Natural Pet Care* says, "Long a folk remedy, cider vinegar has been shown to improve the health of dairy cows, horses, dogs and other animals. It reduces common infections, aids whelping, improves stamina, prevents muscle fatigue after exercise, increases resistance to disease and protects against food poisoning. . .it normalizes acid levels in the stomach, improves digestion and the assimilation of nutrients, reduces intestinal and fecal odors, helps cure constipation, alleviates some of the symptoms of arthritis and helps prevent bladder stones and urinary tract infections."[43] So if Rover or Muffin is ailing, try spiking their water bowl with a shot of apple cider vinegar.

If you have varicose veins or restless leg syndrome, spraying on full strength apple cider vinegar may help. It helps the burning of hemorrhoids (swab full strength with a cotton ball). Dab underarms as a natural deodorant. It stops Athlete's Foot. Mix with water to treat yeast infections. These are simple things that you can try, and if it works on these problems, maybe it works on the bigger ones too. For more about apple cider vinegar, check out Dr. Jarvis' book *Folk Medicine* or the great book by Patrick Quillin, *Honey, Garlic & Vinegar: Home Remedies & Recipes*.

There are a few variations to the Total Health Drink worth mentioning, the most important one involves adding garlic. As you'll see, garlic is another natural food that helps with a myriad of diseases and making it a daily part of your diet may help improve your health markedly. The vinegar-garlic-honey drink (VGH) can be made simply by putting one cup apple cider vinegar, one cup raw honey, and 8 cloves garlic into a blender. Mix on high for a minute and pour into a glass (not plastic) container. Seal and leave in the refrigerator for five days. Take two tablespoons in a glass of water once or twice a day, preferably before meals.

Other variations are to add a couple sticks of cinnamon and/or some chopped ginger to this mixture as it sits in the refrigerator. Cinnamon is believed to strengthen the cardiovascular system, lower cholesterol, improve blood sugar and insulin sensitivity, help with respiratory problems, improve brain function, reduce arthritis pain, improve digestion, and even reduce the proliferation of leukemia and lymphoma cancer cells. I discuss the amazing benefits of cinnamon in other chapters. Ginger is believed to relax blood vessels, stimulate blood flow, relieve pain aid digestion, help with motion sickness and nausea, and inhibit vomiting. Ginger is also an anti-inflammatory, which means it may be useful in fighting heart disease, cancer, Alzheimer's disease, and arthritis.

TV and Weight Gain

Watching television can contribute to weight gain and health problems in everyone, regardless of age. William Dietz, M.D., head of clinical nutrition at New England Medical Center Hospital in Boston says that television viewing is the second most important predictor of adolescent obesity behind childhood obesity. A child who watches four or more hours of television a day has twice the risk of obesity than the child who watches less. Dietz attributes this to a decrease in physical activity and an increase in eating while watching TV.(44)

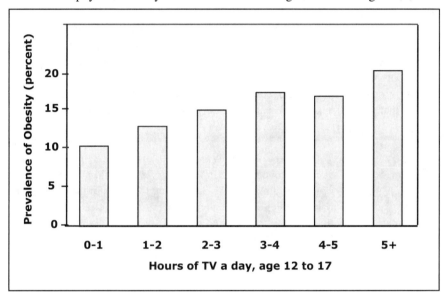

Figure 1

Television and Obesity: A child who watches four or more hours of TV a day has twice the risk of being obese.

Street play – which is sometimes not an option given today's legitimate safety concerns – can scarcely compete with the hypnotic lure of the screen. The prevalence of day care, after school care, and even latchkey kid situations make television an all too convenient "activity."

Unfortunately, there's nothing active about it. The American Academy of Pediatrics confirms "Increased television use is documented to be a significant factor leading to obesity."(45) What's more, the *Journal of American Medical Association* showed that children lost weight, and lost inches around the midriff, if they simply watched less television.(46) Another study by the American Heart association showed that people who spend at least two and a half hours a day watching TV and who eat fast food twice a week are three times as likely to become obese than those who eat out only once a week and watch less than an hour and a half of TV a day.(47)

To better realize the overall impact television has on the lives of our children, consider these sobering statistics:

- The national average for all children is more than three hours of TV per day – about 21 to 28 hours a week. This translates into 20 percent of their waking hours glued to the tube. That doesn't include time watching video movies, surfing the Internet, playing video games or watching music videos. By age 70, today's typical American child will have spent seven to 10 years watching television. The average American child views 20,000 television ads per year (2,000 of them for beer and wine).
- Children as young as three are influenced by pressure from ads.
- Young children are not able to distinguish between commercials and television programs. They don't recognize that commercials are attempting to sell then something.
- In one year's time of average viewing, the child will be exposed to more than 14,000 sexual references. Twenty one hours a week of viewing will show them one sexual reference every five minutes.(48)

In 1999 the American Academy of Pediatrics (AAP) made the recommendation that children younger than two years old should not be allowed to watch television at all, stating that it may stunt the development of their brains. The emotional and intellectual development of young children depends upon interaction with adults. When children watch TV that is lacking. (49)

The academy explains, "Pediatricians should urge parents to avoid television viewing for children under the age of two years. Although certain television programs may be promoted to this age group, research on early brain development shows that babies and toddlers have a critical need for direct interactions with parents and other significant caregivers for healthy brain growth and development of appropriate social, emotional and cognitive skills. Therefore, exposing such young children to television programs should be discouraged." The academy goes on to advise parents to limit all children's TV viewing to one to two hours of "quality programming" per day: "Time spent with media often displaces involvement in creative, active or social pursuits."

Besides weight gain, the American Academy of Pediatrics also blames TV for some of the violence exhibited by some children. "More than 1,000 scientific studies and reviews conclude that significant exposure to media violence increases the risk of aggressive behavior in certain children and adolescents, desensitizes them to violence, and makes them believe that the world is a 'meaner and scarier' place than it is." In 1995, the academy said, "by age 18 the average American child has viewed an estimated 200,000 acts of violence on TV alone. Video games increase that number. . . Although media violence is not the only cause of violence in American society, it is the single most easily remediable contributing factor."

Food for Thought

My drama professor in college said that theater is a reflection of life – a reflection, not a cause. I have to agree that exposing children to violence can do nothing but harm them, as the studies show, and I would endorse any legislation to limit violence and sex on TV. I need to point out, however, that the reason there is so much violence on TV today is because it sells. It sells because it's what people want to watch. It's what people want to watch because it's what they identify with. They identify with it because they are in fact becoming more violent themselves. There are many reasons for this tendency toward violence, as we'll see. These reasons are not just psychological and sociological, but biochemical and physiological as well. Mainstream theater, movies, and TV are reflecting what our society is becoming – one of decreased morals, sick and aggressive minds, and sick bodies.

An American child has viewed about 360,000 advertisements before graduating from high school. The AAP states, "In 1750 BC, the Code of Hammurabi made it a crime, punishable by death, to sell anything to a child without first obtaining a power of attorney. In the 1990s, selling products to American children has become a standard business practice." The AAP "...believes advertising directed toward children is inherently deceptive and exploits children under eight years of age" because children who are developmentally younger than eight "are unable to understand the intent of advertisements and, in fact, accept advertising claims as true."(50)

Children age 12 and younger spent or influenced the spending of around $500 billion in 1997. More and more commercials are geared to children to try and get their share of that money.

The American Psychological Association (APA) says in its brochure titled *Violence on Television*, "Violent programs on television lead to aggressive behavior by children and teenagers who watch those programs." This was from a report by the National Institute of Mental Health, a report that confirmed and extended an earlier study done by the Surgeon General.(51)

Other psychological research has shown three major effects of seeing violence on television:

- Children may become less sensitive to the pain and suffering of others.
- Children may be more fearful of the world around them.
- Children may be more likely to behave in aggressive or harmful ways toward others.
- Children who watch a lot of TV are less aroused by violent scenes than those who watch a little. They are bothered less by violence in general and less likely to see anything wrong with it.

In several studies, children who watched a violent program instead of a non-violent one were slower to intervene or call for help when, a short time later, they saw younger children fighting or playing destructively. George Gerbner, Ph.D., of the University of Pennsylvania, has reported that children's TV shows contain about 20 violent acts each hour. (Imagine how many in an adult program.) He also reported that children who watch a great deal of television are more likely to view the world as a mean and dangerous place.

Gerbner's ground-breaking research was done in the early 1980s. Back then there were an estimated 22 acts of violence per hour on TV. Since then the numbers have increased: In 1992 one prime-time show (*Young Indiana Jones*) registered 60 acts of violence per hour; *Cookie's Cartoon Club* averaged 100; *Tom and Jerry* averaged 88; and *Looney Tunes* averaged 80.(52)

In a study at the Pennsylvania State University, close to 100 preschool children were observed both before and after watching television. One group watched cartoons containing much violence, the other group shows that had no kind of violence. Significant differences in behavior were observed in the two groups: "Children who watch violent shows, even 'just funny' cartoons, were more likely to hit out at their playmates, argue, disobey class rules, leave tasks unfinished, and were less willing to wait for things than those who watched the nonviolent programs," Aletha Huston, Ph.D., reported.(53)

A report in *The Christian Science Monitor* reinforces the fact that young children are very impressionable when it comes to watching TV. When a class of two-to five-year-olds watched *Barney*, they sang along, marched along, held one another's hands, and laughed together. The next day the same class watched the aggressive *Power Ranger*. Within minutes they were karate-chopping and high-kicking the air – and one another.(54)

Leonard Eron, Ph.D., at the University of Illinois, found that children who watched a lot of TV violence when in elementary school tended to show a higher level of aggressive behavior when they became teenagers. He and his team of researchers observed a group of youngsters until they were 30. They found that the ones who had watched a lot of TV when they were eight were more likely to be arrested and prosecuted for criminal acts as adults.(55)

Even though some broadcasters do not believe there is enough evidence to prove that TV violence is harmful, scientists do. The 1992 American Psychological Association's Task Force on Television and Society confirms this view in a report entitled "Big World, Small Screen: The Role of Television in American Society." They say that just by limiting the number of hours children watch television will probably reduce the amount of aggression they see. This will help keep the child in a more peaceful, less agitated state – not just at the time, but later on in life.(56)

Parents should also watch at least one episode of the programs their kids are watching. That way they'll know what their children are being exposed to and can talk to them about it. Or, parents can outright ban any programming they deem too offensive and limit viewing to shows that have less or no violence.

Food for Thought

Here's a totally radical recommendation: Sell your TV. Or box it up and put it in the basement. Or put it away somewhere and take it out only for special occasions or emergencies. Can you imagine life without TV? How did the human species make it without *Seinfeld, 60 Minutes, Sesame Street*? They must have been strong individuals back then to be able to function and not get bored out of their skulls. No TV! Augh!

I've had a number of children's books published, and I go to elementary schools to read the books, do a show, and give writing workshops. Invariably, one of the students will ask me how I got started writing. This is what I tell them, and it's absolutely true: After I finished graduate school (in Environmental Sciences and Engineering), I loaded up my 1979 Plymouth Horizon hatchback (the worst car ever built) with just about everything I owned to go off and look for a real job. You know, be a responsible adult and do something with my degree. I crammed that little car to the ceiling. Just when it was totally full with just the driver's seat clear to sit in, I looked down on the sidewalk and saw my little 13-inch black-and-white TV sitting there.

I was tired of packing and didn't want to open a door because everything would have fallen out, so I left the TV with a friend. I got down to Florida (I wanted a job, but you can't forget golf!) and rented an apartment. Those first few days, coming home after job hunting, I found my hand actually reaching out for the TV's On button, even though there wasn't a TV there! You see, I had become conditioned, kind of like one of Pavlov's dogs, to turn on the TV the moment I came home. (I don't think I started salivating, but I can't say for sure.) Well, poverty is good for some things, because I could barely feed myself, so I surely couldn't afford a new TV.

As a kid, I hadn't watched much TV – I was more interested in playing outside than watching something inside. But from what I've learned from researching this book, if I had watched more TV as a kid, maybe I wouldn't care so much about sports or learning or anything else for that matter. Anyway, to keep myself from climbing the walls, I started to read. Yes, read. I read *Moby Dick, War & Peace, Crime & Punishment, The Castle*.

Then, one night, I picked up a pen, I put it on the paper and out came a paragraph. It was sorrowful and depressing – just like those books. It was bad writing, really, bad. But, I kept doing it anyway. One thing led to another, and I started writing a novel. Then a couple years later, a book for kids (not as depressing as most literature), which eventually got published. The moral of the story is that I became a writer because I didn't have a TV. It's amazing what you can do when you don't have one. It's amazing what you *want* to do when you don't have one.

When I go to schools now and tell this story, I ask the kids what they think it would be like to not have a TV. I get groans of agony in reply. So, I dare you. I double dare you. Turn off the TV. Put it away. Find out what life can be like. It won't just be good for you, but more so for your kids. Just remember, you'll go through a withdrawal period, so brace yourself.

I remember reading about a study once years ago where researchers wanted to see how TV was affecting us. So they had a small community go off TV cold-turkey for about a month. What happened was very interesting. The first several days after taking away all the TVs, crime went up. But after a short while, the community settled down to become more peaceful than when they had TV. The researchers likened it to coming off drugs. There is an initial "withdrawal" period, followed by better health. You can't go wrong watching less TV.

It's not just the content on TV that's a problem; it's the very nature of the TV itself. TV puts the viewer in an altered state of consciousness similar to a hypnotic state. It has been scientifically shown that as little as 30 seconds induces a semi-hypnotic, sleepiness, or inattentive state of mind.[57] (That's why violence on TV works so well – those kinds of images keep the watcher awake.) Humans are more open to suggestion in this state – which the advertisers love.

Since the image on the screen is ready-made, our minds do not have to create it's own as is done in reading. This has lead psychologist Bruno Bettelheim to say, "TV traps the fantasy, it doesn't free it. A good book motivates thinking and simultaneously frees it." Valdemar W. Setzer, Ph.D., a professor of Computer Science, has studied and published on the problems of the influence of TV, video games, and computers on children for almost 30 years. He says, "If you wish to develop your thinking, do reading. If you wish to impair your thinking, dampening it more and more, watch TV."[58]

Not only that, but cathode-ray tube TVs give off low levels of radiation. Some researchers believe that prolonged exposure can cause a host of problems including insomnia, lack of attentiveness, hyperactivity and discipline problems, lack of ability to concentrate, and possible cancer risks.

The pioneer of time-lapse photography and photo biology, John Ott, performed some interesting tests on the effects of exposure to television radiation and biological functioning. He used white laboratory rats in his experiment. Two rats were placed in each of two cages, directly in front of a color TV. The set was turned on for six hours a day and 10 hours on Saturday and Sunday. One cage was shielded from the TV tube with black photographic paper, and the other cage was shielded with one-eighth inch of lead shielding. The sound was turned off and the rats couldn't see the. What Ott observed was that the rats protected with only the black paper became increasingly hyperactive and aggressive within three to 10 days. After that, they became progressively lethargic. At 30 days they were extremely lazy and it was necessary to push them to make them move.

The rats shielded with lead showed some similar patterns of behavior, but they took longer to manifest and were not as severe. Dr. Ott noted that there was another TV (black-and-white) in the area – approximately six feet away, which at the time was considered a safe distance – that was unshielded. He concluded that the lethargic behavior of the shielded rats was probably due to the exposure from the second set. His experiment was repeated three times with different rats, and the results were the same in each experiment. The unshielded rats, when exposed to both the color and black-and-white TVs, were even more severely impacted. All the young rats in one of the cages died within 10 to 12 days. Autopsies were performed, and microscopic investigations indicated brain tissue damage in several instances.

Also of note is what happened in a room nearby – about 15 feet away from the color set. This other room had been used for animal breeding purposes successfully for more than two years. But immediately after the color TV was placed in the adjacent room, the breeding program was completely disrupted. Litters of rats that had been averaging eight to 12 young dropped to one or two, and many of those did not survive. It took approximately six months for the breeding program to return to normal after the color TV was removed.(59)

These experiments were performed around 1965. And you may be thinking that since then, we've gotten wiser and have made televisions cleaner. After all, we have regulatory agencies to protect us. At the time of Dr. Ott's experiments, the National Committee on Radiation Protection and the International Commission on Radiation Protection set a limit of 0.5 mr/hr (5 millirems per hour, a standard way to measure radiation) measured at 5 centimeters from the surface of the set. Sadly but not surprisingly, this standard has not changed.(60) That's more than 35 years with the same standard, despite evidence that it causes harm.

Consumer advocate Ralph Nader spoke up in the '70s to the Senate Commerce Committee: "The standards are too low. Millions of people are being exposed to the risk of physical, genetic, and eye damage." It is important to note that flat panel TVs incorporating Liquid Crystal Displays (LCD) or Plasma displays are not capable of emitting x-radiation. As such these products and are not subject to the FDA standard and do not pose a public health hazard. So one of these types of TVs is better than the CRT type.

Video Games

Although there has not been any conclusive research done on the effects of video games, it's safe to say that playing them is not the healthiest activity a person, especially a child, could undertake. These games often present extremely violent, bloody, and sometimes sexually explicit scenarios that, considering the research done on TV shows, may carry over into life and encourage violent and uncaring behavior. Indeed, John Naisbitt, in his book *High Tech, High Touch:Technology and our Search for Meaning*, tells us that the youngsters who committed the crimes at Littleton, Colorado and West Paducah, Kentucky, actually trained and practiced their acts on video games.(61)

Dr. Setzer says that "…the prolong use of these games can cause, mainly upon children, a number of physical and psychological problems which may include the following: obsessive, addictive behavior; dehumanization of the player; desensitizing of feelings; personality changes; hyperactivity; learning disorder; premature maturing of children; psychomotor disorders; health problems due to lack or exercise and tendonitis; development of anti-social behavior; loss of free thinking and will."[62]

Only time and further research will tell just how harmful these games can be on our children But since so many companies are making so much money selling them and the demand for them is so high, there has been no push to find out if or to what degree they may be harmful.

But while we're waiting for research to catch up with life, use your own common sense. Do you really think sitting around and blowing things and people up on a screen is helping him or her become a mentally healthy and well-balanced child? Instead of letting your child play a video game alone, why not break out the good old *Monopoly*, *Scrabble* or other board game and have some fun with him or her. You can find the time to do this by not watching TV! Go ride bikes or something. You hardly ever see kids on bikes anymore.

CHAPTER III

Cancer

The quality of life and life expectancy in the U.S. has undoubtedly improved over the last century. In 1900, the life expectancy was just 47 years, now it's 71.

Food for Thought

The modern medical establishment and drug/vaccine manufacturers are quick to take credit for our increased life expectancy. Although it's true that medical advances have kept pace with life expectancy and the quality of life, to say they are the cause of them is not true.

The main reason people live longer now in the U.S. than a century ago is due to one simple, overlooked reason – electricity. Electric power plants were first brought on line in the late 1800s (Westinghouse Electric Company was organized in 1886), and the more widespread electricity's uses and accessibility became, the less punishing life got. Life expectancy hasn't increased because of medical advances, drugs, medical technology, vaccines, or even nutrition (the food in 1900 was purer and more nutritious than it is today), but simply because the cruel hardships of simple survival were alleviated due to the machines and conveniences made possible with the advent of electricity.

People point to places like Africa and how so many people are dying or suffering there because of lack of food, medicines, and vaccines. The truth of the matter is, if these communities had electricity, the quality of life and the life expectancy of their people would skyrocket, just as it did in the U.S. a century ago. Modern medicine, drugs, and vaccines, along with some byproducts of technology, have not only made less of a contribution to improving our life than they're given credit for, but are creating problems mankind has never faced. Some of these problems are affecting you directly, some will affect your children, and some are threatening our very existence as a species, as you will see.

To assess the present-day health of our society and determine if it is improving or declining, let's examine the occurrences and severity of chronic, long-term illnesses starting with cancer. Acute diseases are transient and less indicative of an overall systemic breakdown; I think of them as a snapshot of health that may not tell the whole story. They're more difficult to get reliable long-term tracking information on simply because many acute illnesses never need hospital care and are otherwise seldom reported. Although some may argue that many chronic, degenerative diseases are a result of genetic factors, many researchers and health care professionals believe that even if an individual has an inherent predisposition towards a specific illness, the disease will not manifest from this tendency alone.

Food for Thought

We create in our bodies and minds the soil for diseases to take root and grow. We are responsible for our health, or lack there of – even if we have a predisposition towards a certain illness. The human body is incredible and, if properly maintained, can overcome and reverse most infirmities. Modern science might point to genetics as a contributing factor of certain diseases, but it admits that the causes of most degenerative diseases are, to them, unknown. For example, 85 percent of women who develop breast cancer have no known family history of the disease. (1)

Even if genetics did play a role, this still can be overcome or at least ameliorated – something I've done in my own life. My grandmother and other relatives had diabetes, and I was borderline diabetic for several years. Now I have normal blood sugars and am in no danger of developing diabetes, due in large part due to changing my diet over 20 years ago. I have a much stronger system now than when I was in my twenties and thirties when I was eating pizza five nights a week and hamburgers from fast-food restaurants for lunch every day. If I had continued abusing my body in that way, I feel confident that I would now be in need of daily insulin injections or worse.

If you take care of yourself within the laws of nature, genetic weaknesses will be held at bay. In fact, you'd probably regenerate and get biologically younger.

Dorland's Medical Dictionary, defines cancer as "any malignant, cellular tumor. . ." A tumor is defined as "1. swelling, one of the cardinal signs of inflammation; morbid enlargement. 2. neoplasm; a new growth of tissue in which cell multiplication is uncontrolled and progressive." A malignant tumor is "one having the properties of invasion and metastasis and showing a high degree of anaplasia." A benign tumor is "one lacking the properties of invasion and metastasis and showing a lesser degree of anaplasia than do malignant tumors." (anaplasia – loss of differentiation of cells and of their orientation to one another and to the axial framework and blood vessels, a characteristic of tumor tissue.) (2)

Cancer is a cell or cluster of cells that is out of control. A cancer cell replicates without the cellular mechanisms intact, which tells it to differentiate into the correct kind of cell (if healthy, a liver cell replicates to form new liver cells, a skin cell will replicate to form new skin cells, etc.). What's worse, it doesn't know when to stop replicating. A cancer cell is a cell that has gone haywire and is totally confused. It's the ultimate expression of a cell that has lost its integrity and health. Essentially, cancer is evidence of a system that has broken down completely. The cancer not only starts and spreads, but is unchecked by other healthy cells because those cells are too weak to overcome the aberrant ones.

A cancer cell is close to extinction. That's why it replicates so voraciously. When an organism is stressed it reproduces faster and more often, attempting to ensure its own kind does not perish. (Interestingly, that same principle relates to humans overall; as our species has become stressed, we are seeing changes in fertility characteristics such as women menstruating sooner, earlier pregnancies, multiple births, and so on. More on that later.)

It is generally accepted that all of our bodies produce some number of cancer cells every day. If the body is healthy and strong, these aberrant cells are consumed up by phagocytes (the garbage men in our blood), killed or generally rendered harmless and disposed of easily. Only when the total body system is in such a state of internal degeneration will normal cellular processes be overcome by uncontrolled cellular processes. Notice the word "internal." Someone may look healthy, but inside, his or her cells are scrambled and weak.

In 1900, there were 64.0 deaths reported from "cancer and other malignant tumors" per 100,000 people of all ages and races in the U.S. In 1948, that number had risen to 134.9, and by 1989, the figure was 199.99.(3) Between 1950 and 1988, for U.S. whites, incidences of all forms of cancer rose by 43.5 percent and age-adjusted cancer mortality (deaths) increased by 2.9 percent.(4)

Now, every hour, about 156 people in the U.S. will learn they have some form of cancer. Cancer caused about 559,650 deaths in 2007. Cancer is now the number one killer among Americans under the age of 85. It's estimated that from birth to death, one male in two will die from cancer, and one female in three will die from it.(5,6)

In 1998, approximately 12,400 children younger than 20 years of age (which make up nearly 30 percent of the U.S. population), were diagnosed with cancer; and 2,300 died. Overall, cancer is the second leading cause of death among children after accidents. The probability of developing cancer prior to age 20 varies slightly by sex. A newborn male has 0.32 percent probability of developing cancer by age 20, (a one in 300 chance). Similarly a newborn female has a 0.3 percent probability of developing cancer by age 20 (a one in 333 chance).(7,8,9)

Table 1 shows the incidence rates and the 20-year trends from the period 1973-1992. As you can see, in 1973-1974, the incidence of cancer in ages 0 to 14 years old was 12.9 per 100,000 children, and in the 0 to 19 age group, the incidence was 13.8 per 100,000.(10)

Table 1

Age-Adjusted Cancer SEER Incidence Rates* and 20-Year Trends, 1973-92
by Primary Cancer Site, All Races, Males and Females

	Ages 0-14 Ages			Ages 0-19		
	Average Rate**		% Change	Average Rate**		% Change
	1973-74	1991-92	1973-92	1973-74	1991-92	1973-92
All Races	12.9	13.9	8.4	13.8	15.9	15.0
Whites	13.3	14.4	8.7	14.2	16.5	16.1
Blacks	10.3	12.1	17.4	11.1	12.7	14.7
Bone, Joint	0.7	0.7	3.6	0.8	0.9	10.8
Brain, Nervous	2.4	3.3	35.4	2.2	3.1	39.8
Hodgkin's	0.7	0.5	-25.8	1.3	1.4	11.6
Kidney, Renal	0.7	0.8	13.3	0.6	0.6	12.8
Leukemias	4.3	4.1	-4.2	3.8	3.7	-2.7
Acute Lymphoncytic	2.7	3.2	14.7	2.3	2.7	15.1
Non-Hodgkin's Lymphomas	0.8	0.9	12.1	0.8	1.0	32.4
Soft Tissue	0.7	0.9	24.9	0.8	0.9	14.5

* SEER Program. Rates are per 100,000 and are age-adjusted to the 1970 U.S. standard standard
  population. Each rate has been age-adjusted by 5-year age groups.

**The Average Rate is the Average Annual Rate over the specified two-year period.

By 1991-1992, the incidence had increased to 13.9 percent in the 0 to 14
age group and 15.9 percent in the 0 to 19 age group. Therefore, there was an 8.4
percent increase in the younger age group and a 15.0 percent increase in the age
group through 19 years old. That is most definitely a significant rise in both age
groups, and is not due to just statistical variability or probability.

The National Cancer Institute (NCI) reports that the incidence (per 100,000
children) of many childhood cancers has increased steadily during the period
1973-1990. All childhood cancers combined have increased at the rate of 0.9
percent per year. Brain cancer and central nervous system cancers have
increased at 1.8 percent per year. Leukemias have increased at 1.8 percent per
year. Non-Hodgkin's lymphomas have increased at 1.4 percent per year. Kidney
cancer has increased at 1 percent per year.[11] The data from another survey by
the National Cancer Institute are similar. Figures 2 and 3 show the overview of
childhood cancer patterns from this study.[12]

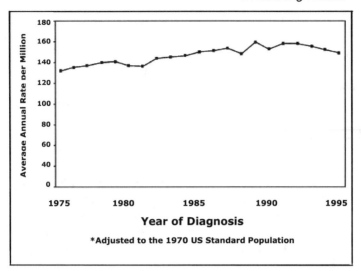

Figure 2

Trends in the age-adjusted* SEER incidence and U.S. mortality rates for all childhood cancers age <20, all races, both sexes,1975-1995

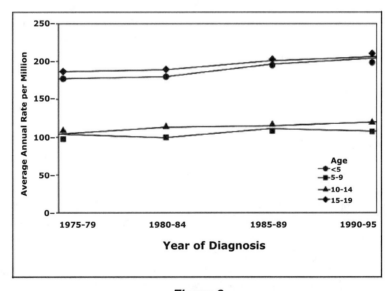

Figure 3

Trends in age-specific incidence rates for all childhood cancers by age, all races, both sexes, SEER, 1975-1995

Again, childhood cancer is on the rise. Of course, part of the increase results from better diagnosis and better recording of cases by state and federal agencies. But the SEER report recognizes that "taken together [changes in record keeping] cannot explain the magnitude of the increases that have been observed over the last several decades."[13]

In adults, cancers occur after a delay of seven to 20 years (or more) between the time of exposure to cancer-causing agents and the manifestation of a cancer. However, in the case of childhood cancers, these delays are often much shorter. That makes it seem as if many childhood cancers occur in children who are somehow predisposed to getting the disease. If they are exposed to a carcinogen before or shortly after birth, their disease manifests quickly. Perhaps the predisposition is inherited, or it may be caused by something in the environment.[14] Whatever the reasons, we are breaking down sooner. Cancer is becoming an epidemic not just for the population at large, but for children too. Our overall health is impaired, allowing cancer cells to flourish and take over. Consider that the severity of a carcinogen (poison) is dose dependant, so children get higher body weight adjusted doses of every poison they consume. This includes pesticides, herbicides, fungicides, cleaning chemicals, chlorine and fluoride in our water, even chemical flame retardants in their bedding and clothing.

Why is cancer increasing at all, among adults and children alike; and why is it affecting people at younger and younger ages? The second question will be discussed more thoroughly later. The answer to the first question may not be obvious to the traditional medical and scientific community, but is readily apparent when you just look at our history, society and environment.

Causes of Cancer

There are a myriad of reasons people get cancer – from alterations in the foods we eat and nutritional problems to the chemicals and impurities in our environment. The list of causative agents seems almost endless and sometimes it may appear as if there's no way to avoid cancer.

However, we are not predisposed to cancer. Many of the causes can be eliminated or lessened simply by changing our lifestyle. In fact, a recent study reported in the *New England Journal of Medicine* examined 44,788 pairs of twins and found that environmental factors such as diet and lifestyle are a much better indicator of cancer risk than genetics.[15] There's one estimate that as many as one-third of cancer cases in the U.S. are a result of obesity and lack of physical exercise.[16] You can do much to protect yourself from cancer (and any other disease for that matter) if you live properly and take precautionary measures. The first step to doing so is to know the enemy.

Chemicals

Since the 1940s, tens of thousands of new chemicals have been introduced into our lives. About 80,000 chemicals are now produced in North America and a thousand new chemicals are introduced each year. Over 3,000 chemicals are added to our food supply and 10,000 solvents, emulsifiers and preservatives are used in food processing. The production of synthetic materials increased from 1.3 million pounds in 1940 to 320 billion pounds in 1980. The health effects for a majority of those compounds are unknown. Only a small percentage of these chemicals have been tested for their effects on the central nervous system.[17]

Don't hold your breath if you expect better testing for adverse health effects of chemicals. John Wargo, Ph.D., of Yale University comments, "Thousands of synthetic chemicals need to be tested to understand their toxicity. By the time the federal government completes these tests, my children will have children." Wargo, one of the country's top experts on toxic chemicals, goes on to give us some sage advice, "It is just common sense to reduce exposure to toxic substances. Eat low on the food chain, test your water, buy organic food when possible, renovate [your house] with special care, and don't allow smoking around children."[18]

But is there proof that these chemicals cause problems in humans? Many people think that modern synthetic chemicals pose little or no risk. But one study of members of the American Chemical Society (ACS) revealed that chemists die at unusually high rates from cancer of the pancreas and lymph system and female chemists had an elevated risk of breast cancer. The study also revealed that chemists tend to commit suicide more than other people do. In another study of 347 white female members of ACS who died between 1925 and 1979, there were increases in breast cancer, ovary, stomach, pancreas, lymphatic, and hematopoietic blood-forming) cancers. Suicide among those women was five times higher than other U.S. white females.[19,20]

In a study reported in the *Journal of Occupational Medicine,* employees of a large pharmaceutical company revealed an increase in the occurrence of several kinds of cancer (lung, skin, brain) among males and an increase in leukemia, breast, and large-intestine cancers in females. Another study, of Exxon employees, revealed an increase in leukemia and lymphatic cancers among scientists, engineers, and research technicians, as compared with managerial employees who had less potential for chemical exposure.[21,22]

Adults are harmed by if they are overly or consistently exposed. The risk of these kinds of exposures to children is probably less, but they are still exposed to chemicals during day-to-day activities. The evidence shows that minimizing exposures to any unnatural chemicals may help reduce the chances of cancers later in life.

As the use of chemicals in our society increases, so do the occurrences of brain cancer. Table 2 shows the increase over a 35-year period. The steady increase in brain cancer is true for all industrialized countries (who use various chemicals consistently). In addition, there are similar increases occurring in children, so the increases are not just an effect of aging.

Table 2

Number of Brain Cancers (23)

Year	Per 100,000 Population
1940	1.95
1945	2.25
1950	2.90
1955	3.40
1960	3.70
1970	4.10
1975	4.25

A study reported in the *British Medical Journal* in 2004 estimated that perhaps 75 percent of most cancers are caused by environmental and lifestyle factors, including exposure to chemicals. A report in the Columbia University School of Public Health went even further, estimating a whooping 95 percent of cancer is caused by diet and environmental toxicity.(24)

Pesticides

Pesticides have been used for centuries. They were mostly natural ones until World Wars I and II, when synthetic chemicals were first manufactured for warfare. This proved to be the watershed for the modern agri-chemical industry since these chemicals later ended up on the farm to control pests. Why? Because these chemicals kill. In fact, one of the reasons the use of chemical pesticides were encouraged and touted was because the chemical companies wanted to find a use for all the leftover chemicals used for warfare after the wars. Instead of having to dispose of these poisons, they found a way to make a profit from them. (As we shall see, not only do they do this with pesticides, but with other deadly things as well.)

German scientists, while experimenting with nerve gas during World War II, synthesized parathion, the first organophosphate insecticide. It was first marketed in 1943 and is still widely used today. In the 1950s and 1960s, these kinds of chemicals became major pest control agents. By 1996, an estimated $26 billion worth of pesticides were used around the world. In 1939 Swiss chemist Paul Muller discovered the deadly properties of DDT. (He later won a Nobel Prize for this.)(25)

The term *pesticide* includes more than just insecticides, which is what most people think of when they hear the term. A pesticide is any substance intended to control, destroy, repel or attract a pest. They may be natural (for example, a living, pest-destroying organism such as *Bacillus thuringensis*) or synthetic – like most of the pesticides we are familiar with.

Pesticides, due to their widespread use and mobility in the environment, are major players in the toxic chemical debacle. A National Institute of Health Sciences research project found that in a large random sample of the general population, DDT was evident in 100 percent of the blood samples at an average level of 3.3 ppb (parts per billion). Chlordane (used for termite control, which seeps up into the living airspace) was found in 95 percent of the population. Other pesticides were also found in significant amounts, many of the type used on food.[26]

Each year some 3.5 billion pounds of industrial toxins and one billion to two billion pounds of pesticides are released into the environment in the United States alone, according to the EPA. Millions of Americans are being exposed to chemicals whose effects are unknown. Eighty percent of the chemicals now in use have never been tested for their carcinogenic, neurotoxic, immunotoxic or other toxic effects.[27]

Considering the lethal properties of such chemicals, pesticides being a major player, you would think their use might decline in inverse proportion to what we learn about them. But consider:

- There are 400 pesticides currently on the market that were registered before being tested to determine if they caused cancer, birth defects or wildlife toxicity.
- The amount of time it takes to ban a pesticide in the U.S. using present procedures is 10 years.
- There are 107 active ingredients in pesticides found to cause cancer in animals or humans. Of these, 83 are still in use today.
- There are 14 pesticides found to cause reproductive problems in animals.
- Thirty-8 percent of all food samples tested by the FDA in 1980 contained pesticide residues. Of the 496 pesticides identified as likely to leave residues on food, the percentage, which FDA tests can routinely detect, is only 40 percent.
- Nationally, the EPA estimates that one out of every 10 public drinking water wells contains pesticides, as well as over 440,000 rural private wells. At a minimum, 1.3 million people drink water contaminated with one or more pesticide.
- Fifty percent of the U.S. population gets its water supply from ground water. Some 14 million people in the U.S. routinely drink water contaminated with carcinogenic herbicides. Seventy-four different pesticides documented by the EPA were present in ground water in 1988, in 32 states. Forty-six percent of all U.S. counties containing ground

water are susceptible to contamination from agricultural pesticides and fertilizers.

- The highest rate of chemical-related illnesses of any occupational group in the U.S. is among farm workers, with approximately 300,000 cases reported each year. There are an estimated 10,400 cancer deaths related to pesticides each year.(28,29)

In April 1999, researchers in Switzerland reported that the rain falling in Europe contained such high levels of pesticides that the rainwater would be illegal if it were supplied as drinking water. It's contaminated with atrazine, alochlor and other common agricultural poisons sprayed onto crops.(30)

Atrazine is a weed killer used on 96 percent of the corn grown in the U.S. It was introduced in 1958 and some 68 million to 73 million pounds were used in 1995 alone, making it the best-selling pesticide in the nation. But it may kill more than pests. It interferes with the hormone systems of mammals, and two studies have suggested that it causes ovarian cancer in humans. The EPA lists it as a "possible human carcinogen." Atrazine is found in much of the drinking water in the Midwestern U.S. And is measurable in corn, milk, beef, and other foods.(31)

Childhood leukemias, lymphomas, neuroblastomas, and brain cancers have all been linked to pesticides as dozens of studies have shown. Considering this fact, there is a conspicuous absence of information on pesticide exposures and toxicity relating to children.(32)

Consumer Report magazine announced that many fruits and vegetables in the U.S. carry pesticide residues that exceed the limits that the EPA considers safe for children and that even one serving of some fruits and vegetables can exceed safe daily limits for young children. The U.S. Department of Agriculture took 27,000 food samples from 1994 to 1997 and looked at foods children are most likely to eat. Almost all the foods tested for pesticide residues were within legal limits, but were frequently well above the levels the Environmental Protection Agency says are safe for young children.(33)

Organophosphates (such as methyl parathion) are neurological poisons and work the same on humans as they do on insects. This insecticide accounts for most of the total toxicity on the foods that were analyzed, particularly peaches, frozen and canned green beans, pears, and apples – many foods children commonly eat. Late in 2000 the EPA stated that methyl parathion posed an "unacceptable risk" but that it had not taken any action to ban it or reduce its use. Another interesting point the *Consumer Report* study found was that U.S. grown foods had, in almost every case, higher pesticide levels than imported foods and more toxic ones at that.

Food for Thought

Some say that pesticides are needed to feed the world. If it weren't for them, they argue, we couldn't grow enough food for everyone, and farming would be too labor-intensive, thus making food too expensive. One researcher estimates that if it weren't for pesticides, we would still have 10 percent to 12 percent of the population working on farms rather than the mere 2 percent now needed to produce enough food to sustain the U.S. population. (Would that be so terrible?)

Consider that since the early 1930s the federal government has maintained a price support program, paying farmers not to grow certain crops, with the intent of keeping the price of food artificially high. The logic here is that since U.S. agriculture is so productive, that without price supports, the abundance of crops coupled with the law of supply and demand, would drive the price of food so low that many farmers couldn't survive, which ultimately might endanger the nation's food supply. Price supports started a decade or two before chemical pesticides made the scene in any significant amount. It seems to me that if we were producing so much food back then without pesticides, so much so that we had to pay farmers not to grow food to keep the prices high, the crops must have been doing just fine without the "help" of toxic chemicals. Also, there are now many farmers that use strictly "organic" methods to grow food. Yes, the "organically raised food" is a bit more expensive. But if all the farms operated this way, would not competition and the law of supply and demand bring down the price of the food?

It's ironic that the manufacturers and sellers of pesticides say that there would not be enough food were it not for pesticides and mass starvation might result. But in a few years we may all starve anyway because while there may be plenty of food, none of it will be edible due to the poisons. Do you doubt this? Then why is it that the occupation with the highest rate of chemical poisonings is farming?

Children are exposed to pesticides in many ways besides from food: pet collars; flea, tick and lice shampoos; pesticides used on lawns; in the garden; and around the home. Pesticides tend to settle on the floor, where children mostly play. A recent study revealed a strong relationship between brain cancers and compounds used to kill fleas and ticks.[34]

One study of chlorpyrifos (trade name *Dursban*) residues in a home showed that after treatment and a recommended ventilation period (on the government-approved label), pesticide residues were detected on the surfaces of children's plastic and cloth toys for two full weeks. Chlorpyrifos is one of the most commonly used pesticides in the United States. It is a potent nerve poison. One fifth of an ounce is all that's needed to kill an adult.[35]

In a study published in the November 1996 issue of *Environmental Science and Technology*, it was reported that outdoor pesticides, once carried inside on shoes and pets, could linger for long periods. The pesticides attach to house dust and accumulate in carpets, upholstered furniture, draperies, and on household surfaces. Since they are now protected from sun, rain, wind, and temperature extremes, the outdoor pesticides, which only last days or weeks outdoors, can persist for years. While exposure levels may be below the limit established by the World Health Organization for adults, the risk levels for children have not been established. Vacuuming only eliminates about one third of the contamination. If you use these products, it's good to remove your shoes at the door, and leave the pets outside.(36) The best thing is to avoid exposing your beloved pet to chemical pesticides – use natural products.

Chlorpyrifos is the common pesticide for flea treatment. Richard A. Fenske, Ph.D. An assistant professor at Rutgers University, conducted a study that showed that after recommended procedures were followed in applying the pesticide to carpets in an unoccupied apartment, levels of the pesticide in the "infant breathing zone" were ten times above the legal limit after seven hours and over three times the legal limit after 24 hours. Pesticide applicators typically state it is safe to return home "several hours" after the application. Please consider that the "legal limit" is not necessarily the actual limit at which adverse effects would not occur.(37)

According to the *Journal of the National Cancer Institute,* pet dogs exposed to the weed killer 2,4-D are dying of cancer at twice the normal rates. Dogs walk across or roll in herbicide-treated lawns and then ingest these toxic chemicals when they lick their coats or paws. The most popular lawn-care products contain 2,4-D.(38) Of course, children play on lawns too, so they will come in contact with the chemicals outside, and also track them into the house.

In 1993 the National Academy of Sciences released its long-awaited report on the health hazards of pesticides to infants and young children. They stated that pesticides are harmful to the environment and are known or suspected to be toxic to humans regardless of age. They are neurologically toxic, and can cause cancer, reproductive dysfunction, and dysfunction of the immune and endocrine systems.(39)

No allowable daily intakes have been calculated for infants, but recall that infants are much more susceptible to toxic chemicals than adults because their kidneys, liver, enzyme systems, and blood-brain barrier are not fully developed. In addition, a newborn has very little body fat available for storage, so any fat-soluble chemicals (pesticides are fat soluble) are circulated in the blood throughout the body for longer periods, thus possibly impacting other organs.

About 600 million pounds of 2,4-D are spread on American soil each year by homeowners and farmers. (Interestingly, federal law does not allow exact data to be gathered.)(40) It's used by homeowners to control crab grass and dandelions and by farmers on potatoes, tomatoes, rice, corn, sorghum, and other crops to keep weeds down. Again, this deadly chemical has a wartime connection: 2,4-D was mixed with 2,4,5-T to create *Agent Orange* and was used from 1962 to 1971 during the Vietnam War to defoliate the jungle where the Vietcong were living. But they were not its only victims. T*he American Journal of Public Health* reports that Vietnam veterans are 70 percent more likely to father children with one or more major birth defects compared with men with no military service.(41)

Throughout the U.S., approximately 75 percent of houses built before 1988 contain air levels of the pesticide chlordane, a common pesticide used for termite control. Thirty-four percent contain levels over the safety limit of 5 micrograms per cubic meter of air (set by the National Academy of Sciences).(42) An estimated 10 million to 20 million U.S. residents could be breathing chlordane levels that exceed the recommended safe limit. Chlordane contamination is linked to childhood cancers and blood disorders. David Ozonoff, Ph.D., of the Boston University School of Public Health, says, "A national program for monitoring all homes treated is urgently needed to detect persistent contamination." He went on to say, ". . .It should also be noted that commercial chlordane formulations contain carcinogenic 'inert ingredients' and contaminants, such as propylene oxide, hexachlorobutadiene, and carbon tetrachloride, apart from some 40 other ingredients so far undisclosed by the manufacturer, formulators, and applicators of chlordane/heptachlor."(43)

In 1987, 250 adults and children were exposed to chlordane when building surfaces and soil around their apartment complex were sprayed. Subsequent testing showed many negative effects upon mental function from low levels of air chlordane in their apartments. Test scores for reaction time, balance, and memory were lower and scores were worse for depression, anger, vigor, fatigue, and mood states. Also, these chlordane-exposed people had more asthma, allergies, chronic bronchitis, wheezing, headaches, and indigestion. The researchers wrote, "Examination of subjects exposed in their homes to chlordane. . .showed significant, and we suggest important, impairment of both the neurophysiological and psychological functions including mood states. These impairments include probably irreversible dysfunction of the brain. . .chlordane use should be prohibited worldwide."(44)

Americans put about 62.7 million pounds of pesticides and 278.5 million pounds of antimicrobials (disinfectants) into their homes each year. A recent study estimated that between 78 percent and 97 percent of families (in the Midwestern U.S.) use pesticides in and around the home. A study in Jacksonville, Florida, detected pesticides in the air in 100 percent of the homes.(45) And it's not just around the home that pesticide use is a problem: A study by Yale University researchers and Environment & Human Health Inc. found that 87 percent of schools apply pesticides on school grounds and in classrooms, often while children are on the premises.(46)

Farmers have an increased incidence of certain kinds of cancer (soft-tissue carcinomas such as non-Hodgkin's lymphomas and malignant lymphomas, the same type of cancer the dogs got when exposed to treated lawns). These cancers are on the rise in the general population as well. In fact, non-Hodgkin's lymphomas (NHL) were the second fastest-growing type of cancer in the U.S. in the 1980s and 1990s, increasing at the rate of 3.3 percent per year between 1973 and 1991. Two well-known Swedish scientists, Mikael Eriksson and Lennart Hardell, published a study in March 1999 showing that non-Hodgkin's lymphoma (NHL) is linked to pesticide exposure. One of the herbicides linked to NHL by this study is *Roundup* (glyphosate), a popular herbicide promoted as a safe spot-killer for weeds.

A previous study in 1998 implicated *Roundup* in hairy cell leukemia (cancer of the blood-forming organs). Several other animal studies have shown that *Roundup* can cause gene mutations and chromosomal damage.[47,48] Jonathan D. Buckley, Ph.D., of the University of Southern California in Los Angeles conducted a study that showed that children whose mothers used pesticides in the home once or twice a week were nearly two and a half times as likely to have non-Hodgkin's lymphoma. If the pesticides were used on a daily basis, the children were seven times more likely to get this kind of cancer. Pregnant women exposed to pesticides by professional exterminators in their homes were three times more likely to have a child with that cancer and children directly exposed to pesticides were just over twice as likely to develop the disease. This from the December 2000 issue of the journal *Cancer*.[49]

A very interesting article about pesticides and aggression was published by the *Environmental Research Foundation* on April 29, 1999. It linked aggression with the use of pesticides. One study the article cited was a five-year-long investigation that looked at the possible effects of low levels of insecticides, weed killers, and artificial fertilizers on the behavior patterns in the test animals. The study concluded that:

> [The] combinations of these chemicals – at levels similar to those found in the ground water of agricultural areas of the U.S. – have measurable detrimental effects. . .[There were] effects on the endocrine system (thyroid hormone levels) and the immune system, and reduced body weight, from mixtures of low levels of aldicarb and nitrate, atrazine and nitrate, and atrazine, aldicarb and nitrate together. . .increased aggression from exposure to atrazine and nitrate, and from atrazine, aldicarb and nitrate together. . . Some, though not all, studies have shown that attention deficit and/or hyperactivity disorders in children are linked to changes in the levels of thyroid hormone in the blood. Children with multiple chemical sensitivity (MCS) have abnormal thyroid levels. Furthermore, irritability and aggressive behavior are linked to thyroid hormone levels. . .[50]

A recent study of four- and five-year-old children in Mexico specifically noted a decrease in mental ability and an increase in aggressive behavior among children exposed to pesticides. This study reported,

Some valley children (exposed to pesticides) were observed hitting their siblings when they passed by, and they became easily upset or angry with a minor corrective comment by a parent. These aggressive behaviors were not noted in the pesticide-free-foothills children. The pesticide-exposed children had far less physical endurance in a test to see how long they could keep jumping up and down; they had inferior hand-eye coordination; and they could not draw a simple stick figure of a human being, which the upland children could readily do.(51)

Americans are searching for the causes of violence in their society. Some blame a decline in religious upbringing and others point to the fact that many times both parents work and no one is minding the kids. Violent movies and violence on TV, extremist Internet sites, and readily available cheap guns all contribute. But no one seems to be asking whether pesticides, fertilizers, and other toxins may be affecting our children's mental and emotional balance and social adjustment. Former U.S. Surgeon General C. Everett Koop comments, "Regarding violence in our society as purely a sociologic matter, or one of law enforcement, has led to an unmitigated failure. It is time to test further whether violence can be amenable to medical/public health interventions."(52)

Nutritionist David Getoff has found that the specific causes of aberrant behavior in his young patients include many different poisons and other triggers. Depending on the specific child, he says it is generally one or more of the following: Nutrient (vitamin or mineral) deficiencies; fatty acid deficiencies; environmental chemicals; food chemicals such as colorings; preservatives and artificial sweeteners; foods themselves such as wheat, gluten, pasteurized dairy, sugars, soy foods, and others.

Monsanto, the company that produces *Roundup*, has been working on genetically engineering crops such as potatoes, corn, and soybeans to withstand the effects of *Roundup*. The goal is to create crops that are not affected by *Roundup* so that unusually large quantities of this pesticide can be applied to eradicate weeds without harming the crops. It's estimated that 20 million more pounds of toxic herbicide per year are being sprayed on American soybean fields because of this. More pesticide sales means increased profits. In 2000, Monsanto's total sales were $5.5 billion, and $2.6 billion of this was from the sale of herbicides and pesticides like *Roundup*.(53)

Genetic modification (GM), also called genetic engineering (GE), is where certain genes of one plant are transferred into another plant in order to have that second plant express certain traits. Some traits aren't expressed right away – they may be latent for a dozen generations. Those traits may be harmful to humans. We, then, become the experiment.

Genetic modification of crops is becoming widespread in America – more than 58 million acres are now planted with GM crops. In 1996, that figure was just six million (most all soybeans are now genetically modified). But not everyone agrees it's beneficial. Japan and most European countries are opposed to the sale of GM produce. Switzerland destroyed 500 tons of chocolate when they learned it contained GM soy lecithin. All GM foods sold in the European Union (EU) must be labeled and the entire EU and India have stopped allowing experimentation with GM foods in the field until more is known about long-term effects. Thailand and Sri Lanka have taken it a step further and banned GM foods completely. Americans have expressed concern too. A petition with 500,000 signatures was presented in Washington D.C. in June 1999, that demanded congress and the FDA require GM foods be labeled. So far, no response. The manufacturers of GM foods say they are safe and even beneficial. How can they say that when no long term studies have been done?

There is one bright spot in all this madness. Gerber, the nation's largest baby food manufacturer said in 1999 that it was going to stop using GM foods.[54] That's good, since we not only don't know enough about GM foods, but also so much more pesticide is used on them that they cannot be any better for your child.

Amazingly, there's more to fear in a pesticide than the active ingredient alone. Of the 600 million pounds of 2,4-D used in the United States each year, 60 million pounds of it are active ingredients (i.e., 2,4-D) and about 540 million pounds of it are inert ingredients. For example, an inert ingredient may be an oily substance that prevents rain from washing the poison away. A typical pesticide is 1 percent to 20 percent active ingredients and 80 percent to 99 percent inert ingredients.

The U.S. EPA Office of Pesticides and Toxic Substances lists 2,000 chemicals that have been approved for use as inert ingredients. Those so called "inert" ingredients can include such known poisons as carbon tetrachloride, chloroform, chloroethane, xylene, cadmium, and lead. Federal pesticide law does not require chemical companies to disclose what those inert ingredients really are. More shocking than that is that federal law levies a $10,000 penalty for any government employee who reveals the make-up of inert ingredients in pesticides.[55] If that's not all, a little known exemption in the RCRA (the nation's basic hazardous waste law) allows hazardous wastes to be "recycled" into pesticides as inert ingredients. Therefore, it's legal to put known carcinogens, mutagens, and teratogens into pesticides that will be sprayed all across the country.

How does the EPA account for this? EPA press officer Al Hire told a reporter that allowing recycled hazardous waste in pesticides is "a way of disposing of hazardous materials."[56] No one will ever know that the thing they use to get rid of their dandelions not only contains the pesticide (bad enough by itself), but has other carcinogenic ingredients as well. Considering our children's playing, getting in the dirt, touching their mouths, noses and eyes, their risk of exposure to these kinds of recognized carcinogenic compounds is increased.

Several studies of laboratory animals have reported that DDE (a breakdown product of the pesticide DDT) can interfere with normal sexual development of males and can cause enlarged prostate glands. Alligators in Florida exposed to similar chemicals were reported to have much smaller than normal penises.(57,58)

In another study, test animals were exposed to different pesticides typically used in agriculture and lawn care – *Lasso* (containing alachlor), *Basalin* (containing fluchloralin), and *Premiere* (containing dinoseb and Maneb-80). The test animals were shown to have over 50 percent more activity (they were considered hyperactive) following a single exposure. The researchers said, "The results of this study suggest that at least some herbicides, in addition to pyrethrins, organophosphate, and carbamate pesticides, can produce behavioral manifestations following accidental exposure. . .The effects of the pesticides on activity also support the hypothesis that these agents may affect the central nervous system."(59)

Philip J. Landrigan, chairman of the department of community medicine at the Mount Sinai School of Medicine in New York City, says:

> Disease caused by toxic chemicals in the environment is a substantial. . .cause of morbidity [illness] and mortality [death] in the United States and around the world. Public health workers and the makers of public policy must recognize that toxic chemicals in the environment are important, widespread, proven causes of human disease. Each year preventable exposures to chemical toxins sicken and kill thousands of persons of all ages in the United States and around the world. These hazards must be confronted. They cannot be wished away. Reduction of exposures to chemical toxins will prevent thousands of deaths and will improve the quality of hundreds of thousands of lives.(60)

Food for Thought

We are led to believe that if a product is sold to the general public, it must be safe. If we follow the label directions, we should be okay. But that is clearly not the case. There are strong political pressures from the manufacturers of these products to keep this information from getting out. Although in some instances the data are incomplete, there is sufficient proof that many chemicals do indeed contribute to cancer.

It's very similar to what happened with the tobacco industry. For years the tobacco companies said no proof existed that their products caused cancer or were addictive. They kept studies that showed that they actually were to themselves under lock and key. Since then there have been all kinds of lawsuits claiming the opposite, and the courts have agreed with the plaintiffs, awarding the victims huge settlements.

I believe the same kind of scenario will be played out with pesticides. Are the companies that make them going to come out and say, "Hey, our products kill people and give dogs and children cancer!" I don't think so. But maybe someone will be brave and take the pesticide manufacturers to court because their child got brain cancer. That will get it onto the evening news. It's our job, like it or not, to change our world into a safe and healthy one. Discontinuing the personal use of pesticides is a good step.

Household Products

We know that chemicals in the home such as pesticides are potential health hazards. However, many other products you may use around the house and yard without thinking twice can be dangerous to you and your child. And these can add up to creating a toxic living environment. How toxic? A 15-year study found that women who were homemakers had a 54 percent greater risk of developing cancer than women who worked outside the home due to continuous exposure to household cleaners, chemicals, and pesticides.[61] (Who said being a mom was easy and safe?) And the EPA rates indoor air quality among the top five threats to human health.[62]

The average American home has three to 10 gallons of hazardous materials stored in it. In 1998 there were more than one million incidents reported to poison control centers related to household chemicals – 220,000 of them specifically related to cleaning products.[63] In all, over 90 percent of all reported poisonings occur at home, and the leading cause is household cleaners.[64] Short-term acute effects such as irritation and burning can be suffered from ammonia, chlorine bleach, and other common chemicals, and ingestion of chemical products can lead to sickness and death. So make sure all chemical products are put out of reach of inquisitive toddlers and children and be sure to know what to do in case of a poisoning.

The danger of chemicals does not stop there, however. These chemicals seep into the air, making the average American home a quite toxic place to breathe. The EPA has found that indoor air contains two to five times more pollution than outdoor air. In fact, the Consumer Product Safety Commission found that in the houses they tested, the outdoor air contained less than 10 volatile organic compounds (VOCs), while the indoor air contained 150 VOCs![65] These VOCs come from a number of sources, not just household cleaners. Many long-term chronic problems can manifest from exposure to the volatile solvents found in cleaners and other chemicals that get into your airspace. These chronic problems include,

- Neurological difficulties such as fatigue, memory problems, personality changes, headaches, sleep disorders, coordination difficulties, visual problems, and sexual dysfunction.
- Asthma. Sensitive young lungs are damaged by prolonged exposure to the chemicals in the air.
- Liver and kidney damage. These two organs are the ones most responsible for detoxification. If they are impaired, the body has

difficulty eliminating toxins, which can lead to numerous health problems.
- Reproductive damage.
- Multiple Chemical Sensitivity (MCS). MCS is a recently defined condition where the person is extremely sensitive to a great number of chemicals found in air, food, water, and those that can be absorbed through the skin. It is thought to result from both acute and chronic chemical exposure.

Remember, children are especially susceptible to chemical exposure due to their developing respiratory and immune systems. If you have any chemicals in your house, not only should you get them out of the reach of children, but keep them sealed up so the fumes don't escape. Better yet, put them in a separate building away from the house (not in an attached garage). This includes paint, paint thinners, strippers and other solvents, gas and kerosene cans, lubricants, cleaners, and anything else that has a chemical smell or has warnings on the label.

Speaking of an attached garage, it's a potential source of significant air pollution in your house. Every time you open the door leading to the garage, the pollutants from car exhausts and any chemicals stored in the garage come into the house. Consider sealing it off with tape and using the front door. Inconvenient, I know, but if someone in your family is sensitive and having problems, it's worth it. For the elderly, the car exhaust and petroleum chemicals that come from a garage have been implicated in the development of Alzheimer's disease. Clearly, chemicals in the air will not do a body good, no matter what the age.

Think twice about storing chemicals under the sink. The chlorine in that scrubbing powder not only gets through your skin as you clean the pots and pans, but also gets into the air and circulates throughout the house. It may not be noticeable, but even tiny concentrations can have effects. This goes for the automatic dishwasher soap and laundry bleach too. Oven cleaners, drain cleaners, and floor and furniture polishes are extremely toxic when ingested, and they pollute the air. Switch to more natural products without chlorine or volatile organics in them or at least put these products in air-tight containers for storage.

Products such as mothballs, glass cleaners, floor and furniture polish, rug and upholstery cleaners, oven cleaners, and air fresheners are not only toxic if ingested but also pollute the air. Table 3 shows simple ways to get around using these.

You should be aware that wall-to-wall carpeting could be especially problematic. New carpeting emits chemicals such as formaldehyde for years. The carpeting holds in most of the dust, food, pesticide residues dragged in on shoes, and harbors dust mites. Even with vacuuming and shampooing (most carpet cleaners have toxic chemicals too), the carpeting will still be contaminated and emit toxins. This is especially bad for children who play on the carpeting. Many experts advise taking out the carpeting altogether and replacing it with nontoxic flooring and using area rugs that can be washed. Remember, your child is probably being exposed to carpet toxicity in day cares and schools. The less they're exposed to at home, the better. Companies that sell non-toxic carpeting are:

www.ecobydesign.com, www.greenbuildingsupply.com, www.earthweave.com.

Table 3

Alternatives for Toxic Household Products (66)

Product	Potential Health Effect	Suggested Alternative
Air Fresheners	Irritant, toxic to liver and kidney, affects lung function	Open window, open box of baking soda, simmer cloves, grow house plants such as spider plants to help detoxify the air
Floor & Furniture Polish	Cancer, birth defects, fetal toxicity, lung effects, cardiovascular effects	1 part lemon oil to 2 parts olive or vegetable oil, vegetable oil soap
Mothballs	Cancer, skin irritant, lung effects, kidney and liver damage, nerve damage	Cedar chips, lavender, aromatic herbs and spices
Glass cleaners	Skin irritant, cancer, corrosive	Use ¼ to ½ cup white vinegar to 1 quart warm water, wipe with newspaper
Rug & Upholstery	Cancer, irritant, kidney damage, nerve damage, corrosive, fetal toxicity, reproductive toxicity birth defects	Baking soda or cornstarch on rug, then vacuum: replace wall-to-wall with washable area rugs.

If you have hardwood floors, use a water-based floor finisher. If using polyurethane finishes, be sure you open all the windows and have the house well ventilated for a few days afterward.

Perchloroethylene is a chemical used in rug and upholstery cleaners and in dry-cleaning and is hazardous if inhaled. People who work in dry-cleaning stores have been shown to have a 25 percent greater chance of dying from cancer than the general public.(67) Do your best to avoid using cleaners with this chemical and to purchase clothes that don't require dry-cleaning. If you do have things dry-cleaned, let them air out outside or somewhere else so the fumes don't come into your house.

One simple way to clean up the air in your house is by having numerous houseplants. They absorb many of the pollutants that are in the air and emit oxygen. The best species to clean the air are golden pothos, nepthylis, spider plant, snake plant, aloe, and philodendron. One plant per 100 square feet is a good rule of thumb. Don't put them in the bedrooms, however, since at night plants use up oxygen and give off carbon dioxide. Getting a good air filter/purifier is not a bad idea either.

Another area of concern is playground equipment, decks, and picnic tables that kids play on. Pressure-treated-wood is treated with chromated copper arsenate. Children playing on this kind of lumber can absorb dangerous amounts of arsenic. These chemicals leach out into the surrounding soil, which they may get on their hands and into their mouths. Keep your child off and away from these, and replace any home equipment with nontoxic alternatives.

Other items that are a serious health risk to your baby are baby-bottle nipples and pacifiers. Many are made of polyvinyl chloride (PVC), which leach harmful chemicals such as phthalates. These have been shown to increase the risks of cancer later in life. Replace these with silicone nipples and pacifiers. They can be found at most major department-store chains or at www.newbornfree.com, www.healthychild.org and www.thesoftlanding.com.

Organically grown food is not just more nutritious, but cleaner. But if you eat conventionally grown food, be sure to wash it well. There are fruit and vegetable cleaners that are supposed to remove the pesticides, but they work no better than common dishwasher soap. Soak produce in water with apple cider vinegar added. Since much of the pesticides used on crops end up in the soil, they end up in the food itself, which cannot be washed off, yet another reason to eat organic. The foods shown to accumulate pesticides the most are apples, grapes, green beans, peaches, pears, spinach, and squash.

As you can see, staying home is oftentimes a hazardous proposition. Cleaning up your household environment will definitely help keep you and your family healthier and happier.

Diet & Our Food Supply

Since the cells in your body are composed of the substances you put in your mouth, if you put the wrong food in, your cells will have the wrong building blocks to work with. This will cause them to be weak, inefficient, and stressed. Conversely, the right foods will allow your cells to be constructed from the right materials and will function correctly.

One of the worst things you can put in your mouth as far as cancer is concerned, is sugar. It's a major food for cancer cells. In fact, cancer cells thrive on it. Is this a new discovery? No. In 1931 Dr. Otto Warburg was awarded the Nobel Prize for discovering that cancer cells thrive on sugar.

This is because cancer cells metabolize through fermentation, and fermentation requires sugar. Fermentation is an anaerobic process (no oxygen involved), unlike normal respiration that requires oxygen. So it's not surprising that cancer cells hate oxygen. In fact, a popular alternative cancer therapy is oxygen therapy where the body is flooded with oxygen. Dr. Warburg found that he could create cancer by lowering the oxygen content in a cell to 35 percent and he could reverse cancer by increasing the oxygen content. (See the chapter on asthma for a breathing method that will get more oxygen to your cells.) So healthy cells get their energy from oxygen, cancer cells get theirs from fermentation which requires sugar.(68) Eating sugar just encourages cancer to form, and if you have it already, to flourish.

Sugar causing cancer is not just theory. A study reported in the *Journal of the National Cancer Institute* shows that women who consumed a high glycemic load diet (a diet high in carbohydrates, sucrose, and fructose – i.e. sugars) were nearly three times more likely to develop colon cancer.(69)

In a study of 80,000 men and women between 1997 and 2005, those who drank soft drinks at least twice a day had a 90 percent higher risk of developing pancreatic cancer than those who didn't drink them at all. People who added sugar to food or drinks (like coffee) at least five times a day had a 70 percent higher risk of this cancer.(70) So cut down and eliminate sugar, and you'll greatly cut down on your chances of getting cancer.

Another thing that cancer loves you to do is to eat cooked foods. This is again related to oxygen. Cooking destroys not only a lot of vitamins, but it also destroys enzymes. Enzymes are needed by the body for a multitude of reasons, one of which relates to how red blood cells clump together. If the enzymes aren't there, the blood cells will clump more, and won't be able to fit through tiny microcapillaries. This causes many anaerobic (low or no oxygen) areas in the body, thus encouraging cancer.

To avoid or reverse cancer, it's best to stop eating sugar (and all starch based carbohydrates like pasta, breads, etc., since they are essentially made of two sugar molecules bound together), and cooked foods. Aajonus Vonderplanitz, Ph.D. reports that he has successfully reversed cancer in many of his clients by putting them on a no-sugar, all raw food diet. He contends that:

> Cancer is basically the body's inability to discard dead tissue. Healthy young cells mutate into cells which collect and contain dead cells, forming tumors. Building a tumor is a means of isolating dead cells into a localized area. Once the dead cells are isolated, and if the body gets the nutrients it needs, the body can gradually dissolve the tumor and eliminate the by-products. There are three factors to address when eliminating and healing cancer. The first is to stop eating dead food [cooked foods] that weakens or kills cells with toxicity and debris. Avoiding cooked meat of all kinds is paramount because so many active and volatile toxins are its byproduct. The second is to fill the blood and body with raw

fats that will bind with dead cells and carry them out of the body, or at least will neutralize toxicity, so that tumors will cease to grow. . .The third is to dissolve tumorous tissue as safely as possible by eating fresh raw citrus or other fruit that is appealing, raw meats and other raw foods.(71)

Food for Thought

Eating raw food, especially raw meat is probably a new concept for you. You may be fearful of food poisoning and bacteria. These issues will be addressed in a later chapter. Suffice it here to say that these fears are largely unwarranted. Dr. Vonderplanitz has been consuming raw meat, (fish, beef, chicken, lamb, eggs) for over 25 years. He has cured himself and many of his clients of a host of illnesses, cancer being one of them. Thousands of his clients eat raw meat regularly with no ill effects. Yours truly has been following many aspects of his diet (I still have the occasional pizza. Give me a break, I'm Italian!) for almost 10 years now with great success. It may seem like a drastic measure to eat all or mostly raw food, but if you have cancer or some other disease, wouldn't drastic steps be needed to reverse it? After all, chemotherapy, radiation, and surgery are all even more drastic, uncomfortable, and expensive.

Food Additives

The regulation of food additives in the U.S. began in 1938 under the Federal Food, Drug, and Cosmetic (FD&C) Act (that created the FDA). This Act gave the FDA authority over food and food ingredients and defined requirements for truthful labeling of ingredients. The Food Additives Amendment to the FD&C Act, passed in 1958, requires FDA approval for the use of an additive prior to its inclusion in food. It also requires the manufacturer to prove an additive's safety for the ways it will be used. Unfortunately, all substances that the FDA or the U.S. Department of Agriculture (USDA) had determined were safe for use in specific food prior to the 1958 amendment were designated as "prior-sanctioned" substances and grandfathered in as acceptable no matter what future research found. The problem here is that these prior-sanctioned substances may not, indeed, be safe. Examples of prior-sanctioned substances are sodium nitrite and potassium nitrite (used to preserve luncheon meats), substances that have come into question many times over the years.(72)

The FDA estimates that there are more than 3,000 different additives, mostly synthetic chemicals, used in our foods – only 2,000 of which the FDA has chemical and toxicological information on. The other 1,000 the FDA has only administrative and chemical information on.(73)

Table 4 shows a very partial list of some food additives (dyes) and their potential health effects. These additives do not increase shelf life. They do not make the food more nutritious. They don't even make it taste better. They're all for appearance.

You may remember when FD & C Red dye No. 2 dye was removed from general use because it caused cancer in lab animals. But there are many other questionable coloring agents still widely in use. Many of these dyes, according to the FDA's own information, are allowed to contain various toxic metals including mercury, lead and cadmium and arsenic.

Table 4

Food additives and their health effects (74)

Additive	Health Effects
FD&C Red No. 2	Angioedema (swelling of the heart), cancer
FD&C Red No. 3	Thyroid tumors, chromosomal damage
Citrus Red No. 2	Cancer in animals
Allura Red AC	Tumors/lymphomas
FD&C Yellow No. 5	Allergies, thyroid tumors, lymphocytic lymphomas chromosomal damage, trigger for asthma, hives, hyperactivity
FD&C Yellow No. 6 (Sunset Yellow)	Allergies, kidney tumors, chromosomal damage, abdominal pain, vomiting, indigestion
FD&C Green No. 3 (Fast Green)	Bladder tumors

It's quite unrealistic to think that all the additives used in foods are 100 percent safe and do no harm. Food additives are chemicals not natural to our body. They're not used as fuel and are not needed for any cellular processes and just get in the way. Many studies indicate that many additives may be cancer causing or cause behavioral or other problems. Even if the additive is not outright poisonous or cancer-causing, it's not a food and therefore only a burden the body must get rid of or store – oftentimes depositing it in fat cells.

It's interesting to consider how the FDA approves a food additive for use. The following is a section of text taken straight out of the FDA/IFIC Brochure titled "Food Additives." I've added emphasis to those phrases I find most alarming:

How Are Additives Approved for Use in Foods?

To market a new food or color additive, a manufacturer must first petition FDA for its approval. Approximately 100 new food and color additives petitions are submitted to FDA annually. . .

A food or color additive petition must provide convincing evidence that the proposed additive performs as it is intended. Animal studies using large doses of the additive for long periods *are often necessary* to show that the substance would not cause harmful effects at *expected levels of human consumption.* Studies of the additive in humans also *may be* submitted to FDA.

In deciding whether an additive should be approved, the agency considers the composition and properties of the substance, the amount likely to be consumed, its probable long-term effects and various safety factors. *Absolute safety of any substance can never be proven.* Therefore, FDA must determine if the additive is safe under the proposed conditions of use, based on the best scientific knowledge available.

If an additive is approved, FDA issues regulations that may include the types of foods in which it can be used, the maximum amounts to be used, and how it should be identified on food labels.

Federal officials then *carefully monitor the extent of Americans' consumption* of the new additive and results of any new research on its safety to assure its use continues to be within safe limits.

In addition, FDA operates an Adverse Reaction Monitoring System (ARMS) to help serve as an ongoing safety check of all additives. The system monitors and investigates all complaints by individuals or their physicians that are believed to be related to specific foods; food and color additives; or vitamin and mineral supplements. The ARMS computerized database helps officials *decide whether reported adverse reactions represent a real public health hazard* associated with food, so that appropriate action can be taken.(75)

I would like to discuss each italicized section to help you realize just what we're dealing with here:

"Animal studies *are often* necessary to show no adverse effects." That really means that they are not always necessary, and a food additive may be approved with no toxicological or epidemiological studies (animal testing).

". . .the substance would not cause harmful effects at *expected levels of human consumption.*" So if someone consumes more than the expected level, they may get sick? Well, yes. As an example, let's look at sulfites, a common food additive. The above-referenced brochure comments on sulfites as follows: "Sulfites added to baked goods, condiments, snack foods and other products are safe for most people. A small segment of the population, however, has been found to develop hives, nausea, diarrhea, shortness of breath or even fatal shock after consuming sulfites. For that reason, in 1986 FDA banned the use of sulfites on fresh fruits and vegetables intended to be sold or served raw to consumers.

Sulfites added as preservative in all other packaged and processed foods must be listed on the product label." In the case of sulfites, it took people dying to change the regulation, and since they're still in some foods, the possibility exists others may still have severe reactions.

"Studies of the additive in humans also *may be* submitted to FDA." "May be" means "a manufacturer has permission to." So it's not required to have any information on the effects of a proposed additive on humans to get FDA approval, but the FDA is giving permission for someone to submit the information if they so choose.

*"Absolute safety of any substance can never be proven." S*o what the FDA does is look at "relative" safety. Then, it all becomes a matter of opinion as to what is safe.

"Federal officials then *carefully monitor the extent of Americans' consumption* of the new additive. . ." I would believe that it's pretty much impossible to track the consumption of FD&C Red No. 3 among our population and see who is consuming it and what effects, acute (short-term) or chronic (long-term), it may be having. The "monitoring" is really a case of disaster regulation. When a disaster occurs, like when people start dying from ingesting too many sulfites, then and only then is the regulation changed. Essentially, what is occurring is that the U.S. population has become the lab test animals.

But back to the FDA's words: "The ARMS computerized database helps officials *decide whether reported adverse reactions represent a real public health hazard* associated with food, so that appropriate action can be taken." In many cases, adverse reactions may not be recognized as coming from a food additive.

How many people would attribute their allergies or asthma to FD&C Yellow No. 5? Then, there's the subjectivity of the officials to determine if reported reactions represent a real public health hazard. Just look at what happened in 2008 with all the deaths of our beloved pets from the melamine added in China to make the protein levels test higher in dozens of brands of pet foods. The FDA finally did some investigating but has yet to pass any substantial regulations to protect us from more of these types of deadly poisoning problems.

Food for Thought

There are two major points I'd like to make using food additives as the example. First, it's virtually impossible to effectively regulate substances used as food additives. Any additive may have adverse effects – either acute or chronic – on certain people. The FDA or any regulatory agency simply cannot ensure that anything used in food is safe. It then becomes the responsibility of the consumer to determine if a certain food is safe for his or her own consumption. The regulations are based on "the population at large," so if someone is overly sensitive, he or she may have an adverse reaction, where most people do not. Too bad for the sensitive individual.

Second, you must understand the human body and how it works to fully appreciate why any additive is really deleterious. If the body cannot use a substance as a nutrient, it sees it as a waste. The more polluted a body becomes, the more likely it will fail to function to its optimum level or will function incorrectly. Considering that, it's not a mystery at all why the body breaks down, gets cancer or becomes ill whether physically, mentally, or emotionally.

The FDA, like most individuals, views the human body in shades of gray, where really the body operates more as black or white. The FDA believes that if a substance does not cause apparent and obvious negative effects, then it is having no negative effect. That is simply not true. Even if a substance does not cause an obvious health problem, if the body is not using it as a nutrient, then it's really a pollutant that will rob the body of energy and cause long-term problems, premature aging, and disease.

It's all a matter of energy dynamics. Your body takes in fuel, nutrients, air, water, and sunlight and converts them into usable energy. That energy is used to operate the muscles, nerves, brain, and so on. There is not an endless supply of energy – it is limited. We eat food and get a certain amount of energy from it. That energy is either used for movement, regeneration and repair, or waste disposal. The more used for waste disposal (getting rid of unusable dyes and other additives, not to mention other pollutants we must expel), the less is available for movement and regeneration and repair . The less available for regeneration and repair, the less regeneration and repair occur – and the more susceptible we become to lack of energy, diseases, and systemic breakdowns.

It's not unlike the operation of a car engine. If the engine oil gets dirty, if the spark plugs are fouled, if the gas and air filters are clogged, is the car going to operate at peak efficiency, or is it more likely to sputter and break down? If waste cannot be eliminated, the body tucks it away somewhere – usually in soft tissue or fat. Over time, these accumulations build up and can cause problems. For example, the intake of the wrong kind of calcium – one being dicalcium phosphate which is used in many health supplements as a binding agent – cannot only interfere with nutrient absorption, but also contribute to deposits of inert calcium in joints and arteries leading to arthritis and arteriolosclerosis.

We do not live in some magic never-never land. With all the science that we use to determine health effects, we are assuming that dyes, additives, preservatives, and other toxins are somehow magically removed or rendered harmless.

Another analogy can be made to computers. Over time, a computer accumulates a lot of unnecessary fragments of information (waste), which slows it down. If you don't defragment it (get rid of the waste), given long enough, the computer will crash completely. Same with the human body. A computer operates digitally: Every switch in the computer is just an on/off switch, either yes or no. The human body is the same. Every substance is either good or bad. Good if it gives energy. Bad if it robs us of energy. Keep this in mind when making decisions on what you put into it.

Aspartame

Aspartame is an artificial sweetener (more than 200 times sweeter than sugar) used in diet sodas, "lite" yogurt and ice cream, sugarless gelatin desserts, and a number of other products. It's the technical name for the brand names *NutraSweet, Equal, Spoonful, Indulge, Canderel, Benevia,* and *Equal-Measure.* It was until recently, the most popular artificial sweetener on the market (replaced by *Splenda*), with sales of more than $100 million a year. In 1987, the last year that *NutraSweet* publicized its records, Americans consumed around 17,100,000 pounds of aspartame. Now our estimated consumption is over 25 million pounds per year.(76) Aspartame is known to cause brain tumors along with a long list of other problems, as we'll see. So it's appropriate here to discuss it at length, not just how it relates to tumors.

Aspartame was discovered by accident in 1965 and approved for use in dry goods in 1981 and carbonated beverages in 1983. It had been approved for use as early as 1974, but objections from neuroscientist John W. Olney, Ph.D., and consumer groups made the FDA revoke its approval, which was later reinstated. Aspartame has been called "by far, the most dangerous substance on the market that is added to foods."(77,78) In all, there have been more than 90 different documented symptoms. Many of these reactions are minor, but some are quite serious. A February 1994 Department of Health and Human Services report lists many reactions to aspartame, two of which are seizures and death.

Mary Nash Stoddard is the founder of the Aspartame Consumer Safety Network and author of a book about aspartame (*Deadly Deception*). She's a recognized expert on aspartame and is a board member of the National Natural Foods Association and a former judge on the State of Texas Board of Adjustments. Way back in 1995 she spoke out against aspartame. She said that at that time, about 78 percent of all "Adverse Reaction" complaints to the FDA concerned aspartame, and at one time, the figure was 85 percent. She called this "a well-hidden secret." She went on to say:

> Aspartame not only causes individual symptoms, it can mimic entire syndromes! For example... it can mimic the symptoms of CFIDS [chronic fatigue and immune deficiency syndrome]. It can also cause grand mal seizures. According to H.J. Roberts, M.D., it can cause decreased vision, pain in the eyes, decreased tears, ringing in the ears, hearing impairment, headache, dizziness, and unsteadiness, confusion, memory loss, drowsiness, sleepiness, slurring of speech, numbness and tingling, tremors, depression,

irritability, aggression, anxiety, insomnia, phobias, heart palpitations, shortness of breath, high blood pressure, nausea, diarrhea, abdominal pain, itching, hives, menstrual changes, weight gain, hair thinning and hair loss, urinary burning and frequency, excessive thirst, fluid retention, bloating, increased infections, and even death. . .Five deaths were reported prior to 1987. We don't know the number since then. . .(79)

Stoddard sees big money behind the approval of the artificial sweetener. After removal from the market, she says aspartame was finally approved again, but not without supposed payoffs and other questionable political occurrences. Even though the FDA approves a substance, it may not be as safe as it sounds. There's big money involved here, and big money has a tendency to sway some people into twisting the truth. One example is how Dr. Arthur Hull Hayes Jr., as the commissioner of the FDA, approved *NutraSweet* for soft drinks. Two months later, he took a position with a subsidiary of the company that manufacturers aspartame (Monsanto) as the senior medical advisor in their public relations firm to the tune of $1,000 a day. Just one isolated incident? Stoddard had this to say:

Watch out diabetics! The NutraSweet Company has given money, money, money to the American Diabetes Association. And remember when you hear a registered dietitian say aspartame is safe for pregnant women, children, and everyone else, the registered dietitian's professional association has been given $75,000 to expound on the virtues of aspartame. The American Dietetic Association has even stated that the *NutraSweet* Company writes their Fact Sheets. Aspartame approval and persistence on the market has everything to do with money and politics, and almost nothing to do with science and reason. Even the FDA's own reviewers were against aspartame until those political [and] financial events I've mentioned. There are reports that many research reports to justify aspartame's use were poorly conducted and outright fraud. Senator Edward Kennedy said, "the extensive nature of the almost unbelievable range of abuses discovered by the FDA on several major Searle products is profoundly disturbing."(80) [Searle Pharmaceuticals manufactures *NutraSweet*.]

Aspartame is made up of three chemicals: aspartic acid (40 percent), phenylalanine (50 percent), and methanol (10 percent). It's considered by many to be a "chemical poison." Russell L. Blaylock, M.D., a professor of Neurosurgery at the University of Mississippi medical school and author of the book *Excitotoxins: The Taste That Kills*, cites almost 500 scientific references that show how excess excitatory amino acids (aspartic acid and glutamic acid found in the popular flavor-enhancer MSG) are causing serious chronic neurological disorders and other acute symptoms. The effects of aspartic acid together with glutamic acid are cumulative – meaning that when both are taken together, their individual adverse effects are multiplied.(81) So don't drink a diet soda when you're having Chinese food.

Blaylock says that too much aspartate or glutamate in the brain kills certain brain cells because it stimulates the neural cells to death. The blood-brain barrier (BBB) normally, but not always, protects the brain from toxins. During childhood, the BBB is not fully developed, and aspartate or glutamate can get into the brain. Therefore, children and fetuses are especially vulnerable. Even in adulthood, excess aspartate and glutamate can seep through the BBB causing damage. And there are some parts of the brain that the BBB does not fully protect. The areas of the brain most affected are the hypothalamus, medulla oblongata, and corpus striatum – each intricately involved in regulating various processes in the body.(82)

Blaylock goes on to say that excessive buildup of phenylalanine in the brain can cause seizures or even schizophrenia. When aspartate and glutamate are in the brain, they slowly destroy neurons. They are silent killers: the majority (more than 75 percent) of the brain cells in a particular area are killed before any clinical symptoms of a chronic illness are evident. Long-term exposure to these excitatory amino acids can contribute to multiple sclerosis, ALS, memory loss, epilepsy, Alzheimer's disease, Parkinson's disease, hypoglycemia, AIDS, dementia, brain lesions, neuroendocrine disorders, brain tumors, mental retardation, lymphoma, birth defects, fibromyalgia, and diabetes.

Ingesting aspartame can lead to excess levels of phenylalanine, an amino acid that's normally found in the brain. People with a genetic disorder called phenylketonuria (PKU) are especially susceptible to this (sometimes causing death), but people without PKU can also be vulnerable. Also, excessive levels of phenylalanine in the brain can cause serotonin levels to decrease, which can lead to depression.

In testimony before the U.S. Congress, Dr. Louis J. Elsas, M.D., professor of pediatrics at Emory University for 25 years, showed that a high blood level of phenylalanine can indeed be concentrated in parts of the brain, and is especially dangerous for infants and fetuses.(83) Even a single dose of aspartame can raise the blood level of phenylalanine. He said,

> First of all, in the developing fetus. . .the mother is supplying that fetus with nutrients. And if she were dieting, let's say, and increasing her blood phenylalanine uniquely by taking *Crystal Lite* or *Kool-Aid*, or any of the various diet foods now, to maintain her weight, and increased her blood phenylalanine from its normal 50 to 150 μmoles/liter [micromoles per liter] by chronic ingestion at 35 milligrams of aspartame per kilo per day – which everyone agrees could be reached – the placenta will concentrate her blood phenylalanine twofold. So the fetal blood circulation to her baby in utero is now 300 μmoles [of phenylalanine per liter]. The fetal

brain then will increase further that concentration into the brain cells of that baby two to fourfold. Those are neurotoxic levels in tissue culture and in many other circumstances.(84)

Dr. William M. Pardridge, M.D., a Professor of Medicine, says that increases in phenylalanine concentrations in the blood of the pregnant mother can cause a drop in the IQ of the child born of that mother and a lowering of the higher cognitive function (the ability to make key decisions). Another study by Elsas showed that "there are quantitative changes in the human electroencephalogram when the blood phenylalanine is raised threefold – something that clearly will happen in children who consume nearly five servings per 50-pound body weight." (An electroencephalogram, or EEG, is a devise to measure the electrical activity of the brain. Variations from a normal reading indicate the brain has unbalanced and unhealthy electrical activity. For your info, an ECG or EKG is an electrocardiogram that measures the electrical activity of the heart.)

One account of harmful aspartame use is worth noting. John Cook was drinking six to eight diet drinks every day. He started experiencing memory loss and frequent headaches. Then came wide mood swings and violent rages. Even though he didn't have PKU, a blood test revealed his phenylalanine blood level was extremely high. Cook showed abnormal brain function and brain damage. When he went off aspartame, his symptoms improved.(85)

Food for Thought

Since a large percentage of people, our young included, are now overweight, many drink diet sodas trying to cut calories. This leads one to wonder if some of the violent acts we see may be partially due to the neurological effects of aspartame.

Ten percent of aspartame is wood alcohol or methanol, a deadly poison. It's caused skid row alcoholics to end up blind or dead. Methanol is released in the small intestine when aspartame is digested. Absorption is sped up when aspartame is heated because free methanol is then created. That's what happens when you make sugar-free *Jell-O* (or when aspartame-containing products are stored above 86° F). Yet, in 1993, the FDA approved aspartame as an ingredient in numerous foods that are typically heated above 86 degrees F. Mary Nash Stoddard has this to say about aspartame and methanol:

> Among other things, [aspartame is] about 10 percent methanol (wood alcohol), famous for causing blindness in alcoholics. In the body, methanol metabolizes into formaldehyde, a neurotoxin; formic acid, a venom in ant stings; and diketopiperazine, which causes brain tumors in animals. It's so bad that in July of 1983, the National Soft Drink Association

presented official objections to putting aspartame in beverages. I'll read you one of their objections: "It is well established under Section 402(a)(3) that a food which contains a decomposed substance. . .is subject to seizure by FDA." It's thoroughly established that after a number of weeks and at temperatures over 86 degrees F, there's no aspartame left in a soft drink, only breakdown products. So, why isn't FDA seizing it under Section 402(a)(3)?. . .Aspartame was originally approved in 1974, but when the brain-tumor issue arose, the approval was withdrawn. . .Many of the test animals fed aspartame developed large tumors. These were actually cut out, and the animals returned to the study. In some cases, the tumors weren't even examined for malignancy, and the tumors weren't reported to FDA. In several cases, animals were reported as dead and later reported as alive again.[86]

Food for Thought

In 90 non-industry-sponsored studies of aspartame, 83 identified one or more problems with it. Of the seven studies that did not find a problem, the FDA conducted six of them. (Soon after the FDA approval of aspartame, numerous FDA officials went to work for the aspartame industry.) Of the 74 industry-sponsored-studies of aspartame, 100 percent of them claimed there were no problems with it. Some of these experiments lasted a grand total of one day. Monsanto (makers of aspartame) funded a study on the possible birth defects caused by aspartame. When preliminary data showed damaging information in the study, funding was stopped.[87,88,89] By the way, there are currently class action law-suits being filed against Monsanto concerning aspartame. (www. holisticmed.com for more information.)

Regular table sugar is bad for you, but aspartame goes beyond the hazards of sugar – in some cases causing severe changes in the brain's activity. In an independent double-blind study in children with generalized absence epilepsy, a single dose of aspartame worsened the EEG spike wave discharges that indicate a seizure's severity. The authors concluded, "Aspartame appears to significantly increase the duration of time that children with absence epilepsy have spike wave on their EEG. In this study, the children spent 40 percent more time in spike wave after aspartame than after sucrose." Simply put, children with epileptic tendencies will be more likely to have a seizure if they ingest aspartame.[90] Of course, the proponents of aspartame will cite different research. However, those studies are hopelessly flawed. For example, one study reported aspartame didn't increase the likelihood of seizures, but 16 of the 18 subjects were on antiseizure medication during the study, and the study consisted of only a single dose of aspartame.[91]

An EPA assessment of methanol says it "is considered a cumulative poison due to the low rate of excretion once it is absorbed. In the body, methanol [breaks down] to formaldehyde and formic acid; both of these metabolites are toxic." They recommended a limit of 7.8 mg/day of methanol. A one-liter (about one-quart) bottle of an aspartame-sweetened beverage has about 56 mg of methanol in it. Someone who drinks four one-liter bottles a day consumes as much as 250 mg of methanol daily, or 32 times the EPA limit.(92)

Concerning formaldehyde, ". . .formaldehyde formation from aspartame ingestion is very common and does indeed accumulate within the cell, reacting with cellular proteins (mostly enzymes) and DNA (both mitochondrial and nuclear). The fact that it accumulates with each dose, indicates grave consequences among those who consume diet drinks and foodstuffs on a daily basis." Formaldehyde also causes retinal damage, is a known carcinogen, interferes with DNA replication, and causes birth defects.(93)

The best known effects of methanol poisoning are eyesight problems, which may include misty or blurry vision, progressive contraction of visual fields, retinal damage, and blindness. Other symptoms include headaches, ear buzzing, dizziness, nausea, gastrointestinal disturbances, weakness, vertigo, chills, memory lapses, numbness and shooting pains in the extremities, behavioral disturbances, and neuritis.

Some fruit juices and alcoholic beverages contain small amounts of methanol. However, in these cases ethanol (another alcohol) is also present. Ethanol is an antidote for methanol toxicity so its presence essentially cancels out the methanol.

Diketopiperazine (DKP) is another byproduct of aspartame metabolism. It has been implicated in the occurrences of brain tumors and uterine polyps. In 1981, an FDA statistician named Satya Dubey stated that the brain tumor data on aspartame indicated it was so bad that he could not recommend its approval. Aspartame has caused large brain tumors in animal experiments at a dose that could be considered within the Acceptable Daily Intake of humans.

The late Adrian Gross, Ph.D., a former FDA toxicologist, testified before Congress that aspartame was capable of producing brain tumors:

> In view of all these indications that the cancer-causing potential of aspartame is a matter that had been established way beyond any reasonable doubt, one can ask, what is the reason for the apparent refusal by the FDA to invoke for this food additive the so-called Delaney Amendment to the Food, Drug, and Cosmetic Act? Is it not clear beyond any shadow of a doubt that aspartame had caused brain tumors or brain cancer in animals, and is this not sufficient to satisfy the provisions of that particular section of the law? Given that this is so (and I cannot see any kind of tenable argument opposing the view that aspartame causes cancer) how would the FDA justify its position that it views a certain amount of aspartame (50 mg/mg body-weight) as

constituting an ADI [Allowable Daily Intake] or "safe" level for it? Is that position in effect not equivalent to setting a "tolerance" for this food additive and thus a violation of that law? And if the FDA itself elects to violate the law, who is left to protect the health of the public?(94)

Between the years 1973 and 1990, the incidences of brain tumors in people over 65 years of age increased 67 percent. Brian tumors in all age groups have jumped by 10 percent.(95) The researchers of study on the carcinogenicity of aspartame reported in the *Journal of Neuropathology & Experimental Neurology* concluded:

> . . .the artificial sweetener aspartame is a promising candidate to explain the recent increase in incidence and degree of malignancy of brain tumors. . .An early animal study revealing an exceedingly high incidence of brain tumors in aspartame-fed rats compared to no brain tumors in concurrent controls, the recent finding that the aspartame molecule has mutagenic potential, and the close temporal association.(96)

Aspartame was introduced into U.S. foods and beverage markets several years prior to the sharp increase in brain tumor incidence and malignancy. Aspartame was approved for use in 1974, revoked, and then approved again in 1981. Officials say it's safe, but what do you think? Are those few calories you save by using aspartame products really worth a brain tumor? Besides, studies clearly show that the people who consume aspartame sweetened foods do not generally lose any more weight than those consuming foods sweetened with sugar.

The American Diabetes Association (ADA) recommends aspartame to people with diabetes. But according to research conducted by H.J. Roberts, M.D., a diabetes specialist who is also a member of the ADA and an authority on artificial sweeteners, aspartame can lead to clinical diabetes, causes poorer diabetic control for those on insulin or oral drugs, leads to the aggravation of diabetic complications such as retinopathy, cataracts, neuropathy, gastroparesis, and causes convulsions. When patients avoided aspartame, Roberts saw "Dramatic improvement. . .and the prompt predictable reoccurrence of these problems when the patient resumed aspartame products. . ."(97)

Roberts states: "I regret the failure of other physicians and the American Diabetes Association to sound appropriate warnings to patients and consumers based on these repeated findings which have been described in my corporate-neutral studies and publications."(98)

Ralph G. Walton, Ph.D., conducted a study to see what the effects of aspartame are on people with mood disorders. Symptoms got so bad that the Institutional Review Board forced him to stop the study. Walton said, "Individuals with mood disorders are particularly sensitive to this artificial sweetener; its use in this population should be discouraged." Walton later stated, "I know it causes seizures. I'm convinced also that it definitely causes behavioral changes. I'm very angry that this substance is on the market. I personally question the reliability and validity of any studies funded by the NutraSweet Company."(99) (By the way, when Walton tried to buy aspartame from *NutraSweet* for his study, they would not sell it to him. He had to get certified product somewhere else.) (100)

Food for Thought

Antidepressants such as *Prozac* (along other drugs to control schizophrenia and seizures) are selective serotonin reuptake inhibitors (SSRIs). That means that they allow serotonin to hang around in the blood longer, thus promoting a better mood. If aspartame decreases the level of serotonin, then more *Prozac* will be needed to maintain the level of serotonin in the blood. The drug companies win twice. They manufacture and sell the aspartame, which leads to depression, and then they manufacture and sell the remedy, SSRIs. Pretty tricky, don't you think? And since *Prozac*, *Zoloft*, and *Paxil* (all antidepressants) cause weight gain, people taking them may turn to diet sodas and foods with aspartame in them thinking they will help keep the weight off. So, the more diet foods and drinks they consume, the more of these drugs they need (and the greater the chances of adverse reactions).

The ADA is not the only organization approving aspartame. The Epilepsy Foundation is also promoting it as safe. Yet at the Massachusetts Institute of Technology, 80 people who had suffered seizures after ingesting aspartame were studied. It was concluded that "These 80 cases meet the FDA's own definition of an imminent hazard to the public health, which requires the FDA to expeditiously remove a product from the market."(101) One of the first studies performed on aspartame was in 1969 by Harry Waisman, Ph.D., who studied its effects on infant primates. Out of the seven infant monkeys, one died after 300 days and five others had grand mal seizures.(102)

The U.S. Air Force magazine *Flying Safety* has published articles warning about the many dangers of aspartame, cautioning that its ingestion can make pilots more susceptible to seizures and vertigo. Other magazines echo that warning, among them, *National Business Aircraft Association Digest*, *Aviation Medical Bulletin* (1988), *The Aviation Consumer* (1988), *Canadian General Aviation News* (1990), *Pacific Flyer* (1988), *General Aviation News* (1989), *Aviation Safety Digest* (1989), and *Plane and Pilot* (1990). More than 600 pilots have reported symptoms from aspartame including grand mal seizures in the cockpit.(103)

Aspartame is everywhere: breath mints, cereals, sugar-free chewing gum, cocoa mixes, coffee beverages, frozen desserts, gelatin desserts, juice beverages, laxatives, multivitamins, sports drinks, milk drinks, pharmaceuticals and supplements, shake mixes, soft drinks, tabletop sweeteners, tea beverages, instant teas and coffees, topping mixes, wine coolers, puddings, chewing gum, candy cough syrups, yogurt, and others. You may wonder why aspartame is used in all these products. Do you think the reason could be because it's cheaper than sugar? In closing this section, I quote an adult victim of aspartame poisoning:

> I know that the average consumer has a devil-may-care, something's-gonna-kill-me attitude. . . but they don't realize that before *this* stuff kills they are going to have a miserable declining existence with *lots* of pain and other problems (not to mention cancer, tumors, and maybe even Alzheimer's or similar things) before death solves the problem.(104)

Food for Thought

In some cases children that have already suffered from aspartame toxicity have had similar toxic reactions to aspartame and some people suspect products that contain aspartame are not labeled as such. If that is happening, it is clearly against the law. To be safe, you may want to purchase products from a health food store, since it is less likely that those products contain aspartame. Some health food stores refuse to even sell products containing aspartame. Many health food companies are quite vigilant since they were born out of a concern for health and the environment. For an excellent documentary on aspartame, check out the DVD *Sweet Misery: A Poisoned World* (you can find it on Amazon.com).

Splenda

Splenda is a relatively new artificial sweetener that's now being used in food. It has gained great popularity very quickly since its introduction in 1998 when the FDA granted approval for it to be used in a wide variety of food products. Now it's the number one artificial sweetener on the market (about five billion packets are consumed each year – that's 9,000 a minute!), replacing *Equal* (aspartame) in the top spot. Promoters say it's better than other artificial sweeteners because it leaves no bitter aftertaste, does not raise blood glucose levels, has a longer shelf-life than aspartame, and remains stable at high temperatures so it's better in baked goods. It's 600 times sweeter than sugar, looks like sugar and tastes like sugar.

No, "it's not sugar," as the advertisements joyfully exclaim. It's worse. *Splenda* is the brand name for sucralose (trichlorogalactosucrose) and is produced by chlorinating sugar (sucrose). If you remember anything about pesticides, many are also chlorinated carbon compounds (DDT being one of them). One report states: "Sucralose may be more like ingesting tiny amounts of chlorinated pesticides. . ." These tend to accumulate in body fat. Since as much as 40 percent of sucralose is absorbed by the body, there's a good chance that some of it will end up there, toxifying the body.(105) Chlorocarbons have long been known for causing organ, genetic, and reproductive damage.

Although the FDA has approved sucralose and the manufacturer says that there are no health hazards associated with it, not everyone agrees. Most European countries have not yet approved it and animal research studies indicate sucralose has caused: shrunken thymus glands; enlarged liver and kidneys; aborted pregnancy; decreased fetal body weights; reduced growth rate; diarrhea; and decreased red blood cell count. These studies have been short-term studies. There have been no long-term studies on sucralose to date.

Although the manufacturer boasts that sucralose has a purity of about 98 percent, what's in the other 2 percent? Heavy metals like lead and arsenic, methanol, triphenilphosphine oxide, and other toxins. As with the case of aspartame, sucralose is metabolized in the body into other substances that can be harmful in their own right. So as far as sweetening your food, you should use something better. Something that nature provides. Something like raw honey. Of course, honey has calories. But if you change your diet to a healthy, nutrient dense one, you will lose weight naturally, without having to subject yourself to the poisons in artificial sweeteners.

Most common forms of cancer

According the American Cancer Society, the most common forms of cancer in 2008 (and new cases per year) are:

1. Nonmelanoma skin cancer (1 million new cases)
2. Lung cancer (more than 215,00 new cases)
3. Prostate cancer (186,000 new cases)
4. Breast cancer (over 182,000 new cases - female)
5. Colon and rectal cancers (nearly 149,000 new cases)
6. Bladder cancer (nearly 69,000 new cases)
7. Non-Hodgkin Lymphoma (over 66,000 new cases)
8. Melanoma (over 62,000 new cases)
9. Kidney (renal cell) (over 46,000 new cases
10. Leukemia (over 44,000 new cases)
11. Endometrial cancer (over 40,000 new cases)
12. Pancreatic cancer (over 37,000 new cases)
13. Thyroid cancer (over 37,000 new cases) (106)

The top four kinds of cancer are covered here. However, you'll see there's a common theme in the discussions that shows how virtually any cancer may be avoided or even reversed. In fact, the fundamentals I espouse in this book are the same for virtually any kind of disease. Life is life, and it generally and consistently responds to specific conditions. Improve the conditions, and you improve life.

Before we get into the top four cancers, here are a few interesting *fast-facts* about cancer:

- Omega-3 fatty acids have been shown to stop the spread of liver cancer.(107)
- Those who eat five slices of white bread a day are almost twice as likely to develop kidney cancer compared to those who ate one and a half slices. Those who ate a high proportion of poultry, meat, and vegetables had a lower risk of getting kidney cancer.(108)
- Phytochemicals in broccoli and cauliflower are powerful anti-cancer foods.(109)
- Acrylamide is a carcinogen created when starchy foods are baked, roasted, fried, or toasted. Women with increased acrylamide in their blood had doubled the risk of breast cancer.(110) Common foods high in acrylamide when cooked these ways are potatoes, chips, French fries, grains, bread crust, toast, roasted breakfast cereals, processed snacks, coffee (roasted coffee beans), and even coffee substitutes based on chicory.
- People who eat bacon five times a week or more are almost 60 percent more likely to develop bladder cancer due to the nitrosamines in the bacon.(111) Another study showed that eating a lot of processed meats such as hot dogs and sausage increased the risk for pancreatic cancer by 67 percent.(112)
- Ninety percent of oncologists (doctors who treat cancer) said that if diagnosed with cancer, they would not take the very same chemotherapy they tell their patients to take.(113)
- Honey, propolis, and royal jelly (products from the honey bee) have been shown to stop tumors from developing or spreading in test mice. The leader of the research team, Dr. Nada Orsolic, said, "The intake of honey-bee products may be advantageous with respect to cancer and metastasis [secondary cancers] prevention."(114)

Skin Cancer

The most common kind of skin cancer, nonmelanoma skin cancer (NMSC) kills relatively few (about 1,500) people a year. Compare that with breast cancer killing over 40,000 women a year and prostate cancer killing 30,000 men a year, and although NMSC is serious and prevalent, it is not as life threatening. Melanoma is a less common form of skin cancer, but is much more deadly, killing roughly 8,000 people a year. Not surprisingly, people who get skin cancer are more than twice as likely to get other forms of cancer.(115) That shows that someone who gets cancer has problems, not just of the skin in this case, but of the whole body as well.

NMSC cancer is becoming more prevalent. One study showed that over a 22 year period (1970-1992), there was a three-fold rise in the number of patients with basal cell carcinoma and a 10-fold rise in the number of patients with squamous cell carcinoma.(116) Another study reported that the incidences of NMSC have increased in both men and women younger than the age of 40, and this is a marked increase since the 1970's.(117) NMSC is cancer that forms in basal cells (small, round cells in the base of the outer layer of skin) or the squamous cells (flat cells that form the surface of the skin). Melanoma (cancer of the melanocytes – skin cells that make pigment), and neuroendocrine carcinoma (cells that release hormones) are the other two prevalent forms of skin cancer.

Most basal cell and squamous cell skin cancers can be cured if found and treated early enough. Signs of skin cancer are easily noticed on the surface of the skin and include a sore that doesn't heal, a change in an old growth like a birthmark or mole, appearance of a firm, red lump, waxy lump, or a lump that bleeds or develops a crust or scab. The area may get dry or itchy or turn into a brown patch that is rough and scaly.

Surgery is the normal treatment for this kind of skin cancer, and many skin cancers can be removed quickly and easily. Sometimes traditional treatments involve chemotherapy, radiation or lasers. Of course, there are side effects and drawbacks to each.

Most people believe that sunlight causes skin cancer, specifically the ultra-violet portion (UV) of the light. We are cautioned not to go outside without sunscreen, sun glasses, and proper clothing. But is sunlight really such a hazard? A discussion of light and how it affects biological systems is in order to see if we can tell what is really to blame.

Light and Health

Phillip Hughes, Ph.D., a specialist in neurological sciences, physiology and psychology, says:

> Along with food, air and water, sunlight is a most important survival factor in human life. Solar radiation activates other important biochemical events in our bodies involved in endocrine control, timing of our biological clocks, entrainment of 24-hour circadian rhythms, immunological responsiveness, sexual growth and development, regulation of stress and fatigue, control for viral and cold infections, and dampening of functional disorder of the nervous system.(118)

It's only logical, then, that under natural light or an artificial source that duplicates natural light, there is less human fatigue and stress and better visual acuity and production. Yet, we're indoors most of the day where we are not only being deprived of natural sunlight, but are also being subjected to regular fluorescent lighting, with its very distorted spectrum that contributes to health and behavioral problems. Not to mention that many adults and children go home and sit in front of the TV. A double whammy; we're not getting the natural light we need, and instead, come home to be bombarded with low level radiation and artificial light.

Dr. John Ott started researching light back in the 1950s when Disney hired him to produce the first time-lapse photographs of flowers growing. During the course of making the plants grow, he discovered that they would only flower and grow normally under certain lighting conditions. As he learned more, he expanded his investigations on the effects light and certain kinds and quality of light have on animals and humans. He showed that it can indeed be dramatic.

In experiments on first grade students in Sarasota, Florida, researchers found that children in a classroom with cool-white fluorescent lighting were more hyperactive than students in another classroom with full-spectrum fluorescent tubes that duplicated natural sunlight. "Under the standard, cool-white fluorescent lighting, some first graders showed nervous fatigue, irritability, lapses of attention and hyperactive behavior," says Ott. "Within a week after the new lights were installed, the children settled down and paid more attention to their teachers."[119]

The Fort Worth, Texas, school system was one of the first to install fluorescent lighting years ago in a dozen schools. But they soon removed them because of all the complaints of eyestrain, headaches, and other health related problems. Ott demonstrated that radiation from regular fluorescent lights can grossly weaken muscle strength and affect both academic achievement and behavior. Fluorescent lights can cause eyestrain, headaches, insomnia, irritability, hyperactivity, fatigue, and increase dental caries. Dr. Fritz Hollowich showed that exposure to cool-white fluorescent lights resulted in the release of the stress hormones ACTH and cortisol. Under full-spectrum lights, this did not occur.[120]

The Greek athletes used to sunbathe naked before competitions because they believed it increased their strength. Without natural light, our whole endocrine system suffers since light directly influences both the pituitary gland and the pineal gland. The pituitary gland is often referred to as the "master gland" since it is the prime regulator of the whole endocrine system.

The pineal gland is instrumental in setting and controlling sleep cycles and our body's internal clock. It also produces a hormone called melatonin that helps us to fall asleep at night, and helps regulate estrogen production. Not enough melatonin, and estrogen levels rise. The over-abundance of estrogen in the system has been correlated with a high incidence of female type cancers such as breast and uterine cancers. Not enough sunlight means too much melatonin is produced which causes too much estrogen. So women, if you want to cut down on your chances of breast or uterine cancer, get some pure, unfiltered sunlight.

Without question, adequate exposure to ultraviolet light is required for maximum health. It's needed to convert nutritional precursors to active forms of vitamin D, which the body needs to perform many healthy functions including the development and maintenance of strong healthy bones. Consider one study by British researchers that demonstrates the importance of adequate sunlight (containing UV rays), in children's bone development. The study was performed in two areas of India: downtown Delhi, where there was significantly more haze and less sunlight; and Gurgoan, which had less haze with more sunlight. The researchers measured serum levels of calcium, vitamin D, and other markers of bone growth in 56 children. Children who lived in hazier downtown Delhi with less exposure to sunlight had a lower mean level of vitamin D, which would impact bone growth and development. The researchers concluded that children living in more polluted and high-haze areas should be offered vitamin D supplements.[121]

Vitamin D deficiency is not only a problem in other nations, but in the U.S as well. Rickets, a bone-softening condition in children that was common years ago, was becoming so rare in the United States that the government stopped keeping statistics on it. It's been making a comeback in recent years however, and is now affecting more and more youngsters. Government officials attribute the comeback to three things: the popularity of milk substitutes such as soy that lack certain nutrients; the failure to supplement breast milk with vitamin D; and a lack of sufficient childhood exposure to sunlight. Vitamin D deficiency has also been linked to increased risk for colon carcinoma.[122]

Sunlight is not just important for a growing child, but the amount of it the mother is exposed to during pregnancy has been found to affect the baby's height later on in life: the more sunlight the mother receives, the taller the person will grow.[123]

A vitamin D deficit in the mother can also affect the child's brain development. Children whose mothers took cod liver (rich in vitamin D) during pregnancy scored significantly higher on IQ tests at four years of age than children whose mothers did not take the oil. Another study showed that low maternal vitamin D increases the risk of a child developing schizophrenia later in life.[124,125] Human breast milk is often deficient in vitamin D because the mother is deficient too, and so the baby does not get enough of it. Lactating mothers need at least 3,600 IUs of cholecalciferol (the natural form of vitamin D) to maintain their own and their infant's vitamin D levels. This is about 10 times what the federal government says a lactating woman should have. Moreover, Professor Robert Heaney of Creighton University Medical Center – a world renowned expert on vitamin D, found that normal adults need 10 times more vitamin D than the government recommends. This is especially true of black people, who were found to be 10 times more likely to be vitamin D deficient (more sunlight is needed the darker the skin).[126]

Food for Thought

Dr. Mercola, a physician who also has one of the most popular health websites on the internet (www.mercola.com) has this to say about our governments' vitamin D policy:

"Although we know of no vitamin D scientist in the nation who believes the government's current guidelines, the guidelines remain and the result is widespread vitamin D deficiencies in the American populace, especially among blacks and very especially among black neonates. Furthermore, our government knows that vitamin D is crucial for neural development. Nevertheless, the government refuses to act. Why?"

Mercola and many top scientists including those from the Vitamin D Research Council believes that as many as 70 percent of Americans are vitamin D deficient. This may result in many health problems since vitamin D helps regulate calcium metabolism, bone health, and cell growth.

Michael Holick, Ph.D., M.D. is one of the world's foremost authorities on vitamin D and author of the book titled *The UV Advantage*. He shows that there are links between vitamin D deficiency and breast cancer, prostate cancer, ovarian cancer, and colon cancer. Lack of vitamin D can also play a major toll in the development of diabetes, especially if one was deficient of it as a child.(127)

Vitamin D is produced by the body when it's exposed to natural light. Dr Holick says: "The notion that we have to protect ourselves from the sun all the times is misguided and unhealthy." Our irrational fear of the sun is causing thousands of premature deaths each year." He estimates that 27,500 American women die prematurely every year from breast cancer caused by vitamin D deficiency. Dr. Holick says that for every 55 to 60 men who die of prostate cancer due to underexposure to sunlight, one dies from overexposure; and you are three times less likely to die of colon cancer if you have healthy levels of vitamin D.

We produce quite a bit of vitamin D when exposed to natural sunlight – as much as 20,000 units in 20 minutes in the summer. But when vitamin D is produced by the body as a result of sun exposure, it's never toxic, no matter how much we produce because any excess will be destroyed by the sun itself. But if you take it internally in a pill or liquid, you can overdo it. It's hard to get enough vitamin D from the diet - you'd have to drink 200 glasses of vitamin D fortified milk to get enough. That's why it's best to get your vitamin D the way nature intended - through sun exposure. But in the winter this may not possible in many places, so it's best to supplement with good cod liver oil (see the Resource Guide).

Start sun exposure slowly, just 10 minutes a day, and work up to more. The last thing you want to put on your skin is sunscreen, because it not only doesn't stop skin cancer, but is made of toxic chemicals that get absorbed into your skin (the skin, by the way, is the body's largest organ). The incidence of skin cancer has increased as the sales of sunscreen have increased. If you're afraid of too much sun, wear light clothing and a hat or spread on some coconut oil - it's a great natural sunscreen. Getting sun will help you become healthier, happier, and less likely to get cancer. Please let your kids get sun without sunscreen too. An excellent book that tells of the importance of natural sunshine is *The Healing Sun* by Dr. Richard Hobday.

Zane Kime, M.D., tells of a rabbit study that showed that the animals kept in dim light were more susceptible to cancer. An increase in the light resulted in a decrease in cancer. Another study in Russia was undertaken to prove that UV rays induced cancer. However, much to the researchers' surprise, the lab animals living under lights with UV rays, as compared with those living under fluorescent lights, developed significantly *less* cancer.(128)

An article in the journal *Cancer*, reported that there is an inverse relationship between cancer mortality in the U.S. and the levels of ultraviolet B exposure (UV-B gives you a tan and is blocked by sunscreen, glass, glasses, and contact lenses). In all, 13 kinds of cancer showed this inverse relationship: the strongest correlations were with breast, colon, and ovarian cancers. Cancers of the bladder, uterus, esophagus, rectum and stomach showed correlations also.(129) This clearly shows that the less sun you get, the more your chance of getting cancer becomes. This is true even for melanoma, the deadly skin cancer.

Research has shown that people who get regular sun exposure as part of their jobs are less likely to get melanoma than people who work inside all the time.(130) Lifeguards in Australia exhibit the country's lowest rates of melanoma, while office workers have the highest.(131) A study by the U.S. Navy found that melanoma occurred more often in sailors who worked indoors all the time, and those who worked outdoors had the lowest incidence of melanoma. Interestingly, melanoma often appears on parts of the body that are seldom exposed to sunlight.(132)

I'm not saying a lot of sun cannot cause problems – too much of it can. Overexposure to UV rays *can* cause tissue damage (sunburn). Overexposure to *anything* can be hazardous. But consider that people of generations ago who worked the land under the hot sun did not have sun block or sun glasses, and cancer was rare.

Ott tells an interesting story about some members of a Congolese tribe that had suddenly developed cancer when the disease had been previously unknown to them. The natives, who wore nothing but loin cloths, had recently taken to wearing sunglasses as a symbol of status. Dr. Ott speculates that the lack of full-spectrum light entering the eye was the cause of their cancer.(133) With that in mind, it's a good idea to get some unfiltered sunlight into your eyes (don't look at the sun directly) by taking off your glasses or removing your contacts every now and then.

Food for Thought

There's a kind of contact lense most people don't know about that allows your eyes to get unfiltered sunshine all day. That's because you wear them at night while you sleep! They are hard, gas-permeable contact lenses specifically shaped for each eye that changes the shape of the cornea to give you correct vision. (They work for nearsighted and astigmatic eyes.) When you wake up, you remove them, and your cornea stays the same, corrected shape for between one and three days. Very cool.

If you don't want to get laser surgery, which I don't recommend because of the small but significant chance of problems, these contacts are great. It's called Orthokeratology (non-surgical cornea reshaping) and it's been around for decades and is FDA approved. Check out www.ortho-k.net.

During winter months or if you cannot get adequate sunlight, you can purchase specially designed full-spectrum lighting that is very close to sunlight. These lights are sold to combat Seasonal Affective Disorder (or SAD), a condition that shows similar symptoms to depression and that manifests in people in northern latitudes who do not get enough sunlight. The best of these lights I have found that include UV light come from Full Spectrum Solutions (www.FullSpectrumSolutions.com)

What we eat has a much bigger influence on whether or not a person develops melanoma. Studies have shown that there was a 40 percent reduction in melanoma in those who ate fish regularly. This is because of the high content of omega-3 fatty acids which tend to inhibit cancer growths. Conversely, omega-6 fatty acids tend to stimulate cancer growths. Omega-6's are found in vegetable oils like corn oil, and safflower oil. Omega 3's are found in cod liver oil, salmon oil, meat, fish and some nuts and seeds.(134)

The ability to use sunlight to produce vitamin D decreases with age. It's estimated that as much as 95 percent of those over 50 years have a vitamin D deficiency.(135) So the elderly should be certain to consume enough of it through supplementation (especially in the winter) and get some sunshine every day. The *American Journal of Clinical Nutrition* correlated widespread vitamin D deficiency with osteoporosis, heart disease, rheumatoid arthritis, multiple sclerosis, diabetes as well as cancer. Your risk of dying from colon cancer, breast cancer, prostate cancer and ovarian cancer goes down when your vitamin D levels go up.(136,137)

Light-skinned people have less of the skin pigment melanin than dark skinned people, and can synthesize vitamin D from sunlight six times faster. Therefore, it's not surprising that blacks need to get more vitamin D from their diet. In fact, one study said that African-American women should take at least 2,000 IU of vitamin D daily, and some who are vitamin D deficient may need as much as 4,000 IU.(138) The study said that African-Americans simply cannot get enough vitamin D by following the RDA guidelines, and should take 2,800 IU. The current RDAs for vitamin D are: 200 IU for children and adults, 400 IU for adults between 50-70, and 800 IU for adults over 70 (that are definitely too low).

You can overdose from too much vitamin D (from supplements), so be careful. That said, one researcher said, "Worrying about vitamin D toxicity is like worrying about drowning when you're dying of thirst." One report in the *American Journal of Clinical Nutrition* reported that people could take 10,000 IU of vitamin D every day, month after month safely, with no evidence of adverse effect. Someone would have to consume 50,000 IU a day for several months before hypercalcemia (the first signs of vitamin D toxicity) might occur.(139)

The sure way to tell if you're getting enough vitamin D is to test your blood level before you start supplementing. The researchers are not in total agreement but they are generally telling us that an optimal level is most likely between 50 and 60ng/dl. Anything less than 8 ng/ml is severely deficient and will cause rickets.

Since there are two kinds of blood tests for vitamin D, be sure to get the one that tests 25(OH)D or 25-hydroxyvitamin D. It takes about 1,000 IU of vitamin D to increase blood levels by 10 ng/ml. You can find places on the internet that sell test kits for vitamin D. These sites have them: www.directlabs.com, www.ZRTlab.com.

There are two kinds of vitamin D supplements too. Be sure to get the natural kind, Vitamin D_3 (found in cod liver oil), and not the synthetic D_2. Any supplementation should be done under the supervision of your health care professional.

Where else can you find vitamin D? One tablespoon of cod liver oil has about 1360 IUs; 3 ounces of herring has 1383 IU; 3½ ounces of sardines has 270 IU; 3½ ounces salmon has 360 IU; 3 ounces tuna has 200 IU; 3½ ounces oysters has 640 IU; One egg yolk has 25 IU; One ounce Swiss cheese has 12 IU.

Food for Thought

It's important to realize that cod liver oil also contains vitamin A, which is a necessary nutrient too, but can be toxic in high amounts. Some researchers fear that taking a lot of cod liver oil may lead to vitamin A toxicity. However, if the cod liver oil contains naturally occurring vitamins A and D, the vitamin A will not be toxic except in cases where vitamin D is deficient. Vitamins A and D work synergistically; if you take large amounts of vitamin A without vitamin D, you may develop symptoms of vitamin D deficiency. If you take large amounts of vitamin D without vitamin A, you may develop symptoms of vitamin A deficiency. So it's vital that you consume ONLY the brands of cod liver oil I recommend that are known to have the right balance of these two important nutrients.

One of the reasons cod liver oil has come under attack concerning the vitamin A toxicity issue is because most cod liver oil on the market is actually deficient in vitamin D because the deodorization process many manufacturers use actually strips vitamin D from the oil. In addition, many brands remove the naturally occurring vitamins, and then add in synthetic versions of A and D, which are toxic.

Older studies showing the benefits of cod liver oil used oil that had not been deodorized and that contained natural vitamins in normal amounts. Over-processing to make the oil more appealing has not only made most brands ineffective, but potentially harmful. Another fear of cod liver oil is that it contains mercury, since fish are known to have high levels of it. However, mercury accumulates in the protein portion of fish, not in the oil, and repeated testing has shown that the amounts of mercury (and PCBs) in cod liver oil are undetectable.[140]

Nutritionist David Getoff adds that he almost always has his patients on BOTH extra D and extra A. Although as fat soluble nutrients, it is possible to get too much of them, it is not easy or likely to do so. David recommends to those who are worried about vitamin A toxicity, that they get a current copy of the physician's main reference book called the MERCK Manual and read the section on vitamin A. It clearly shows how tremendously high the doses must be in order to cause a problem. In addition, unlike the sometimes deadly side effects of drugs, it also clearly shows that the effects of too much vitamin A immediately goes away as soon as the extra vitamin A is discontinued, and there are no lasting effects.

Another point to keep in mind is that for the body to properly utilize vitamin D, adequate magnesium is necessary. If it isn't available, you may experience heart flutters or constipation. I discuss magnesium in depth in later chapters and show you the best kind and where to purchase it.

If you need more vitamin D than what you can get from cod liver oil (based on blood tests), you can purchase vitamin D by itself.

Places on the internet with good vitamin D are lifespannutrition.com and bio-tech-pharm.com.

The farther north you live, naturally, the less sun you get especially in winter. If you live above 30 degrees latitude, you should supplement your diet with vitamin D from September through April. If you don't get out much even during the summer, you might need to supplement all year round. Tanning beds are not acceptable as a means of getting your daily dose of vitamin D (they provide high levels of UV-A and very little UV-B, which is what you need to synthesize vitamin D).

Food for Thought

Instead of exposure to sun or UV rays, could it be that other factors are making us generally more sensitive and skin cancer is manifesting due to different reasons? In a 1965 research study, Dr. Frederic Urbach et al., concluded that, "more than one-third of all basal cell carcinomas occurred on areas receiving less than 20 percent of the maximum possible ultraviolet dose. This suggests that some factor in addition to ultraviolet radiation plays a significant role in the genesis of basal cell carcinoma."[141] Our overall health and vitality, or lack thereof, plays a significant role in whether we get cancer – skin or any other kind.

Speaking of overdoing it, one study that has contributed to our fear of UV rays was titled "Phototherapy Exposure Tied to Retinal Damage."[142] In that experiment, newborn piglets were exposed to a bank of 10 high intensity 20-watt fluorescent lights filtered to deliver only UV light (this is the equivalent of 300 foot candles of light). One eye was held open and dilated for 72 hours straight and the other covered with a patch. It's not surprising that the eyes not protected showed retinal damage. The conclusion was that light with UV rays is bad and causes damage. That's like holding a piglet under water for 10 minutes and saying water is dangerous.

In his classic book *Health and Light*, John Ott shares a couple stories about how ultraviolet light can affect health. The manager of a certain restaurant that used black lights (UV rays) to set the desired mood said that he had essentially the same group of men working for him as he had when they had opened the restaurant 18 years before. He said that the ultraviolet lights had been in use continually during that time, and that the health record of his men had been so consistently excellent that the manager of the hotel had checked into the situation, with medical supervision, to try to determine why this particular group of men was always on the job, even during flu epidemics, when other departments in the hotel would be short-handed because of employees' illness. . ."These men working in the restaurant seemed to be a particularly happy group – courteous and efficient, and all seemed to get along well together. . .Not one of them wore glasses. . .and none had ever complained of any eye problems or discomfort as a result of the ultraviolet light."

At the Seaquarium in Miami, Dr. Ott noticed a similar black light ultra-violet light over some of the fish aquariums. He said, "I learned that these lights had originally been placed over some of the aquariums for decorative purposes, to give the fish an eerie but attractive appearance. . .[The curator] told me that the added black light seemed to solve one of their main problems in keeping fish healthy. This was a condition of exophthalmus, or pop-eye, recently identified as due to a virus. I was told that it is rare that any aquarium fish are troubled with exophthalmus when kept in an outdoor aquarium under natural daylight and nighttime conditions. Another problem of fin-nipping also disappeared under natural conditions. . ."(143) The "fin-nipping" is obviously an aggressive behavior. Could some of the increase in aggression of adults (and children) is due to a lack of a vital nutrient – that being full-spectrum light with the UV included.

People in Denmark eat more herring (the richest source of vitamin D) than anyone in the world, and they're consistently ranked as the happiest, most fulfilled people.(144) Maybe a simple nutrient can make a difference in our happiness. I'll even take it a step further: The lack of vitamin D could be causing not just unhappiness, but some of the aggression and violence we see all too often these days. By the way, the USA ranked 23rd in happiness.

Diet seems to be the key in the development of skin cancer, rather than getting too much sunlight. A study in Australia found that a high-fat diet does not increase the risk of skin cancer (both non-melanoma and melanoma). In fact, the results showed that the higher the fat intake, the lower the risk of non-melanoma.(145) I already mentioned the importance of consuming the proper ratio of omega 6 to omega 3 fatty acids, and omega 3s are known to fight cancer in their own right.

The bottom line to avoiding skin cancer is two-fold: get some unfiltered sunshine and/or take vitamin D supplements; and eat the right kind of (raw) and adequate amounts of good quality fat.

Food for Thought

Donald Miller, M.D., a cardiac surgeon and Professor of Surgery at the University of Washington in Seattle, is another proponent of vitamin D. He says,

"The U.S. government and its citizens currently spend $2,000 billion dollars ($2 trillion) on 'health care,' each year. The cost of taking 5,000 IU supplement of vitamin D every day for a year is $22.00. [Probably higher now.] The cost for 30 million Americans taking this supplement would be $6.6 billion dollars. The number and variety of diseases that vitamin D at this dose could prevent, starting with a 50 percent reduction in cancer, is mind-boggling. If everyone took 5,000 IU/day of vitamin D, the U.S. 'health care' industry would shrink. It would no longer account for 16 percent of the gross domestic product."[146]

Dr. Miller also comments on the role of vitamin D in multiple sclerosis (MS), of which 500,000 Americans suffer from. Researchers have shown that the risk of MS decreases as the level of vitamin D in the blood increases.[147] People living at higher latitudes have a lower risk of MS and people who live below 35 degrees latitude have a lower risk.[148]

Grandma's advice to take your cod liver oil every day doesn't seem so crazy now, does it? Listen to grandma! She was a good woman who probably knew more about how to stay healthy than most doctors do today.

Lung Cancer

Lung cancer is the leading cause of cancer deaths in the U.S for both men and women. It claims more lives each year than colon, prostate, breast and lymph cancers combined. One in 14 men and women will be diagnosed with lung cancer at some point in their lives. In 2008, 114,690 men and 100,300 women will be diagnosed with it and 161,840 will die because of it.[149]

Lung cancer typically doesn't cause signs and symptoms in its earliest stages, but rather after it has advanced. Symptoms may include: a new cough that doesn't go away, changes in a chronic cough, coughing up blood, shortness of breath, chest pain, wheezing, and hoarseness.

The cancer starts in the cells that line your lungs, and can occur in non-smokers as well as smokers. Smoking damages the cells that line the lungs that are full of blood vessels and lymph vessels. This gives cancer cells easy access to travel to other parts of your body. This is why lung cancer may spread to other parts of your body before you even experience any signs or symptoms, and sometimes is detected elsewhere before even being detected in the lungs.

Other risk factors besides smoking include exposure to radon gas, exposure to asbestos and other chemicals (arsenic, chromium, nickel, tar soot), excessive alcohol use, exposure to second hand smoke, and a family history of lung cancer.

A woman who smokes the same amount as a man has a greater chance of getting lung cancer. Researchers believe that this is because women inhale more than men, are less likely to quit, and estrogen may play a role in making them more sensitive to the cancer-causing substances in the smoke. Recently it's been determined that even women who have never smoked are now getting lung cancer more often. In 2005, 10 percent of men with lung cancer have never smoked, but 20 percent of women who have the disease never smoked. Lung cancer currently kills about 15,000 non-smoking women each year. The disease remains as deadly now as it was 30 years ago, and only 15 percent of lung cancer patients survive as long as five years.(150)

The typical way to screen for lung cancer is through taking chest X-rays or CT scans (computerized tomography). Others include an MRI (magnetic resonance imaging), PET scan (positron emission tomography), bone scans, and tissue samples for a biopsy. But none of these are conclusive in determining if someone has cancer or not. In fact, frequent screening with chest X-rays was shown not to reduce the odds of dying from lung cancer and could even lead some people to undergo unnecessary treatments for lung tumors that would never have been fatal.(151) The world expert in low level radiation was John W. Gofman, M.D. His vast amount of published scientific research clearly showed that the more X-rays a person gets, the more they have an increased risk of cancer due to the well documented cumulative effect of radiation.

Treatments for lung cancer include surgery, chemotherapy, radiation therapy or targeted drug therapy. A combination of these may be used depending on how far advanced the cancer is. Surgery options include removing small sections of the lung (wedge resection), an entire lobe of one lung (lobectomy), or the whole lung (pneumonectomy). Chemotherapy includes drugs administered intravenously or orally over weeks or months, with breaks in treatment so that your body can recover from their toxic effects. Radiation therapy includes external beam radiation, or implanting seeds with radioactive material inside the body near the cancer. Drug therapy includes using the drug Bevacizumab (*Avastin*), which carries a risk of severe bleeding, or Erltinib (*Tarceva*), which may produce skin rashes and diarrhea.

Of course, no one wants to loose a lung or part of a lung, and radiation and drugs have nasty side effects. The best way to beat lung cancer is to avoid it in the first place, and following the dietary and life-style changes detailed throughout this book will help you do that. There are, however, a few specific things that can help.

Avoiding and Surviving Lung Cancer

One thing that has been shown to increase the survival rate of lung cancer victims is, not surprisingly, sunshine. As you read in the section on skin cancer, vitamin D is a powerful anti-cancer agent. One study showed that lung cancer patients who were operated on during the sunny time of year had a higher survival rate, and those who had surgery during the sunniest time of year and took vitamin D supplements more than doubled their chances of survival beyond the five-year mark (72 percent survival rate) compared to patients who had surgeries in the winter and took less or none of the vitamin (30 percent survival rate). Those who had the highest intake of vitamin D were 28 percent less likely to die.(152)

But not all supplements are good for you. One study found that high doses of vitamin E in supplemental form increased cancer risk by 28 percent, and smokers were at particular risk.(153) If you think you need more vitamin E, eat some nuts or leafy green vegetables, and buy organic food that is richer in vitamins.

A substance in tangerines and oranges (a flavonoid), has been shown to inhibit lung cancer cells effectively.(154) But don't try to get this from store-bought orange juice. There may be some in there, but commercial orange juice is contaminated with mold from damaged fruit, and pasteurized, which destroys many of the beneficial qualities. Eat fresh, organic oranges or tangerines or make your own juice.

The trace element selenium was first associated with cancer risk in the late 1960s. Areas that have moderate to high soil selenium levels were shown to have lower mortality rates for cancers of the lung, colon and rectum, bladder, esophagus, pancreas, breast, ovary, and cervix.(155) This study reported that selenium of 200 mcg per day decreased the overall incidence of all cancers by 35 percent and cancer mortality by 50 percent. Another study showed that low selenium contributes to the risk of lung cancer especially if they smoke.(156). The richest source of selenium is brazil nuts, with shelled nuts having 12 to 25 mcg of selenium. I go into more detail on selenium in the chapter on prostate cancer.

Research at Penn State College of Health and Human Development stated that a compound in garlic (diallyl trisulfide or DATS) slowed and even killed human lung tumor cells (and cancer cells in the colon and skin). Another compound (S-allylysteine or SAC) interfered with breast tumor cells in rats. John Milner, one of the researchers and head of Penn State's Department of Nutrition said, "Clearly we are learning that there is more than one mechanism by which garlic can reduce cancer. Our studies and others have shown that compounds in garlic can block the irritation phase of cancer as well as the subsequent promotion phase."(157)

Garlic cannot only helps with lung cancer, but it is becoming recognized as being able to inhibit the growth of cancers of the digestive tract too. A study published in the *American Journal of Clinical Nutrition* found that people who consumed garlic regularly have about half the risk of getting stomach cancer and two-thirds the risk of colorectal cancer as people who eat little or no garlic. The researchers said, "There seems to be a strong, consistent protective effect for people who are regular garlic consumer." Fresh, raw garlic is most effective, whereas pills and powders are not.(158) A study in France found that increased garlic consumption was associated with a significant reduction in breast cancer.(159) A study reported in *Cancer Epidemiology Biomarkers & Prevention* showed that the risk of pancreatic cancer was 54 percent lower in people who ate larger amounts of garlic compared wit those who ate lower amounts.(160)

Research is also showing garlic can help leukemia, melanoma, and neuroblastoma.(161) One small study reported in the *Archives of Dermatological Research* indicated that the application of garlic extracts to some skin tumors may help. Applying ajoene (a sulfuous chemical found in garlic) to the skin for a month markedly decreased the size of tumors in 17 of 21 patients. The tumors shrunk as much as 88 percent.(162)

Researchers believe that it's the high content of sulfur containing compounds that are responsible for the medicinal properties of garlic. Other foods with similar sulfur compounds are onions, chives, leeks, and scallions. Garlic also contains arginine (see male virility section), selenium, flavonoids, and olgosaccharides. Half a clove to two cloves of garlic a day is the recommended amount to eat to see the beneficial effects.

Another natural food that is proving to fight cancer is vinegar. I already discussed it in the chapter on obesity, and I'll get into specific research on it concerning heart disease later, but for now, there are several studies I want to bring to your attention. It's been shown to not only inhibit cancer cells from proliferating, but it has been shown to stimulate apoptosis (the mechanism that allows cancer cells to die), stimulate natural killer cells, prolong life span due to tumor regression, and has antioxidant properties that protect against cancer.(163,164,165,166,167,168,169,170) Remember, the only kind of vinegar you should use is raw, unfiltered apple cider vinegar.

Food for Thought

You may think I'm being overly optimistic thinking garlic, vinegar, nuts and other natural things can prevent or reverse cancer. But please consider a few things. One: If you don't discontinue doing what is causing cancer or other diseases in the first place, nothing is going to stop them from starting or spreading. That's why I go into such detail on the environmental causes of disease – to alert you to the things you need to avoid. Two: Many drugs are modeled after compounds found in nature. But since these can't be patented, the drug companies make small changes to the compounds so they can be. That way, they can make it an exclusive product and make money. Three: For some reason people in our culture believe that technology is better than nature. If something hasn't gone through some complicated process in a lab or a high-tech machine hasn't been used, most think the treatment can't be nearly as powerful or as effective as something from the grocery store or back yard garden. Granted, natural remedies sometimes work slower than drugs or technology, but they don't have the side effects. And, as I've said and will continue to remind you, when you alter your lifestyle to eliminate the things that are making you sick, and replace them with things that nourish and nurture you (like garlic, vinegar, organic food and so on), you're getting *double goodness* that actually increases the effectiveness exponentially.

If you do get lung cancer, it's bad news. As I said, most people don't survive more than 5 years (the average age of people who get lung cancer is 71), and even detecting it is unlikely.(171) Obviously, avoiding lung cancer is the best thing to do. The two major causes of lung cancer are smoking and radon gas, so let's look at both.

Smoking

Smoking may not only causes lung cancer and heart disease, but a host of other health problems. I will discuss most of them here, including how smoke can affect children, babies and even fetuses not just in the short run, but for the rest of their lives. If you have a teenager, having them read this may help them realize how important it is to never start.

The Centers for Disease Control and Prevention says that tobacco use is the nation's leading cause of death, accounting for about 430,700 of the more than two million annual deaths in the U.S. One in every five deaths in the U.S. is caused by tobacco use, which accounts for more than $50 billion a year in medical expenditures and another $50 billion in indirect costs.(172,173) Smoking among adults has dropped dramatically between 1965 and 2000 – from 42 percent to 22 percent – so these numbers should be coming down.(174)

Heart disease, lung cancer, emphysema, and throat cancer in adults are all the obvious results of smoking. But smoking can and does effect the whole body and all the biochemical processes in the body. It affects blood sugar which affects energy levels and thinking capability. In fact, one reason people crave a smoke is because it temporarily raises the blood sugar level, giving that person a pick-me-up. This can have direct consequences to the liver and pancreas. And as we'll see below, smoking can have serious effects on children as well, setting them up for health problems immediately and later in life.

Parental smoking contributes to 150,000 to 300,000 respiratory infections in babies causing 7,500 to 15,000 hospitalizations a year. The effects of smoking by the parents not only can affect the infant, baby, and child, but can also affect future children in the womb and even before conception.

Donna E. Shalala, Ph.D., the Secretary of the U.S. Department of Health and Human Services says, "Today, nearly 3,000 young people across our country will begin smoking regularly. Of these 3,000 people, 1,000 will lose that gamble to the diseases caused by smoking. The net effect of this is that among children living in America today, 5 million will die an early, preventable death because of a decision made as a child."

An estimated 4.5 million (20 percent) of youths age 12 to 17 years were smokers in 1995, while 48 million (24.7) percent of adults age 18 years and older currently smoke – 27.6 percent of men and 22.1 percent of women.(175) Data suggest that smoking prevalence may be increasing among young adults, especially girls.

Ninety percent of smokers begin before age 20, 50 percent begin by age 14 and 25 percent begin by age 12. Since 1991, past-month smoking has increased by 35 percent among eighth graders and 43 percent among tenth graders.

Between 1988 and 1996, among adolescents 12 to 17 years old, the incidence of initiation of the first use of tobacco increased by 30 percent and of first daily use increased 50 percent. An estimated 4.1 million teenagers are smokers in this age category.(176)

The health risks of young people smoking are the same as those found in adults: death from cancer, heart and cardiovascular disease, and emphysema. There's evidence that those who begin smoking before they're 20 years old have the highest incidence and earliest onset of both coronary heart disease and high blood pressure.(177)

In fact, it's been shown that cigarette smoking by children or their exposure to smoke initiates events that lead to coronary artery disease, cancer, and chronic obstructive pulmonary disease. Smoking in children (or exposure to smoke) also changes the serum lipoproteins in the blood and increases platelet aggregation. It causes injury to the endothelial cells (the cells lining the blood vessels), which is thought to be the primary initiating event of atherosclerosis; pathological changes of the endothelial cells have even been observed in the umbilical arteries of infants born to mothers who smoke.(178)

In January 1993, the EPA officially declared environmental tobacco smoke (ETS) a known human carcinogen. It is now classified as a Group A carcinogen, known to cause cancer in humans – in the same category as asbestos and other hazardous substances. The EPA's report called ETS a serious and substantial health risk for nonsmokers, particularly children.(179) ETS contains more than 4,000 chemicals and at least 40 known carcinogens. Nicotine is the addictive drug in the smoke and leads to acute increases in heart rate and blood pressure. Exposure to ETS causes about 10 times as many deaths from heart and blood vessel diseases as does cancer. ETS is also associated with acute middle ear infections, tonsillectomy, cancer in childhood, slower growth, adverse neurobehavioral effects, colds and sore throats, and meningococcal infections (infections of the meninges of the brain).(180)

Nine million American children under five years of age live in homes with at least one adult smoker, so they breathe secondhand smoke regularly. Children who are exposed to secondhand smoke are more likely to have upper respiratory problems, including infections, bronchitis, asthma, pneumonia, wheezing, more throat infections, and even more ear infections. Indeed, children newborn to five years old who are exposed to maternal smoking are over twice as likely to develop asthma compared to those free from exposure. A study in Italy of almost 19,000 children ages six and seven and more than 21,000 adolescents ages 13 and 14 showed parental smoking dramatically increases the incidences of asthma in children. It's estimated that 15 percent of asthma cases in children and 11 percent of wheezing cases among adolescents are attributable to parental smoking. "There is no question that a parent who smokes – especially a mother – puts her child at risk of asthma," says Norman H. Edelman, M.D., a consultant for the American Lung Association.(181) A report by the California Environmental Protection Agency estimates that parents who smoke each year cause 8,000 to 26,000 new cases of childhood asthma in the U.S. And make existing asthma worse in 20 percent of the two to five million children who already have the disease. The children of parents who smoke compared with children of nonsmoking parents have increased frequency of respiratory infections, increased respiratory symptoms, and slightly smaller rates of increase in lung function as the lung mature.

A child's lungs undergo important growth and development during the first two years of life. If an infant regularly breathes secondhand smoke, it may stunt lung growth and may cause a permanent decrease in lung function – affecting his respiratory health for the rest of his life.

If parents smoke in their home or car, their children breathe in their second-hand smoke. The nicotine from that smoke can be measured in the child's urine. Secondhand smoke contains harmful chemicals such as arsenic, cyanide, tar, formaldehyde, carbon monoxide, carbon monoxide, benzene, and nicotine.(182)

Children are especially vulnerable to respiratory hazards – their airways are smaller than adults, they breathe more rapidly and inhale more pollutant per pound of body weight than adults and they often spend more time engaged in vigorous activities. The Centers for Disease Control gives these statistics:

- Children with parents who smoke suffer excessive and unnecessary colds, flu, bronchitis, and pneumonia.
- More than 10 million children (31.2 percent) are being exposed to cigarette smoke in their homes.
- Children exposed to smoke miss more than 28 million days of school a year, one third more than kids from smoke-free homes.
- These children have 1.7 million more colds and acute respiratory infections – 10 percent more than kids who are not exposed, and suffer over 10 million days a year of restricted activities such as missing sports practice – 21 percent more than unexposed kids.(183)

Children in homes with low income and educational levels are far more likely (48 percent) to be exposed than kids in homes with high income and educational levels (28 percent).

Smoking can cause problems even before the child is born. Smoking by the mother during pregnancy is responsible for 14 percent of premature deliveries,

30 percent of low-birth-weight babies, and 4,600 infant deaths per year. Mothers who smoke 10 or more cigarettes a day during pregnancy cause as many as 26,000 new asthma cases a year among children. Nicotine makes the mother's blood vessels smaller, so less nourishment, water, and oxygen gets to the fetus. Poisons in the smoke reach a baby through the mothers' placental bloodstream and later through breast milk. The nicotine in the smoke also raises the blood pressure and slows the heartbeat of the fetus, which can damage the baby's blood vessels and heart, even before birth. Maternal smoking increases the likelihood of SIDS by more than three times.(184)

A study by a team of researchers at the University of Southern California indicated that cigarette smoke damages the unborn babies' lungs at crucial points in their development leading to reduced lung capacity in later life. Passive smoking after birth had the same effect, but was not as marked as the damage done during pregnancy. The airflow was significantly impaired in the small airways of children whose mothers had smoked. Frank Gilliland, Ph.D., warned that the long-term effect for children whose mothers smoked during their bodies' development could be obstructive pulmonary disease, lung cancer, and cardiovascular disease.(185)

In fact, a study at Ohio State University suggests that the effects of environmental tobacco smoke linger long after that child has left home and is no longer exposed. It showed that children who were exposed to high levels of ETS growing up maintained higher blood pressure, mean arterial pressure, and resting heart rate, and heart rate during psychological stress compared to students who grew up with low levels of ETS. One of the researchers said, "We've learned that children who grow up in a smoking household will have small but long-lasting negative effects on their health. You don't have to be the one smoking, but you can still vicariously suffer some of the effects."(186)

Clive Bates, director of the British group Action on Smoking and Health, comments, "When babies are exposed to the chemicals in cigarette smoke while still in the womb, it is just about the nastiest form of passive smoking imaginable and it looks as though it does lasting damage. It's hard to think of a more pervasive and pernicious assault on the health of the most vulnerable infants."(187)

Smoking by the mother during pregnancy has been shown to increase the risk of miscarriages, premature birth, stillbirths, and death in the first few weeks of life. Nicotine, carbon monoxide, and polycyclic aromatic hydrocarbons are known to cross the placenta and have been identified in newborns of smokers. Carbon monoxide likes to bind with hemoglobin, which reduces the capacity of the blood to adequately transport oxygen to the fetus. The placental blood flow is reduced due to fewer fetal capillaries with smaller diameters, which is believed to slow fetal growth. Studies have shown that these effects can take place even if the mother doesn't smoke, but if the father does and the mother is exposed. Pregnant smokers have a higher incidence of the placenta rupturing (called placenta previa) and premature rupture of the membranes. Anencephaly, a congenital absence of the brain and the spinal cord because the cranium does not close properly, is also higher in babies whose mothers smoked during pregnancy.(188,189)

Several studies have shown that birth weight is decreased by an average of about 200 grams in infants whose mother smoked throughout pregnancy. A low-birth weight baby is two to four times more likely to be born to a smoking mother than one who does not smoke.(190) A normal weight for a new born is considered 2,500 grams or more. Smoking increases the risk by more than 50 percent in light smokers and over 100 percent in heavy smokers that their baby's weight will be less than that. Such babies are more likely to be stillborn, to need intensive care in the hospital, or to die in infancy.(191)

In an Australian study of over 8,500 women, children of women who smoked during pregnancy were far more likely to suffer middle ear infections or ear surgery by age five than children of mothers who did not smoke while pregnant.(192) 7 percent of ear infections in children are attributed to exposure to tobacco smoke. Ear infections cause most of children's hearing loss.

Research shows that mothers who quit smoking during pregnancy may decrease the risks of potential health problems in their newborns. But even if a woman stops smoking during pregnancy and resumes later, her baby is twice as likely to die from SIDS. If a mother smokes and breastfeeds, her baby gets nicotine with every meal. Nicotine stays in the breast milk for up to five hours after smoking. Smoking can also decrease the quantity of breast milk and can change its quality and may lead to the necessity of early weaning.

Perinatal mortality (occurring at about the time of birth) is 25 percent to 56 percent greater in infants of mothers who smoke than those who do not. There are also higher mortality rates in infants of fathers who smoke.(193)

Food for Thought

Here's a risk I bet you haven't thought of: children can become sick from swallowing cigarette butts. In 1995 there were 7,917 reports of potentially toxic exposures from swallowing cigarettes among children six years of age or younger, with the greatest risk among the ages of six months to one year old. Reactions included depressed breathing, irregular heartbeat, and convulsions.(194)

SIDS is greater in infants exposed to tobacco smoke in utero (as a fetus), and postnatally (after birth) than those with only postnatal exposure. If a mother smokes during pregnancy and after birth, her child is three times more likely to die of SIDS than nonsmokers. If the mother smokes only after the child is born, the child is two times more likely to die of SIDS. Smoking by the mother during pregnancy may result in chronic fetal hypoxia (lack of oxygen), which can impair the normal development of the central nervous system. Nicotine has been shown to cause necrosis (cell death) of cells in the brain stems of fetal rats.

Abnormal cell growth in the respiratory centers in the brain have been found in some cases of Sudden Infant Death Syndrome, possibly resulting from exposure to the poisons in smoke.(195)

The lead and carbon monoxide in the tobacco smoke inhaled by the mother can damage the baby's brain, leading to developmental, learning, and behavioral problems. Children of mothers who smoke during and after pregnancy are more likely to suffer from hyperactivity and impairment in school performance and intellectual achievements than children of non smokers.(196)

Sharon Milberger, M.D., of the Pediatric Psycholpharmacology Unit at Massachusetts General Hospital in Boston, says that exposure to nicotine, the most potent psychoactive component of tobacco, causes damage to the brain at critical times in the developmental process. Research has reported that 22 percent of the children with ADHD had mothers who smoked during pregnancy while maternal smoking occurred in only 8 percent of the healthy group. ADHD and behavioral and cognitive disorders from smoking causes detrimental changes in the dopamine delivery system in the brain and causes fetal hypoxia when the fetal brain does not get enough oxygen. The study, reported in the *American Journal of Psychiatry,* states that "it is now believed that the human fetus is actually exposed to a higher nicotine concentration than the smoking mother [and] chronic exposures during pregnancy, especially those producing hypoxia. . .are most associated with neuropsychiatric impairment." The study also noted that the ADHD children whose mothers had smoked during pregnancy had significantly lower IQs than those whose mothers did not smoke.(197)

Children from mothers who smoked during pregnancy are more likely to commit crimes later in life. One study reported, "Our results support our hypothesis that maternal smoking during pregnancy is related to increased rates of crime in adult offspring." Although the researchers admitted that there is not enough evidence to add prenatal smoking to the list of established risk factors for adult crimes, the statistics showed that more than a quarter of the men whose mothers had the highest levels of smoking and delivery complications with their births were arrested for a violent crime as an adult. The researches did note that mothers who smoke during pregnancy are often young women who have had previous misconduct problems, so there may be an inheritability of misconduct problems.(198) (Or maybe *their* mothers smoked too.)

The reasons children and adolescents start smoking have to do with being accepted by one's peers, asserting independence, feeling attractive and glamorous and signaling maturity. Children who have a low self-image and are less academically successful have fewer skills to cope with social pressures to smoke. Girls who smoke tend to have good social skills, whereas boys do not; and girls may also believe that smoking helps them to control their weight. Adults who smoke are more likely to have a lower income and lower educational level than those who don't smoke.

Teenagers who smoke are 56 percent more likely to suffer serious sleep disturbance, and teens who smoked a little were 20 percent more likely to have mild insomnia, according to a study appearing in *Pediatrics*. The exact mechanism is not understood, but nicotine, the addictive drug in tobacco, is a stimulant that may keep them awake.(199) Lack of sleep, of course, can lead to a host of behavioral and physiological problems, and this applies not just to children.

Nicotine can keep adults awake too, which may affect their mood, work performance and thinking ability. In fact, Thomas Edison would not hire anyone who smoked because he felt that smoking clouded their thinking process. He was also the first to claim that cigarettes caused cancer not so much because of the tobacco smoke, but because of the acroline that was emitted when the white cigarette paper burned.

Cigarette smoking appears to be a gateway to drug and alcohol use. Twelve- to 17-year-olds who smoked cigarettes in the previous 30 days were about three times more likely to have consumed alcohol and eight times more likely to have smoked marijuana, and 22 times more likely to have used cocaine in the past 30 days. Those who use drugs rarely do so *before* smoking cigarettes. The CDC says that youths ages 12 to 17 that smoked were about eight times as likely to use illicit drugs and 11 times as likely to drink heavily as nonsmoking youths. A young person who uses tobacco daily is likely to become addicted to nicotine, and to get a young person to stop smoking is difficult.(200)

Food for Thought

It's no coincidence that the time people start smoking is one of the most tumultuous times of their lives – adolescence – when there are significant physiological, psychological, and social changes taking place. Young people are in a most vulnerable position and are attempting to come to grips with their own bodies and lives. Those who feel most secure emotionally will be less likely to start smoking to fit in with the crowd, to show their independence or to rebel against authority. A loving environment in the home is important to establish this attitude, and that begins with a healthy environment. It's been shown that children from lower income families are more likely to start smoking and lower-income families oftentimes do not get proper nutrition. When a child is not fed adequately, numerous deficiencies may result, leading to less than ideal behavior. Could the development of an inadequate self-image and need for stimulation from cigarettes be a result of having an undernourished and underdeveloped brain?

Protecting your child from smoking isn't easy. Besides the peer pressure to start smoking, the tobacco industry spends $6 billion a year advertising and promoting their products in the U.S. One study found that 30 percent of three-year-olds and 91 percent of six-year-olds could identify "Joe Camel" as a symbol of smoking. (This kind of advertising – blatantly targeting youngsters with cartoon characters – is now illegal in the U.S.) (201) The tobacco industry must recruit 5,000 new young smokers every day to maintain the total number of smokers, and advertising is an effective way to do this. They have also targeted women more in recent years, introducing different brands that appeal to their sense of independence and sexuality. They have been successful as evidence in the increase in women smoking. Lung cancer has become the leading cause of cancer death among women, having increased by nearly 400 percent in the past 20 years. More than 145,000 women die every year from smoking-related diseases. As former U.S. Surgeon General Antonia Novello said, "The Virginia Slims Woman is catching up to the Marlboro Man."(202)

On the bright side, those who quit smoking decrease their risk of heart disease by half after one year off cigarettes. After 15 years, the risk of heart disease is similar to that of people who've never smoked. The body can regenerate itself. In five to 15 years off cigarettes, the risk of stroke returns to the level of those who've never smoked.(203)

Radon Gas

Radon is a radioactive gas that you can't see, taste, or smell, and is the second leading cause of lung cancer in America. It claims about 20,000 lives every year.(204) Radon comes from the natural decay of uranium that's found in nearly all soils, and may move up through the ground into your home. Any home can have a radon problem, so it's a good idea to test yours to see. There are inexpensive radon test kits available at hardware stores. For more in this, go to www.epa.gov/radon or call your local health department or state radon office.

Another thing that's been shown to introduce cancer-causing chemicals into the home or workplace is plug-in air fresheners. Experts believe these unnecessary but popular devices cause formaldehyde to accumulate in the air, and formaldehyde causes cancer.(205) If you have a radon problem, you can fix it. Fixing the average house of radon gas problems costs about $1,200. Considering radon can cause cancer, it would be a good thing to check into.

Prostate Cancer, BPH, & Male Virility

The prostate gland is a small gland that's part of the male reproductive system. It secretes much of the liquid portion of semen, the milky fluid that transports sperm through the penis during ejaculation. It's located just below the bladder in front of the rectum, and encircles a section of the urethra (the tube that carries urine from the bladder out the penis). During ejaculation, semen is secreted by the prostate through small pores in the walls of the urethra.

Interestingly, the prostate gland is in a continual state of growth throughout a man's life. So it's not surprising that the older the man, the more the prostate will be a problem. In young men, the prostate gland is usually healthy and not large enough to cause problems. The three most common prostate problems are inflammation (prostatitis), prostatic enlargement (benign prostatic hyperplasia or BPH), and prostate cancer.

Inflammation of the prostate causes it to enlarge. Not surprisingly, prostatitis can cause difficult or painful urination that feels like burning, and a strong and frequent urge to urinate, which results in only small amounts of urine sometimes accompanied by pain in the lower back or abdomen.

Benign Prostatic Hyperplasia (BPH)

BPH is an enlarged prostate due to excessive growth of tissue. This tissue is noncancerous, or benign, and why it occurs is still not known. By age 60, more than half of all American men have at least microscopic signs of BPH. By age 70, more than 40 percent will have enlargement that can be felt on physical examination.[206]

A man with BPH finds it hard to initiate the flow of urine, and it may be just a dribble. He may need to urinate frequently or have a sudden, powerful urge to urinate. He likely has to get up several times a night to urinate, or have the feeling that the bladder is never completely empty. Straining to empty the bladder is not advisable, since it can harm the muscular walls of the bladder and damage the kidneys. BPH can eventually weaken the bladder, and once the bladder is damaged, it's virtually impossible to repair. A weak bladder can lead to other complications such as bladder stones and bleeding. In severe cases, the man may need to be catheterized; a procedure in which a tube called a catheter is inserted through the penis into the bladder to allow urine to escape.

The prostate in a healthy young male is about the size of a walnut. By the time a man is 40 years old, the prostate may already have grown to the size of an apricot. By age 60, it could be as big as a lemon. One doctor said, "You know the old saying about death and taxes – two things in this life we can be sure of. But for American men age 50 and over, I must, unfortunately add another certainty: prostate problems."[207]

BPH is detected by a physical exam called a "digital rectal examination" where the doctor inserts his finger up the rectum to feel the elasticity and size of the prostate. The source of many locker-room jokes, it's not a fun experience. Urinalysis is done to check for bleeding or infection, and a blood test called a prostate-specific antigen (PSA) test may be run to see if cancer of the prostate is present. Oftentimes, X-rays, and ultrasound may be used, although according to federal guidelines, these add nothing to the decision as to what form of treatment should be used. These tests, although unnecessary, are routinely used by two-thirds of urologists, which add up to tens of millions of dollars every year.[208]

About half of the men with BPH develop symptoms serious enough to warrant treatment. But consider that BPH is not an indication of or precursor to prostate cancer, and it doesn't increase your chances of prostate cancer either. We'll examine ways to improve prostate health towards the end of this section. But for now, some remedial actions to take include limiting fluid intake in the evening, especially beverages that contain alcohol or caffeine, taking time to empty the bladder completely when urinating, and not allowing long intervals to pass without urinating. Another helpful thing to know is that over-the-counter cold and flu medicines can cause increased urinary retention, hindering the ability to urinate, so it's best to avoid them.[209]

Medical treatments for serious cases of BPH include drugs and surgery. Drug therapy for BPH started in the early 1990s. There are two classes of drugs that can increase urine flow, but in different ways.

Alpha adrenergic blockers (or alpha-1 blockers), originally used for the treatment of high blood pressure, relax smooth muscles in the muscular portion of the prostate and the area where the urethra comes out of the bladder. Generic drug names are phenoxybenzamine, prazosin, tamsulosin hydrochloride (*Flomax*), and terazosin. Side effects include dizziness, fatigue, and headaches. One of these drugs, trade name *Hytrin* (terazosin), is being prescribed, but there's no knowledge of its long-term effects. But since alpha adrenergic blockers have been used for some time now for the treatment of high blood pressure, we do know one of their ugly side effects – impotence. If your blood pressure is normal and you take a drug that lowers blood pressure, then the drug could cause your blood pressure to drop to a dangerously low level. Other side effects of *Hytrin* are weakness, fatigue, headaches, edema, palpitations, nasal congestion, sleepiness, decreased libido, and blurred vision.

Another class of medicine used for BPH is enzyme inhibitors and include dutasteride (*Avodart*) and finasteride (*Proscar*). They block the enzyme called 5-alpha-reductase, which is necessary to change testosterone (the male sex hormone) into another hormone called dihydrotestosterone, or DHT. It's believed that DHT causes the prostate to enlarge. Merck & Company, its manufacturer, admits that it takes a full 6 months of continual use for this drug to work, and that although it may shrink the prostate, symptoms of BPH may not go away. In addition, once the patient stops using it, its effects wear off, and men who start may have to take this medicine for the rest of their lives.[210] This drug has also been used to stimulate hair growth in men, but at smaller doses.

Typical side effects of *Proscar* and *Avodart* include back pain, decreased libido, decreased volume of semen, diarrhea, rash, itching, hives, dizziness, headache, and impotence. Women are warned to not even handle the pills, since that can cause birth defects in a male fetus (it causes changes in the genitals of the fetus). Another interesting side effect is these drugs may cause a man's breasts to enlarge. A statement on the *Proscar* website says, ". . .some men may have breast enlargement and/or tenderness. You should promptly report to your

doctor any changes in your breasts such as lumps, pain, or nipple discharge."
(That sounds worse than having to pee every two hours!)

Food for Thought

William Campbell Douglass, M.D. says the following about *Proscar* and the prostate in his report *Prostate Problems: Safe, Simple, Effective Relief.* . .

"But in fact, studies reported in the *New England Journal of Medicine* indicate that *Proscar doesn't work at all.* There is also a possibility that the drug is carcinogenic. Wouldn't that be something? A 'cure' approved by the FDA that gives you cancer.

But here's the really sleazy part of this story: Saw palmetto berries, in the form of an extract called LSE seronoa, are just as effective as *Proscar* in inhibiting the conversion of testosterone to DHT, maybe more so. The herb is nontoxic and costs a third as much as *Merck*'s drug. But the Food and Drug Administration rejected an application to have the extract approved as an over-the-counter treatment for BPH. Although the saw palmetto extract has been used for BPH since 1905, and is listed in all the pharmacopeias, the *Physician's Desk Reference* (until 1948, when it was quietly removed), and all the pharmacy texts, the FDA declared the herb to be an 'unapproved new drug!'. . .

Get some saw palmetto berries and make a tea out of them (weak at first to test your sensitivity, then gradually increase the strength) or make an 'infusion' (prolonged soaking in water) and keep it refrigerated. [Be sure you get organically grown berries.] Drink the tea or the infusion, one cupful, three times a day. There is scientific evidence for this treatment. Saw palmetto berries inhibit the enzyme 5-alpha-reductase, and a low activity of this enzyme is associated with a reduced risk of prostate cancer. This berry is also effective in the treatment of benign prostatic hypertrophy, which is not always so benign in its effects."

Dr. Campbell also recommends to empty the bladder as fully as possible when urinating (do not strain, though), avoid long intervals between urination, and to use parsley as a "prostate herbal" and to make a tea of it - "the stronger the better" and add lemon for taste. (Even better, just make some fresh parsley juice using a good juicer.) (211)

According to one herbal website, there have been over a dozen clinical studies involving almost 3,000 men showed that saw palmetto can markedly alleviate BPH symptoms without decreasing the man's libido like prostate drugs do.(212) Saw palmetto is effective in 90 percent of patients suffering from BPH within the first year of treatment compared to less than 50 percent for patients taking finasteride (*Proscar*). And since saw palmetto prevents testosterone from converting to DHP, it has been (anecdotally) reported to stop hair loss and trigger hair growth. There are no known side effects to saw palmetto (it's even OK for women to handle the berries).

The berries were used as food by the Seminole Indians in Florida, and have also been used to ease upset stomachs and insomnia. In the early part of the 20th century, it was commonly recommended as a treatment for BPH and chronic urinary tract infections. It's still being used for prostate problems in Europe, even though here in the U.S., most doctors will probably tell you it's ineffective and recommend the emasculating, poisonous, possibly carcinogenic, drugs.

Prostate Cancer

In the mid-80s, the number of men diagnosed with prostate cancer was about 90,000 per year. By 1997, that figure had risen to an estimated 209,000. In 2006, the number of men being diagnosed with it is around 220,000 per year with 30,000 of them dying from the disease.

The explosion of prostate cancer from the mid-80s to mid-90s is attributed in part to better detection methods. In addition to the digital rectal exam, doctors began using a blood test called the prostate-specific antigen (PSA), which detects a protein produced by prostate cells and is normally present in small quantities in the blood. Often it is elevated when cancer is present, but can also be elevated in some benign disorders of the prostate – so it's not a foolproof test.[213] It's interesting to note that the researcher who developed the PSA test, is so unhappy with the inaccuracy of his test, that he wishes he had never developed it. He has made this statement due to the fact that a large percentage of men undergo surgery based on their PSA number, only to find out that in fact they do not have prostate cancer. However, I believe that a true increase could very well be the case, considering that other degenerative diseases are also on the rise and that one theory of why men get prostate cancer in the first place is because of toxins in our environment – specifically, chemicals and estrogenic pollutants (xenoestrogens). Prostate cancer is the second most prevalent cancer in men (skin cancer is first), and it's estimated that one American male in 10 will get it.[214]

The average age of diagnosis of prostate cancer is age 72. More than 75 percent of prostate cancer cases are in men age 65 or older with only 7 percent occurring in men younger than age 60. African-American men have the world's highest incidence of prostate cancer – a full 33 percent greater than a white American man. Smoking is another risk factor as is eating processed foods. But the actual cause of prostate cancer is presently not known.

Although many men may end up getting prostate cancer, for many of them, it will surface when they are in their 70s and 80s and the cancer is usually slow growing. The Federal Consumer Information Center says a man with the low-grade localized disease "is much more likely to die of other causes than of prostate cancer."(215) In fact, seven out of 10 men diagnosed with prostate cancer (in Canada) die from other causes.(216)

PSA, when elevated above 4ng/mL (nanograms per milliliter), can indicate prostate cancer. This screening test is recommended by the American Cancer Society and the American Urological Association to be performed yearly on men age 50 and over. But other research indicates that anyone with lower PSA levels (below 1.9 ng/ml) the recommendation is to be tested every two years.(217)

As mentioned above, the PSA test is unreliable. There are often false positives and false negatives, so one cannot be sure either way. If a doctor sees a positive high level, he/she may be inclined to treat it with drugs or want to perform surgery, when these may not really be needed. Plus, the doctor may want to poke around to get a biopsy, and this in itself may actually spread the cancer (disturbed cancer cells reproduce faster). Dr. Campbell says, "under no circumstances should you permit your doctor to perform a needle biopsy on the tumor. Such a biopsy can only help to spread the cancer throughout your system. A needle, no matter how small, is basically a knife, and when the needle passes into the gland, it is cutting tissue, which, if cancer is present, can spread the tumor. A cancer that is localized in the prostate is a problem, but it can be controlled. Once the cancer branches out, your chances of survival drop to below 20 percent."(218)

There's a new way to test for prostate cancer that you won't hear about in the mainstream – Power Doppler Sonography (PDS). It's very advanced ultrasound that can produce a detailed image of the body's internal structures and has a much higher resolution and the ability to highlight areas of blood flow in dense or soft tissue, allowing tumors or inflammation to be viewed and measured clearly. In addition, the 3D version of PDS can detest the spread of cancer through the margins of the prostate (or breast in breast cancer). One study reported in the *British Journal of Urology* showed that this kind of screening only misses 1 percent of prostate cancers.(219) Prostate sonograms are safe, painless, and inexpensive. Unlike other screening methods, they can be repeated as often as necessary to closely monitor areas of concern and assess treatment efficacy. For these reasons, sonograms have been found to be a more effective alternative to biopsies in detecting prostate tumors, and better than MRI and PET/CT Scans as a means for tracking these tumors. PDS can also be used to monitor inflammation and tumors in the breast and other parts of the human body (see breast cancer chapter). To learn more and where you can get a sonogram, check out www.cancerscan.com and www.phoenixsonograms.com.

Food for Thought

The cancerscan.com website is that of Robert L. Bard, M.D., who is one of the best known and highly regarded leaders in the field of sonography. He has experience using sonography in just about every area of the body, and tells me that he can now detect skin cancer (melanoma) and other cancers accurately and early. He is also working to find alternative treatments to treating cancer. Sonography detects 40 percent more invasive cancers than mammograms. When combined with Doppler imaging, it is also excellent at finding the most aggressive tumors that grow so quickly they need a larger blood supply (these are called *interval* cancers).(220) I believe that sonography will become the method of choice in the not-to-distant future for detecting both prostate and breast cancer for several reasons: It is very accurate, it's easy to do and doesn't take long, it's non-invasive, inexpensive, and does absolutely no harm to the patient in any way.

However, the traditional medical community will be reluctant to switch to it because they make so much money using the other, more profitable diagnostic methods. But eventually, people will wake up and start demanding it. I hope you will be one of the first.

There are four stages to prostate cancer: A through D. (This is also called the Gleason Curve.)

Stage A: This stage is difficult to diagnose since the number of cancer cells are so few, even with the PSA test. There are no symptoms with this stage, and it's really not worth worrying about. Intervention might do more harm than good.

Stage B: This is when a tumor is present, but it's still confined to the prostate. The symptoms for this stage cancer are the same as BPH, or no symptoms at all.

Stage C: The tumor is no longer confined to the prostate gland, and it likely has spread to the testicles. Symptoms may increase plus pain in the prostate.

Stage D: Here the cancer has metastasized (spread throughout the body). There's pain in the pelvis, lower back and upper thighs.

If a cancer is detected, a prostate acid phosphatase test (PAP), also sometimes called the prostate specific acid phosphatase test (PSAP), may be done to see if the cancer has spread. But unfortunately, this test isn't fool-proof either: 25 percent of patients with stage D prostate cancer have a normal PAP level.(221) If you have Stage C, you need to take action, but not necessarily drugs or surgery.

Food for Thought

Dr. Campbell recommends getting a second and even third opinion on the kind of treatment your doctor recommends if you have prostate cancer, and to get these opinions from doctors in different towns. He says doctors don't want to offend a colleague they know with a different diagnosis. Good advice for any medical situation (and many legal situations too!). He also says not to let a doctor pressure you into quick surgery. Since the vast majority of prostate cancers are slow moving, you should have plenty of time to make a decision or pursue other treatment options. Another doctor who has done extensive investigation into prostate cancer is Isreal Barkin, M.D., F.A.C.S. His website is www.pcref.org.

Although a standard way to treat prostate cancer in its early stages is with surgery, there's no hard evidence that it's any more effective than waiting and seeing if the condition gets worse (which may include drug therapy). In fact, doing nothing at all seems to be just as effective as surgery or radiation treatments as far as survival rates go, an opinion echoed in the *Journal of the American Medical Association.*[222] That's because prostate cancer is not only slow growing, but usually stays within the confines of the gland itself for many years. Surgery, especially in an old man who probably has other health issues, could be harmful and even fatal due to blood clots or the cancer spreading triggered by the surgery itself.

Prostate surgery can often lead to unwanted problems. Dr. James Talcott found that of 282 patients who had prostate surgery, within a year of their operation, 41 percent of them had to wear diapers because of chronic leaking from their bladder. Other research showed that 60 percent of the men who had prostate surgery were impotent 18 months after the surgery, and 8 percent had complete urinary incontinence. Dr. Talcott says, "Patients need to know what they are in for. We need to prepare them for the bad things that may befall them." I suspect that few doctors actually do.[223,224]

This is not to say that surgery is never needed. If the cancer is at Stage C, it may be. Removal of the prostate could save your life (although it will destroy your sex life) and extend it many years. But I think you should check out alternative methods first. If you follow the recommendations in this book, hopefully, you will never get prostate cancer.

Another form of mainstream treatment is radiation. The main problem radiation is that it kills good cells along with the cancer cells. Nausea, diarrhea, and rectal bleeding may result also. It's another treatment better off avoided.

It's been shown that testosterone, the male sex hormone, encourages the growth of prostate cancer. So testosterone deprivation, or ablation, is used to treat prostate cancer. To do this, the testicles are removed, since testosterone is made in them. Besides the obvious inconveniences of being castrated, this treatment has been shown to negatively affect memory. Interestingly, theories are that lack of testosterone affects the hippocampus – the part of the brain implicated in Alzheimer's disease.[225] On the other hand, some experts note that younger men, who generally have much higher testosterone levels, have a far lower rate of prostate cancer. So more needs to be learned.

Men with advanced prostate cancer are also treated with hormone suppressing drugs – specifically testosterone suppressing drugs called luteinizing hormone-releasing hormone (LHRH) agonists. LHRH agonists are just as effective as surgical removal of the testicles in eliminated the production of testosterone. But who wants to be castrated, either literally or by drugs?

In addition, LHRH agonists present another set of hazards. The major side effect is, of course, impotence. Then there's the increased risk of bone fractures (researchers found these drugs account for about 3,000 fractures a year) due to the fact that testosterone is necessary for maintaining bone density.(226) Using LHRH agonists may also cause hot flashes (just like a woman, since now the man has no testosterone to counteract the female hormone estrogen – which is naturally present in small amounts in men), loss of mental sharpness and loss of muscle mass and strength. Then there's the fact that LHRH agonist treatment does not cure prostate cancer anyway. The only real "cure" for prostate cancer, according to the traditional medical community, is achieved by surgery or radiation.

If all these treatments tend to frighten you, I don't blame you. It's bad enough realizing you're getting old and you can't pull the trigger like you used to, but realizing you may need to wear diapers, be castrated, or even die is enough to make you think outside the box. So here are a number of natural, non-invasive, virtually harmless ways to address prostate problems, including cancer.

How to Improve Your Prostate and Avoid Cancer

The medical community will tell you they don't know what causes prostate cancer. But if we look at the research, we can get a pretty good idea. Dr. Al Sears says,

> If you listen to the AMA, you'd think that every man in every nation on earth gets prostate cancer at one time or another. The truth is shockingly different. Prostate cancer is nearly entirely absent in parts of Asia and some third world countries. But if that Chinese man moves to America? You guessed it. His risk rapidly catches up to the average American born man. . .
> Prostate disease, in fact, appears to be largely the result of modern technology – toxins we take into our body from artificial foods, from polluted air and contaminated water. . .(227)

So the first thing to do is to realize that prostate cancer is not an inevitable part of getting old. There are many things you can do to prevent it and even reverse it:

Lose weight. Being overweight or obese is really bad for the prostate gland. It increases the likelihood and severity of BPH and cancer. But going on a low-fat diet is not the answer. One study published in the *Journal of Clinical Oncology* showed that a low fat diet did nothing to stop the onset of prostate cancer.(228)

Get enough iodine. Japanese men have much lower rates of prostate cancer than American men, and when they move to the U.S., their rates or getting it go up. Dr. David Brownstein believes this indicates that prostate cancer may develop due to a deficiency of iodine, which is much less likely on the Japanese diet than the American diet. I discuss iodine in depth in the chapter on breast cancer, which everyone should read.

Get enough sunshine and vitamin D. A study reported in the *Journal of the National Cancer Institute* showed that men with the highest levels of vitamin D were the 17 percent least likely of getting cancer and 29 percent less likely to die of it. High levels of vitamin D were very protective against digestive system cancers (colon cancer), with 1,500 IU daily associated with a 43 percent reduction in the risk of developing such tumors and a 45 percent lower risk of dying of them.(229) Taking cod liver oil is fine, but getting unfiltered sun on your skin is better. Dr. William G Nelson of Johns Hopkins University says that men and women should get at least 1,000 IU of vitamin D (in the form of D_3) a day.

Curb alcohol consumption. Too much alcohol wreaks havoc on your prostate. A little red wine (from organically grown grapes with no sulfites added) is OK and may even be beneficial. But other kinds of alcohol are bad.

Exercise regularly. I highly recommend you get on the exercise program I discussed in the section on heart disease. It's a short duration, high intensity program that has been shown to build muscle and lose weight (if needed) than any other program I've seen.

Stop taking drugs. That includes prescription and over-the-counter drugs. Of course, discontinue them under a doctor's supervision and improve your diet at the same time. Drugs easily irritate the prostate gland and negatively affect your overall sexuality. Antihistamines and blood pressure medications are particularly injurious. If you recently developed BPH after just starting a drug treatment, chances are the drugs caused it.

Stop consuming pasteurized dairy and calcium supplements. Reports at the Annual Meeting of the American Association for Cancer Research showed that men with high consumption of pasteurized dairy products had a 30 percent higher chance of getting prostate cancer. Those who took calcium supplements had about three to four times greater chance.(230) This may be because the form of calcium in pasteurized dairy or supplements may impair vitamin D metabolism, which is important for proper cell metabolism. Unpasteurized dairy is fine and actually good for the prostate.

Stop consuming sweetened foods and drinks. Sugar accelerates cancer and may even cause it. Eliminate sugar and artificial sweeteners.

Do not barbecue meat. When meat is charred at high temperatures, a compound called PhIp is formed that has been shown to cause cancer in rats. PhIP can initiate prostate cancer and increase its growth. Heterocyclic amines are also formed when meat is cooked at high temperatures when grilled or barbecued, and these are also potent cancer-causing substances. There's less harm done to the meat if you sear it on the outside and leave the inside lightly cooked or rare – the rarer, the better.

Don't smoke. Men who have smoked are about two and a half times more likely to have prostate cancer spread outside the prostate (when they get it) than men who have never smoked. Smoking makes prostate cancer or BPH more severe. The more a man smokes, the more likely the disease will advance. Researchers believe that the carcinogens in cigarette smoke promote prostate cancer.(231)

Avoid pesticides and added hormones. Farmers (not organic farmers) have a 14 percent greater chance of developing prostate cancer due to frequent handling of pesticides.(232) Pesticides are deadly (that's why they're used) and tend to accumulate in tissues like the prostate. Avoid them as much as possible. Hormones found in meat, poultry, and dairy (added to increase production) cause the prostate to grow. Dr. Al Sears says that being exposed to hormones (estrogens) ". . .relentlessly signals their prostates to grow. It causes feminization, weakness and fatigue and worsens the loss of virility. . . But now men are living longer yet losing virility young than ever. This combination of trends is creating a whole generation of 'avirile' tired old men. And some of them aren't that old. The fast pace of this trend occurring in younger and younger guys is alarming."(233) How to fight these unnatural chemicals? Dr. Sears recommends eating cruciferous vegetables, which contain a compound that when metabolized by the body, inhibits cancer cells.

Natural Fixes for the Prostate

Tomatoes are good for the prostate. Men who consume two or more servings of tomato sauce each week were 23 percent less likely to develop prostate cancer.(234) Tomatoes (in any form – cooked, fresh, dried, juiced) contain the antioxidant lycopene, which is believed to be responsible for this effect. Lycopene comes in supplement form, but it's best to get it from food. Other foods high in lycopene include watermelon, apricots, and grapefruit.

Cruciferous vegetables (broccoli, cabbage, cauliflower, kale, mustard greens, radish, bok choy, and Brussels sprouts) are good for the prostate. Men who consumed three or more servings of cruciferous vegetables a week had a 41 percent lower risk of prostate cancer than men who ate less than one serving per week. Cruciferous vegetables are rich in a substance called isothiocyates that detoxifies carcinogens.(235) Interestingly, fruit consumption had no effect on prostate cancer.

Cruciferous vegetables also tend to neutralize the estrogenic effect of chemicals and hormones in our food, which signal the prostate to grow. The breakdown of cruciferous vegetables produces a compound called diindolylmethane (DIM), which when added to prostate cancer cells in lab trials, reduced them by 70 percent.(236)

Eating broccoli and tomatoes together seems to have an even greater effect than consuming them separately. Dr John Erdman at the University of Illinois said, "Separately, these two foods appear to have enormous cancer-fighting potential. Together, they bring out the best in each other and maximize the cancer-fighting effect."(237) As part of Erdman's research, he looked at the effect of lycopene, the compound in tomatoes thought to affect the prostate. He found that lycopene alone had no effect, but tomato powder with its full range of vitamins and nutrients of normal tomatoes, were effective. (Yet another reason not to take isolated supplements.)

Vegetables from the *Allium* family also help cut prostate cancer risk. These include onions, garlic, scallions, shallots, and leeks. A study in China showed that men who ate these foods daily had a 33 percent less risk of getting prostate cancer. China men have the lowest rate of prostate cancer in the world, and these foods are staples in the Chinese diet.(238) I've discuss other benefits of garlic in the chapters on diabetes, heart disease, Alzheimer's disease, and breast cancer.

Food for Thought

Tomatoes, onions, garlic. . . Sounds Italian to me. Learning the health benefits of these foods makes it easier for me to explain (and excuse) my old pizza addiction. Yes, yours truly was hopelessly addicted to pizza for many, many, years (when I was young and didn't know any better). It all started in undergraduate school when we would order a late-night *Dominos* pizza after studying. Our cafeteria food was awful, and nobody else delivered to the dorms, so pizza was it. Then after college, while I was deciding whether to get a real job or go to graduate school, I delivered pizzas for *Dominos*. We got free pizza every night we worked, and got discounts if we ever bought one. I was probably eating pizza for dinner five nights a week.

By the way, I was a pretty good delivery boy. I still hold the record for number of pizzas delivered in one night – 119 – at the store I worked at. I made $120 that night including wages, tips, and commissions (that was big money in 1979). It could be a frightful job sometimes, though. Once I walked into an apartment and a guy standing besides the door pointed a shotgun at my head and pulled the trigger. Of course, it wasn't loaded, but I just about passed out. All the people in the apartment thought it was the funniest thing they ever saw. I would have dumped the pizza on the guy's head, but he was holding a gun, so I thought better of it. One night one of my coworkers was hijacked along with the four pizzas he was delivering and the hijackers drove him out into the middle of a corn field, forced him to take off all his clothes except his socks, and left him there. He made it to a house and got help and he was OK, but not surprisingly, he quit the next day. (So be nice to your delivery person – it's a dangerous job.)

When I started to change my eating habits, I found it hard to leave pizza alone. I woke one night, hungry and unable to go back to sleep, and of course, I started thinking about my favorite food. It was three in the morning, and I didn't have anything in the house to make a pizza with, so instead, I got up and read pizza recipes imagining how good one would be. That's pretty serious.

Maybe there was something about the pizza that my body was craving. The sauce, the garlic, the onions. I just read that garlic is high in selenium, and selenium is good for your energy and mood (not to mention it helps prevent cancer). James G. Penland, a USDA psychologist found that men who boosted their intake of dietary selenium felt less anxious and more energetic, confident, and agreeable. Another study showed that increased selenium lifted the mood of both men and women.(239) Maybe Italian men are such good lovers because all the garlic they eat makes them so agreeable!

But seriously folks, selenium could be important in the development of prostate cancer. Larry C. Clark, Ph.D. of the University of Arizona did extensive research on selenium to see if it affected cancer rates – prostate cancer in particular. He stated that taking a modest dose selenium supplement decreased prostate cancer by 69 percent, colorectal cancer by 64 percent, and lung cancer by 39 percent.(240,241) That's pretty impressive. But while checking this research I found the disturbing news that Dr. Clark died at the tender age of 51 from – you won't want to believe it – prostate cancer. That kind of throws a damper on it, doesn't it?

As part of his research, Dr. Clark had volunteers take selenium in supplement form, so I would imagine he followed his own advice. There are a couple things we might learn from all this: I have no doubt that selenium is important for health. There's research showing that a deficiency of it may play a role in diabetes, Alzheimer's disease, cancer, thyroid function, heavy metal toxicity, arthritis, asthma, and mood. But, taking a selenium supplement is not a magic bullet that will by itself prevent prostate cancer or anything else. As much as we want one little pill that will make everything all right, life just doesn't work that way. Taking selenium, or anything else in supplement form, is a compromise, and may contribute to biochemical imbalances we can never pinpoint or make allowances for. That's why food is your best supplement. Foods have the minerals and vitamins we need in packages that our body understands and can use. So if you want to increase your selenium intake, which may be wise, get it from food. Foods that are high in selenium include sunflower seeds, nuts (especially Brazil nuts and walnuts), garlic, meat, organ meats, and seafood (especially swordfish, tuna, and oysters). But keep in mind that swordfish and tuna have high mercury content, so eat these only rarely.

Another mineral that reduces the risk of prostate cancer is boron. One study showed that men who consumed the most boron reduced the incidence of prostate cancer by as much as 64 percent. They did this by eating boron rich fruits (plums, red grapes, apples, pears and avocadoes) and nuts.(242) What's more, another study showed that boron can shrink existing prostate tumors by between 25 percent and 38 percent, and decrease PSA readings by up to 88 percent.(243)

Consuming more omega-3 fatty acids has been shown to help prevent prostate cancer from spreading, and conversely, omega-6 fatty acids (as in vegetable oils) were shown to increase the spread of prostate tumor cells into bone marrow.(244) The omega-3s tend to block the harmful effects of the omega-6s, so it's important that you consume enough of them. Conversely, too much omega-6 fat interferes with the functioning of omega-3s, and can lead to inflammation and heart disease. The best source of omega-3s is krill oil, fish and fish oils, nuts and seeds, and grass fed beef. One note on the beef: If the cattle are raised on grain as is typically done in commercial production, the meat has 20 times greater ratio of omega-6 fat than you need and an overall deficiency of omega-3s. So if you eat commercially raised beef, you need to get your omega-3s from somewhere else, and you need to get even more of them to counteract the omega-6s.

Some vegetarians believe that getting their omega-3s from flax seed oil instead of from animal sources is good enough. However, often times the kind of omega-3 (ALA) predominant in flax seed oil is not adequately converted into the required omega-3 fats DHA and EPA, which provide the anti-cancer benefits. This is especially true in people who have impaired health. In addition, a study published in the *American Journal of Clinical Nutrition* showed that ALA actually stimulates the growth of prostate cancer. So taking flax seed oil is not the best way to get your omega-3s. Researchers also found that EPA and DHA help reduce the risk of prostate cancer specifically.(245) So it's important to consume DHA and EPA directly (fish, krill oil, or fish oil).

Vitamin D is also being proven to be important for prostate health and even the reversal of prostate cancer. It's well established that prostate cancer is more prevalent in men who live in northern climates where there is less exposure to ultraviolet light from the sun (that produces vitamin D in the skin). African-Americans whose skin contains the pigment melanin that filters out significant amounts of the ultraviolet rays are also more prone to prostate cancer.

The lead researcher for a study on vitamin D and prostate cancer at Harvard University School of Public Health said, "Our findings suggest that vitamin D plays an important protective role against prostate cancer, especially aggressive disease. This research underscores the importance of obtaining adequate vitamin D through skin exposure to sunlight or through diet, including food and supplements."(246) Men in this study with the highest levels of vitamin D had significantly lower overall risk (45 percent) of prostate cancer, including aggressive prostate cancer.

Consider that normally, over 85 percent of vitamin D is synthesized in the skin due to exposure to natural light. Specifically, vitamin D is synthesized from

7-dihydrocholesterol in the skin (notice that this is a derivative of cholesterol) under the influence of UVB radiation in sunlight. Sunscreens block UV radiation, so it's best not to use them. Cod liver oil (but not fish oil) has substantial amounts of vitamin D and should be included in the diet unless enough sunlight is being received throughout the year. Please see the section on skin cancer for precautions for taking cod liver oil.

There is some evidence that vitamin E supplements may reduce the risk of prostate cancer.(247) However, one study published in the *Annals of Internal Medicine* reported that "Those who take greater than 400 IU of vitamin E a day are about 10 percent more likely to die than those who do not."(248)

There is no doubt that vitamin E is necessary for health and the health of the prostate. But taking it in supplement form is not the best way to get it. Nutritionist Aajonus Vonderplanitz has this to say about vitamin E:

> The worst-case example of a toxic supplement is vitamin E. Most vitamin E is the byproduct of the film-development and film-process industry. Because the chemical waste (tocopheral) is similar in molecular structure to natural vitamin E (d-alpha tocopheral) it is called vitamin E and sold as a supplement. In reality, those manufacturers make profits instead of paying fortunes to the hazardous disposal of their toxic waste. [Similar to fluoride from aluminum and fertilizer manufacturing being used in water supplies.] In other words, profiteers make money by seducing us into purchasing and ingesting toxic waste. Vice versa, foods rendered into waste products after vitamins and other nutrients are chemically extracted, are then made into foods, such as chips and cereals, or animal fodder. . .Even natural vitamin E has to be either heat-processed or solvent-extracted. Heat-processing destroys vitamin E and solvent-extraction causes destruction and low-grade poisoning.(249)

Foods high in vitamin E are nuts (especially almonds), seeds (especially sunflower seeds), spinach, mustard greens, turnip greens, chard, peppers, and olive oil. Since vitamin E is easily damaged by oxidation, exposure to air (keep the olive oil tightly capped) should be avoided and for the same reason, the nuts should be raw, as roasting or cooking would oxidize (destroy) most of the E. Chickens, turkeys, and cattle that are raised organically have higher amounts of various nutrients, especially trace minerals such as selenium, zinc, boron, etc. Grass fed beef as well as eggs from organic free range hens, have much higher levels of the healthy omega 3 fats. Meats, including grass fed red meats and poultry contain little or no vitamin E.(250)

Consuming enough vitamin E will go a long way towards protecting you from skin cancer since it protects the skin from many of the damaging effects of ultraviolet radiation. In addition, those who consume adequate amounts of vitamin E have up to a 50 percent reduced risk of developing bladder cancer.(251)

This is especially important for men, since bladder cancer is the fourth leading cancer killer among men, and kills 12,500 Americans annually.

A vitamin E deficiency often results in digestive system problems where nutrients are poorly absorbed from the digestive tract. This can encourage celiac disease (a digestive disease that damages the small intestine and interferes with absorption of nutrients – aggravated by ingesting products with gluten such as wheat, rye and barley), and diseases of the pancreas, gallbladder, and liver. A vitamin E deficiency can also cause peripheral neuropathy, where there is pain, tingling and loss of sensation in the arms, hands, legs, and feet. (If you feel you must supplement with vitamin E, David Getoff says the best brand is *Unique E*.)

David Brownstein, M.D., believes that sufficient levels of iodine are also critical to prevent prostate cancer. I go into iodine in depth in the section on breast cancer.

The prostate gland normally contains one of the highest concentrations of zinc than any other organ in the body. Zinc is a mineral that's helps regulate cell division, growth, wound healing, and proper functioning of the immune system. It's vitally important for the maintenance of the health of the prostate gland, but its exact function in the prostate is still unclear. Prostates that have cancer also have low levels of zinc, and a zinc deficiency increases a man's risk for cancer.[252] But zinc supplements have been shown to not decrease the incidence of prostate cancer. In fact, a study at the National Cancer Institute found that men who took more than 100 milligrams of zinc a day were twice as likely to develop advanced prostate cancer, especially if they had taken it for 10 years or more, compared with those who took no zinc supplements.[253] However, when zinc is consumed as part of food, it is beneficial to the prostate, and increasing dietary zinc is associated with a decrease in the incidence of prostate cancer.[254]

Those on a vegetarian diet are much more likely to be zinc deficient, since the best sources of zinc are red meat, seafood (especially oysters) and liver. Milk and other dairy products have zinc (remember, only unpasteurized dairy, please), as do brewer's yeast, wheat germ, and especially oysters. For women, zinc is needed for vaginal lubrication, which decreases as they age. So women should increase their zinc intake as they age too. Iron supplements will decrease the absorption of zinc, so no more *Geritol* unless you have had a ferritin test, which proves that you are truly in need of supplementary iron. Check with your doctor.

Low zinc levels in elderly men are also correlated with osteoporosis, which makes them vulnerable to hip and other fractures.[255] So it's no surprise that men with prostate cancer also tend to have significantly lower bone density than men without prostate cancer.[256]

The recommended daily allowance of zinc is 11 mg/day for men and 8 mg/day for women. But if you eat the foods you should, you won't need to worry about getting enough in your diet. Zinc is often found in throat lozenges because it's believed to fight the common cold, but there's no convincing evidence to this effect. So don't take those, because the added zinc might add to prostate problems. On the other hand, a large percentage of people test as being low in zinc, and only the *zinc taste test* or an *intracellular zinc test* are accurate for this nutrient. To take the zinc taste test, there's a solution called *Zinc Tally* you hold in your mouth for a minute. If it doesn't taste metallic after several seconds, you're probably zinc deficient. You can order it online at www.thewayup.com. *Zinc Tally* is also a good liquid zinc supplement.

Since it is well accepted that the government's daily recommendations for nutrients are barely adequate to prevent disease and not in any way sufficient to attain or maintain optimal health, many do indeed need more zinc. So seek out the foods that can supply this nutrient and if you take a supplement, do not take doses as high as 100 mg per day or more unless a health practitioner whom you trust has shown you to be deficient with a valid test.

Another food good for the prostate gland is pumpkin seeds. Not surprisingly, they are high in zinc and omega-3 fatty acids. They were used in the early 1900s to treat enlarged prostate symptoms and other urinary tract complaints. One man reported, "When I was diagnosed with an enlarged prostate, a friend encouraged me to eat pumpkin seeds regularly. Three months later, I no longer wake up in the middle of the night to urinate."[257]

Pumpkin seeds have also been reported to be beneficial for improving sex drive, decreasing inflammation due to arthritis, and may decrease the risk of certain cancers.[258,259,260] The recommended amount of pumpkin seeds is a handful (about an ounce) three or four times a week. You can grind them up and sprinkle them on food, or just snack on them. I recommend they be organic, raw, and unsalted. It's best to store them in a refrigerator in an airtight container.

Food for Thought

Here's a tasty salad that will do wonders for your prostate gland. Vegetable ingredients (should be organically grown): lettuce and greens, celery, tomatoes, broccoli florets and/or cauliflower, and onion.

Dressing: ¼ to ½ cup apple cider vinegar; a couple tablespoons of sparkling mineral water; 1-2 tablespoons raw honey and/or bee pollen; fresh ground pepper; ½ clove garlic; other spices if desired. Put all ingredients into blender and blend. Pour over salad. Pumpkin seeds, sunflower seeds, walnuts, and Brazil nuts can be added to the salad - ground up and sprinkled over it. They should be raw, unsalted, and organic if possible. An hour latter, you could have some raw oysters. They're not only going to help your prostate, but your sex drive too.

You'll notice there is no oil in the above recipe since oil and vinegar simply don't mix well, and oil may coat the vegetables, which may impede digestion. Try it and see if your digestion is better. However, if you want to use oil, it's fine, and should do you no harm. Organic extra-virgin olive oil is best.

Another food that's great for your prostate (and everything else) is bee pollen. It is chock-full of vitamins, minerals (zinc), antioxidants, good fats, enzymes, and bioflavonoids. One study reported that men who took bee pollen for four months had a 78 percent improvement in urinary flow, had decreased residual urine and a reduction of prostate volume.(259) A study in Japan reported an overall success rate of 80 percent for improvements in urinary function.(260) Not just that, but bee pollen improves fertility. It's reported that it helps sperm swim faster and last longer – they're more motile and viable. I discussed bee pollen in detail in the chapter on obesity.

Male Virility

Why are men getting BPH, prostate cancer, and are having difficulty having sex? Humans aren't the only ones having sexual kind of problems – other species are too. Some male alligators' penises are shrinking, so much so that the gators are sexually incompetent. Male bald eagles have decreased sperm counts, and male fish are showing feminine characteristics.(261) These aberrations are hardly because these animals aren't taking the right drugs. They, like us, are being exposed to agents in our environment that are causing the problems.

A recent USGS (U.S. Geological Survey) study analyzing water samples found ". . . Traces of at least 11 compounds linked to birth control and hormone supplements." These compounds are almost identical to estrogen, and when they get into the male body, emasculating and other things – such as smaller penises, sex reversal in fish, and early puberty in children – occur.

Synthetic estrogens are all over the place. They're not only in many drugs, but in the wastes of drug manufacturing, which end up in drinking water. They're in pesticides, plastics, dental sealants, and some food cans. They're used in cattle and chicken feed because they encourage weight gain, and since the estrogens are very stable compounds, they get passed on to us who eat the hormone laden meat.(262)

If they cause animals to gain weight, what do you think they do to humans who consume them? You guessed it. . .they cause you to pack on the pounds. These compounds are so resistant to environmental break-down, they can survive for decades without losing their biological effect. They're also fat soluble (termed *lipophilic* from *lipo* – fat and *philic* – loving), so they accumulate in fat cells and are very difficult to excrete from the body. They tend to cause an extra layer of fat under your skin, which makes you appear "doughy," and even can cause a gradual enlargement of the pectoral muscles until they resemble a woman's breast. (Smaller penises and bigger breasts do not make the man!)

It used to take a year to fatten a chicken enough for market. Now, with growth stimulating hormones (mostly estrogen), it takes a mere three months. The FDA says that these hormones are safe, but there's no evidence to back that up and a lot to show that they're not. Some cattle ranchers even implant more hormones into the muscle tissue of the cow to get an added boost of hormones. This can cause the animal to have hormone levels three hundred times higher than even what the FDA approves.

These hormones are not just bad for you, they are disastrous to your sex drive and reproductive capabilities. High estrogens levels in men can cause the prostate gland to swell and cause BPH, muscles to weaken and atrophy, make you moody, and encourage weight gain. High estrogen also changes your ratio of testosterone/estrogen, which is an indication of your "manliness." Blood tests can be used to determine your total estrogens (which should be below 100 pc/dl) and testosterone levels (healthy levels are between 650 to 850 ng/dl). Most men should have a T/E ratio of at least 4 to 1. More "manly" ratios are 8 to 1, and sometimes athletes get it to 10 to 1. (Please note that many health care professionals are using 24 hour urine tests and saliva tests, which have completely different numbers and ranges.)

The more testosterone you have compared to estrogens, the more "manly" and sexual you'll be. So it's important to keep estrogens out of your body, while boosting things that increase testosterone levels. This is especially important as you age because the body tends to produce less and less testosterone, especially after the age of 40. Remember, cruciferous vegetables are very good at getting estrogens out of the body, so regular consumption of them is a good idea. In fact, my nutrition-expert friend David Getoff says that they're so good at getting the estrogens out, some of his women patients who eat a lot of them have to be put on supplemental estrogens.

Other things you can do to limit estrogen exposure are: drink pure water to avoid pesticides; wash fruits and vegetables; avoid processed meats; have regular bowel movements since the longer you wait, the more estrogens are absorbed; eat hormone-free and free-range meat and poultry; avoid alcohol and drugs, since they impair liver function which is needed to eliminate estrogens; and eat other estrogen inhibiting foods such as onions, green beans, cabbage, berries, citrus, pineapples, grapes, melons, pumpkin seeds, squash, pears, and figs.

Testosterone is not just good for your sex life, it protects you from a number of diseases such as heart disease; stroke; Alzheimer's; osteoporosis; Type II diabetes; depression; fatigue; and obesity (especially around the mid-section). High testosterone levels boost confidence, assertiveness, bravery, and valor. Men with higher levels of testosterone are more likely to be in positions of power and victorious on the playing field. Karlis Ullis, a medical director at UCLA says,

> Testosterone is a near magic substance that makes a man a man. There is no other substance on the planet, natural or man made, that can have such profound affects. It can restore or boost sex drive in men of virtually any age. It can decrease fat tissue and increase muscle tissue. It can sharpen the mind and build

confidence. It can increase overall energy levels and boost mental acuity.(263)

Obviously, it's imperative for men to have adequate levels of testosterone – not just for a good sex life, but to make it as a healthy, confident, sharp, and manly man. So how do we get more of it? We have to do the things that allow and encourage the body to make it naturally.

High-fat diets have been cursed by the medical establishment and media for over 30 years. But one study showed that switching from a high to a low fat diet actually lowered testosterone levels in men by 10 percent. That may be good news for the makers of *Viagra*, but not for the regular guy.(264)

Testosterone is a hormone, and hormones are built from cholesterol. I discussed fat and diet in detail in the chapter on heart disease. Low fat diets typically mean the diet is high in carbohydrates, which causes a spike in insulin production (leading to diabetes and the stimulation of the feminizing effects of estrogen) and body fat production. So the first thing you should do to increase your testosterone level is to get off of a low fat diet. As I've been saying, it's best to consume fat that hasn't been cooked or heated. Raw coconut oil, raw eggs, raw butter, raw fish, and even raw meat are good. Remember to get organically raised food to keep the xenoestrogens down.

Another thing you can do to increase your testosterone level is to exercise regularly in the correct ways. (See the chapter on cardiovascular diseases) Proper exercise stimulates testosterone production, which in turn increases your sex drive. It also can stimulate the production of human growth hormone (HGH), which is responsible for rejuvenating and repairing all the tissues in your body. One of the consequences of aging is a steady decline in HGH, which results in wrinkles, energy decline, excess fat gain, and loss of muscle tone. However, if HGH is replenished, strength, sexual capacity, and physical function all improve.(265) It has been shown that heavy, gut wrenching exercise can create a surge of HGH. But you need to be in good physical shape to do that level of exercise, and don't do it without proper medical supervision. One of your goals, however, is to get to the point of being able to do really heavy-duty exercises. Consuming more protein (rather than starches) also increases the levels of HGH – so a proper diet is important too. (Remember, some carbohydrates such as broccoli, asparagus, and other vegetables are healthy, but starches, like bread, pasta, rice, sugar, are not.)

A common problem with men these days is what's called erectile dysfunction (ED), which is when a man cannot get an erection, or loses his erection at some time during sex. It affects more than 30 million U.S. men, and is more common in the U.S. than any other country. More than one third of men regardless of age may experience it at some time, and more than half of all men over the age of 50 experience it.(266)

That's depressing news: and depression is actually one factor that may contribute to ED. We'll see later that depression is a result of other problems, most of which are physiological and biochemical, so if a man takes care of himself, it will not only help lift his depression, but will help lift his equipment also.

Not surprisingly, almost all antidepressant drugs can cause ED. Many blood pressure drugs, indigestion drugs, antihistamines, muscle relaxants, and sedatives can contribute to it also. (If a guy needs a good reason to believe what I've been saying all along that drugs are evil, this may finally convince him.) So see if you're taking any of these, and consider getting off of them with your doctor's supervision.

One class of drugs that really wreaks havoc with the male libido is statin drugs. Of course, a TV ad shows the football coach all happy now that he's taking *Zocor*. But I wonder if his wife is really happy about it, because as far back as 1996, there have been reports of statins – especially *Zocor* – causing ED. Studies have shown that most men who came off *Zocor* were soon able to have normal erections. If they were put back on it, they again developed ED.[267] Why would this be? It's because statin drugs prevent the body from making cholesterol, which as you now know, is the building block of testosterone. No testosterone – no erection.

Food for Thought

Having ED may be a blessing in disguise, since it is oftentimes an indicator of heart disease. Since erections are a result of blood flowing into the corpus cavernosa of the penis, circulation problems could cause it. In fact, arteriosclerosis is the most common cause of impotence in North America.[268] One study found that 64 percent of men who had a heart attack had ED before the event.[269] If you're having some trouble getting it up, it may be a wake-up call to change your lifestyle. You can use the recommendations I make in this section as a fairly quick and easy test. Try them for a couple or three months. If you see improvement in the bedroom, which I suspect you will, you may then feel confident enough to try other recommendations given throughout the book. You may find, that as un-cool or un-technical as natural solutions are, they can make your life a heck of a lot better – for a lot less money and hassle.

Besides cholesterol, another important building block of sex hormones is protein. A high protein, low starch diet will do great things for your sex drive and performance. Red meat is important since it contains creatine, which gives you strength and energy. It's also high in Coenzyme Q_{10} (CoQ_{10}), which is essential for heart health.

Wild fish (not farm raised), eggs, dairy, nuts, and seeds will all help put the fire back in your love life (remember, all are better raw). Egg yolks have all the required fat soluble vitamins (A, D, E, K), iron, and omega-3 fat. Egg whites have all the water soluble vitamins and have what is considered one of the highest quality proteins on earth.

Food for Thought

If you ever saw the first *Rocky* movie, you may remember a scene where *Rocky* (Sylvester Stallone) is training for his big fight. He wakes up, gets out of bed, cracks about a dozen eggs into a jar, and drinks them down in one shot. He didn't poach them, fry them, scramble them, or make an omelet out of them – just chugged 'em down. He knew what he was doing. . .because eating eggs this way – *Rocky Style* – will give your muscles bulk and definition and improve your strength much better than any kind of cooked egg. Forget all those protein powders that are usually loaded with soy protein (bad, bad, bad) and other marginal ingredients. Eat the real thing to get ripped. . .raw eggs. If you think you can't because they're gross, well, just how tough are you?

Walnuts and almonds are the most nutritious nuts, with omega-3s, vitamin E, potassium and other minerals. Others are brazil nuts, pecans, and macadamias. I already discussed the benefits of pumpkin seeds and sunflower seeds, which not only help your prostate, but your sex drive too.

A food that's often times called an aphrodisiac is oysters. Oysters have a lot of zinc, which helps increase testosterone levels. They also help with a woman's vaginal lubrication. Celery is also sometimes considered an aphrodisiac.

Food for Thought

I've heard that in order to perform better, male adult film stars eat a bunch or two of celery before they perform. Not just a couple stalks – the whole bunch. I don't have any journal studies to validate this, but it stands to reason because celery contains androsterone, a hormone that helps reinforce the libido (it's a weak androgenic steroid hormone). Snacking on raw celery and even indulging in a bunch before sex, may make a bunch of difference in your performance. Juicing celery is good and recommended too, but eating the whole plant is also needed for maximum effectiveness. (Of course, overindulging in anything may not be good, so monitor how you feel.)

Almonds, walnuts, pecans or some other nut, and celery are a great sex-enhancing snack. Ditto for oysters and celery together. You'll find that celery helps with the digestion of these high protein foods because it contains a high amount of chlorine. Chlorine (as chloride in the body), aids in protein digestion by contributing to the synthesis of gastric hydrochloric acid. Chloride is necessary for the manufacture of glandular hormone secretions, and helps prevent the buildup of excessive fat, which explains why celery is oftentimes used as a food to encourage weight loss. Don't think you need to eat regular table salt to get chloride, however. I discuss the problems with salt in the chapter on cardiovascular disease.

It's best to get your sodium already in bioactive form from foods like celery. I discuss celery in more depth in the chapter on cardiovascular disease. It is truly a wonder and I feel one of the most important foods you can eat since it improves so many bodily functions.

Back to virility. Olive oil raises the estrogen level in women (reportedly without raising cancer risks), which will increase her sex drive. Garlic improves blood circulation – the Greeks and Egyptians used it to improve sexual performance. Avocados contain vitamin E that boosts fertility in males, improves sex drive, arousal, and orgasms. I've heard that eating avocados and oranges together for a couple days really revs up your sex drive. Shrimp contains phenylalanine, an amino acid that increases both desire and alertness. Pecans are rich in arginine, which helps hormone levels and sperm counts and keeps sperm upwardly mobile. Even tomatoes (known as the "apple of love,") are packed with magnesium (and potassium) that is calming and helps with stamina.

Smoking constricts your blood vessels, and there's two decades of evidence indicating that it can cause impotence.(270) Caffeine also constricts blood vessels, so it won't help either. A drink or two may be all right, but anything more, and habitual use of alcohol, is not recommended if you want good sex. Of course, exercise is essential for blood flow and sexual activity. Speaking of smoking, celery is thought to be good for detoxifying many of the pollutants associated with cigarette smoke.

Viagra, Cialas, and other ED drugs work by increasing the concentration of nitric oxide (NO – a neurotransmitter) in the blood, which allows the dilation of blood vessels, especially those associated with erections. These drugs work by inhibiting the enzyme responsible for the natural degradation of NO, allowing NO to stay in the bloodstream longer and thus have a greater effect on the blood vessels. (This is similar to how serotonin reuptake inhibitors work on serotonin to improve mood.)

Sounds good, and these pills do in fact work. But one survey showed that more than half the men taking *Viagra* stopped after 3 years because it stopped working. And, more than 30 percent of men find that they had to increase the dose to twice as much to achieve the same effect as when they first started taking it.(271)

Food for Thought

The incidence of adverse reactions for *Viagra* is reportedly small (less than 5 percent). But some of them can be very serious and even deadly (I've included the package insert below which details all the hazards). Conversely, I've never heard of anyone dying from eating oysters or celery. The only contraindication to *Viagra* is the use of nitrates (sublingual nitroglycerin, long acting nitrates, nitrate pastes). Several patients have fainted while using nitrates and *Viagra* because of a drop in blood pressure.

Adverse Reactions listed on Viagra package insert: Cardiovascular and cerebrovascular: Serious cardiovascular, cerebrovascular, and vascular events, including myocardial infarction, sudden cardiac death, ventricular arrhythmia, cerebrovascular hemorrhage, transient ischemic attack, hypertension, subarachnoid and intracerebral hemorrhages, and pulmonary hemorrhage have been reported post-marketing in temporal association with the use of VIAGRA. Most, but not all, of these patients had preexisting cardiovascular risk factors. Many of these events were reported to occur during or shortly after sexual activity, and a few were reported to occur shortly after the use of VIAGRA without sexual activity. Others were reported to have occurred hours to days after the use of VIAGRA and sexual activity. It is not possible to determine whether these events are related directly to VIAGRA, to sexual activity, to the patient's underlying cardiovascular disease, to a combination of these factors, or to other factors (see **WARNINGS** for further important cardiovascular information). **Other events** Other events reported post-marketing to have been observed in temporal association with VIAGRA and not listed in the pre-marketing adverse reactions section above include: **Nervous:** seizure and anxiety. **Urogenital:** prolonged erection, priapism (see **WARNINGS**) and hematuria. **Special Senses:** diplopia, temporary vision loss/decreased vision, ocular redness or bloodshot appearance, ocular burning, ocular swelling/pressure, increased intraocular pressure, retinal vascular disease or bleeding, vitreous detachment/traction, paramacular edema and epistaxis. Non-arteritic anterior ischemic optic neuropathy (NAION), a cause of decreased vision including permanent loss of vision, has been reported rarely post-marketing in temporal association with the use of phosphodiesterase type 5 (PDE5) inhibitors, including VIAGRA. Most, but not all, of these patients had underlying anatomic or vascular risk factors for developing NAION, including but not necessarily limited to: low cup to disc ratio ("crowded disc"), age over 50, diabetes, hypertension, coronary artery disease, hyperlipidemia and smoking. It is not possible to determine whether these events are related directly to the use of PDE5 inhibitors, to the patient's underlying vascular risk factors or anatomical defects, to a combination of these factors, or to other factors.

Arginine is an amino acid that has been linked to the release of HGH, greater muscle mass, rapid healing from injury, reversal of atherosclerosis, proper mental function, and increased sexual potency.[272] It's also necessary for the production of NO. So if you have an arginine deficiency, you get a NO deficiency, and you get no erection. Arginine may be helpful in treating sterility in men since it has been shown to increase sperm count, and has also been noted to increase libido and induce erections.[273,274,275]

Arginine plays a vital role in protein metabolism and energy production since it stimulates the enzyme that starts the urea cycle, which converts toxic ammonia (a waste product of glucose metabolism) to urea which is less toxic and which is then eliminated by the kidneys. Since arginine helps blood vessels relax, it may be helpful in treating cardiovascular conditions such as angina, heart failure, peripheral vascular disease, vascular headaches, and atherosclerosis. So having enough arginine in your system is really important. Dietary sources of arginine are meats; dairy products; coconut; raisins; chicken; nuts (walnuts, filberts, pecans, almonds, Brazil nuts); and seeds (sunflower, sesame). Arginine is made from aspartic acid, so having aspartic acid is necessary too. Dietary sources of aspartic acid are meat, poultry, dairy, and sprouting seeds. Symptoms of aspartic acid deficiency are fatigue and depression.

Enhancing your sex life naturally will naturally enhance your whole life, without any nasty side effects.

Breast Cancer

Breast cancer is the most common cancer among women in the U.S. with an estimated 240,510 new cases in 2007: Every 3 minutes a woman is diagnosed with breast cancer). It's the second leading cause of cancer deaths among women with 40,460 deaths in 2007, whereas there were 71,930 deaths from respiratory system cancers (lung, bronchus, and larynx). African American women are more likely to die of breast cancer than white women. Breast cancer incidence in women has increased from one in 20 in 1960 to one in eight today. It's not very well publicized, but men can get breast cancer too. An estimated 2,000 men will get breast cancer in 2007, and 450 of them will die from it. There are currently about 2 million breast cancer survivors in the U.S.[276,277]

As with many diseases, the medical community does not know what causes breast cancer. Risk factors of developing it include early puberty, late childbearing, obesity, use of oral contraceptives, no experience breast-feeding, heavy alcohol consumption and smoking. The biggest risk factor is age, since most breast cancers occur in women over the age of 50, and women over 60 are at the highest risk.[278]

The most common sign of breast cancer is a new lump or mass in the breast. A lump that is painless, hard, and has uneven edges means its likely cancer, but sometimes the lumps can be tender, soft, and rounded. Other signs include a swelling of part of the breast; skin irritation or dimpling; nipple pain or nipple turning inward; redness or scaliness of the nipple or breast skin; a clear, bloody, or yellow discharge from the nipple; and a lump in the underarm area. Cancerous breast lumps are firm and do not shrink and expand with the menstrual cycle. While most lumps are not cancerous, any breast abnormality should be brought to the attention of a doctor.

Clinical ways of detecting breast cancer include mammograms (an X-ray that detects abnormalities) and biopsy (a tissue sample is taken that is analyzed in a lab). A mammogram does not show whether you have cancer or not – it just shows overly dense tissue that may be cancerous. A biopsy is necessary to determine if the aberrant cells are cancerous. Denser breast tissue, as found in younger women, makes it harder to get an accurate mammogram. So for women under the age of 40 mammograms may not show much of anything.

There are five stages of breast cancer – 0 through IV – ranging from the cancer cells remaining inside the breast duct without invading normal breast tissue, to the cancer spreading (metastasizing) to other parts of the body. Conventional treatments include surgery, radiation therapy, chemotherapy, hormone therapy, and biological therapy. Oftentimes more than one of these therapies is used. The choice of treatment depends on the stage of the disease.

Each of these treatments along with their hazards are presented below. Later on I will discuss alternative ways to address breast cancer, but for now, let's look at what a woman would be looking at if she addressed breast cancer in the conventional, mainstream way.

Food for Thought

As with my recommendation in the prostate section, you should always get a second opinion if diagnosed with cancer. The misdiagnosis rate for breast cancer is high – around 30 percent using mammograms. It's best to get a second opinion from a doctor in a different city, since doctors don't want to offend a colleague they know with a different diagnosis. Yes, this actually happens. You can call 1-800-4-CANCER for help with finding another doctor.

I realize that getting breast cancer is very, very frightening. The 5 year survival rates range from 100 percent for Stage 0 and I, to just 20 percent for stage IV (Stage II – 92 percent; Stage III – 81 percent; Stage III – 54 percent)(279)

So if you get breast cancer, according to conventional medical statistics and using only conventional treatments, you have a pretty good chance of not being here 5 years after you're diagnosed. That's scary. It's so scary that most women do what the doctor says, even if it means having their breasts removed. It's hard to blame them. The mystique that doctors and the medical community have woven over the past 100 years has taken firm root in our minds. According to them, only they have the answers, only they have the cure.

Hopefully, you don't currently have breast cancer. If that's the case, you have a great opportunity to change the path you're on to ensure you'll never get it. If you do have breast cancer, changing your path is still a good idea. It may cause remission, or at least it will make the likelihood of recurrence less and recovery easier. If you have been diagnosed with breast cancer, consider this: It was reported in the *Archives of Surgery* that women who had undergone needle biopsies had a 50 percent greater risk of the cancer spreading to the lymph nodes, thereby reducing the subject's chance of survival. This suggests that disrupting a cancerous tumor with a needle may raise the risk of it spreading.(280) Just like with prostate cancer, it appears that leaving the tumor alone is better than sticking or cutting it.

Surgery for Breast Cancer

Surgical treatments for breast cancer can be divided into two classes: breast-sparing or mastectomy. Breast-sparing surgery includes a lumpectomy (removal of the malignant tumor only); segmental mastectomy; and partial mastectomy. Mastectomy surgery (where the whole of one or both breasts is removed) includes mastectomy (removal of the whole breast); a modified radical mastectomy (removal of breast and lymph nodes under the arm); and a radical mastectomy (removal of breast, lymph nodes and chest muscle).

Surgery is the most common treatment for breast cancer, and usually it's performed along with chemotherapy or radiation treatments before or afterwards. Obviously, losing part or all of a breast is a definite negative side effect along with any other side effects from surgery, chemo, or radiation. Many women who are told they could have breast-sparing surgery surprisingly opt to have a radical mastectomy anyway, thinking it will stop the chance that the cancer will reoccur or any cancer that was missed would spread.

Radiation Treatments

Radiation therapy uses high-energy rays of ionizing radiation to kill cancer cells (among other cells). Radiation therapy can be used before surgery to shrink the size of the tumor or after surgery to kill off any remaining cancer cells and (supposedly) stop any potential spread of cancer.

There are two types of radiation: external where the radiation comes from a large machine outside the body; and internal, where a radioactive substance is placed directly in the breast for several days. Side effects of radiation therapy include red, dry, tender, itchy, and weepy moist skin. Extreme fatigue is common and can last for a long time – sometimes years.

Chemotherapy Treatments

Chemotherapy uses anticancer drugs to kill cancer cells, administered as a pill or by injection so these drugs travel throughout the body. The side effects are vast and depend on the type of drug, amount taken and the length of treatment. Temporary side effects include fatigue, nausea, diarrhea, vomiting, loss of appetite, hair thinning and loss, being more prone to infections, and mouth sores. Changes in the menstrual cycle may be temporary or permanent, and low blood cell counts are typical.

Premature menopause and infertility (because the drugs damage the ovaries) are potential permanent complications and are more likely as a woman gets older. Rapid bone loss is a potential complication as is permanent heart damage. Getting pregnant while receiving chemotherapy could lead to birth defects.

Chemo brain may occur, meaning a decrease in mental function, concentration, and memory lasting up to a couple years after treatment. Rarely, one to two years after chemo, the drugs may cause acute myeloid leukemia – a life threatening cancer of the white blood cells. Generally, women who have received chemotherapy do not feel as healthy as they did before treatment, even years after the treatment has stopped. Fatigue is the biggest complaint.[281] There are some drugs that supposedly stop or lessen some of the side effects of chemotherapy.

Undoubtedly, chemotherapy is hazardous and uncomfortable. After all, its whole intent is to kill cells. Dr. Douglass has this to say about chemo and a possible alternative:

Chemotherapy is the greatest crime committed by modern medicine. It is so illogical that I sometimes find it hard to believe that trained physicians from accredited universities subject cancer patients to its destructive effects. If the cancer is relatively benign, the chemotherapy will often "work" – despite the toxic nature of the treatment. But if it's benign, why put your body through chemotherapy when there are safer, nontoxic methods available that can produce even better results?(282)

Dr. Douglass goes on to tell of a man who was diagnosed with an aggressive form of non-Hodgkin's lymphoma, who conquered his cancer not by chemotherapy, but by changing his diet. This cancer survivor followed the nutritional principles of the Price-Pottenger Foundation or Weston A. Price Foundation, which are very similar to recommendations in this book.

Food for Thought

One overlooked hazard of getting cancer is that of developing a potentially fatal blood clot deep inside your leg. This is called deep vein thrombosis (DVT), and is the second leading cause of death among cancer patients. (A blood clot is a *thrombus*.) For people fighting some kinds of cancers, more than half died because of DVT. The risk of developing DVT for people taking chemotherapy drugs is twice as high as people free of cancer.

Complications from DVT blood clots kill around 200,000 people a year in the U.S., which is more than AIDS and breast cancer combined. The classical symptoms of DVT include pain, swelling, and redness of the leg and dilatation of the surface veins. In up to 25 percent of all hospitalized patients, there may be some form of DVT, which often remains clinically unapparent

Typical treatment to prevent DVT is to administer anti-coagulation drugs like heparin or warfarin. But these also have their side effects. Following the recommendations for diet, exercise, rest, sleep, breathing and others that I make throughout this book should keep you safe from blood clots, since your overall health, and thus the health of your blood, will be just fine.

By the way, warfarin (trade name *Coumadin*) was originally used as a rat poison and is still in the same class of drugs (coumarins) as the contemporary rodenicides used today. They all interfere with blood coagulation by inhibiting vitamin K metabolism. Understandably, the side effects of warfarin are hemorrhaging (bleeding), coughing up blood, blood in the stools, bleeding from the nose and gums, and even death.

Hormone Therapy

Hormone therapy or hormone treatment is used to add, block, or remove hormones in the body. Since certain hormones can attach to cancer cells and cause them to multiply, controlling the hormones might possibly control the cancer. The female hormones estrogen and progesterone can promote the growth of some breast cancer cells – so by blocking the production of these hormones, the cancer may not grow. (Hormone therapy for breast cancer is not the same as hormone replacement therapy, or HRT, used to treat the symptoms of menopause. More on that later.)

Hormone therapy consists of drugs (e.g., Tamoxifer, Fareston, Arimidex, Aromasin, Femara, Zoladex) to inhibit estrogen and progesterone. Sometimes surgery is used to remove the ovaries since they are the main supplier of estrogen. So a woman who has gone through menopause would not need that surgery since the ovaries produce less estrogen after menopause.

The drug most commonly used in hormone therapy is Tamoxifen (*Nolvadex*). It's a pill that's been used for breast cancer for 25 years, and is a type of drug called a selective estrogen-receptor modulator (SERM). It blocks estrogen from attaching to the estrogen receptors on cancer cells, and this prevents estrogen from exerting its growth stimulating effect on these cells thus conceivably halting the cancer.

The side effects of Tamoxifen are oftentimes similar to the symptoms of menopause – hot flashes and vaginal discharge. But other side effects include irregular menstrual periods, headaches, fatigue, nausea, vomiting, vaginal dryness and itching, irritation of the skin around the vagina, and skin rashes. More serious side effects are the formation of blood clots in the veins – most often in the legs and lungs. If one of these clots becomes loose, it could travel to the brain causing a stroke, or to the heart causing a heart attack.

Tamoxifen can cause cancer of the uterus, so it's recommended that women on this drug get regular pelvic exams and report any unusual activity such as bleeding in the vaginal area to their doctor. It's still possible to become pregnant while taking Tamoxifen (or any of the other drugs), and the drug may harm the fetus.

Biological Treatment

Biological therapy involves using a drug called Trastuzumab (*Herceptin*), a monoclonal antibody given intravenously that blocks a certain protein that slows or stops the growth of cancer. The side effects of this drug are fever, chills, weakness, nausea, vomiting, diarrhea, headaches, or rashes. In addition, it may cause heart damage that may lead to heart failure, and affect the lungs causing breathing problems. If that occurs, a doctor should be seen immediately. The benefits of this drug have been greatly manipulated to make it appear very helpful but the true statistical research show otherwise. Check out www.CancerDecisions.com

Food for Thought

Here's a question that most doctors and cancer treatment professionals wouldn't really appreciate, but needs to be asked: Why is it that even with surgery, chemo, radiation treatments, and the use of mammograms, the survival rates of breast cancer patients has not improved over the last 70 years?(283) With all the research going on and all the teases from the media about how science and technology is getting closer to a cure, why are just as many women dying of breast cancer as ever before?

Mammograms for Diagnosis of Breast Cancer

Mammograms are the most popular screening tool used by doctors. A mammogram involves firmly (and painfully) pressing your breast up against a plate and taking X-ray pictures of it from several angles. A survey in 2004 showed that nearly 90 percent of women who had no signs of the disease got screening mammograms, and most felt it would be irresponsible for a midlife woman not to.(284) Women are constantly admonished by the press, TV, medical establishment, and loved ones to get a mammogram "just to be safe." After all, the American Medical Association, American Cancer Society and just about any doctor says a mammogram is the best way to catch breast cancer before it kills you.

True? Some other experts don't think so. Dr. Anthony Miller, Professor Emeritus at the University of Toronto, conducted a major study of mammography, studying 90,000 women in their 40s and 50s who had mammograms during breast exams or breast exams alone. He found that mammography helped detect more and smaller cancers, but did nothing to reduce death rates. In one part of the study, 105 of 25,214 women who had mammograms had died, and 107 of 25,216 women who had not had mammograms (just physical and self-exams) had died at the 13-year follow-up. This large sample and closely controlled study clearly shows no advantage to mammograms as far as death rate goes.(285,286,287)

Food for Thought

In response to learning that results of the study conduced by Dr. Miller mentioned above had been published in the *Journal of the National Cancer Institute*, Dr. Mercola, a well respected medical doctor, had this to say:

"Well now, here we have it: mammograms don't work. This is not published in some 'rinky-dink' journal or press release. This is from the National Cancer Institute. Their analysis confirms what we have suspected for some time that mammograms are not a good idea. Most physicians recommend them for fear of being sued by a woman who developed breast cancer after which he did not advise her to get one. Now natural medicine physicians can rest comfortably and encourage women to get a thorough breast examination for abnormalities, as well as perform frequent self-examinations."(288)

Allan Spreen, M.D. has another interesting comment:

"Back in my pathology residency, we examined cancerous breast tissue under the microscope. It was quite shocking to see, but many times I found a track of cancer cells extending out from the main tumor in a straight line. I came to find out this track of cancer cells was actually from a previous needle biopsy! Biopsies can actually disturb a tumor on a molecular level, pulling cancer cells into healthy breast tissue. I always felt a mammogram could do the same thing. A mammogram creates such intense pressure to the breast tissue (not to mention the radiation showered on the breast), it's possible that cancer cells could become dislodged."(289)

Another study published in the *Archives of Internal Medicine* in 2008 showed something even worse: mammograms actually increase breast cancer rates. Over 220,000 women were studied, and the women who had regular mammography screening (twice a year for six years) had a 22 percent higher rate of breast cancer than women who had but a single mammogram at the end of the six year period. The authors said, ". . .it appears that some breast cancers detected by repeated mammographic screening would not persist to be detectable by a single mammogram at the end of six years. This raises the possibility that the natural course of some screen-detected invasive breast cancers is to spontaneously regress." Meaning, the body can sometimes (and more than rarely) rid itself of cancer cells on its own.(290) Given half a chance, the body can do miraculous things. A Swedish study published in the *The Lancet* reported that the death rate from breast cancer among women under 55 was 29 percent higher in the group that had been screened with mammography compared to the unscreened control group. In addition, women in their 40s and 50s who had yearly mammograms actually had a 36 percent to 52 percent increase in breast cancer mortality.(291)

Mammograms aren't even reliable. In a Swedish study of 60,000 women, 70 percent of the tumors detected by mammography weren't tumors at all. Of the 5 percent of mammograms that suggested further testing, about 93 percent were false positives (showing cancer when there really was none).(292) Estimates are that 70 percent to 80 percent or all positive mammograms do not, upon biopsy, show any presence of cancer.

According to the National Cancer Institute, there is a high rate of missed tumors in women ages 40-49, resulting in 40 percent false negative test results (not showing cancer when there really was cancer). The National Institutes of Health admit that mammograms miss 25 percent of malignant tumors in women in their 40s, and 10 percent of malignant tumors in older women.(293,294,295)

Here's something else to think about: About one in four modern breast cancer diagnoses (using mammography) determine that the cancer is the slow developing ductal or lobular carcinomas (those that are *in-situ* – tumors still confined inside the ducts or lobules), which only become malignant, according to one report I read, about 2 percent of the time.(296) Another doctor said that between five and 20 percent of these kinds of cancers are malignant.(297) But oftentimes women are panicked into getting a mastectomy in these cases, when close monitoring would be sufficient. After all, only two out of 100 of these kinds of tumors become life threatening.(298) A thorough evaluation by you, your doctor, and a qualified oncologist is needed, and you need to get the real story on just what kind of tumor you have. Don't be afraid to ask questions and be demanding. It's your life.

Why might mammograms actually cause or worsen breast cancer? Two reasons: First, as Dr. Douglass says, "In what I call the 'compression syndrome,' the act of squeezing and compressing the breast in order to get good images during mammography may activate and spread an otherwise contained or localized mass of cancerous cells."(299) A tear in the tissue can cause a "leak" in the tumor, which allows the malignancy to spread and spread faster. In the old days, doctors were advised that breast lumps should be handled with care to prevent any such leak. Now? During a mammography, the breast is hardly handled with care. So in the same way that disturbing the prostate gland in a man might cause cancer cells to be activated, disturbing a woman's breast could activate the cancer too.

Second, the radiation used during a mammogram may cause the cancer. John W. Gofman, M.D, Ph.D., was a world renowned expert on radiation and Professor Emeritus in Molecular and Cell Biology at the University of California, Berkely. In his landmark book *Preventing Breast Cancer*, he states, "Our estimate is that about three-quarters of the current annual incidence of breast cancer in the United States is being caused by earlier ionizing radiation, primarily from medical sources."(300) His data show that the more mammograms a woman is subjected to, the greater her chances of getting breast cancer:

Age range	Number of Mammograms	Chance of Breast Cancer
30-34	1 exam	1 in 1,100
	5 exams	1 in 220
35-49	1 exam	1 in 1,900
	10 exams	1 in 190
50-64	1 exam	1 in 2,000
	15 exams	1 in 133

Dr. Gofman says that: radiation is a proven cause of human breast cancer; a woman's breast is more vulnerable to radiation than other parts of her body;

breast irradiation during infancy and childhood increases the rate of breast cancer in adulthood; and, there is no safe dose of radiation – every exposure creates an increased rate of cancer in a population of cells.

A highly regarded group of health care analysts at the Cochrane Centre in Copenhagen, Denmark analyzed seven of the biggest and best studies on mammography screening. Their conclusion was that the best trials failed to show a significant reduction in breast cancer mortality. Even more, they said that because of mammographic screening, there are more breast cancer diagnoses and women of all ages undergo 31 percent more partial mastectomies, 20 percent more mastectomies and 24 percent more radiation treatments that do nothing to extend their lives.(301)

Dr. Gofman goes further, saying that medical radiation is a highly important cause, and probably the principal cause, of cancer mortality in the U.S. during the 20th Century. (Medical radiation includes X-rays, CT scans, and fluoroscopy.) He also says that medical radiation, even at very low and moderate doses, is an important cause of death from Ischemic Heart Disease due to it causing mini-tumors in the smooth muscles of the heart.

The Lancet reported that since mammographic screening was introduced in 1983, the incidence of ductal carcinoma in situ (DCIS) (which represents 12 percent of all breast cancer), has increased by 328 percent – 200 percent of this increase they conclude was due to the use of mammography.(302) These reports are compelling, to say the least, and hopefully will make you think twice before getting another X-ray, no matter where on your body or for what reason.

Alternatives to Mammograms

There are other tests that are being used as alternatives to mammograms. Two of them I do not recommend, two of them I do.

The AMAS (Anti-Malignant Antibody Screen) is a simple blood test that the originators claim can detect cancer cells of any type originating anywhere in the body. There is only one lab in the country doing the test (the people who say the test works) and the literature, testing, and validation of this test is inconclusive and sketchy. Personally, I don't recommend it.

Then there's the new-fangled genetics testing that supposedly can reduce a woman's risk of developing cancer. However, these tests are not only expensive, but very limited and focused for certain genes such that it's estimated that perhaps just 1 percent of women without a family history of the disease would benefit from them.(303)

An alternative to mammograms that I do believe is effective, noninvasive and much safer is called thermography. This is not a blood test, but a way to detect possibly cancerous tissue by measuring infrared heat from the body. (A biopsy is necessary to determine if it's truly cancer.) It does not use any radiation.

One study showed that thermography had an over 95 percent predictive value and has revealed the presence of breast cancer despite normal reports from a mammogram (mammograms miss 10 percent of breast cancers).(304) Another study reported that thermography can detect 86 percent of non-palpable breast cancers and up to 15 percent of cancers that were not visible by mammography.(305) Thermography can detect a pathologic state of the breast up to 10 years before a cancerous tumor can be found by any other method, and has the ability to detect fast growing aggressive tumors.

The thermography test costs about $195 and some insurance companies cover the procedure. I think you'll see it become more and more popular as the years progress and people finally wake up to the fact that mammograms are not that good and can even be harmful. To find a doctor near you who uses thermography, or for more information, go to www.breastthermography.com. At the very least, if you think you must get mammograms, you could still get them, but less often, and use thermography to test the other times.

Another new test for breast cancer is Power Doppler Sonography (PDS) (also used to detect prostate cancer). It's very advanced ultrasound that can produce a detailed image (sonogram) of the body's internal structures and has a much higher resolution and the ability to highlight areas of blood flow in dense or soft tissue, allowing tumors or inflammation to be viewed and measured clearly. It can detect twice as many breast cancers as mammography and a study reported in the *British Journal of Urology* showed that this kind of test only misses 1 percent of prostate cancers.(306) Sonograms are safe, painless and inexpensive. Unlike other screening methods, they can be repeated as often as necessary to closely monitor areas of concern and assess treatment efficacy. For these reasons, sonograms have been found to be a more effective alternative to biopsies in detecting prostate tumors, and better than MRI and PET/CT scans as a means for tracking these tumors. PDS can also be used to monitor inflammation and tumors in the breast and other parts of the human body. To learn more and to find out where you can get one done, check out www.cancerscan.com and www.phoenixsonograms.com. Many health insurance companies are paying for these.

Food for Thought

I mentioned sonograms in the prostate chapter and highlighted the work of Robert L. Bard, M.D., who does these for both prostate and breast cancer. He is one of the world experts on cancer detection using this new, non-invasive, and incredibly accurate screening method. He says,

"About 25 percent of proven cancers will remain inactive in the breast and not grow or metastasize even in the absence of medical treatment. Many cancers are very low grade and grow slowly over 5-10 years before turning highly malignant. . .Some cancers grow rapidly and are highly malignant. These tumors seem to be best diagnosed by sonograms because sonography can detect a malignancy when it is ¼ inch in size and is highly accurate especially in high risk patients with lumpy breasts where mammograms are of limited diagnostic value. . .The combined use of breast sonograms with Doppler blood flow study will provide early detection of most highly malignant cancers resulting in life saving early diagnosis and sparing the patient radical surgery. . .Sonography detects 4 times as many cancers as physical examinations and twice as many cancers as mammography."(307)

Ladies – it's simple. Don't do the mammogram, go get a sonogram!

Causes of Breast Cancer

Before we get into specifics, there's a comment by Peter Montague, editor of *Rachel's Environment & Health News* I want to share:

> The medical establishment dominated by male doctors pretends that the breast cancer epidemic will one day be reversed by some miracle cure, which we have now been promised for 50 years. Until that miracle arrives, we are told, there is nothing to be done except slice off women's breasts, pump their bodies full of toxic chemicals to kill cancer cells, burn them with radiation, and bury our dead. Meanwhile, the normal public health approach of primary prevention languishes without mention and without funding. We know what causes the vast majority of cancers: exposure to carcinogens. What would a normal public health approach entail? Reduce the burden of cancer by reducing our exposure to carcinogens. One key idea has defined public health for more than 100 years: PREVENTION.(308)

Although the medical establishment insists they don't know the cause of breast cancer (so they can continue to get funding for their drug research), it is fairly obvious if you review the scientific literature. I believe that most breast cancers are caused by exposure to chemicals, endocrine-disrupting chemicals, drugs, and ionizing radiation. Other causes could include deficiencies in selenium and iodine as well as over consumption of sugars and processed starches.

Chemicals

A Japanese women living in Japan has about one quarter the risk of getting breast cancer has her American counterpart. When Japanese women move to America, by the second generation, their risk of breast cancer has risen to "normal" American levels. We must conclude that something in the environment and diet, not genetics, is at work here.

In Israel, deaths from breast cancer in young women less than 44 years old in the 1960s and 1970s began to sharply increase. Then, the death rate from breast cancer in women 44 or younger dropped between 1976 and 1989: but the death rate among older Israeli women continued to rise. That was an unusual pattern. Was there an explanation?

There was. In the 1970s, measurements of three carcinogenic pesticides in cow's milk and human milk in Israel found levels five to 1,000 times higher than in the U.S. These contaminants were Lindane (since banned in U.S.), DDE (a chemical created when DDT breaks down in the environment) and alpha-BHC. Cow's milk and human tissues were all found to be heavily contaminated with these. Finally, in 1978, after public protests, Israel banned these pesticides. By 1980, breast milk contamination had dropped 90 percent or more among the Israeli women.(309)

Could these pesticides have caused the unusual breast cancer pattern in Israel? Many scientists think so. A recent study in America showed women with breast cancer have significantly elevated levels of DDT, DDE, and PCBs in their fat compared to women who do not have cancer.(310) The incidence of breast cancer goes down when a woman exercises on a regular basis, and eats more green vegetables and fiber.

Food for Thought

The connection between breast milk and toxicity is not intended to discourage you from breastfeeding your baby. Breast feeding gives an infant immunity against gastrointestinal diseases and respiratory infections, offers protection against food allergies, provides emotional bonding between mother and child, and is really the right food for the baby. Prepared formulas and baby foods are usually even more contaminated than mother's milk.

Human breast milk can also be affected by pollution. Scientists first discovered human breast milk was contaminated with DDT in 1951. DDT, like many other chlorinated organic chemicals (pesticides), is soluble in fat but not very soluble in water. So when it enters the body, it's not easily excreted and builds up in fatty tissue. Breast milk contains about 3 percent fat and fat-soluble chemicals collect there. So, if the mother is contaminated and she breastfeeds her baby, the baby gets contaminated too.

In 1975 the EPA conducted a study of the milk of American women. Taking samples from more than one thousand women and analyzing them for only a few pesticides, they found DDT in 100 percent of the samples, PCBs in 99 percent, and dieldrin in 83 percent. All three are considered probable carcinogens by the EPA.(311)

Until early 1999, pesticides had never been measured in the amniotic fluid of pregnant women. (The amniotic fluid is what the fetus floats in the womb prior to birth.) But in June 1999, researchers in the United States and Canada found p,p'-DDE (a breakdown byproduct of DDT), in 30 percent of the women examined. The concentrations of p,p'-DDE found in the amniotic fluid are a real concern. Of the various health problems associated with these chemicals, developmental abnormalities of the male reproductive tract, suppression of immune function, development of the brain, and neurobehavioral problems in children are of major concern because they are irreversible. DDE is known to interfere with male sexual development by deactivating the male sex hormone, testosterone.(312)

Endocrine-disrupting Chemicals

Hormones and growth factors act as chemical messengers in the body and are important in the normal growth and functioning of cells and tissues, including breast tissue. However, they can also play a role in the development of cancer, especially when they come from external and unnatural sources.

There is much evidence that links breast cancer to "xenoestrogens," chemicals strange or foreign to the human body that mimic or interfere with the body's natural estrogen, the female sex hormone. Indeed, many common industrial chemicals and pesticides mimic these hormones and thus interfere with fundamental bodily processes. DDT, methoxychlor, benzene, and others can act like sex hormones and interfere with fundamental biological processes such as reproduction in wildlife and humans. It is believed that xenoestrogens stimulate the growth of cells in the breast, possibly giving rise to cancer.(313)

From epidemiological studies (studies of diseases in the human population), there's evidence that exposure of females to xenoestrogens while in the womb can increase their risk of breast cancer as adults. Not only that, but if a male is exposed to these same chemicals while in the womb, it reduces his ability to produce sperm later in life. It's estimated that the average male today produces only half as much sperm as his grandfather did, and exposure to environmental toxins may well be the cause of this decline. (If this decline were to continue at historical rates, humans in industrialized countries would have difficulty reproducing themselves by about the year 2020.) There is also evidence that prostate cancer, the second leading cause of cancer deaths in the U.S. for men, (lung cancer is number one), is linked to these xenoestrogens.(314)

There are probably hundreds of substances that mimic naturally occurring hormones from pesticides, cleansers, solvents, plasticizers, surfactants, dyes, cosmetics, PCBs, and dioxins.

Hormone Replacement Therapy

Hormone Replacement Therapy (HRT) is designed to ease the transition through menopause and lessen symptoms such as hot flashes, vaginal dryness, mood swings, sleep disorders and decreased sexual desire. Drugs for this use include the hormones estrogen and progesterone (usually synthetic progestin), which are usually administered by pill, patch, or vaginal cream. The most popular brand name is *Prempro*. Estrogen is oftentimes used alone, the most popular brand name being *Premarin*.

A large-scale study on the combination drug using estrogen and progesterone (*Prempro*) was started in 1993 by the National Institutes of Health (NIH). By 2002, the study was halted three years early because so many women were having serious health problems, most notably, an increased rate of breast cancer.

The results of the study showed that women taking these drugs experienced: 26 percent increase in breast cancer; 41 percent increase in strokes; 29 percent increase in heart attacks; twice as many blood clots, and; 22 percent increase in total cardiovascular disease.(315) Other health problems in study participants included coughing up blood, vision problems, nausea, hair loss, headaches, depression, decreased libido, weight gain, and fatigue.(316)

Food for Thought

Since 1942 when these drugs were introduced, the estrogen in *Prempro* and *Premarin* has come from the urine of pregnant mares (female horses). To get the urine, the mares are forced to stand in stalls less than five feet wide 24/7 with urine collection devices strapped to them. They are unable to turn, lie down, or exercise, and the devices strapped to them can cause infections and chafing. In the last months of their eleven-month pregnancy, the mares are put out to pasture to have their foals (baby horses). Then, they're put in a herd with a stallion so they become pregnant again as soon as possible, and their foals are taken away from them even if they're not fully weaned. Once pregnant again, it's back into the pee barn so more urine can be collected.

Besides the cruel treatment of the mares, the foals are oftentimes slaughtered and their meat shipped to Europe and Japan (I guess they eat horse meat there, maybe unknowingly). When the mare can no longer get pregnant, she is slaughtered too. All told, it's estimated that over the years, the production of these drugs has cost the lives of over a million horses.(317) Besides these drugs being bad for the women who take them, realize that every time they're prescribed, untold misery is inflicted on those poor horses.

But will that stop the manufacturer, Wyeth, from promoting these products? Hardly. After all, they make about $1 billon a year from the sales of *Premarin, Prempro*, and two other drugs along the same line, *Premphase* and *Prempac*. In fact, Wyeth has successfully lobbied (January 9, 2008) the FDA to ban the use of the natural hormone estriol in estrogen medications. Estriol, a *bioidentical hormone*, has been used successfully for years without major health problems. But when Wyeth's profits dropped more than 57 percent ($2.07 billion in 2003 to $800 million in 2004) after the above mentioned study was released showing serious side effects of these drugs, they had to do something!

Concerning treatment for menopausal symptoms, Dr. Mercola says, "If you are going to use hormone replacement therapy, clearly bioidentical hormones are the way to go and an absolute no-brainer if one has had a surgically induced menopause."(318) Bioidentical hormones are those that are made to be the same as the hormone your body would have produced. This is as opposed to using a synthetic or horse hormone.

It's estimated that in 2002, 22 million women were taking *Premarin* for menopausal symptoms. But when the study mentioned above was released that year showing the link between HRT and all those other health problems, not surprisingly, many women stopped taking it. (This study funded by the National Institute of Health as part of the Women's Health Initiative was cut short because of the higher incidences of health problems the participants were having.)(319)

What happened? Breast cancer rates in America declined by 7.2 percent the year after the study was published (14,000 fewer women were diagnosed with the disease in 2003). The symptoms of menopausal may include hot flashes, vaginal dryness, mood swings, sleep disorders and decreased sex drive – all discomforts to be sure, but usually not life threatening (as are the problems with the drugs).

About 30 percent of American women over the age of 50 have taken HRT between 2000 and 2005.(320) That's a lot of women. The study was conducted on 161,809 women ages 50-79, from 40 different medical centers – a pretty good size study. Once again, a drug is shown to cause more problems than it fixes.

Food for Thought

Hormones are big business. It all started back in 1934 when American drug companies began selling synthetic hormones to be used in cosmetics, drugs, food additives, and animal feed. The best known of these hormones is diethylstilbestrol (DES). It didn't take long to realize it could cause cancer: In 1938 and again in 1941, studies were reported by the National Cancer Institute that showed DES caused breast cancer in rodents. But DES is 400 times as potent as natural estrogen and can be made very cheaply, so instead of banning its use because it caused breast cancer in women, the FDA, bless their hearts, approved its use in 1941.

Since then, DES has been used as a morning after pill to prevent pregnancy, to prevent miscarriages, and as a breast-enlarging cream. As early as 1947, adverse effects of DES were reported among U.S. women who ate chicken treated with this hormone. In 1971, human cancer from DES was confirmed, and it was banned from meat in 1973. But other growth hormones are now used instead to fatten animals. These hormones are used to promote cell and tissue growth, and cause weight gain. (You wonder why so many people are fat? The hormones end up in *us*.) So is it really surprising that they would also promote cancer cell growth?

Not everyone thinks that hormones are good – Europe will not allow U.S. meat be imported because of the U.S.'s ubiquitous use of hormones in animal feed.(321)

Concerning chemicals, Europe has eliminated 900 compounds for use in beauty products due to their suspected role in causing cancer, genetic mutations, and reproductive disorders. They banned the use of phthalates (a chemical used in plastics and resins) in nail polish in 2004. Europe has also restricted the use of six phthalate compounds in toys. Although manufacturers in the U.S. said they would limit their use in toys voluntarily, they are still being used today.(322)

Common characteristics shared by many women who end up developing breast cancer include: early menarche; late menopause; late childbirth and no children or the birth of few; lack of breast-feeding; obesity; a high fat diet; being tall; taking oral contraceptives; cancer of the ovaries or uterus; and excessive use of alcohol.

"What is the message running through all of these risk?" ask Dr. Janet Sherman, author of *Life's Delicate Balance – The Causes and Prevention of Breast Cancer*. "Hormone, hormones, and hormones. Hormones of the wrong kind, hormones too soon in a girls' life, hormones for too many years in a woman's life, too many chemicals with hormonal action, and too great a total hormonal load."(323)

Excess Weight

Weight gain during adult life, especially after menopause, increases the risk of breast cancer, and weight loss after menopause decreases the risk of getting it. There's between a 4 percent and 24 percent higher risk of breast cancer for women who have gained at least 2 kg of weight since age 18. Researchers said ". . .we estimated that 15 percent of post-menopausal breast cancer cases in our population may be attributable to weight gain of 2.0 kg [4½ lbs] or more since age 18 years and 4.4 percent attributable to weight gain of 2.0 kg or more since menopause."(324)

Deodorants and Cosmetics

Of special concern are findings that makeup and underarm deodorants and antiperspirants can increase the risk of developing breast cancer. Both products often contain parabens (a preservative found in lotions, shampoo, sunscreen, skin foundation, bath gels and deodorants), that has been shown to act like a weak estrogen. Parabens have been found with regularity in breast tumors, and are thought to have estrogenic effects in estrogen-sensitive human cells (which breast cells are). Notably, 60 percent of all breast tumors are located in the upper-outer quadrant, nearest the underarm where deodorants are typically applied.(325)

One researcher, Dr. Kris McGrath, showed that women who shaved at least three times a week and applied antiperspirants at least twice a week were almost 15 years younger when diagnosed with cancer than women who did neither. Dr. McGrath believes that's it's the aluminum in the antiperspirant that is the culprit. Usually they don't penetrate the skin, but when the skin is freshly shaven, they do.(326)

Food for Thought

For a natural deodorant, take a lemon wedge and rub under the arms. Adding a little ginger helps too. If you must use store-bought antiperspirants, please get one that doesn't contain aluminum, since it is believed to contribute to Alzheimer's disease. Since sweating is one of the body's main methods of detoxification, and since the breast is immediately adjacent to the underarms, it may be that reducing the detoxification (sweating) in this area could easily increase breast cancer. Use a nontoxic *deodorant* and NOT an *anti-perspirant*.

Cosmetics are typically not only laden with parabens, but contain phthalates too. These chemicals have been linked to certain birth defects and also can disrupt the natural hormones balance in the body, which may in turn increase the risk of breast cancer.

Not only that, but a study by Dr. Janet Gray at Vassar College suggests that women who begin using makeup at an earlier age and in greater amounts may have an increased risk of developing breast cancer later in life. It appears that shampoos and other hair care products, especially those marketed to the African-American community, are the worst offenders. These products have extracts from placentas (to strengthen hair and reduce breakage), which contain adult hormones like estrogen.(327)

Dr. Gray says, "Adolescence is the time when breasts are developing, so this is clearly a time when exposure matters for developing breast cancer 20 to 30 years later." For a list of cosmetic product that are supposed to be free of these chemicals, go to www.safecosmetics.org.

Antibiotics, Aspirin, Antidepressants, and Smoking

A study reported in the *Journal of the American Medical Association* states that antibiotic use is associated with an increased risk of breast cancer, and the more antibiotics used, the more the risk increased. The study of over 10,000 women found that those who took antibiotics for more than 500 days (or had more than 25 prescriptions for the drugs over a period of 17 years or so) had more than twice the likelihood of developing breast cancer compared to women who didn't use any antibiotics.(327a) Even if a woman had between one and 25 prescriptions over the same period, they are one-and-a-half times more likely to get it. Researchers aren't sure why, but the evidence is compelling.

Food for Thought

Personally, I don't find it surprising that antibiotics use can lead to cancer, be it breast or any other kind. Antibiotics kill (they are poisons, after all) bacteria which, believe it or not, help to keep our bodies clean of metabolic wastes and toxins from the outside world. I go into more detail about this in the chapter on vaccines.

A study of 114,000 women in California showed some alarming trends in those who took aspirin and/or ibuprofen and the development of breast cancer. The daily use of aspirin for five years or more caused a dramatic increase in breast cancer, and those taking ibuprofen every day for at least five years increased a woman's chances of developing breast cancer by 50 percent compared to those who did not use the drugs regularly.(328)

How about antidepressants? Women taking paroxetine (*Paxil*) were shown to have a seven-fold increased risk of breast cancer in one study.(329) Women taking tricyclic antidepressants (TCAs) were found to have about twice the risk of developing the disease.(330) These findings have been known since 2000, but has the general public, or even the doctors prescribing these medicines, heard about them?

Smoking, not surprisingly, can increase the risk of developing breast cancer too. Women who were current smokers had about a 30 percent greater chance of getting this cancer than those who had never smoked. But, the good news is, there's no evidence of significantly increased breast cancer risk among women who had previously smoked but had quit.(331)

Bras

A husband and wife team of medical anthropologists has done intriguing research they say indicates that wearing a bra can cause breast cancer and fibrocystic breast disease. Sydney Ross Singer and Soma Grismaijer surveyed 4,730 women to determine their bra-wearing habits and incidences of diseases. They found that women who wore their bras 24 hours a day had a three out of four chance of developing breast cancer. Women who wore bras more than 12 hours a day had a one in seven chance. Those who wore one less than 12 hours a day had a one in 152 risk, and women who wear bras rarely or never had a one in 168 chance of getting breast cancer.

Although this study was not a scientifically controlled study, the results are compelling. Singer and Grismaijer believe the pattern is due to the constricting nature of the bra, which hinders or stops lymph flow. Lymph is the garbage-disposal system of the body, and is totally dependant on movement since there's no pump for it. If the breast and surrounding tissues are bound tight, they're not able to receive the gentle massage during everyday movements and walking that move the lymph and help cleanse the tissues. The lymph fluid accumulates in the breast tissue and this accumulation leads to breast tenderness, pain, and ultimately the fluid turns into cysts.

There are reports that within days or weeks of stopping wearing a bra, the breast tissue is allowed to flush out the excess fluid, the cysts disappear and the breast pain and tenderness go away. Singer and Grismaijer say that getting rid of the bra has resulted in over 95 percent recovery of pain and cyst problems.(332) Therefore, it's probably best not to sleep in a bra, and perhaps wear one less during the day if possible. Singer and Grismaijer wrote a book that discusses this in detail titled *Dressed to Kill*, that you can find on the internet.

Most bras are made of fabric that contains petrochemicals. Having that next to your skin for hours on end can't be good. When you do wear a bra, try to have it be of natural fibers.

Food for Thought

Not surprisingly, the American Cancer Society (ACS) debunked Singer and Grismaijer's research because it ". . .was not conducted according to standard principles of epidemiological research and did not take into consideration other variables, including known risk factors for breast cancer."(333) OK, maybe it wasn't the perfect study. (Which one is?) But the research at least points to a possible contributing factor for breast cancer. So with such compelling evidence, why doesn't the ACS design and conduct a study that meets their criteria so we can see if maybe something as simple as wearing a bra less than 12 hours per day could make a difference? Simple: It won't make them money.

I'm not sure if it's just human nature or the "powers that be'" are intentionally twisting things so the innocent and trustworthy keep following their dogma, but the end result is us spending money in directions that have in the past, not proven fruitful. How many times do we hear: "We're getting closer to a cure. We need to do more research to find out. It may be a virus, it may be genetics, we just don't know. We need more money to do the research to find out. Please give to _____"

So millions of well intentioned Americans give millions of dollars a year to the cancer foundations, heart foundations, diabetes foundations, and countless others. There are walkathons and pink ribbons and teddy bears for sale with funds going to medical research. And what does this research do? Aside from a few token studies on nutrition and environmental factors, the overwhelming bulk of the money for research goes into answering one question. . ."what drug can we invent, patent and sell to treat it?"

By now you probably realize I'm not a pro-drug kind of guy (a bit of an understatement!), and I believe that some of the tactics the drug companies use are downright evil. Concerning medical research, they are very, very, tricky. They actually have good natured Americans finance drug research when they participate in and donate to these "find-a-cure" campaigns. They don't use the profits they make selling the drugs (sometimes, a drug will sell for 200,000 times what it costs to make), instead, they get you to wear out your sneakers to earn them even more money to use for research. (On the bright side, at least you're getting some exercise.)

Sorry to be a kill-joy, but every time you see that pink ribbon and all those people marching for a cure, they're doing no such thing. They're unwittingly marching to ensure that the researchers keep researching, the drug companies keep selling drugs, and the doctors keep prescribing, zapping, and cutting. The public surely doesn't know what's really going on, and most doctors, researchers, and even drug salespeople (I know some pharmaceutical reps and they're all very nice) are well intentioned people. But they simply don't realize that what they're doing – looking for a "cure" through drugs or medical technology – doesn't, and will never, exist.

Why? First, drugs don't heal. They can't – only the body can heal. Drugs just alter and alleviate symptoms (at the expense of the overall health of the body). Second, drug companies and researchers make their living from sick people. Why should they find a cure when they make so much money chasing one? So they'll say they're making advances and things are better than they used to be and the cure is just around the corner. It's not. As I show time after time in this book, the health of Americans is getting worse and worse. (Partly because of all the drugs we're consuming. Heck, drug residues are now even in our water supplies.)

This "we-need-drugs" mindset has to change. There are TV drug commercials for prostate problems, depression, impotence, osteoporosis, cholesterol, heart conditions, colds, flu, heart-burn, allergies, bi-polar disorder, bladder weakness, cervical cancer, even restless legs. A friend of mine made the observation that this generation of kids who are exposed to this drug media blitz, will, by the time they are adults, think it's perfectly natural to have these diseases and that the only way to treat them is with drugs. All this advertising is not just to sell drugs now, but to brainwash all the children and teens into believing that taking them is as normal a way of life as washing your hair. (Have you noticed all the cartoon characters like butterflies or cute bumblebees in the ads? Just like Joe Camel cigarettes years ago before he was banned.) Inculcation (repeated exposure) works. . . Adolph Hitler said, "Tell a lie long enough, loud enough and often enough, and people will believe it." Look what he was good for.

It's sardonically amusing to me when a politician gets up and says something like, "I'll make sure that all Americans, especially the elderly, can get the drugs they need!" Like he's doing us a *favor*? Like that's one of our unalienable rights? Some day, some brave soul will get up and say, "My dear Americans. We need to rebuild America from the ground up. If elected, I will make sure that our farmlands are replenished with all the minerals they need to grow healthy and nutritious crops; for as Pulitzer Prize winning author and agriculturist Louis Bromfield said, '. . . one of the great problems of American agriculture [is] the decline of human stock through the decline in fertility and mineral content of the soil itself. *"Poor land makes poor people"* is a saying every American should have printed and hung over his bed.'(334) I will ensure that every one of us, young and old alike, can get inexpensive organically raised food, meat without hormones, eggs from free-range hens, raw milk and wholesome cod liver oil a-plenty. I'll get the additives, artificial sweeteners, and preservatives out of our food supply and make sure that we, and especially our children, are not forced into being shot up with poisons. I'll make it possible for you to have the time to get adequate sunshine and plenty of exercise. If I'm elected, I pledge to you to take all the money that goes into drug research and development and spend it on cleaning up our food supply and the environment and making sure all products are non-toxic. My fellow Americans, deep down in your hearts, you know. . .you *know*. . . that only nature can heal and it is our unalienable right to be given the opportunity to simply allow it to do so. We've been deceived by the greedy and power-hungry for too long! It's time for a change – a REAL change, literally from the ground up! It's time to rise up and say no more! No more deception! No more lies! No more weakening of the American body and spirit just to make a buck! If you are strong enough, brave enough, resilient enough and insightful enough, you'll see that the natural way is the only way to true health and happiness. Yes, if you're brave enough, you can rise above the pain and suffering. You can rise up and ensure that your children and future generations will be able to claim our God-given right – our right to natural and everlasting health! Then, and only then, will America be restored to greatness!" (Applause, applause.)

Avoiding Breast Cancer

Sunlight and Vitamin D

People who live in warm and sunny climates have less risk of developing some cancers, and it's been documented that people in northeastern states have a higher mortality rate from breast, colon and other types of cancer than people living in southern states. The death rate is directly related to the amount of solar radiation received, and the closer you get to the equator, the lower your risk of breast-cancer death.(335,336,337) Now researchers are trying to determine just how much vitamin D is needed for breast cancer prevention. Cedric Garland, DPH of the University of California San Diego suggested in the American Association for Cancer Research annual meeting in 2006 that increasing intake of vitamin D can lower the chance of developing breast cancer by 10 percent to 50 percent.(338)

The average vitamin D intake in the U.S. is 320 IU/day, which is only about one tenth the amount to be associated with a 50 percent reduction of breast cancer incidence. "We believe that higher doses of vitamin D will product proportionate reductions in the incidence of breast cancer. . .It's nearly impossible to get enough vitamin D in your diet alone," Garland says. An 8-ounce glass of milk contains only 100 IU of vitamin D and a serving of cereal has 20 IU. He recommends taking 1,000 IU of vitamin D (in the form of D_3, not D_2), especially during the winter months. By comparison, someone who spends 10 to 15 minutes in the sun on a sunny day without sunscreen can absorb 2,000 to 5,000 IU of vitamin D if 40 percent of the body is exposed. (339,340)

Researchers in Canada have also shown vitamin D to be important in breast cancer prevention, and found that exposure to sunshine early in life (especially between the ages of 10 to 19) had a significant effect on whether a woman gets breast cancer later in life. "Current thinking is that exposures during adolescence or before a full-term pregnancy may have a greater effect, as that is when breast tissue is going through the most rapid development," Dr. Knight says. In addition, taking vitamin D-rich cod liver oil between ages 10 and 19 reduced breast cancer risk by about 35 percent later in life.(341)

Magnesium

Magnesium is critical for the proper function of the endocrine system, which makes and balances the hormones that play such an important role in breast cancer genesis. Specifically, if the body does not receive enough magnesium, the delicate balance of hormones will suffer. And since about 75 percent of all breast cancers are stimulated by estrogen, it's important that it be maintained at its proper level.

Magnesium is necessary for the production of cholesterol, from which all the sex hormones (estrogen, testosterone) as well as aldosterone and DHEA (dehydroepiandrosterone) are made (another reason you need cholesterol). It's vital for the proper function of the pituitary gland (the *master gland*), which helps balance hormones, and the pineal gland, which helps regulate sleep. Since an overabundance of estrogen is a primary cause of breast cancer, it's important to keep all the hormones in balance.

Since magnesium is instrumental in the regulation of hormones, it not only plays a role in breast cancer, but is also important during menopause. During menopause, the natural secretion of estrogen is decreased, and signs of aging and discomfort are common. Dr. Norman Shealy, an expert on anti-aging, says he has found that through the transdermal (across the skin) use of magnesium, women have reported complete abatement of menopausal symptoms and some have even returned to their menstrual cycle.(342)

This improvement did not occur when magnesium was taken orally, but by spreading a product called *magnesium oil* on the skin and letting it soak in. It's been reported that serum magnesium levels can be raised higher and faster using this product since it doesn't cause diarrhea as large oral doses of magnesium does. In addition, magnesium oil contains magnesium chloride, the form of magnesium the body assimilates most readily. (See the Resource Guide)

Dr. Melvyn R. Werbach believes that borderline magnesium levels seen in premenstrual syndrome (PMS) can explain most of the symptoms associated with it. Double-blind studies have shown that magnesium supplementation has relieved these symptoms. Dr Werbach says that a marginal deficiency of magnesium can deplete levels of dopamine, impair estrogen metabolism, increase insulin secreting and cause the enlargement of the adrenal cortex, which produces many hormones including sex hormones, stress hormones, and blood-sugar hormones.(343)

It's estimated that up to 80 percent of American women experience hot flashes or other symptoms of menopause vs. just 10 percent of Japanese women. It's thought that this is probably due to the fact that the Japanese eat so much seaweed, which is very high in magnesium.

Since a magnesium deficiency can cause blood vessels to go into spasm thus causing a menstrual migraine, additional magnesium can help delay or eliminate these headaches. Magnesium taken orally during the last 15 days of the menstrual cycle has been shown to sometimes prevent these types of migraines.(344) Of course, each woman's body is different and has different needs, so there's no guarantee just taking a few magnesium pills will prevent a headache. Based on the research, using the magnesium oil is much more effective than oral supplementation. In fact, Dr. Sircus says that only one-third to one-half of dietary magnesium is absorbed into the body, and we need about 1,000 mgs a day just to keep up with daily demands. So he highly recommends using the magnesium oil to obtain this kind of intake.

Eating a diet high in magnesium (drinking fresh vegetable juices) and avoiding things that rob your body of magnesium (alcohol and all drugs) is still the best way to go. All in all, magnesium is a great mood enhancer, muscle relaxant and even helps in temperature regulation (helps those hot flashes). So it may be helpful to give nature's tranquillizer a try.

Iodine

Animals in an iodine deficient state are more likely to develop breast cancer, and the longer the diet is deficient in iodine, the more likely it will develop.(345,346,347) An iodine deficiency also encourages breast tissue to respond more to estrogen, which, we know, will increase the likelihood of cancer.(348)

Unfortunately, the American diet is lacking in iodine, and the recommended daily allowance (RDA: 150 mcg/day for adult male to 290 mcg/d for lactating woman), many experts now believe is too low. Dr. David Brownstein, a leading proponent of iodine, says, "Iodine deficiency, coupled with exogenous estrogens from the diet (e.g. hormones fed to animals) or chemicals in the environment (e.g., phthalates from plastics), could explain the epidemic of breast cancer that is occurring in this country (as well as in many other western countries)."[349]

I already mentioned that the Japanese eat a large amount of seaweed, which is rich in magnesium. Seaweed is also one of the best sources of iodine, allowing the Japanese to consume about 13.8 mg of iodine per day. This is 100 times more than the U.S. RDA for iodine. Japanese women have remarkably lower levels of breast cancer (and endometrial and ovarian cancers as well). Further, when Japanese women move to the U.S., their rates of mortality from breast, endometrial and ovarian cancer increases. Other studies show that countries with higher intakes of iodine have lower rates of breast cancer (and goiter); and countries with lower intakes of iodine have higher incidences of breast cancer (and goiter).[350]

In contrast, the average daily intake of iodine in the U.S. is just 240 micrograms (or 0.24 mg) of iodine, which is less than 2 percent of what the Japanese consume.[351] Dr Donald W. Miller, Jr., noted that about 15 percent (one in seven) women in the U.S. probably suffers from iodine deficiency and one in seven American women now develop breast cancer. Thirty years ago, only one in twenty women developed breast cancer, and the consumption of iodine was significantly greater.

These observations are consistent with medical research. Studies show that high intake of iodine is associated with low incidence of breast cancer, and low intake of iodine is associated with high incidence of breast cancer.[352,353]

Is there a connection between iodine consumption and breast cancer? Many experts now believe so. But it's not like this link is anything new: The relationship between low iodine levels and breast cancer was noted in modern medical journals as early as 1960, and the first time iodine was used to treat breast cancer was in 1896.[354,355]

Breast tissue is one of the body's main storage and utilization sites for iodine. But since the thyroid gland is the organ that uses and needs iodine the most, when the diet is deficient in iodine, the thyroid gets it first, and the breast tissue (and other tissues) has to wait. Since iodine is so important to proper functioning of breast tissue, a supply that more than meets the needs of the thyroid gland is needed. How much is this? Brownstein says adults should consume between 6 mg and 50 mg of iodine per day.

Besides cancer, iodine is important in another disease of the breast, which may turn into cancer – that being fibrocystic breast disease. This disease has increased from 3 percent in the 1920s to 90 percent of women today. The symptoms include fluid-filled cysts, fibrosis with tenderness and breast pain that lasts more than six days during the menstrual cycle. In short, there are lumps that are hard and painful.

Russian researchers reported that 71 percent of women who had the disease were healed by taking 50 mg per day of potassium iodide (KI). Other studies in America found similar findings (70 percent success rate) when iodine was given in therapeutic amounts.(356,357,358)

Dr. Brownstein also reports that iodine is extremely effective in treating and preventing fibrocystic breasts, and that iodine has been the most researched mineral in treating this disease. He says that after iodine supplementation is started, women typically see a rapid improvement with the cysts and pain disappearing within a few months. If there's no improvement by then, then the disease is probably caused by other factors.(359)

Guy Abraham, M.D., Jorge Flechas, M.D., and David Brownstein, M.D. started what they called the Iodine Project in 2003 to study the effects of higher than normal consumptions of iodine. In this study, volunteers took 12.5 mg to 50 mg of iodine a day (those with diabetes took 100 mg/day). Patients reported a greater sense of well being, increased energy, lifting of "brain fog," need for less sleep, improved skin complexion, more regular bowel movements, feeling warmer in cold environments, reversal of fibrocystic disease, less need for insulin for diabetics, hypothyroid patients needing less thyroid medication, migraine relief and relief of fibromyalgia symptoms. Although the results are not yet conclusive, they also noted a reduction in the incidence of breast cancer.(360) The authors say that it's hard to overdose on iodine, and ingestion of up to 5 grams a day have shown no ill effects for short periods. But, some people are oversensitive to it, so any supplementation should be done under the supervision of a health care professional.

There are different kinds of iodine. The drug-store tincture of iodine should never be taken internally. The forms that can be taken orally are potassium iodide (KI), super-saturated potassium iodide (SSKI), Lugol's solution (a combination of iodide and iodine, which some doctors think is better than taking iodide alone), Iodoral (Lugol's solution in pill form), and nascent iodine (an atomic from rather than the molecular form the other forms are in – supposedly easier to absorb and what I recommend). Again, only take iodine supplements under the supervision of a health care professional since too much can cause hyperthyroidism and goiter although overdosing is rare. Also, if you have had a history of goiter or other thyroid problems, or are currently taking thyroid medication, only take iodine supplements under a doctor's care.

A simple, but not that precise way to see if you're low on iodine is to do the iodine patch-test. Get a bottle or Tincture of Iodine (the original orange-colored solution, not the clear solution and not *Povidone* Solution) from the drug store. **Warning: Do NOT take this internally. This is NOT the same as SSKI or Lugol's Solution, so do not use it the same way. Tincture of Iodine is for external use only!**

Paint a patch of it an inch wide by about 3 inches long on the underside of your forearm or on your abdomen or inner thigh. Do this right before you go to bed. In the morning, look at the patch and notice if there's any color left – it may be grayish, yellow or bright yellow orange (like when you first painted it). If there's no color left at all, then you are definitely iodine deficient. If there's color left, observe it during the day to see if and when it leaves. The quicker it leaves, the more deficient in iodine you are. If all the color isn't gone by bedtime, you're not iodine deficient.

You can also get the iodine-loading test done that is much more accurate. It involves taking a dose of iodine and seeing how much is excreted the next morning. You can order the test kit for this from FFP Labs at (877) 900-5556 or www.helpmythyroid.com (828) 684-3233.

Foods rich in iodine include seafood, vegetables grown in iodine rich soils, seaweeds of all kinds, milk (sometimes), yogurt, eggs, strawberries, and raw sunflower seeds. The best source to get iodine is from wild-caught saltwater fish and shellfish. You can figure that 4 - 6 ounces of fish per day will supply you with about half the RDA of 150 mcg. About 2 grams of iodized salt will supply the RDA. Another good source of iodine is seaweeds (kelp, dulse, nori). However, these are also sometimes high in arsenic (which is bad), and have a high salt content. So if you think you might need more iodine, supplementation may be the best way to go. Remember, many researchers consider the iodine RDA too low, so you probably need more in your diet.

Certain foods contain *goitrogenic* compounds – so named because they encourage goiter by blocking the absorption or utilization of iodine. These include cruciferous vegetables (cabbage, broccoli, Brussels sprouts, and such), soybean products, peanuts, mustard and millet. So if you're trying to increase your iodine, or you have thyroid problems, cutting back on these foods is advisable. Cooking these foods is believed to eliminate their goitrogenic effects.

Iodine metabolism is dependant on the trace mineral selenium, (discussed in the chapter on the prostate gland), so adequate supplies of it must be available. Vitamin A, E, and zinc deficiencies can exacerbate the effects of iodine deficiency. So you can see that a nutrient dense diet is necessary to ensure iodine utilization. Some drugs and food coloring agents also have a negative effect iodine metabolism.

Severe iodine deficiency during pregnancy or infancy causes cretinism, a condition characterized by hypothyroidism. This can lead to the failure of the thyroid gland or severe mental retardation, stunted physical growth, deafness, and spasticity. If discovered in its initial stages, cretinism can be corrected with iodine supplementation. Breast milk contains iodine and lactating women require extra iodide. Dr. Flechas believes that since iodine is so important to the developing fetus and for the first three years of life, the mother should supplement her diet during pregnancy and, if nursing, for the first two years after pregnancy.(361) Goiter or thyroid nodules can be detected with a thyroid ultrasound.

Food for Thought

Iodine consumption in the U.S. has plummeted over the last 30 years. This is chiefly due to two factors: One: Since 1924, iodine has been added to regular table salt (providing 76 mcg of iodine per gram of salt) to decrease the number of people getting goiter (disease of the thyroid gland). But over the last 25 years, those who use iodized table salt have decreased their consumption of it by 65 percent due to concerns that salt raises blood pressure. In addition, about 45 percent of American households buy salt without iodine added and some health-conscious people now buy sea salt, which, surprisingly contains only trace amounts of iodine. So if you use sea salt, you need to get your iodine somewhere else.

Since vegetables grown on land only contain trace amounts of iodine (0.001 mg/g vs. 0.5-8.0 mg/g in marine plants), and there is insufficient iodine in meat and dairy, supplementation, I believe, is warranted. The kinds of diets that may cause iodine deficiency are diets without ocean fish or sea vegetables, diets without enough iodized salt, diets high in bakery products that contain bromide (see below), and vegan and vegetarian diets. It's interesting to note that salt restrictive diets are more prevalent in the elderly and that 25 percent of the people over age 60 will become senile as a result of hypothyroidism, which, you know, may be a result of iodine deficiency. So people in the very age group that needs iodine the most may be being told to avoid the condiment that usually supplies it.

Two: In the 1960s and 1970s iodine was added to commercial baking products as a dough conditioned, but in the 1980s it was replaced with bromine due to concerns the high levels of iodine (there was about 150 mcg of iodine in one slice of bread) would cause malfunctioning of the thyroid gland. But there's a problem with that: Bromine (in a class of elements called *halogens*, as are iodine, chlorine, and fluorine), competes with iodine in the body. So it interferes with iodine utilization in the thyroid as well as wherever else iodine is used and concentrated (e.g. breast tissue). For this reason, bromine is known as a goitrogen (promotes the formation of goiter). Not good.

Bromine is itself a toxic substance that the body has absolutely no use for and, is a known carcinogen to the breast. And yet they add it to bakery products??? Come on. Those donuts don't sound as appealing now, do they?

And men, don't think you're immune from the ravages of iodine deficiency. Dr. Brownstein says that iodine deficiency is a major cause of prostate cancer in American men. The same pattern of cancer of the prostate in Japanese men vs. American men is similar to that of breast cancer in Japanese women vs. American women; and Japanese men who move to the U.S. start getting prostate cancer just like the American men.(362)

Bromine (or in its reduced form of bromide) is pretty nasty stuff. It can cause you to feel dull and apathetic and make it difficult to concentrate, causes depression, headaches, and irritability. It's used to fumigate crops, as an antibacterial agent for pools and hot tubs and used to kill termites and other pests. Besides being used in the baking industry, it's also used in the production of vegetable oils (brominated vegetable oils), which are oftentimes used in soft drinks and sports drinks. In fact, bromine toxicity has been reported from the ingestion of *Mountain Dew, AMP Energy Drink*, and some *Gatorade* products.(363) I ask you, doesn't anyone at the FDA read these reports??? How can something that's used to kill boll weevils and termites be allowed in sports drinks and soda pop? And we wonder why our youth can't get motivated to do anything. One more thing on bromine – it once was used in many medicines, but was removed because of its known toxicity. But it's still in some medicines to treat asthma (inhalers) and bladder dysfunction. Go figure.

Fluoride is another halogen that is evil. (I had evil on my mind since I just mentioned boll weevils.) You'll learn all about fluoride in the chapter on osteoporosis. It also competes with iodine, so it can cause thyroid problems. It's a major ingredient in antidepressants such as *Paxil*, and it's been documented that women on the SSRI antidepressants that use fluoride have in increased risk of breast cancer.(364) That's not to mention that fluoride is added to our water supply, toothpaste, and mouthwash under the mistaken belief that it strengthens teeth. Instead, it's helping to create an iodine deficiency that's leading to epidemics in breast and prostate cancer.

While we're at it, we might as well look at the last halogen on the list, chlorine. Now *chloride*, is abundant in the body: There's a lot of it naturally in the extra cellular fluid, and it's needed to help break down protein during digestion. But *chlorine* is toxic, and has been linked to birth defects, cancer, reproductive disorders, and immune system breakdown.(365) (See chapter on birth defects.) Since our drinking water is treated with chlorine to disinfect it, we're exposed to it quite often. If that's not enough, you can always get more of this yummy toxic compound by using *Splenda* (sucralose), the sugar-substitute that is nothing but chlorinated table sugar. (They joyously proclaim in their ads – "It's NOT sugar!" No, it's even worse!)

Some other good things about iodine:

Iodine is a potent anti-oxidant, much along the lines of vitamin C. Iodine induces apoptosis, which is programmed cell death. Why is that good? Because when cells keep growing uncontrollably without dying in their normal lifecycle as they should, cancer results. So iodine is an anti-cancer agent.

Iodine removes toxic chemicals and biological toxins from the body. It rids the body of toxic fluoride and bromide, and even mercury and other heavy metals.(366) Iodine is needed by the main thyroid hormones, T_3 and T_4, and if there isn't enough of it, hypothyroidism will result. Oftentimes, reversing an iodine deficiency can correct a hypothyroid condition. Albert Szent Gyorgi (1983-1986), the physician who discovered vitamin C and winner of the Nobel Prize, has said, "When I was a medical student, iodine in the form of KI was the universal medicine. Nobody knew what it did, but it did something and did something good. We students used to sum up the situation in this little rhyme: If ye don't know where, what, and why. . . Prescribe ye then K and I"

Doctors used to prescribe iodine for many diseases, and in large doses. The 11th edition of the *Encyclopedia Britannica* published in 1911 stated regarding iodine salts (like potassium iodide), ". . .they possess the power of driving out impurities from the blood and tissues. Most notably is this the case with the poisonous products of syphilis. This disease yields in the most rapid and unmistakable fashion to iodides, so much so that the administration of these salts is at present the best means of determining whether, for instance, a cranial tumor be syphilitic or not."(367)

Doctors used to use potassium iodide in doses starting at 1.5 gm to 3 gm and even up to 10 gm a day. Gram amounts of KI are still being used by dermatologists to treat inflammatory dermatoses. They start with an iodine dose of 900 mg/day, followed by weekly increases up to 6 grams a day as tolerated. Side effects of too much iodine generally don't happen and if they do, are mild: acne;, metallic taste in mouth; sneezing; excess saliva; and frontal sinus pressure.

Remember the ways to tell if you actually need iodine: the simple patch test described above, and a lab test you can get via Jorge D. Flechas, M.D. It costs about $90 and involves a urine sample. To order go to www.helpmythyroid.com or call (828) 684-3233. For more on iodine, I recommend the book by Dr. Brownstein, *Iodine: Why You Need It, Why You Can't Live Without It.*

Maybe we need more iodine than the typical diet supplies. Maybe it can help you avoid breast cancer, prostate cancer, fibrocystic breast disease, or hypothyroidism. Maybe something so simple – supplying the body with the raw materials it needs to function properly – is all we need to do to stay healthy.

Diet

Broccoli, Brussels sprouts, kale and cauliflower contain a compound that can inhibit the growth of cancer cells, including breast cancer. It's been shown that organically grown vegetables contain higher levels of the cancer-fighting class of compounds called flavonoids. This was reported in the *Journal of Agricultural and Food Chemistry*, the *Journal of the American Chemical Society*, the world's largest scientific society.(368,369)

There's evidence that women who consume foods rich in omega-3 fatty acids over many years may be less likely to develop breast cancer, and the risk of dying from breast cancer may be significantly less for those who eat a lot of omega-3s from fish and brown kelp seaweed (common in Japan). The research shows that the balance between omega-3 and omega-6 fatty acids (which should be 2:1) is an important role in the development and growth of breast cancer. Eating fish or taking a good fish oil supplement certainly can't hurt.

As with any cancer and any condition of ill-health, sugar in any shape or form should be avoided. In addition, consumption of a lot of sweet or starch food all at once causes a spike in insulin secretion, which is thought to accelerate the growth of breast cancer cells. Cinnamon has beneficial effects cinnamon has on blood sugar levels, so even though there's been no research on cinnamon as far as breast cancer is concerned, it stands to reason that if a spike in insulin accelerates the growth of breast cancer cells, consuming cinnamon might help in this regard. Garlic also has been shown to retard breast cancer growth. A study in France reported in the *European Journal of Epidemiology* showed breast cancer risks for 345 women decreased the more they consumed garlic and onions.(370)

There have been claims that soy offers protection against breast cancer. But, as we're learning, soy may be good for fixing nitrogen in soil, but nature didn't intend it for human consumption (more later). An article in the *Journal of Nutrition*, reported there were no significant differences in breast tissue density (an increase in breast tissue density is associated with increased risk for breast cancer) between women who consumed soy regularly over a two year period and those who didn't. In fact, women who consumed more soy during their lives had a higher percentage densities than women whose diet included little soy.(371)

Researchers have reported that women who ate flame-broiled meat more than twice a month had an increased risk of developing breast cancer. Not just that, but women who consumed the most well-done meat compared to those who ate less-cooked meat were twice as likely to develop breast cancer.(372) The problem comes from cooking meat at high temperatures (by any method), and by charring the meat during grilling. Charred meat contains heterocyclic amines, which are believed to promote many types of cancer, not just breast cancer.

A study at the Harvard Medical School said that giving girls under five years old one portion of chips (fried) increases their risk of developing breast cancer later in life by 27 percent. Deep frying is the culprit here, so I'm sure that French fries (a favorite food of kids), would probably do the same thing.(373)

It's also thought that breast tissue is especially vulnerable to damage from the carcinogens in tobacco smoke during puberty when breast cells are actively dividing. Second hand smoke exposure during this time may increase the risk of breast cancer later.

Exercise

Exercise is important to avoid breast cancer, if you have breast cancer, and recovering from breast cancer. One study of 65,000 women showed that high levels of physical activity from ages 12 to 22 had a 23 percent lower risk of getting breast cancer risk before menopause (one-quarter of all breast cancers are diagnosed in women before menopause). The lead investigator Graham Colditz, M.D., Dr. P.H said, "We don't have a lot of prevention strategies for premenopausal breast cancer, but our findings clearly show that physical activity during adolescence and young adulthood can pay off in the long run by reducing a woman's risk of early breast cancer."[374]

Another study showed that women who have had breast cancer and walk or did the equivalent of walking at a pace of 2-3 mph improve their survival rate (compared to inactive women) depending on how long they exercised: one to three hours/week resulted in a 20 percent lower death rate; three to five hours/week decreased the risk of death by 50 percent; and five to eight hours/week resulted in a decrease in death rate of 44 percent. After 10 years, of the women who exercised about half an hour per day (three to five hours per week), 92 percent were still alive. Of those who got less than an hour a week, only 86 percent were still alive.[375,376]

Two of the best exercises you can do to help avoid breast cancer is swimming (try to do it in water that is not chlorinated) and arm circles (hold your arms out like you're flying and circle them around). This is because these exercises move the areas right next to your arm pits where major lymph glands are. As you move these areas, the lymph circulates better and any toxins in these areas are removed. Breast cancer is much more serious when it spreads into the lymph glands, so doing these exercises greatly improves your chances of avoiding the cancer or reversing it, and it may help counteract the effects of wearing a bra.

Breast Implants and Breast Cancer

Currently, about 300,000 women a year (about two million since it started in 1962), have had breast augmentation surgery. Eighty percent of these surgeries are for purely cosmetic reasons, while 20 percent are for breast reconstruction after breast cancer. The first implants used in 1962 when this surgery began, were filled with silicone. So many problems occurred with them that the leading manufacturer at the time, Dow Corning Corp. faced 19,000 lawsuits related to their silicone implants, resulting in its filing for Chapter 11 bankruptcy in 1995.

Subsequently, silicone implants were banned by the FDA, being replaced with saline ones. But in 2006, the FDA reversed its stance and has approved them for use in women over the age of 22. Dr. Sidney Wolfe, who works for Public Citizen, a national non-profit public interest organization, said, "In terms of adverse safety and health information known at the time of approval – such as high rates of rupture, the need for repeat surgery and clear evidence of lymph node infiltration and damage by leaked silicone – silicone gel breast implants are the most defective medical device ever approved by the FDA. The approval makes a mockery of the legal standard that requires 'reasonable assurance of safety'" (377)

But do breast implants cause breast cancer? They do interfere with mammograms, preventing about 10 percent of the tissue to be adequately scanned. (Of course, you should never get a mammogram, but use thermography or sonography instead.) The pressure exerted on the implant during the test may in fact rupture the implant.

It appears that there's no real difference in breast cancer incidences or mortality between women who have breast implants and those who don't.(378,379) But this research also showed that women who have had the surgery (strictly for cosmetic reasons), had two to three times higher rates for brain and respiratory cancers.(380) Another study of 23,500 women found that women with breast implants had a suicide rate 73 percent higher than women in the general population.(381) The researchers think that the high suicide rate is due to the type of women who gets the surgery, not to the implants: the psychological profile of women who receive breast implants is characterized by lack of self-confidence, low self-esteem and more frequent mental illnesses such as depression.

CHAPTER IV

Cardiovascular Diseases

Heart Disease

Heart disease or cardiovascular disease has been the perennial most potent killer of Americans every year since 1900 (except for the year 1918), although cancer is now killing just about as many.

Food for Thought

Actually, *cause of death* statistics can be misleading since only one cause of death is generally listed on a death certificate. This means that if an individual had an advanced case of cancer (that would have caused their death within the next 12 months), but died of heart disease first, only cancer is listed on their death certificate. What does this mean? We're probably in worse shape than these simplistic statistics indicate.

In 2002, cardiovascular diseases claimed 927,448 American lives (that's 38 percent of all deaths and one death every 34 seconds) and 70,100,000 Americans had one or more forms of cardiovascular disease.

Cardiovascular diseases are:

- High blood pressure (65 million Americans have it)
- Coronary heart disease (13 million Americans have it), including
    - Myocardial infarction (heart attacks: 7.1 million Americans have had one)
    - Angina pectoris (chest pain: 6.4 million Americans have it)
- Stroke (5.4 million Americans have had one)

Nearly one in three adults has high blood pressure, and 30 percent of these don't realize it. From 1992 to 2002, the death rate from high blood pressure increased 26.8 percent, and the number of deaths rose 56.6 percent. People with lower educational and income levels tend to have higher levels of blood pressure (as they are more likely to smoke and eat junk food).[1]

Normal resting blood pressure is 120/80. The upper number is the systolic pressure, or the pressure in the arteries when the heart beats. The lower number is the diastolic pressure, or the pressure in the arteries in between heartbeats. If your pressure is over 140/90, you are considered to have high blood pressure.

How do you know you're at risk for heart disease? Here's a few ways to assess your cardiovascular health to determine if you're at high risk for heart disease:

- If your systolic blood pressure is above 140 mm HG.
- If you smoke or have smoked in the last five years.
- If your resting heart rate is above 70 beats/minute.
- If after exercise your heart rate does not drop by 12 beats or more after one minute of rest.
- If your gums bleed when your brush your teeth.
- If your waist size in inches is greater than ½ your height in inches.
- If your resting oral temperature is between 98.4 and 98.8 degrees Fahrenheit (women should measure temperature on the second or third day of their period after the flow begins). Taking your temperature indicates if your thyroid is functioning correctly. A lower than normal temperature indicates low thyroid function (hypothyroid), which will cause abnormal lipid metabolism, which affects the cardiovascular system. Such a large percentage of the public now has a lower than normal (98.6°F) body temperature, that the medical establishment has considered lowering what is considered normal. Just one more way in which medicine can mislead us as far as what is believed to be healthy. This temperature change is possibly due to the reduced thyroid function and metabolism caused by the high levels of numerous toxic substances in our bodies.

Cardiovascular disease is the greatest killer of women, killing one every minute. Women are two to three times more likely to have coronary heart disease after menopause than before menopause. Cardiovascular disease also ranks as the number two killer of children under age 15: In 2002 about 210,000 cardiovascular procedures were performed on children. Congenital cardiovascular malformations are the major cause of problems in children.

About 6.4 million adults suffer from chest pains and 400,000 new cases of it occur each year. Nearly one in three adults has high blood pressure. Each year, 500,000 new people have a stroke and 200,000 have a second or third. Females account for 61.5 percent of all stroke victims. The direct and indirect costs of these diseases cost America $393.5 billion in 2005.[2]

Food for Thought

Eating fresh, raw (preferably organic) grapefruit or fresh squeezed grapefruit juice or fresh cucumber and cucumber juice helps lower blood pressure. Fresh garlic helps to normalize blood pressure, whether it's low or high. As early as the 1920s, studies have shown the beneficial effects of garlic on the cardiovascular system, as have recent studies.[3,4,5]

A study published in the *Journal of Complementary and Integrative*

Medicine said,

"Garlic is well reported to scavenge oxidants, increase super oxide dismutase, catalase, glutathione peroxidase, and glutathione levels, as well as inhibit lipid peroxidation and inflammatory prostaglandins. . .Garlic has been shown to inhibit LDL oxidation, platelet aggregation, arterial plaque formation, decrease homocysteine, lower blood pressure, and increase microcirculation, which is important in diabetes, where micro vascular changes increase heart disease and dementia risks."[6]

One study showed a reduction in systolic pressure, while others showed significant decreases in diastolic pressure with garlic consumption.[7]

Having a salad with fresh cucumbers, tomatoes, onion, broccoli, and celery (lots of good minerals) every day for lunch would help keep your blood pressure in check. Add some fresh raw nuts or seeds to this salad, and you have a nice nutritious, filling lunch. Make a dressing with organic cold-pressed olive oil, organic apple cider vinegar, fresh ground pepper, some mineral water, ½ clove garlic, sliver of ginger, and raw honey.

Starting your day with a glass of fresh squeezed grapefruit juice is good (no store bought juice). Please note, that consuming grapefruit may cause prescription drugs to have more of an effect, so check with your physician before you drink the juice or eat many grapefruits.

A study published in the journal *Circulation* reported that patients eating large amounts of almonds (a quarter of their total daily caloric intake) reduced their low density lipoprotein (LDL) by over 9 percent. Four tablespoons of honey (should be raw) in 2 glasses of water was shown to improve the antioxidant levels in blood, which helps with heart health.[8] Remember, most honey is heated, which ruins its nutritional value. Be sure to use raw honey. (See Resource Guide)

Although there is no clinical proof that apple cider vinegar brings down blood pressure in humans, there are numerous studies that point in this direction.[9,10,11] Apple cider vinegar is rich in potassium, which is known to lower blood pressure. There are so many reports or apple cider vinegar helping the heart and circulation that it's definitely worth considering it. Certainly, replacing your commercial, pasteurized, filtered vinegar with the wholesome kind can't do any harm. Natural, raw honey is also believed to be very beneficial for the cardiovascular system. Dr. Rubaiul Murshed, a Healthcare Management Specialist, says,

"Pure honey improves cardiac activity. It has a very useful effect on the weakened heart muscle in various types of cardiac diseases. It causes veins to expand and improves circulation through coronary arteries. The heart muscle works continuously and needs glucose. . .Honey contains a unique mixture of glucose and fructose that are quick and easy to absorb. it does not cause the sudden drop in blood sugar that is associated with refined sugars. Make a paste of honey and cinnamon powder, apply on bread or tea and take it regularly for breakfast. It reduces the cholesterol in the arteries and saves the patient from heart attack. Regular use. . .strengthens the heartbeat. . .the arteries and veins, which lose their flexibility. . .get revitalized. If two tablespoons of honey and three teaspoons of cinnamon powder mixed in 16 ounces of water are given to high cholesterol patients, it reduces the level of cholesterol n the blood by 10 percent within 2 hours."(12)

Congestive heart failure (CHF) is when the heart can't pump enough blood to meet the body's needs. It's one of the most common, costly, disabling and deadly diseases affecting more than 4.8 million Americans. Every day, 139 people die from CHF in the U.S. – that's almost 50,000 people a year. A full 10 percent of people over the age of 70 have CHF. "Once diagnosed with CHF, patients have a one in three chance of dying within one year, and a two in three chance of dying within five years."(13)

The major causes of CHF are narrowed arteries that supply blood to the heart, hypertension, heart valve disease, heart defects and disease of the heart muscle itself (cardiomyopathy). The early symptoms of CHF are shortness of breath, cough or a feeling of not being able to get a deep breath. So it's not surprising that many people think there's something else wrong, say, a breathing problem, unrelated to the heart. If you notice that mild exercise causes shortness of breath, you may have CHF. But, there may in fact be a breathing problem, that being, exercise induced asthma. So both need to be considered. (See the Asthma chapter.)

When CHF worsens, fluid backs up into the lungs and interferes with getting oxygen into the blood, which will cause difficulty breathing at rest (dyspnea) or at night (orthopnea). Sleeping can be improved by using several pillows or sleeping in a recliner. Swelling may occur in the legs, feet and ankles especially after prolonged sitting or standing.

The typical treatment of CHF is with drugs. ACE (angiotensin-converting enzyme) inhibitors, beta blockers, digitalis, diuretics, and vasodilators are often prescribed. Some of these may be necessary in crisis situations, but as we will see, there are natural and healthier ways to improve and strengthen the heart.

What causes CHF? Smoking and excessive alcohol consumption are major contributors but also harder drugs like cocaine can cause it. (*Ritalin* is pharmacologically identical to cocaine, so could giving it to kids be setting them up for CHF later in life?) Excess weight, high blood pressure, and having diabetes also stresses the heart, which can lead to CHF.

Food for Thought

It's interesting to note that research published in the *Journal of the American College of Cardiology* showed that CHF patients had higher than normal concentrations of heavy metals in their heart tissues than normal.

Some of these levels were amazingly high. Mercury was 22,000 times higher, antimony 12,000 times higher, and chromium 13 times higher. Patients with less severe heart problems (secondary dysfunction) had lower concentrations of these toxic minerals.[14] While the traditional medical community is pointing its finger at fat and cholesterol (discussed at length below), can it be that the heart muscles are simply being poisoned to death?

Clearly, something is wrong. You hear a lot on the news and in the papers about what causes heart disease and stroke and how to prevent them or lessen the risks. But is it correct and based on good science, or politics and money? We're going to find out.

Traditional medicine points the finger at saturated fat as the main cause of coronary heart disease. It supposedly accumulates and clogs the arteries. Smoking too is correctly blamed for causing a lot of heart and circulatory problems, but for now we will focus on diet.

Saturated fats are solid at room temperature and very stable. They are found in animal fats and tropical oils, and your body manufacturers them from carbohydrates.

Food for Thought

The *saturated* in saturated fats means that the fat molecule is saturated with hydrogen atoms (H), on a chain of carbon atoms (C), with no double bonds. This makes the chain of carbon atoms straight with no kinks, so the fat molecules can stack on top of the other easily. Examples are: butyric acid found in butter: $CH_3-CH_2-CH_2-COOH$ (or $CH_3-(CH_2)_2-COOH$); and stearic acid found in beef: $CH_3-(CH_2)_{16}-COOH$.

An *unsaturated* fat has fewer hydrogen atoms (it's not saturated with hydrogen atoms) in the chain, forcing some carbon atoms to have double bonds (shown by = in example below). This, although I can't show it graphically here, changes the angles of the bonds so that instead of the fat molecule being totally flat, there are bends where the double bonds are. These bends make stacking much less likely. An example is linoleic acid: $CH_3-(CH_2)_5=(CH)-(CH_2)-(CH)=(CH)-(CH_2)_6-COOH$.

When the bends in an unsaturated fat molecule are such that both ends of the molecule point in the same direction, let's say up, that molecule is in the *cis* configuration (*cis* from the Latin meaning *same.*)

If an unsaturated fat is hydrogenated (e.g. partially hydrogenated vegetable oil), or subjected to very high heat (482º F), the *cis* configuration is changed to a *trans* configuration causing the molecule to no longer have the same bend in it (*trans* from Latin meaning on the opposite side). This causes the *trans* fat to be pretty much straight and no longer bent. *Trans*-fats stack differently, causing a change in the melting point of the fat.

Where a cis-fat melts at 55º F (liquid at room and body temperature), the trans-fat version melts at 111º F (solid at room and body temperature). *Trans*-fats are broken down slower than *cis*-fats by enzymes in the body. Since a major fuel of the heart is fatty acids, an abundance of *trans*-fats may lower the ability of the heart to perform. So no matter what they tell you about margarine and other hydrogenated products being "heart-smart," you now know that this is not true at all.

Unnatural *trans*-fats are stickier than *cis*-fats, causing blood platelets to stick together more, increasing the likelihood of clotting, which may cause blockages in the blood vessels leading to heart attacks and strokes.

Since cell membranes throughout the body are largely composed of fat molecules, when *trans*-fats take the place of *cis*-fats in the membrane, the permeability of the membrane increases, making it possible for some things that are suppose to stay inside the cell get out, and some things that are suppose to stay outside the cell get in. This may lead to decreased cell viability and increased allergic reactions. About 95 percent of *trans*-fats in the diet come from partially hydrogenated vegetable oils.

Back in the 1950s it was first proposed that saturated fats and cholesterol in the diet cause coronary heart disease. The vegetable oil industry latched on to this idea and helped promote it as dietary gospel. They pointed to some studies that supposedly proved this hypothesis, but close inspection of these studies didn't show this correlation at all. One of the studies was The Framingham Heart Study. However, the director of the study said, ". . .the more saturated fat one ate, the more cholesterol one ate, the more calories one ate, the lower the person's serum cholesterol. . .we found that the people who ate the most cholesterol, ate the most saturated fat, ate the most calories, weighed the least and were the most physically active."[15]

Other evidence that saturated fats don't cause heart disease abounds, including numerous studies that show there is no relationship between high saturated fat diets and heart disease. One study in Britain of several thousand men asked one group to reduce saturated fat and cholesterol in their diets and to stop smoking. After one year, this group had 100 percent more deaths than the group that continued to eat a diet high in saturated fat and continued to smoke. Seventeen hundred patients with hardening of the arteries were surveyed by Dr. Michael DeBakey, the famous heart surgeon who performed the first heart-bypass operation in 1964. (He also operated on John F. Kennedy, Richard M. Nixon, and Lyndon B. Johnson.) He reported no relationship between the level of blood cholesterol and hardening of the arteries.[16]

A study published in the *Journal of the American Medical Association* in 2006 reported there was no benefit found for low-fat diets in preventing cardiovascular disease.[17] Another study published in the *Journal of Clinical Nutrition* found that low-fat diets were associated with 20 per cent lower calcium absorption than higher fat diets.[18] This indicates that a low-fat diet could be harmful for the elderly, considering the prevalence of osteoporosis, or for growing children who need calcium for bone and muscle development. Researchers have also found that people who eat low fat diets have weaker immune systems, and have no improvement in blood sugar levels, insulin levels or blood pressure levels.(19)

Examining certain cultures around the globe echoes these findings. People in northern India consume 17 times more animal fat than people in southern India, but have seven times less coronary heart disease. Eskimos eat a lot of fats from fish and marine animals, yet hardly ever have heart problems. A study of the long-lived people of Soviet Georgia shows that the people who ate the fattiest meat live the longest. In Okinawa, where the average life-span is one of the longest in the world, residents eat a lot of pork and seafood and do all their cooking in lard.(20)

Over the past 80 years, the amount of cholesterol the average American eats increased only about 1 percent, while the amount of vegetable oils we eat (margarine, shortening, refined oils) increased about 400 percent. The amount of animal fat we eat has declined 21 percent between 1910 and 1970. So if animal fats did in fact cause heart disease, we would expect the frequency of heart disease to have gone down. This is clearly not the case. In Japan since WWII, the amount of animal fat and protein the diet has increased while their life-span has gone up. The Japanese diet is typically not low-fat, and they eat eggs, pork, seafood, organ meats, chicken, and beef regularly. The French diet is loaded with eggs, butter, cheese, liver, and meats, so why is the rate of heart attacks for French men half that than American men? (145/100,000 French middle-aged men have heart attacks per year versus 315/100,000 middle-aged American men.) (21)

If you were to examine the plaque inside an artery, it is composed of about 74 percent unsaturated fat and only 26 percent saturated fat. Saturated fat makes up 50 percent of cell membranes, is important for calcium metabolism, protects the liver from toxins and alcohol, and is necessary for enhanced immune system function. To top it all off, the fat surrounding the heart itself is highly saturated and the preferred fuel for the heart is saturated fat. Why would nature do that if it was so bad? Unsaturated fats and polyunsaturated fats are touted as the answer to heart disease, but as the consumption of them increased over the years, so has heart disease. Most of the fats Americans eat these days are polyunsaturated fats from vegetable oils (soy, corn, safflower, and canola). There are three major problems with these fats.

First, they are highly unstable and go rancid easily. When this happens, free radicals form that attack cell membranes and red blood cells and damage DNA/RNA strands. One of the tissues these free radicals damages are the inside of arteries causing small wounds and scratches on the walls, which initiates plaque build up. That plaque will be composed mostly of unsaturated and polyunsaturated fats.

The second major problem with these fats is that they are not balanced correctly when it comes to two essential fats – omega-3 linolenic acid and omega-6 linoleic acid. If there's too much omega-6 fat, prostaglandin synthesis is disrupted, which can result in: the increased tendency to form blood clots; high blood pressure; depressed immune function; cancer; weight gain; infertility; and inflammation. Ideally, our diet should supply an omega-6 to omega-3 ratio of 1:1 (this was what it was in early human history). The typical American diet, however, has a ratio of between 20:1 and 50:1. This paves the way for heart disease. In order to avoid this, you should decrease your intake of fats that contain a lot of omega-6's such as any vegetable oil, and increase your consumption of the omega-3's such as from wild-caught fish and grass-fed beef, fish oil, krill oil and/or cod liver oil.

The third problem with unsaturated and polyunsaturated fats is the high percentage of *trans*-fatty acids in them when they are made into margarine and shortening. They do this with a process called hydrogenation. This turns the liquid oil (usually cottonseed, soy, corn, or canola oil) into a solid at room temperature. *Trans*-fatty acids rarely occur in nature, and are very harmful to the body. The body mistakes them for *cis*-fatty acids – the healthy, natural kind – and when they are incorporated into cell walls, they wreak havoc on the cell's metabolism. Hydrogenated fats are *trans*-fats and are associated with atherosclerosis (hardening of the arteries), diabetes, obesity, immune system dysfunction, low-birth-weight babies, birth defects, decreased visual acuity, sterility, and problems with bones and tendons. *Trans*-fat is the worst kind of fat you can eat, and it's everywhere: French fries; chips; baked goods; and anything made with partially hydrogenated oil, shortening or hydrogenated oil.

Food for Thought

The oils that are used to make margarine and shortening are processed in the cheapest ways possible, which destroys any nutritional value these oils may have had. The corn or safflower seed is first crushed and heated, then squeezed in a press using 10 to 20 tons/square inch pressure. All the while, heat and oxygen are degrading the oils. Then a solvent, usually hexane (a known carcinogen), is used to get the last drops of oil out. The hexane is boiled off, but some is left behind in the final product. BHT and BHA, two preservatives suspected of causing cancer, are added to replace the natural vitamin E that was lost during this torturous processing. During this process, the oils begin to smell rancid so they are then sent to a deodorization plant to burn off the foul smelling molecules while further harming the oils. Now the oils are finally ready to put into bottles or to be partially hydrogenated and made into margarine or shortening and sold to the unsuspecting consumer.

Margarine and shortening are made by taking vegetable oil and mixing it with tiny metal particles, usually nickel oxide. This mixture is pressurized with hydrogen gas after which starch and emulsifiers are mixed in. Then it's subjected to very high heat during a steam cleaning process to remove its unpleasant, rank odor. This looks gray, so the mixture is bleached, dyed, and artificial flavors are added. Finally, the mixture is compressed with high pressure into blocks or tubs.

Sounds like a great natural food, doesn't it? But we've been brainwashed into believing it's better than nature can provide and that eating butter – what it's supposed to replace – is a sin.

Trans-fats also lower your good cholesterol (HDL) and raise your bad cholesterol (LDL) and are known to clog arteries and contribute to Type II diabetes. Even the FDA says to keep your intake of *trans*-fat as low as possible.[22]

A diet composed of saturated and monounsaturated fat (butter, lard, coconut oil, olive oil) is what Americans ate in the early 1900s, and heart disease was rare. Now Americans eat a diet that is as high as 30 percent of calories from polyunsaturates, which is very unhealthy for your heart, brain, and everything else. Research shows that you should not consume more than 4 percent of calories as polyunsaturated fats. Small amounts of polyunsaturated oils are found in legumes, grains, nuts, green vegetables, fish, and olive oil.[23]

Is eating cholesterol a problem? Watching TV makes you think cholesterol is the grim reaper himself, with all the cholesterol lowering medications being advertised. Let's take a closer look.

Cholesterol is a large molecule that is in some animal foods (not vegetable foods), and is manufactured in the liver. It's manufactured there because the body needs it, and needs a pretty good amount of it. Cholesterol is required for a long list of vital operations your body performs every day including:

- Cell membrane integrity.
- Precursor to vital corticosteroids that help us handle stress, protect against heart disease, and cancer.
- Precursor to the sex hormones androgen, testosterone, estrogen and progesterone.
- Bile salts, vital for digestion and assimilation of fat, are made from cholesterol.
- Cholesterol is needed for proper brain function and mood enhancement: low cholesterol levels are found in people who are depressed, violent, suicide, or memory problems.
- Cholesterol is important for the maintenance of the intestinal wall.
- Cholesterol acts as a free radical scavenger and actually protects the heart and blood vessels from damage (inflicted by *trans*-fats).
- Cholesterol is a precursor to vitamin D when the body manufactures it from being exposed to sun. Vitamin D is important for healthy bones,

nerves, proper growth, mineral metabolism, muscle tone, insulin production, reproductive and immune system function.

Think back to the Framingham Heart Study that found that the more cholesterol consumed in the diet, the lower the cholesterol was in the blood. This study showed two important things: That a high cholesterol diet did not cause blood cholesterol to go up; and that the presence of cholesterol in the blood did not cause heart problems. Also consider that mother's milk is very high in cholesterol. Why? Babies need it for proper growth and development of the nerves and brain.

When cholesterol levels go up, it's not because you ate too much of it – it's because the body is producing more of this important substance to help itself heal. An elevated cholesterol level is not necessarily bad, and it is not the *cause* of heart problems. (It's similar to when the body produces a lot of adrenaline in order to handle stress.) So you cannot generally lower your cholesterol by eating less of it or taking drugs. You lower it by avoiding things that create the havoc that the cholesterol has been made to repair – like the damage caused from *trans*-fats and polyunsaturated fats, fried foods, and other denatured foods.

Cholesterol is highly overrated as a risk indicator for heart disease. Brian Vonk, M.D., has this to say about it:

> We get disease if cholesterol is too high or too low. But in the broad range of cholesterol levels from 180 to 240 there is no correlation with heart disease. Below 180 there is increased risk of hemorrhagic stroke, depression, and suicide. Above 240 there is increased risk for cardiovascular disease and ischemic stroke. Over age 70, elevated cholesterol and cardiovascular events no longer correlate. All told, total serum cholesterol alone is a poor indicator of cardiovascular disease. Half of all heart attack patients have normal total cholesterol levels.[24]

Low levels of cholesterol have been linked to stroke, depression, suicide, and aggressive behavior. Some researchers believe that LDL cholesterol levels below 135 are too low and that optimum levels are around 200.[25] But current medical advice says that a total cholesterol level of 200 is too high.

Food for Thought

It's interesting to note that the upper limit of total cholesterol considered normal used to be 220 mg/dL. Now it stands at 200 mg/dl. Simply changing the definition of high cholesterol, millions of Americans suddenly had elevated cholesterol levels – making them candidates for cholesterol lowering drugs.

One under-reported reason cholesterol levels may be high is due to an under active thyroid. This has been known since the 1930s. Once thyroid hormone is normalized, oftentimes cholesterol levels will often normalize as well.(26)

Triglycerides are a form of fat that comes from food and is found in blood. High triglycerides in the blood (above 400 mg/dl) can be a risk factor for heart disease, so it's important to lower them if they are. But how? Mainstream medicine says to cut down on the fat in your diet. But recent research points to the abundance of starches, sugars and alcohol in the diet rather than fat. In a study published in the *American Society of Clinical Nutrition*, the authors state: "Short-term studies consistently show that raising the carbohydrate content of the diet increases serum triacylglycerol concentrations. . .starches, sugars (particularly sucrose and fructose) tend to increase serum triacylglycerol concentrations by around 60 percent"(27)

What happens is that the grain and sugar based carbohydrates you eat get converted to fat, and circulate in the blood. This not only raises blood fat, but the excess fat gets deposited in the body, and you get – fat! So a good way to help your heart, arteries, and eliminate excess body fat is to stop eating these types of carbohydrates (sugar and all white flour products – bagels, bread, pizza, muffins, and so on). There are, however, some very healthy carbohydrates such as broccoli, cauliflower, spinach, asparagus, red peppers, and many other colorful vegetables.

High levels of triglycerides may also indicate liver problems, an under-active thyroid gland, diabetes, pancreatitis, and kidney disease. All these are usually caused by a diet too low in protein and good fats, and too high in the starchy carbohydrates. Conversely, low triglycerides (less than 10 mg/dl) may indicate malnutrition, a diet too low in fat, an overactive thyroid, or mal-absorption.

Food for Thought

With all the talk about low carb, high protein diets, you may be tempted to drink one of those high protein shakes that dieting programs sell or that you get at the health food store. Please realize that none of these concoctions are good, healthy, sources of protein. Most of the time these products are loaded with soy, and other fractionated, highly processed foods. You may be replacing carbohydrates by consuming them, but your liver and kidneys will suffer in the long run because of all the impurities in them.

A rule-of-thumb for consuming anything. . .the less processed the better. Go have a steak, some eggs, chicken, beef jerky, or nuts and seeds. These are less processed foods more in line with what nature intended. Maybe not as cool, but definitely better for you.

While we're on the topic of convenience foods made to look healthy, it's interesting to note that the founder of the *PowerBar* company, nutritionist Brian Maxwell, died of a heart attack at the age of 51. The *PowerBar* he created is loaded with carbohydrates and high-fructose corn syrup is the main ingredient. Yes, it's good for energy production in the short-run, but that ingredient and other highly processed ingredients make this energy bar (and 99 percent of any manufactured energy bar) a hazard to your health. Incidentally, Mr. Maxwell created the *PowerBar* to help him finish running marathon races. He was at one time the third ranked runner in the world. Just goes to show you that exercise is not the only thing, or even the primary thing, that will keep you healthy and that well intentioned and well educated people don't always get things right and don't always know the truth. That's why I highly encourage everyone to stop and evaluated any health information based on their own research, observations, and common sense.

A popular medical treatment for high cholesterol involves using drugs called statins (*Lipitor, Zocor, Mevacor,* and *Pravachol*) which inhibit its production. Statins are so effective in lowering cholesterol, they can lower it by 50 points or more. The medical establishment and media have been so successful scaring people into believing high cholesterol leads to heart attacks that an estimated 16 million Americans are taking *Lipitor*, the most popular of these mediations. The drug companies claim that 36 million Americans are candidates for statin drug therapy.(28)

But there are numerous and serious side effects to these drugs. Muscle pain and weakness or wasting (called *rhabdomyolysis*) is the most common complaint, probably caused because CoQ_{10} is depleted by these drugs. The drug companies claims only two percent of people experience this, but an independent study showed that 98 percent of patients taking *Lipitor* and one third of the patients taking *Mevachor* suffered from muscle problems.(29)

Taking statns for one year was shown to increase the risk of never damage (*polyneuropathy* or *peripheral neuropathy*) by 15 percent, and 26 percent if taken for two ro more years.(30) The nerve damage is considered irreversible, and will likely persist even after the drugs are discontinued.

Ironically, but not surprisingly, satins can lead to heart failure, which has more than doubled since statins were introduced.(31) This is probably due to the inhibition of CoQ_{10}, which the heart needs to work properly. Yet, virtually all patients with heart failure are put on statin drugs, even if their cholesterol is already low. Researchers found that for every point decrease in serum cholesterol there was a 36 percent increase in the risk of death within 3 year.(32)

Another side effect of statins is cognitive impairment. One researcher found that 15 percent of statin patients develop some cognitive side effect. A former astronaut, Duane Graveline, had complete memory loss for a period which was so devastating, that once he discontinued taking *Lipitor*, he wrote a book about it (*Lipitor: Thief of Memory*). Other people report things like arriving at a store and not remembering why they are there, inablility of finding their way home, and forgetting the names of their loved ones. These symptoms occur suddenly and disappear just as suddenly. Other side effects of statins include cancer, depression, dizzyness, and pancreatitis.(33)

Sudden Cardiac Death (a heart attack) is responsible for about 50 percent of all mortality from cardiovascular disease.(34) Many studies show that the intake of fish oil with its omega-3 fatty acids significantly reduces mortality from fatal heart disease. One study reported a more than 30 percent reduction and another found a 45 percent reduction in sudden death in patients consuming omega 3 fatty acids.(35,36) Omega-3's also tend to thin the blood, important for those with heart disease. Fish oil or cod liver oil are high in omega-3s as are nuts, seeds, fish, grass fed beef, and eggs.

A fat that is largely a saturated fat that is good for your heart (and body) and that has received a lot of bad press in recent decades is the fat found in coconuts. The black-eye the press has given coconut oil and the other tropical oil, palm oil, is again based on poor science and deception originating from the vegetable oil manufacturers, specifically, the American Soybean Association (ASA).

Back in the 1980s, the ASA declared war on coconut and palm oil to squeeze them out of the market and replace them with vegetable (soybean) oil. They did this by manipulating research and hiring "experts" to declare that saturated fat is unhealthy for you, especially your heart. Food manufacturers, restaurants, even movie theaters' popcorn makers, switched from coconut oil to vegetable oil, which is hydrogenated and contains a lot of *trans*-fatty acids.

Research abounds proving that coconut oil is good for your heart. Coconut oil has and still is often the main ingredient in baby formula. Not only does research show coconuts to be healthy, but history and other societies who eat them do too. The Pacific Islanders call the coconut tree *The Tree of Life*, and for good reason. The coconut has been a staple in their diet for thousands of years, sometimes accounting for 60 percent of their total caloric intake. So why has heart disease (and other degenerative diseases) been virtually unheard of among those islanders who did or still do eat so much coconut and its fat? Bruce Fife, N.D., in his excellent book *The Healing Miracles of Coconut Oil* responds to those who contend coconut oil is unhealthy and causes heart disease by saying: "The simple fact is that Pacific Islanders who live on traditional diets rich in coconut don't get heart disease."(37)

Weston A. Price, D.D.S., a dentist who traveled the world in the 1930s studying remote societies in search of the cause of dental cavities, examined the peoples of numerous Pacific Islands. He found that those islanders eating their primitive, traditional diets rich in coconuts, rarely had cavities, heart disease or other degenerative diseases. He calculated that they had cavities only 0.3 percent of the time, while those who abandoned their traditional diets in favor of a Western Diet had cavities 30 percent of the time.(38)

Any good farmer or rancher can tell the health of an animal by examining their teeth, since they are an indication of what is going on in their body. Studies show that there is a definite link between heart disease and tooth and gum problems. Robert J. Genco, D.D.S., Ph.D. found that heart disease was three times more prevalent for those with gum disease.(39) One large 1993 study, The National Health and Nutrition Study, which included nearly 10,000 people ages 25 to 74, showed that patients with periodontal disease had a 25 percent increased risk of heart disease compared to people without gum problems.(40) These studies corroborate what we see in the Pacific Islanders – no tooth problems equals no heart problems. By the way, these native Pacific Islanders never brushed their teeth, never flossed, and never used mouth wash. Just as the health of the teeth reflects the health of the body, the health of the teeth is dependent on the overall health of the body. If you eat right, get the right fats, get some exercise and sunshine, your teeth, your heart, and your body will be healthy.

Food for Thought

It's interesting that the Pacific Islanders never brushed their teeth. We scientific Westerners believe that bacteria cause tooth decay and that if we don't brush and floss and gargle, we're going to end up toothless. But this is not what was seen in people who live naturally, eat plenty of saturated fats, and eat little or no refined foods. Dr. Weston Price lived with and studied the people of numerous societies around the world who were still consuming their traditional foods. Like the Pacific Islanders, they had exceptional health and no tooth decay without the benefits of any of our modern dental products. Why didn't those nasty bacteria destroy their teeth? Something to think about and we'll look more at bacteria and just what they do and are responsible for in a later chapter. But understand that, as Dr. William Campbell Douglas puts it, "Your teeth are the window to your body's physical condition. They reflect your general state of health. If your teeth are deteriorating, you are deteriorating. Hardening of the arteries and decaying teeth are part of the same degenerative process. The one you can see, cavities, comes early in life. The other, atherosclerosis – heart attack, is not seen and comes later. They are a continuum – part of the same degenerative process leading to disease and death."(41)

Every cell in your body needs a supply of fuel to keep its engine running. Most often the fuel is in the form of glucose (blood sugar) or fat (in the form of Long Chain Fatty Acids or LCFAs). Glucose requires insulin as a helper to get it into cells. If there's no insulin, or if the cells are not sensitive to insulin, then glucose can't get in and energy production halts. This is what happens in diabetes. LCFAs also need help from enzymes get into the blood stream. So to get either glucose or LCFAs into cells requires both enzymes reserves, insulin and energy expenditure.

But there's a different kind of fat that doesn't require enzymes, insulin or energy expenditure to be absorbed and utilized by the cells. That fat is medium chain fatty acids (MCFAs), found in abundance in coconuts. MCFAs can be absorbed directly into the blood stream and used for energy almost immediately without having to be processed by the liver or digested with enzymes. They are burned as fuel by the cells almost immediately providing an excellent source of quick energy, consequently increasing your overall rate of metabolism. MCFAs aren't converted into body fat or cholesterol either.

Since MCFAs don't require help to get into the cell you get a boost of energy when you eat them. You'll have more energy for daily functions and have better endurance. Several studies with mice show that mice fed MCFAs over an extended period, outlasted other mice in swimming competition.(42)

MCFAs are especially good for people with an under active thyroid. If your thyroid is sluggish, it's hard to get enough energy and it's hard to digest food. You probably have cold hands and feet or failing eyesight and are easily depressed. None of these conditions affected the Pacific Islanders who stayed on their traditional diet of coconut and its oil (and didn't use vegetable oil).

No legitimate research has shown that coconut oil causes heart disease or elevated cholesterol levels and there is now research that indicates that it is actually good for your heart and blood vessels.(43) This is because the MCFAs are burned soon after ingestion and don't cause blood platelets to become stickier, like other fats do. Bruce Fife sums up the health benefits of coconut oil: "Numerous scientific studies, observations of coconut eating populations and even just plain old common sense would tell you that coconut oil. . . is heart healthy. . .Not only does coconut oil not contribute to heart disease or any other health problem it actually provides protection from them. If you want to prevent heart disease you may want to add coconut oil to your diet."

How about eggs? You've heard they're bad for you too. That assertion began in the main-stream media back in the 60s and continues today. However, the truth about eggs and fat are beginning to surface. In a report in the *Journal of the America College of Nutrition*, Clare M. Hasler, Ph.D. said that "eggs are an excellent dietary source of many essential and non-essential components, which may promote optimum health. . .Eggs have not traditionally been regarded as a functional food, primarily due to concerns about their adverse effects on serum cholesterol levels. . .It is now known that there is little if any connection between dietary cholesterol and blood cholesterol levels."(44)

Another article published in the *International Journal of Cardiology*, showed that egg consumption had no effect on total cholesterol or LDL (the bad cholesterol), and that eating eggs every day did not increase the risk of heart attack or cardiovascular disease.(45) Al Sears. M.D., says, "Eggs are the perfect food. I eat them every day. . . They don't even raise your blood cholesterol. The developing embryo needs it to produce sex hormones – and so do you. Eggs do not cause heart disease. In fact, there was never any evidence they did."(46)

The egg is a valuable source of many key nutrients. Eggs have the essential nutrient choline, which is necessary for cell membrane integrity, nerve signaling, lipid transport, and normal brain development in the fetus. In one experiment, rats fed supplemental choline either in utero (while in the womb) or during the first two weeks of life had improved brain function and greater lifelong memory.(47) Thus, the memory of an individual as an adult is greatly influenced by the diet that his or her mother ate during pregnancy. (This research helps validate what I call "The Ancestry Factor" described later.)

Eggs contain vitamins A, D, B_6, E, and B_{12}, C, and people who don't eat eggs are shown to have higher rates of deficiencies in these vitamins. Eggs also contain the important vitamin folate (B_9), which is discussed more below and in the chapter on Alzheimer's disease.(48) Eggs supply lutein and zeaxanthin (these are carotenoids), which are great for the prevention of macular degeneration and cataracts. Eggs are also a great source of high-quality protein, magnesium, potassium and selenium. Selenium is very important for proper heart function: Selenium deficient soils correlate to high levels of heart disease.(49) Good sources of selenium include seafood and Brazil nuts.

Food for Thought

I eat several raw eggs a day (for breakfast) and have done so for over almost 10 years. Not only that, I don't refrigerate the eggs because refrigeration harms certain enzymes in the eggs. People in Europe and South America have never refrigerated eggs. I've eaten eggs that have sat on my counter for more than to a month with no ill effects. My friend, nutritionist David Getoff, says between himself and his wife they consume close to 4 dozen raw eggs a week and have done so for decades.

What about the dreaded *Salmonella*, you may ask? Well, it's not the risk it's made out to be and unless the egg has been damaged, will probably never be a problem. In fact, one researcher says that the chances of getting *Salmonella* poisoning from eating raw eggs is about 0.00003 percent.(50) If there's a crack in the shell, don't eat it. If the whites are real runny, don't eat it. If there's an objectionable smell, don't eat it. If it tastes funny, don't eat it. If you follow those rules, go ahead and eat it.

Some people are allergic to eggs because the eggs are consumed after being cooked. (It's the same with milk allergies and lactose intolerance, as you will see later.) If you eat the egg raw, it's much less likely you'll have an allergic reaction because raw foods contain the necessary enzymes, minerals, and vitamins to digest themselves. It's when these vital components are destroyed by heat that allergic reactions occur because the body can't handle the "sludge" created from the indigestible food. In addition, some people are actually allergic to chemical residues in the eggs, so if you can afford to buy only organic free range eggs, then you can eliminate this problem as well while greatly benefiting your health.

It's important to eat eggs from hens that are free-range (not kept in pens) and are fed organic grain since conventional grain has pesticides that tend to bioaccumulate in the egg. The fat content (omega-3s vs.

omega-6 fatty acids) are also better in organically raised eggs. The egg yolks have all the required fat soluble vitamins (A,D,E, and K), iron, and omega-3 fat. The whites have all the water-soluble B vitamins and are the source of the highest quality protein available.

I get my eggs from a local farmer who never refrigerates them for me. You should too, but that's probably not possible for most of you. The next best thing is to buy organic eggs from the health food store (some supermarkets carry them now) and don't refrigerate them.

Of course, the best way to eat eggs is raw. Just crack them into a glass, break the yolks, and chug them down. They're not bad after you get used to them. Otherwise, put them in smoothies with milk (raw) and honey (raw) and maybe some fruit. Soft boiled is next best, and scrambled is the worst. I do not eat eggs that are cooked.

What happens to eggs when they are cooked is a great illustration of what heat does to a food. A raw egg is runny and slippery and you can suck it through a straw. A cooked egg is thick and congealed. Try to suck it through a straw and you may hurt your cheeks. Why do you think the consistency of the egg changes with heat? It's because the fats become less fluid and the proteins harder. From a simply mechanical point of view, that once slippery food has become one tough hombre that will not only clog a straw, but possibly your arteries as well. When you factor in the fact that vitamins, minerals, and enzymes are destroyed, it just doesn't make sense to subject this marvel of nature to heat.

I know you may not like eating raw eggs. I know it will take courage and spunk. But you won't like a heart attack a heck of a lot more. As a kid your mom probably got some nasty medicine from the doctor and made you take it. You made faces or tried to hide under the covers. But in the end, you opened up and swallowed that yucky stuff. And even still as adults, if "the doctor" tells you to, most people will follow his or her advice, no matter how uncomfortable or sick it makes them. After all, people go through chemo, surgery, barium enemas, spinal taps etc., all because the doctor said so. And those are a heck of a lot less comfortable than eating some raw eggs.

Now if the doctor told you to take this yucky gooey yellowy not-that-great-tasting slop, most people would take it without question no matter how uncomfortable it was. Well, pretend I'm the doctor. "Mr. or Ms. Doe, here's your prescription. Go to the farmer (not the pharmacist), get a couple dozen of these brown or white spheres (they kind of look like pills, but larger), take two or three each day, crack them open and put the contents into a glass and swig them down like a shot of liquor. They only cost a couple or three dollars a dozen and they are about the best thing to take for your heart, nerves, and brain. Now, you may not like the taste at first, but you'll get used to them. It's very important, so off you go. Take two a day and call me next week when you're feeling better." Now THAT would be practicing medicine!

In the "I couldn't have said it better myself" category, in her book *Nourishing Traditions*, Sally Fallon gives an excellent review of different cultures' use of fat in the diet and the incidences of disease:

> . . .a study comparing Jews when they lived in Yemen, whose diets contained fats solely of animal origin, to Yemenite Jews living in Israel, whose diets contained margarine and vegetable oils, revealed little heart disease of diabetes in the former group but high levels of both diseases in the later (The study also noted that the Yemenite Jews consumed no sugar but those in Israel consumed sugar in amounts equaling 20-30% of total carbohydrate intake.) A comparison of populations in northern and southern India revealed a similar pattern. People in northern India consumed 17 times more animal fat but have an incidence of coronary heart disease seven times lower than people in southern India. The Masai and kindred tribes of Africa subsist largely on milk, blood and beef. They are free from coronary heart disease and have excellent blood cholesterol levels. Eskimos eat liberally of animal fats from fish and marine animals. On their native diet they are free of disease and exceptionally hardy. An extensive study of diet and disease patterns in China found that the region in which the populace consumes large amounts of whole milk and had half the rate of heart disease and several districts in which only small amounts of animal products are consumed. Several Mediterranean societies have low rates of heart disease even though fat – including highly saturated fat from lamb, sausage and goat cheese – comprises up to 70% of their caloric intake. The inhabitants of Crete, for example, are remarkable for their good health and longevity. A study of Puerto Ricans revealed that, although they consume large amounts of animal fat, they have a very low incidence of colon and breast cancer. A study of the long-lived inhabitants of Soviet Georgia revealed that those who eat the most fatty meat live the longest. In Okinawa, where the average life span of women is 84 years (longer than in Japan) the inhabitants eat generous amounts of pork and seafood and do all their cooking in lard. None of these studies is mentioned by those urging restriction of saturated fats. . . the French diet is just loaded with saturated fats in the form of butter, eggs, cheese, cream, liver, meats and rich pates. Yet the French have a lower rate of coronary heart disease than many other western countries. In the United States, 315 of every 100,000 middle-aged men die of heart attacks each year; in France the rate is 145 per 100,000. In

the Gascony region, where goose and duck liver form a staple of the diet, this rate is a remarkably low 80 per 100,000. This phenomenon has recently gained international attention as the French Paradox. [The French do suffer from many degenerative diseases, however. They eat large amounts of sugar and white flour and in recent years have succumbed to the timesaving temptations of processed foods.] (51)

Having thick and sticky blood obviously puts you at a higher risk for heart disease and stroke. Many doctors and researchers have recommended people at risk take low doses of aspirin since aspirin does in fact thin the blood. But even low doses of aspirin cause problems. An article in the *British Medical Journal* reports, "We found that no particular dose of aspirin between 75 mg and 300 mg daily currently used in cardiovascular prophylaxis is free of risk of causing bleeding from gastric or duodenal ulcers. Even very low (75 mg) doses of aspirin reportedly caused gastric bleeding in volunteers."(52) If you do or are considering taking aspirin to help prevent heart problems, it's been shown that all you need is one small children's aspirin a day to get all the benefits while decreasing your risk of long-term problems. Better still, take an omega-3 fatty acid supplement (fish oil, cod liver oil) and you'll be doing the same thing as the aspirin while helping a lot of other parts of your body. Eating an adequate amount of certain types of fish and nuts can be very helpful as well, but you can't really know the dose of omega 3s you're getting.

Another safe way to lessen the stickiness of blood is by adding cinnamon to your diet. If blood platelets clump together too much, blood flow can become inadequate. Cinnamon has been well-researched for its effects on blood platelets and prevents unwanted clumping by inhibiting the release of an inflammatory fatty acid called arachidonic acid from platelet cell membranes and reducing the inflammatory molecule called thromboxane A_2. (We need arachidonic acid [it is essential and an important constituent of cell membranes], but its release from platelets initiates inflammation and blood clot formation.) Therefore, cinnamon is also considered an anti-inflammatory.(53) Cinnamon has also been shown to lower cholesterol and triglycerides. More on cinnamon in the Diabetes chapter.

Food for Thought

While doctors will tell a heart patient to take a low dose of aspirin a day to keep the blood thin, they won't tell them that using NSAIDs (non-steroidal anti-inflammatory drugs – aspirin is one) greatly increases a person's risk of developing Congestive Heart Failure (CHF). This was found to be true especially in elderly patients. An article in the *Archives of Internal Medicine* states, ". . .we found that recent use of NSAIDs by elderly patients doubles the odds of being admitted to the hospital with an episode of CHF."(54) Not just that, but the authors estimated that the number of deaths caused by NSAIDs in heart patients could be as large as the number of NSAID caused deaths in gastrointestinal complications. (Which, as already mentioned, is 16,500 deaths a year in the U.S.) Naproxen and other NSAIDs may also exacerbate Parkinson's disease.(55)

Most people have quite a lackadaisical attitude when it comes to aspirin and other over-the-counter drugs. They're encouraged to take them whenever a discomfort arises. After all, what harm will a little aspirin do? But these drugs, just like any other drug, can cause harm. And the older you are, the more likely you'll experience a side effect from them – or even death. So why are the biggest consumers of drugs, and the people who are prescribed the most drugs, the elderly? Doesn't make sense, does it? (But it makes the doctors and pharmaceutical companies a lot of money.)

NSAIDs are known to cause thousands of deaths a year and are sold in every drug store in the country. However, if you get caught using marijuana, which is relatively harmless and is sometimes even used for medicinal purposes, you might get arrested. The Drug Abuse Warning Network did an exhaustive search of medical literature and medical examiners' reports and found no reports of death caused by the consumption of marijuana by itself. As best they can tell, no one has died from an overdose of marijuana alone.(56) Although a plant might give just as much relief as a pill, the drug companies can't own it and control it and thus they can't make nearly as much money from. So the plant is "bad" and will get you in thrown in jail, and the pill is "good" and will get you TV ads.

I in no way am advocating the use of marijuana. Although it might be natural, using it causes problems in the human body. But from purely a health stand-point, I would think a plant would do less harm than a pill from a chemical factory.

Speaking of factories, as an environmental engineer, I had the opportunity to inspect more than a few. The factories and kinds of facilities I saw ran the gamut from metal plating operations, textile mills, and nuclear power plants all the way to chicken processing plants, car washes and Laundromats. I saw quite an assortment of nasty and dirty problems, since my job was to make sure the facilities were kept clean and their wastes were disposed of properly.

One day while in the office, a number of inspectors were comparing notes, and the question was raised which kind of facility we disliked inspecting most. The answer was unanimous – pharmaceutical plants. They were the nastiest, dirtiest, stinkiest, most toxic places we saw, and that's saying something. The one I had to inspect regularly had hoses and cans strewn about, puddles of chemicals, pipes leaking slime. At the end of the employee's parking lot, there were several sprayers that hosed your car off as you left. I asked the vice president why it was there, and he said

> that if you didn't hose your car off at least a couple times a week, it would start to corrode and just melt away because the air around the plant was so caustic. One of the VP's walked with a limp, one had an incessant eye twitch, and there was the story of the man who worked there whose skin turned bright orange (I never met the man, he died before I started going there). There were massive fish kills in the river downstream of the plant and trees around the plant died. We forced them to build berms to control run-off, spend millions to improve their wastewater treatment plant, and do groundwater reclamation. That's not to mention all the air quality control things another department forced them to do. All in all, it was a very toxic and dangerous place. And what did they make there? Heart medicine and anti-inflammatory drugs.
>
>   Seeing what really goes on at pharmaceutical plants and just how drugs are made and what is used to make them made a big impression on me: I haven't taken any kind of drug, pill, potion, or medicine of any kind since then. That was over 30 years ago. It was like pulling the curtain away from the Wizard of Oz – just an imposter with a lot of hot air.

Menopausal and post menopausal women often undergo hormone replacement therapy (HRT) and are told by their doctor that doing so will reduce their risk of cardiovascular disease. But a study published in the *New England Journal of Medicine* showed that HRT actually increases the risk of heart disease.

> . . .the Heart and Estrogen/progestin Replacement Study found that 4.1 years of treatment with. . . estrogen. . .had no overall effect on the rate of nonfatal myocardial infarction or death among women with established coronary artery disease. However, an increased risk of cardiovascular events was associated with the study regimen in the first year. . .(57)

A study showed that HRT significantly increases the risk of stroke too.(58) Ladies, please think twice before taking those artificial hormones. (More on this in the chapter on breast cancer.) Yet another class of drugs, calcium channel blockers, is prescribed to lower blood pressure. However, postmenopausal women taking these medications have been shown to be at twice the risk of dying from heart disease, especially when the woman is also taking diuretics.(59)

I could go on and on with the problems of drugs and their effects on the heart, arteries, and overall body in general, but that would take volumes. I'll just mention one more class of drugs, Cox 2 Inhibitors that wreak havoc with the heart. *Vioxx* and *Celebrex* are the two most widely known. There are reports of nearly 100,000 people having adverse reactions to *Vioxx*, including heart attacks and death, and this lead to it being taken off the market. These drugs effect blood clotting and blood vessel constriction at the expense of pain control for arthritis sufferers.

This is a prime illustration of how drugs rob Peter to pay Paul. Any drug, and I mean *any* drug, works this way. You may get relief from joint pain, but you may also get a heart attack. You may thin your blood, but you may get an ulcer. You may lower your cholesterol (which is an extremely essential nutrient and isn't bad in the first place), but increase you risk of liver problems. Sometimes the cure is worse than the disease. Drugs force your body to respond in a certain way and there is always a side effect. They are *all* toxic and must be processed by the liver and kidneys for elimination, which will eventually wear out these important organs and make them much more susceptible to disease. Your best medicine is proper food and proper lifestyle. Anything else will come back to haunt you.

The mineral magnesium plays another significant role in heart health. Most heart attack victims are deficient in magnesium. In *The Miracle of Magnesium*, Dr. Dean writes:

> . . .magnesium plays a crucial role in the prevention of both atherosclerosis and arteriosclerosis. It maintains the elasticity of the artery wall, dilates blood vessels, prevents calcium deposits and is necessary for the maintenance of healthy muscles, including the heart muscle itself. For all these reasons, magnesium is critical to the maintenance of a healthy heart. . .The very diet that promotes elevated cholesterol also causes magnesium deficiency.[60]

Studies show that communities that use water rich in magnesium have decreased incidences of heart disease. Where calcium in the water is elevated significantly above that of magnesium, so is heart disease. One of the major side effects of heart medication is magnesium deficiency. If magnesium is administered intravenously immediately after a heart attack, the odds of death are decreased 55 percent. When magnesium was administered to patients after a heart attack, the risk of heart failure decreased by 25 percent.[61,62,63] Magnesium has also been shown to aid in heart arrhythmia, rapid heart beats, (atrial tachycardia), premature beats, mitral valve prolapse, and atrial fibrillation.[64] The most common time people suffer heart attacks is in the morning and late afternoon, the same times magnesium levels are their lowest. Stress decreases magnesium levels, which in part explains why heart attacks are brought on by stress. I discuss magnesium in more detail throughout this book, since a deficiency in it may contribute to or even cause so many serious health problems. For now, realize that magnesium is of paramount importance to not only your heart, but your whole body and mind. You can find high magnesium levels in nuts, seeds (especially pumpkin and sunflower), avocados, garlic, onions, shellfish, and green leafy vegetables.

It's interesting to note that as important as everyone thinks calcium is for health, all the muscles in the body contain more magnesium than calcium. Furthermore, calcium cannot do its job correctly if there isn't a sufficient supply of available magnesium. So it's important to have the proper amount of both these minerals in your body for the proper functioning of a host of biological processes. Calcium causes the contraction or tightening of muscles, including the smooth muscles of blood vessels. Too much calcium and not enough magnesium, and you can have sustained muscle contraction, spasms, and even convulsions. This can result in many different problems, including hypertension and various types of muscle cramping.

Food for Thought

One of the most popular heart medications for various reasons (high blood pressure, angina, and some arrhythmias) are drugs called calcium channel blockers (or CCBs, calcium blockers, or calcium antagonists). They prevent the flow of calcium ions into the muscle cells of the heart and blood vessels causing them to dilate and relax.

Sounds good, but as you know, drugs come with side effects. In this case, headaches, swelling in the lower legs, constipation, fatigue, and stomach discomfort may occur. (Actually a good natural CCB is the mineral magnesium.)

As already mentioned, calcium channel blockers were shown to put women at twice the risk of dying from heart disease. The study involved nearly 20,000 postmenopausal women between the ages of 50 and 79 who were being treated for high blood pressure. The researches said their findings probably apply to men as well.[65]

And at the 2000 Congress of the European Society of Cardiology, Dr. Curt Furberg, a well known expert on the effectiveness of cardiovascular drugs, reported that his research showed that patients taking calcium blockers had a 27 percent increase in heart attacks and a 26 percent increase in heart failure compared to patients taking other kinds of drugs for hypertension.[66] Of course, there was an up-roar from the pharmaceutical industry with some of their hypertension experts saying Dr. Furberg's research was "unscientific," "unbalanced," and "outrageous." And why wouldn't they get defensive considering that the sales of calcium channel blockers is about $6 billion annually? But Dr. Furberg's results are not surprising considering heart medications in general often cause magnesium deficiencies.

In a study at the University of Maryland, researchers determined that calcium blockers work differently than once previously thought – operating on a certain part of the cell that is also affected in the same way by elevated concentrations of magnesium.[67] Well how about that? Of course, the drug companies would never encourage you to take your magnesium lest they miss out on $6 billion a year in revenue.

People with high blood pressure are oftentimes be put on a salt restricted diet, and rightly so, because salt may increase blood pressure. Sodium attracts water causing increased volume, which creates more pressure inside the blood vessels. The government has set a tolerable *upper intake level* for salt at 5,800 milligrams a day, but most people consume more than that not just because they sprinkle it on food, but because most processed foods have already had salt added to them.

Food for Thought

Table salt or sodium chloride (NaCl) is composed of sodium and chloride, and some say it's a necessary nutrient. Although we do need sodium and chloride, personally, I do not think any kind of salt (table, sea, rock) is beneficial. Here's why:

Yes, we do need sodium (Na) and we need chloride (Cl), but not in the concentrated forms they are in salt. There are numerous studies that show that the high concentration of sodium in salt cause excess calcium excretion through the kidneys. This, some researchers believe, may be responsible for osteoporosis, especially in elderly women.(68,69,70,71) Here is an excerpt from an article published in the *Journal of Nutrition*:

"This study shows that the loss of bone calcium is proportional to dietary intake of sodium and that even at moderate intakes of sodium there was significant loss of bone. . .Short term human studies and cross sectional studies in humans have shown that high salt intake is associated with increased calcium loss. A significant negative correlation between sodium intake and bone mineral density has been reported. . .This degree of calcium loss can lead to substantial bone loss, especially if the calcium intake is low as in the elderly in whom the absorption mechanism may not be adequate."(72)

What is high intake of salt? The average daily consumption of most people in the U.S. is about 9 to 10 grams, which these studies consider high. Another researcher said that the sodium from table salt causes sodium clumps in the blood, which kill red blood cells. "Four little grains of salt (including sea salt) destroys approximately two million red blood cells. It takes at least three hours to replace the blood cells and about 24 hours to clean out the dead cells. During these processes important nutrients are leached from the blood and body. As a result, salt speeds aging."(73)

"But that's ordinary table salt," some may counter. "Sea salt has many trace elements we need for optimum health." But the fact that sea salt contains trace elements does not change the fact that calcium must be excreted when sodium is excreted through the kidneys. (This is called *obligatory excretion*: when sodium intake is increased, the excess has to be excreted, and when it is, calcium must go with it.) So although sea salt is better because it contains these trace elements, I still believe the overall effect on the body is a negative one, for starters, because of this relationship with calcium.

Paul Bragg, N.D., Ph.D., said that salt interferes with normal digestion because when it's present in the stomach, only half as much pepsin (the enzyme that breaks down protein) is produced, resulting in incomplete and slow protein digestion. This results in putrefaction, gas, and digestive distress.(74)

Another, common sense reason salt is harmful is the fact that it changes the osmotic potential in and around cells. When the concentration of a mineral or minerals is higher on one side of the cell membrane than the other, water will flow to the side with the higher concentration to equalize the concentration on both sides of the membrane (called *osmosis*).

Picture two swimming pools next to each other – one with a salt water concentration of 10, the other with water having a salt concentration of 2. If you connect the two pools with a pipe that has a screen that only allows water through it and not any minerals (called a semi-permeable membrane, which is what the cells in your body have), what will happen is water will flow from the fresh pool to the salty one until the salty side has a concentration of 2 also. You can imagine that it's going to take a lot of water from the fresh water pool to dilute the salty water this much, and that's exactly why you can get so thirsty when you eat salty foods: when your cells become dehydrated, you get thirsty. So really, salt is dehydrating. It causes fluid to be pulled out of your cells to maintain the osmotic balance between intra and extra cellular fluids.

If you consume too much salt (like taking *Epsom* salts [magnesium sulfate], which is a common anecdote for constipation), you may get diarrhea, because all that salt in your stomach gets diluted by water gushing out of your cells to equilibrate the osmolarity between the cells and the fluid in your stomach. (By the way, a lot of sugar does the same thing, and you'll find that most laxatives have a tremendous amount of sugar in them.)

The common recommendation to drink a lot of water (eight glasses a day) is in one way a good recommendation for those on the typical American diet of salty, additive laden, cooked foods. The water will dilute the salt and impurities and tend to flush them out of the body. The bad part is, other minerals that the body needs get flushed out too, resulting in mineral depletions, which, or course, are not good. Plus, the cells get dehydrated which tends to pucker them up. (If you want to look younger, stop eating salt.)

Salt imposes a considerable strain on the body to eliminate it since it is not readily excreted by the body. It tends to accumulate and persist in tissues (in joints causing arthritis), creating the necessity of excess water to dilute it. People who eat salt have in effect too much water (a hidden edema), which, of course, is heavy. When you switch to a healthy diet, that excess water will not be needed, and you will lose weight.

I believe that any food that makes you thirsty is really dehydrating you. If you eat wholesome, mostly raw foods, you'll rarely get thirsty. There's no need to guzzle water if you're on a healthy diet. If you eat right, drink vegetable juice, raw milk, and have the right kinds of fat in your diet (fat lubricates), you will hardly ever need or even want to drink water.

Let's go back to that example of the two swimming pools for a moment. You can imagine that the water that's trying to get to the salty side will exert a pressure, which it does (called *osmotic pressure*), on the screen (the cell membrane). That's why doctors will tell heart patients to cut down on salt: too much of it in your bloodstream will cause more pressure in the blood vessels as the water tries to come through the cell membranes to dilute the salt. If you have headaches, stop eating salt (while changing your diet to a healthier, raw one) and there's a good chance your headaches will diminish or stop: osmotic pressure affects all the blood vessels in your body, your brain included.

Some outdoorsmen will counter that it's natural to eat salt, as evidenced by deer in the wild licking salt licks. However, Dr. Bernard Jensen noted that this only occurs during the dry grass season when chlorophyll is lacking.[75] When the deer have fresh green grass rich in chlorophyll and minerals available, they are not attracted to the salt. This is further evidence that a mineral deficiency causes salt cravings, and a good reason to drink fresh vegetable juice loaded with chlorophyll.

Hold a teaspoon of salt into your mouth, and see how it feels. Salt is irritating, not just to lining of your mouth, but your intestinal tract and nerves. Salt is a preservative because nothing will grow on it – that's why the Great Salt Flats in Utah are lifeless and barren and why the Egyptians used salt for embalming.

Some claim that salt is necessary for life itself and that mankind has used it from the beginning of time. Sodium and chloride are necessary, but not in the lifeless, concentrated form as in salt. Consider that there were several cultures of healthy people that never used salt. The Eskimos, several American Indian tribes, great numbers of tribes in tropical and desert regions have existed for ages without taking salt.[76] Personally, I haven't had a salt shaker in my house for 20 years. It may be difficult to go off salt, but usually after a couple weeks without it while eating healthily, salt cravings go away.

Minerals from cooked foods are less absorbable by the body, so one would tend to eat more to get their mineral requirements met. The minerals need to be added to the body and the best way is to eat fresh unprocessed foods and foods that have plenty of minerals. Fresh raw tomatoes, melons, fresh celery juice or whole celery, and fresh raw fish, especially shell fish, and eggs will correct a mineral deficiency naturally. Another good source is unpasteurized, unsalted cheese eaten along with unpasteurized butter. Meats are also an exceptional concentrated source of quality absorbable minerals. Of course, high quality meats such as grass fed organic beef and lamb are best, but any kind is acceptable. Ideally, you should eat meat uncooked, but rare is the next best. Never eat meat that's been cooked more than rare.

Food for Thought

One study undertaken at the University of Chicago Medical Center, showed that celery is very effective in lowering blood pressure. The researcher's father had a mild case of hypertension, and started eating a quarter pound of celery every day. His blood pressure dropped from 158/96 to 118/82 in a week.

This prompted his son, Mr. QT Le, a medical student at the University, to find out why. He discovered that a compound called 3-n-butyl phthalide (that gives celery its characteristic flavor and smell) was responsible for the improvement. His study findings showed that a small amount of this compound given daily to test animals lowered their blood pressure from 12 to 14 percent.(77,78) A quarter pound of celery is about 4 stalks. Some herbalists recommend 4 - 8 stalks a day to get all the health benefits. ("Four stalks a day keeps high blood pressure away.") Celery is also high in potassium and magnesium, which also tend to lower blood pressure.

It turns out that celery and celery seeds are very beneficial foods, and had been used for centuries for medicinal purposes. The first recorded mention of its medicinal properties dates back to the 9th century B.C., when celery was mentioned by the Greek poet Homer in his epic tale *Odyssey*. The Greeks used celery leaves as laurels to decorate their renowned athletes, and Romans used it as a seasoning. Oriental medicine has used celery for centuries to treat circulatory disorders and high blood pressure.

Elixirs and tonics using them were widely sold in the U.S. during the19th century. Celery acts as a diuretic, helps with menstrual discomfort, calms anxiety, and can improve asthma and bronchitis. In fact, herbalists sometimes recommend celery for the treatment of nervousness and hysteria. Oriental medicine also uses the seeds to treat headaches. It's also been recommended as an antiflatulent and aphrodisiac.

Even though celery is thought to be high in sodium, about 2 stalks worth contains only about 100 milligrams of sodium – will below the 2,400 milligram FDA recommended daily limit. Plus, the sodium is well balanced with potassium, which helps keep body fluids balanced, and celery contains pthalides, which reduce stress hormones and relax the muscles around the arteries. So instead of celery causing fluid retention (which regular sodium found in table salt does), it's actually a diuretic (which decreases fluid retention).

The 3-n-butyl phthalide in celery has been shown to help prevent stroke, improve blood flow to the brain, enhance recovery from stroke, and significantly increase lifespan.[79,80,81,82,83,84,85] Celery is a great source of vitamin C, which is not only a great cold fighter, but has also been shown to reduce the risk of death from all causes including heart disease, stroke, and cancer.[86]

Celery and its seeds help maintain healthy joints due to their anti-inflammatory properties that reduce swelling and pain around the joints. The 3-n-butyl phthalide in celery has been shown to be very effective in decreasing the pain associated with arthritis, rheumatism, osteoarthritis, fibromyalgia, and gout. One study showed that 70 patients suffering from rheumatic pain experienced significantly less pain, more joint mobility, and better overall quality of life.[87] 3-n-butyl phthalide also appears to lower the production of uric acid (after the initial uric acid crystals are dissolved and flushed out), thus greatly improving the symptoms of gout.[88] And there have been no adverse side effects noted in any of the research studies.

There's even evidence that celery seeds can fight cancer. In one study using rats, the researchers concluded, "On the basis of the above results it can be said that *A. Graveolens* [celery seed] is a potent plant against experimentally induced hepatocarcinogenesis [development of liver cancer] in Wistar rats."[89] Celery also contains coumarins, compounds that are believed to help fight cancer, along with other compounds that are believed to detoxify carcinogens, especially those found in cigarette smoke.[90]

3-n-butyl phthalide is unique to celery. As you see, it's really quite a wonderful compound with many health benefits and no known problems. Don't be surprised if a few years from now, you start seeing drugs come out with 3-n-butyl phthalide as the active ingredient since the drug companies are already researching that possibility. But all you have to do is eat 4 - 8 stalks a day, and you'll be getting all the health benefits of this unique compound.

Celery has 18 different amino acids including all eight of the essential amino acids, so it's surprisingly a source of complete protein. And celery and its juice is exceptionally rehydrating since it's high in both water and electrolytes, making it great for those who are physically active. Some day you may see coolers full of celery juice on the sidelines of football games instead of *Gatorade*. Can you imagine. . ."And keeping with tradition, the players just poured the cooler of celery juice on the winning coach! Oh my, what a site!"

Drinking fresh vegetable juice (celery, parsley, zucchini, cucumber etc.) is a great source of minerals, vitamins, and enzymes. Much better than any vitamin pill you could take. It's best to have some raw fat like butter, cod liver, krill oil, or coconut oil, along with the juice because fat allows better absorption of the vitamins and minerals.

Although celery is rich in vitamins and minerals, it would take close to 10 pounds of celery to supply the amino acid protein content of a 4 ounce serving of beef or lamb. So don't go eating celery all day to avoid eating meat. Really, you need both, and they actually complement each other so eating them at the same meal is fine.

Dr. Norman Walker, well known in natural health circles and a huge proponent of drinking vegetable juices, lived to the age of 110. He even developed his own juicing machine that is still sold today. Jack LaLane, a well known physical fitness fanatic has his own juicer too, although it's not nearly as good as the Norwalk Juicer, or the Omega or Green Star Juicers (see Resource Guide). LaLane is well into his nineties and still very active. He celebrated his 90th birthday by pulling several commuter busses tied to a rope! Include celery in your diet every day, and you're going to fight disease and revitalize every cell in your body. Drinking it as part of a vegetable juice drink should become part of your daily routine. (Even more on celery in the chapter on prostate cancer.)

We've all heard about the benefits of exercise when it comes to cardiovascular health, and here's more proof. A study was done on over 7,300 men to see what effect exercise had on heart disease. The amount of benefit depended not on how long they exercised, but on how many calories they burned when they did. Those who burned the most calories a week through exercise had a 40 percent less chance of developing heart disease than men who exercised but burned fewer calories. The researchers also found that the men who participated in intense exercise (running, swimming laps) had a significantly lower risk of heart disease than those who exercised moderately. Walking helped, as did other regular exercise. But the greatest benefit occurred when the exercise was intense and vigorous.(91)

On the other hand, researchers at Harvard studies walking as compared with vigorous exercise in 72,000 women over an eight-year period and found that walking briskly three or more hours a week reduced the risk of coronary events by 30 to 40 percent.(92) Further, they said that vigorous exercise in these women did not decrease the risk of heart problems any more than walking did.

Food for Thought

One study of men said that vigorous exercise was better, and a study of women said it made no difference. Maybe there's a difference in needs for men and women: Perhaps men need short bursts of high-demand exercise and women need a gentler, more consistent form. In any event, everyone needs it. One study showed that for children age 5 to 17, long

walks combined with repetition resistance exercise (weight training) were
the most effective in reducing body weight for overweight kids.(93)

Exercise is also good for your brain. In a study on rats, scientist showed that
rats that exercised moderately had brains that aged only 25 percent as fast as the
brains in rats that did not exercise. They noted that the exercising rats had
healthier DNA and more robust brain cells than the less active rats.(94)

Food for Thought

Although I'm not going to devote much time to discussing exercise in
this book, please don't overlook its importance. Exercise is a key
fundamental to health, and you need to do it consistently for the rest of your
life. Some forms of exercise are better than others as you will see below,
but any exercise is better than nothing. Doing something you enjoy is good
especially if it's outside. Don't use the excuse that you're too old or have
never exercised before so it won't do you any good to start now. Research
has shown that even frail patients of very advanced age improve muscle
strength with regular exercise and people in their 70s regained lost lung
capacity. Balance, strength, and power all improved in elderly people who
exercise, and even the chance of hip fractures from falls decreased
because bones are strengthened from exercise.(95)

We call my Dad The Bionic Man. He's 90 years old and has had a
number of health challenges that required medical intervention. He's had
cataract surgery, has a pacemaker, had trouble with his bladder. When he
was in his 40s, he had all his teeth yanked and got a set of dentures
because his teeth gave him such trouble. Years later, he had heart
problems (teeth problems = heart problems, remember?) and had two
angioplasties and they wanted to perform open heart surgery on him. He
declined, thank goodness, or I doubt he'd be alive today. He's had friends
who got the surgery who didn't last long because they never addressed the
underlying cause of the problem. My Dad and Mom have changed their diet
significantly over the years. They take cod liver oil every day and eat some
fish every week. And they exercise a bunch. Every morning my Mom goes
to the local shopping mall before it opens and walks around and around at
a pretty good clip. My Dad has an elliptical trainer he's almost worn out. He
rides that thing very day. He's also outside a lot in the garden or playing
golf (still!). He doesn't wear sun screen. Although he still wears his
pacemaker, his heart is doing fine and his mind is pretty sharp. So maybe
all that exercise has helped. If you want to last, you need to do it too.

They sell these mini-trampolines that are about 3 feet in diameter. I
suggest you get one and put it in your family room. Whenever a
commercial comes on while you're watching TV, get off your sofa and
bounce on that trampoline. Bounce almost as hard and as fast as you can

for a minute or two. When the commercial is over, go back to the couch. Do this 10 or so times and you'll get in a pretty good work out. So now there's no excuse you don't have the time, These trampolines are great for your heart and lymphatic system, will strengthen your bones and joints, and encourage better circulation to your brain so it will stay sharp.

The best way to exercise to increase your lung and heart capacities, improve endurance, lose weight, get rid of excess fat, and increase muscle mass is through short duration, high intensity activity with rest periods in between. That's why I tell you to bounce almost as hard and fast as you can on that mini trampoline – you need the high intensity, but you don't want to strain anything either. If you are at all unstable, buy the support bar for the rebounder so you can hold on while you are bouncing.

I have to warn you to be sure to work up slowly to higher intensities. It's estimated that 6 to 17 percent of all sudden cardiac deaths occur in association with acute exertion.(96) As you make improvements to your lifestyle, you'll be able to increase your exercise intensity without fear, but if you don't make these lifestyle changes, you may be asking for trouble.

One study analyzed 25 years worth of previously published study results to see how effective dieting and aerobic exercise was for losing weight. Shockingly, those who dieted and exercised lost only a tiny bit more weight than those who dieted alone: 10.7 lbs. lost for the diet/exercise group verses 11 lbs. lost for the diet alone group.(97)

Another study compared people doing long duration cardio exercise with people doing short duration high intensity workouts. The high intensity group spent less time exercising and did half the work as the cardio group and yet they increased their aerobic capacity by 30 percent and lost nine times as much body fat as the cardio group.(98) Almost more importantly, short duration, high intensity workouts increase muscle mass and muscle tone, whereas the long duration, low intensity workouts does nothing significant for muscle mass. Remember, your heart is a muscle.

Dr. Al Sears is a big proponent of these short duration, high intensity workouts. He says that typical aerobics actually accelerate aging. He says, "Do enough aerobics and it will make you sick, tired, and old before your time." Dr. Sears has developed what he calls the PACE program, which stands for Progressively Accelerated Cardiopulmonary Exertion. (Just saying that is a workout!) In a nutshell, you do one minute of high intensity exercise (after a gentle warm-up to loosen your muscles) followed by one minute of rest and recovery. The one minute of exercise is hard enough to give your heart and lungs a challenge. If you feel out of shape, take it easy for the first two weeks, but still push yourself a little. As you work up to more intense periods, you should be working hard enough to work up a sweat over the course of the 10 minute session.

After the one minute of hard exercise (again, the mini trampoline is great for this), slow down to an easier pace of whatever you're doing, and relax. You can stop walking, bouncing, running, or whatever if you want. You want your heart and breathing to start to slow down and recover. You MUST do this recovery, slow-down period. As Dr. Sears says, "Training your body to recover is one of the keys to your success."

Keep alternating high-intensity/rest periods for 10 minutes. If you work up to say 15 to 20 minutes eventually, that's fine. But just 10 minutes of this kind of exercise has been shown to be more beneficial than hours of straight aerobics. Dr. Sears has a CD/video of his program that is really good and I highly recommend it. You can find it at www.alsearsmd.com.

One of the great parts about this kind or exercise is that it takes so much less time than the hour a day or so they say you need if you do straight aerobics. And you actually get a better work out in less time – a win/win deal.

But don't get the idea that just walking, hiking, biking, gardening or other low intensity activities are bad for you. Any movement is good for your circulation and everything else. But aerobics, jogging for long periods, or moderate workouts of any kind for long periods are actually damaging. Ever notice how thin and gaunt long-distance runners look? There's the story of the first marathon runner – a Greek who ran from the coast 24.6 miles to the city of Athens to announce that the Trojan war was over. He got there, blurted out "The war is over," keeled over and died. In recent years I have heard of quite a few marathon runners dying also. On the other hand, look at the body of a sprinter – muscular and strong, not emaciated and weak like a marathoner. Do the short, hard stuff with rests in between (after working up to it), and you'll be much better off. Please check with your doctor before you begin any exercise program.

To sum things up as far as heart health goes, I quote Mary Enig, Ph.D., a world renowned expert on fats and diet:

> The cause of heart disease is not animal fats and cholesterol but rather a number of factors inherent in modern diets, including excess consumption of vegetable oils and hydrogenated fats; excess consumption of refined carbohydrates in the form of sugar and white flour; mineral deficiencies, particularly low levels of protective magnesium and iodine; deficiencies of vitamins, particularly of vitamin C, needed for the integrity of the blood vessel walls; and of antioxidants like selenium and vitamin E, which protect us from free radicals and; finally, the disappearance of antimicrobial fats from the food supply, namely, animal fats and tropical oils. . .
>
> The best way to treat heart disease then is not to focus on lowering cholesterol - either by drugs or diet – but to consume a diet that provides animal foods rich in vitamins B_6 and B_{12};. . . to avoid vitamin and mineral deficiencies that make the artery walls

more prone to ruptures and the buildup of plaque; to include the antimicrobial fats in the diet [e.g. coconut oil, raw butter]; and to eliminate processed foods containing refined carbohydrates, oxidized cholesterol and free-radical-containing vegetable oils that cause the body to need constant repair.[99]

Stroke

A stroke (apoplexy) is a sudden decrease or loss of consciousness, sensation and voluntary motion caused by a rupture or obstruction of an artery of the brain. Hemorrhagic stroke occurs when a blood vessel ruptures within the brain. Ischemic stroke, or cerebral infarction (the more common kind of stroke), results when a blood clot blocks a blood vessel and therefore prevents blood from flowing to the brain. The risk factors, which have been shown to increase the likelihood of a stroke, are:

- High blood pressure (over 140/90 mmHg)
- Diabetes (fasting blood sugar over 126 mg/dl) This test may soon be replaced with the hemoglobin A1C or just HA1C test (a value of 6.5 or above would indicate diabetes)
- Carotid or other artery disease (These supply blood to your brain)
- Coronary heart diseases such as enlarged heart, heart valve disease or congenital heart defects.
- Transient ischemic attacks (TIAs) (These produce stroke-like symptoms without lasting effects.)
- High red blood cell count, sickle cell anemia, high cholesterol, and atrial fibrillation.
- Age. Children can have strokes, but generally the older you are the more likely you are to have a stroke.
- Smoking, excessive alcohol consumption, and poor diet.

More men get strokes, but more women die from them. Women who are pregnant have a higher stroke risk as do women on birth control pills who smoke. Heredity plays a factor since those with a history of stroke in their family are more likely to suffer one too, and African Americans have a much higher risk of death from a stroke than Caucasians do (as they also have higher risks of high blood pressure, diabetes and obesity). If someone has had already had a stroke, their risk of having another one is much greater. If someone has had a heart attack, their risk of suffering a stroke is greater too.[100]

Each year roughly 6 million Americans die as the result of a stroke, which makes it the third greatest cause of death in the U.S. It is also a major cause of serious, long-term disability. Yet most people over the age of 50 don't even realize what a stroke is, what its signs and symptoms are, and how important is to seek immediate medical attention (it should be treated as if someone had a heart attack).(101)

How do you know if you've had or are having a stroke? Here are some of the symptoms:

- Sudden confusion or disorientation.
- Sudden dizziness, loss of balance or coordination.
- Sudden numbness or weakness of an arm, leg, or face, especially on one side of the body.
- Sudden difficulty seeing out of one or both eyes.
- Sudden, severe headache.

Here are three simple questions to ask someone to see if he or she is having or about to have a stroke:
1. Ask the person so smile.
2. Ask the individual to raise both of their arms.
3. Ask the person to speak a simple sentence such as "Mary had a little lamb."

If the person has trouble with any of these tasks, call 911 or take the person to the closest emergency room since prompt diagnosis and treatment can prevent serious consequences including brain damage and death.

The after effects of stroke can be paralysis in many parts of the body, especially in the face or one side of the body. Recovery from a stroke is usually slow and requires a lot of effort. It's best to take steps now to prevent a stroke from ever occurring. So the key to dealing with strokes is not so much with treatment, but with prevention – and this advice applies to those who have had a stroke already since it can help prevent another one and help the person recover quicker and easier.

The best steps to take to prevent a stroke are virtually identical to those to prevent a heart attack (see previous section). Consuming the proper kinds of fat, eating fresh, wholesome food and getting exercise will help lower your risk of developing a stroke.

A recent study showed that a Western diet (of processed foods) increases the likelihood of stroke compared to a more wholesome diet with higher intakes of fruits, vegetables, fish, and whole grains.(102) Another study showed that eating fruits and green or yellow vegetables daily (spinach, carrots, pumpkin, squash) may reduce the risk of stroke by 26 percent.(103)

A 20-year study showed that people who consumed at least 300 micrograms (mcg) of folate per day had a 20 percent lower risk of a stroke and a 13 percent lower risk of cardiovascular disease than those consuming less than 136 mcg of folate per day. Folate is a B-vitamin (vitamin B_9) found in citrus fruits, tomatoes, leafy green vegetables, whole grain products, chicken livers, and beef livers. If you cook your vegetables, most of the folate ends up in the water you throw away since it is water soluble. One of the best sources of folate is chicken livers (cook lightly). Folate is also in bee pollen.

A folate deficiency can turn your skin a grayish-brown color, make you tired and depressed and cause anemia, heart disease, and even dementia. Folate deficiencies are prevalent in the elderly. The American Heart Association recommends adults consume at least 400 mcg of folate and pregnant women consume 600 mcg per day.(104) (See Alzheimer's chapter for more on folate.)

Magnesium is an important mineral for proper blood circulation so it's no surprise that it's vital to maintain the blood vessels in and around the brain. Magnesium has also been shown to slightly help to reduce platelet aggregation, so although it does not thin the blood, it can indeed help promote proper blood flow. It keeps blood flowing while reducing the likelihood of clot formation although not as effectively as fish oils and cod liver oil. It relaxes head and neck muscles, which in turn allow normal blood flow in their associated blood vessels. It also helps to protect the brain from the toxic effects of chemicals.

Carolyn Dean, M.D., N.D., comments about magnesium and our brains:

> With most of the U.S. population deficient in magnesium, many Americans are a greater risk for a host of serious problems, including stroke with severe post stroke complications, depending on the degree of magnesium deficiency; poor recovery from head injury with escalating neurological damage; neurotoxin damage from vast numbers of chemicals in our air, food, and water: seizure disorders; Alzheimer's disease; and Parkinson's disease. These conditions are the neurological equivalent of heart disease. After all, both heart and brain are excitable tissues that give off electrical energy, and both must have magnesium. . .It was determined that the higher the magnesium levels in water, the lower the incidence of stroke. . .Decades of research show that withdrawal of magnesium from cerebral arteries causes them to spasm, whereas elevated magnesium produces relaxation. . . Animal studies show that when there is normal or elevated magnesium in the brain, the damage caused by stroke is reduced and the neurological deficit is lessened.(105)

Magnesium deficiency can also affect the brain in other ways. Twenty-five million Americans suffer from migraines and a magnesium deficiency may be a major reason why. Drs. Bella and Burton Altura have been studying migraines for about ten years. They found that magnesium is often deficient in people with migraine headaches and many other types of headaches. If the deficiency is corrected, most often the headaches stop.(106)

A study at Massachusetts Institute of Technology (MIT) showed that adequate magnesium is needed to allow the neurons in the brain to operate effectively, which enhances memory and learning.(107) Depression, anxiety, and attention deficit disorder may also manifest with a magnesium deficiency. To put it bluntly, without enough magnesium, mental function is stunted.

Food for Thought

Although I normally don't recommend nutritional supplementation, considering the importance of magnesium and the vast amount of research done with magnesium supplementation, I believe its benefits outweigh any problems associated with it. If you were drinking fresh vegetable juice every day and eating nothing but organic foods, you might not need it. But most people can't or won't do that. It's very difficult to get enough magnesium taking oral supplements, since it tends to cause diarrhea in high doses. You can replenish imagnesium faster and easier using a relatively new product called magnesium oil that is absorbed through your skin.

It's best to be tested to see if you're deficient in magnesium. The magnesium test, which most physicians order, is called a "serum magnesium" test. The world expert on magnesium research, Dr. Mildred Selig, M.D., MPH, says this test is useless and will rarely catch those individuals who badly need more magnesium. The Red blood cell (RBC) magnesium test, although not perfect, is a far better test. Aim for a high normal reading in the laboratory range of magnesium. (See Resource Guide)

You should not to take nutritional supplements haphazardly since you may be causing more harm that good. For example, research has shown that people with elevated iron levels in their bodies may be at a higher risk for severe damage to their brain after a stroke. This may be because high levels of iron promote the release of a chemical that kills brain cells.[108] Since most multivitamins contain iron, you may be getting too much of it if you take one of them consistently. Symptoms of an iron overload are abdominal pain, nausea, constipation, and diarrhea. With this in mind, it may be a good idea to stay away from supplements that contain iron – not just because you may be getting too much, but because the inorganic iron in supplements is too reactive in the body when not encased within the heme structure of hemoglobin (as it is when you consume it from red meat).

Being low in iron isn't good either. An iron deficiency may cause fatigue, pale skin, and breathlessness during exercise. A study showed that women who were known to be iron deficient increased their endurance with the proper iron supplementation.[109] Women and growing children are sometimes iron deficient while adult males are usually not. A simple blood test called a *serum ferritin test* can be used to assess your iron level. Anything below 20 indicates an iron deficiency, but some people do not feel their best until they get to 25 or 30. David Getoff adds that he likes to have his patients' ferritin levels between 35 and 70 for long term heath but that many have far higher levels such as 150 to 400. In those cases he tells them to give blood a few times a year until it gets down to the healthy range. Anything above 1,000 mcg/L indicates iron overload. Visit www.askaboutiron.org to learn more about this test.

Extreme cases of iron deficiency result in anemia. This is often triggered in women by menstruation or internal bleeding. Iron is not the only nutrient involved in anemia, however. A deficiency in folic acid, vitamin B_{12} or B_6 may cause it as can bleeding (including internal), hemolysis (destruction of red blood cells), kidney disease, leukemia, multiple myeloma (cancer of the plasma cells), bone marrow failure (bone marrow is where red blood cells are made), and erythropoietin (a certain blood protein) deficiency.

Anemia is a general term that is used to describe a low blood cell count and is the most common blood disorder in the U.S. with 3.4 million sufferers. It occurs more frequently in women than men. Symptoms include feeling tired and weak, headache, dizziness, ringing in the ears, difficulty sleeping, difficulty concentrating, fainting, and breathlessness.

Blood is made up of three different parts – red blood cells, white blood cells, and platelets. Red blood cells are the part of blood that carries oxygen to all the parts of the body. Anemia occurs when there aren't enough of these red blood cells, so not enough oxygen is supplied to the tissues of the body. To see if you're anemic, have a red blood cell (RBC) count blood test done. You can get a RBC test done as part of a complete blood cell count test at www.healthonelabs.com, or ask your doctor. Consider that without the ferritin test, you cannot know if anemia is due to low iron or possibly low B_{12} and folic acid.

Since too much iron can be as bad as too little, it's a shame that most doctors prescribe iron without doing the ferritin test first. Getting adequate nutrition will help prevent or alleviate anemia. The best source of iron is red meat, fish, poultry, beef liver, and chicken liver. Good nutrition is especially important for seniors, since as we age our ability to absorb nutrients from food diminishes. So the older you are, the more likely you are of becoming anemic. Getting checked for it is a good idea, since anemia promotes cancer and dramatically increases the risk of mortality from heart disease.

The importance of the right kind of fat in the diet cannot be overemphasized as far a prevention of strokes or other cardiovascular problems are concerned. A most important kind of fat crucial to human health is the omega-3 fatty acids. Unfortunately, the typical foods we eat simply do not contain enough of them. Not only that, but the ratio of omega-3 fats to omega-6 fats in our diet is unhealthy. This ratio should be anywhere from 1:4 to 1:1, but it is more like 1:20 to 1:40 (not enough omega 3, too much omega-6).

Omega-6 fats (bad fats) are abundant in sunflower, corn, soy, safflower, and canola oils. Omega-3 fats (good fats) are available in extra virgin olive oil, coconut oil, avocados, butter, grass-fed beef, fish, bison, almonds, and walnuts.

A good way to increase your intake of omega-3 fats is to take a tablespoon of cod liver or fish oil a day. Cod liver oil is not only high in omega-3 fats, but also contains vitamin A and vitamin D. You should take cod liver oil during the winter months since you don't get adequate amounts of sunshine for your body to make vitamin D. During the summer months, if you get outside for several hours a week, you can take fish oil, which lacks vitamin D. You can overdose on vitamin D, so if you have any doubts during the summer, stick with the fish oil, not the cod liver oil. That being said, it's now becoming accepted by numerous scientists (see The Vitamin D Council http://www.vitamindcouncil.org) that the vast majority of the public is deficient in this vitamin all year long. That means that there seems to be very good reasons to take cod liver oil all year and not switch to fish oil during the summer months as been previously advised. The only way to really know if your D status is adequate is to have your physician order a 25(OH) vitamin D_3 test for you – with the optimum between 50 and 70 ng/ml. Please refer to the council's web site for current information and understand that different countries use different units of measure for laboratory testing. (Use the brands of cod liver oil I recommend in the Resource Guide)

In a study of post-menopausal women it was discovered that most of them were deficient in vitamin D – even those who were taking vitamin D supplementation.[110] As we age, our absorption of the vitamin D our skin produces decreases, so supplementation becomes even more important for the elderly. And how many older people spend time outdoors these days?

Studies have shown that eating fish just once a month can cut the risk of stroke among men a whopping 40 percent.[111] Other studies show that benefits of fish eating for stroke prevention work for women also. But fish these days has high amounts of mercury. The fish oils I recommend have been tested and have very low levels of mercury, so it may be better to get the beneficial effects of fish by consuming these oils. But I don't think eating fish one a week will do you much if any harm as far as mercury is concerned.

Food for Thought

Eating raw fish may be safer than cooked fish when it comes to mercury. There's evidence that if the fish is not cooked, the mercury doesn't accumulate in the body but just passes right through. I don't have hard research results on this, but it's something to keep in mind. So enjoy the sushi!

CHAPTER V

Diabetes

Diabetes mellitus (Greek for *honey that passes through*) is a group of diseases characterized by high levels of blood glucose resulting from defects in insulin secretion, insulin action, or both. Diabetes can be associated with serious complications and premature death.[1]

Diabetes is a disease of the endocrine system, specifically, a disorder of the pancreas. The pancreas produces hormones that help digest your food, but the pancreas has another important function: it creates hormones that regulate your body's use of glucose, a form of sugar that fuels most of the daily activities of all your body's cells.

The pancreas produces three hormones: insulin, glucagon, and somatostatin. When the concentration of sugar rises in your blood (after a meal), insulin stimulates muscle and fat cells to recover glucose from the blood and store it. Insulin also stimulates storage of excess glucose in the liver in the form of a starch called glycogen.

When more sugar is needed in the blood, the pancreas produces the hormone glucagon to break down glycogen in the liver and turn it back into glucose (blood sugar), which is then released into the blood stream. The third pancreatic hormone, somatostatin, is not so well understood as the other two, but is thought to also help regulate sugar levels in the blood.

When the pancreatic system fails to control glucose properly, the blood can end up containing too much sugar, a condition called hyperglycemia. Eventually, this sugar gets dumped in the urine, so a diabetic's urine sugar will be higher – thus the Greek *honey that passes through*.

Eighteen million adults in the United States have some form of diabetes. That's roughly 8.7 percent of people age 20 years or older. Roughly 210,000 people under 20 years of age have diabetes. Of these 18.2 million people with this disease – it's estimated that almost 5.2 million of them are undiagnosed cases. Many people suffering from diabetes symptoms do not realize they have the disease. There are 1.3 million new cases of diabetes in adults diagnosed each year. In 2000, diabetes was considered a major contributing cause of death in 213,062 people, and was ranked as the sixth leading cause of death. Overall, people with diabetes are twice as likely to die compared with someone who does not have the disease.[2,3]

Diabetes may be underreported on death certificates, both as a condition and as a cause of death. However "I expect diabetes to be one of the major killers of the world in the year 2010," says Jak Jervell, president of the International Diabetes Federation. "What is bothering me is that the developing world will bear the brunt of this increase," referring to people adopting an American lifestyle of fatty fast food with little or no physical exercise.(4)

In 1947 there were about 600,000 cases of diabetes in the U.S. Although the U.S. population has approximately doubled since the 1940s, the number of diabetics has risen more than 20 times.(5,6) Between 1990 and 1998 diabetes in the adult population as increased 33 percent. The CDC is predicting an alarming and steady rise in diabetes in the near future. The highest increase is in young adults between 20 and 30 years of age, which has gone up 70 percent from 1990 to 1998. The American Diabetes Association projects that at a conservative 3.5 percent growth rate, 50 million Americans will have diabetes by the year 2025 – that's one in every five or six citizens.(7)

Diabetes and obesity go hand in hand. According to Dr. Ali Mokdad, a senior epidemiologist at the CDC, the main reason behind the rise of diabetes is a concurrent rise in obesity and the association of obesity and diabetes is as strong as the association of cigarette smoking and lung cancer. Many researchers have noted a relationship between obesity and diabetes in both adults and children – and considered it one of the major contributing causes of diabetes. With roughly 25 percent of U.S. children being overweight or obese, diabetes is concomitantly a major problem. In fact, a study of adolescents in Cincinnati found 92 percent of 1,027 children with diabetes were obese.(8)

Food for Thought

Parents, if your child is overweight, that's not just a problem in itself or something he or she will just grow out of. There's a very good chance he or she will develop diabetes later in life. It's vital that you change your and your child's dietary habits now before it's too late. As more and more people are getting diabetes at a younger age, in the not to distant future, we will see more and more children getting diabetes too (along with other degenerative and emotional disorders).

In both human and economic terms, diabetes is one of our nation's most costly diseases. It's the leading cause of kidney failure, blindness in adults, slow wound healing, gangrene, and amputations. It's a major risk factor for heart disease, stroke, and birth defects, it shortens average life expectancy by up to 15 years, and it costs the nation in excess of $105 billion annually in health-related expenditures. At present, more than one of every ten health-care dollars and about one of every four Medicare dollars are spent on people with diabetes. It's expected that over the next decade, these numbers will grow as the number of people afflicted by diabetes continues to increase at an alarming rate. Since 1981, the death rate due to diabetes has increased by 30 percent.(9)

Diabetes is not just a single disease, but occurs in several forms. The most common forms are Type I (insulin-dependent or IDDM) diabetes, which usually starts in childhood or adolescence (this is also called juvenile-onset diabetes), and Type II (non-insulin dependent or NIDDM) diabetes, which typically affects adults and increased dramatically with age and obesity. As the name implies, IDDM (Type I) requires a person to take insulin, usually by daily injections. About 10 percent of all diabetics have IDDM. NIDDM (Type II) usually appears after age 40 and the people who get it are usually obese. These people do not need to take insulin because the insulin levels in the blood are about normal, but their body seems to be unable to make good use of the insulin. They must control their blood sugar by controlling their diet – not an easy task for someone who already has a weight problem. About 90 percent of diabetics have NIDDM. Whereas one of the first signs of Type I diabetes is a loss of weight, in Type II, it's usually a gain in weight. The main effect of diabetes (any kind) is to cause changes in the body's small and large blood vessels. These changes in turn effects nearly every system in the body:

- Diabetic eye disease (retinopathy) is the most common cause of blindness in working age adults.
- Diabetic kidney disease (nephropathy) accounts for 42 percent of new cases of end-stage renal disease, and is the fastest growing cause of kidney dialysis and transplantation (over 100,000 cases per year).
- Nervous system damage (neuropathy) affects over 60 percent of diabetics, causing numbness or pain in the feet or hands, slowed digestion of food in the stomach, impotence, and other problems.
- More than half of lower limb amputations in the U.S. occur among people with diabetes.
- About 80,000 amputations are performed each year on people with diabetes.
- Heart disease death rates in adults with diabetes are about two to four times those people without diabetes. Premenopausal women lose their protection from heart disease and have even more markedly increased risk.
- High blood pressure affects over 60 percent of people with diabetes. As a result of the combination of hypertension and diabetes the risk of stroke is increased two to four times.
- The rate of major congenital malformations and death of the fetus and newborn are increased three to four times when the mother is diabetic.
- Higher rates of infection, periodontal disease, and many other problems occur in people with diabetes.(10)

I bring the above details to your attention because there are so many people who do not even know they have diabetes. We will go into the symptoms a little later. If, after you read this chapter, you believe you may have diabetes or have many of the symptoms, I suggest you consult a trained health care professional.

It's estimated that one out of every 400 to 500 children in the U.S. has diabetes, which is about 210,000 children under the age of 20. Most of these cases are Type I, IDDM diabetes. It is one of the most frequent chronic diseases in children in the United States. The incidence of IDDM is higher than all other chronic diseases of youth. Much has been written about the frequency of childhood AIDS, which is certainly a major health concern. However, the number of children who develop IDDM each year is about 13,000, more than 14 times that seen for cases of childhood AIDS. The economic impact of IDDM is large, with a cost to age 40 years of almost $40,000 per case.(11)

There are 13,171 new cases of IDDM (juvenile-onset diabetes) a year in people less than 20 years old and 16,542 cases of IDDM in people 20 years old or older. If we compare the 13,171 new cases of IDDM for young people with rates of other diseases, onset diabetes is clearly a major problem: There are an estimated 796 cases of muscular dystrophy a year, 8,829 cases of cancer a year and 2,822 cases of leukemia a year for the same age group. "In the United States. . . rapid rises during certain years and in certain areas. . .may be suggestive of epidemics."(12)

IDDM is largely a disease of children, while NIDDM is largely a disease of adults. However, in recent years more and more children are getting NIDDM. Prior to 1992, only 2 percent to 3 percent of pediatric patients had NIDDM and 97 percent to 98 percent had IDDM. But in a study of youngsters in Cincinnati, Ohio, in 1994, NIDDM accounted for 16 percent of all new diabetes cases. Among diabetes patients 10 to 19 years of age in this study, NIDDM accounted for 33 percent of diagnoses of diabetes that year. This represents a staggering tenfold increase in NIDDM among children in recent years.(13)

The most accepted theory about how diabetes develops is that the repeated and heavy intake of sugar causes the body's energy system to become defective. When sugar enters the bloodstream, the beta cells of the pancreas are signaled to secrete more insulin and they continue to do so until the blood sugar level drops to normal. Repeated intakes of large amounts of sugar forces the pancreas to work overtime to produce more and more insulin. Eventually, the pancreas becomes exhausted and production of insulin slumps. So when children consume too much sugar too often, they will be more likely to wear out the pancreas and the chances of developing diabetes increases.(14)

Another contributing factor to the development of diabetes was brought to light by Walter Mertz, Ph.D., former chief of the U.S. Department of Agriculture's Vitamin and Mineral Research Division. His experiments showed that a shortage of chromium in the diet can bring on diabetes. This is because insulin needs small amounts of chromium to help get glucose through cell walls. Mertz thinks that most adult-onset diabetes results from a diet of chromium-poor, over processed foods. He recommends including chromium-rich foods such as brewer's yeast, beef liver, chicken and various meats, and whole grains in the diet to avoid this problem.

Since epinephrine, a hormone released by the adrenal gland, increases free fatty acids in the blood and turns off the release of insulin, it is thought that continued stress can upset the balance of pancreas hormones and bring on diabetes (epinephrine is released when we're under stress or in *fight-or-flight* situations).(15)

Although excess fat is a contributing cause of diabetes, the traditional medical establishment knows of no biological mechanism to explain just how the presence of this excess body fat might cause diabetes. However, one researcher has a plausible explanation:

W. John H. Butterfield, M.D., Professor of Medicine at Guys Hospital in London, has done experiments to determine why overweight individuals are more prone to developing diabetes. His research showed a striking similarity in how the body handles carbohydrates in overweight individuals and those with diabetes. In the book *Solved: The Riddle of Illness*, authors Stephen E. Langer, M.D., and James F. Scheer write:

> Obese subjects handled carbohydrates almost like diabetics. . . As obesity progresses, less and less insulin reaches the insulin-responsive muscles, so less and less glucose uptake occurs there, making it necessary for more and more insulin to be formed. When obesity increases to certain proportions, the pancreas can't keep up production of insulin to meet demand, and hyperglycemia results. Reversible-obesity diabetes, then, adds up to a breakdown of the body's insulin-glucose economy. Another significant insight of Dr. Butterfield's about the propensity of diabetes in obese people is that body fat competes with muscle for insulin, and fat wins. Then carbohydrates are changed into more fat.(16)

James Anderson, M.D., of the University of Kentucky, says that both obese and lean diabetics are helped with a diet high in fiber. This usually reduces blood fats and the need for insulin. Diets containing large amounts of raw foods, fruits, vegetables, whole grain breads, nuts, and seeds all contain a lot of fiber. Specific foods that have been shown to help are prunes, corn, spinach, fresh peas, sweet potatoes, apples, blackberries, whole wheat bread, broccoli, almonds, raisins, potatoes, zucchini, plums, and kidney beans.

Professor Somasundaram Addanki, Ph.D., of the Ohio State University College of Medicine, says that a high-fiber diet is good not only for managing diabetes, but also for preventing it. Ninety percent of people prone to diabetes can avoid the disorder by not eating the typical American diet high in fat and sugar and low in fiber. Drawing from his own personal experience, he said that he and his wife did not develop diabetes until they came to America from their native India and started eating American foods. He thinks that only about 8 percent of diabetic cases can be strictly attributed to heredity, based on research in Africa and Japan. That theory is backed by the findings that many Japanese living in Japan did not develop diabetes; however, when they moved to Hawaii and started eating American food, they developed diabetes in great numbers.(17)

Although many people believe that heredity plays a major role in diabetes, many researchers now rule this out.

There is a definite genetic component to the development of Type I diabetes and some of these genes are known. . .But genetic predisposition to diabetes is far from the whole story. For one thing there is a high prevalence of these so-called susceptibility genes in the general population, yet this is not reflected in the incidence of the disease. Even in identical twins, one of which may develop diabetes, in about half the cases the other twin, who carries the same genes, does not develop diabetes. Furthermore, in recent years the disease has been increasing in the general population at about 2.5 percent a year.[18]

Do any environmental factors contribute to the development of diabetes? In a study of Vietnam veterans, the level of dioxin levels in the blood correlated with the development of diabetes. The study compared 989 veterans who had participated in Operation Ranch Hand (which sprayed roughly 12 million gallons of Agent Orange over 10 percent of South Vietnam between 1962 and 1971) with 1,276 Air Force veterans who served in Southeast Asia during the same period but did not participate in the herbicide-spraying program. Dioxin was at about 3 parts per million in the Agent Orange.

Blood dioxin levels were significantly higher in the Ranch Hand group, and these men were about 50 percent more likely to get diabetes compared with the control group. The severity of diabetes increased in the Ranch Hand group as the level of dioxin in the blood increased. Also, the time-to-onset of diabetes was shorter among those with more dioxin in their blood. The study found consistent increases in the likelihood of glucose (blood sugar) abnormalities with increasing dioxin levels.[19]

This finding linking diabetes to a chemical like dioxin, which is a known endocrine-disrupting chemical, offers another explanation as to why obesity con-tributes to diabetes. It's well recognized that human fat accumulates toxic chemicals. For any particular chemical, our fat often has a concentration 100 times as high as the concentration found in our blood. It's also known that chemicals can be released from fat to recirculate in the blood stream during times of pregnancy, stress, illness, or fasting. Many fat-stored chemicals are known to interfere with our endocrine systems by mimicking or blocking natural hormones.[20]

So it may not just be the fat that's contributing to more diabetes. It could be that the unnatural, harmful chemicals stored in the fat are causing endocrine problems which leads to diabetes. It would be interesting to find out if years ago, before all these chemicals were introduced, there was the same kind of correlation between obesity and diabetes. If there wasn't, then it very well could be that the chemicals stored in the fat, and subsequently recirculating in the blood, could be responsible for disrupting the endocrine system.

It's also been observed that up to 40 percent of people with diabetes are deficient in the mineral magnesium. In fact, low blood magnesium levels have been used as a marker for diabetes. Low magnesium increases the risk of cardiovascular disease, eye symptoms, and nerve damage in diabetics.[21]

And guess what might cause a magnesium deficiency? Not surprisingly, common table sugar. Sugar is pretty much devoid of minerals (they are left in the molasses during processing), and only 11 percent of magnesium is left in the sugar after it's fully processed. Sugar creates an acidic condition in the body because one of the results of the digestion of sugar is the formation of pyruvic acid – a toxin that must be neutralized by the body drawing out alkaline minerals (magnesium, calcium, and potassium) from bones and muscles. (Now you know why sugar also causes osteoporosis, tooth decay, and muscle weakness.)

Since magnesium is essential in the production of energy from sugar stored in the muscles and liver, if we don't have enough of it, the cells cannot produce enough energy and "believe" they need more sugar. More insulin is needed, and a downward spiral into diabetes begins. Magnesium is also needed in the secretion and function of insulin, and without it, diabetes is inevitable.[22]

Besides being important in diabetes, magnesium is a major cause for concern in a myriad of other diseases and conditions. A magnesium deficiency may result in the following symptoms: Charlie horse; anxiety; depression; neurotic behavior; panic attacks; excessive emotionality; fatigue; muscle weakness; stiff and aching muscles; chronic fatigue syndrome; hyperactivity; angina; stroke; heart disease; hypertension; hypoglycemia; PMS; back pain; aggressive behavior; hiccups; seizures; headaches; insomnia; light-headedness; dizziness; migraines; nerve problems; musculoskeletal conditions; infertility; sensation of a lump in the throat; asthma; kidney disease; liver disease; impaired breathing; pins and needles of the extremities; cramps muscle pains and twitches; abnormal heart rhythm; chest pressure; palpitations; amnesia; Sudden Infant Death Syndrome; osteoporosis; Raynaud's Syndrome; tooth decay; cystitis; and tremor.

It's not surprising a magnesium deficiency can cause so many problems since it's responsible for the correct metabolic function of over 350 enzymes in the body. Magnesium is intricately involved with ATP (adenosine triphosphate) production – the molecule used to produce most of the energy in the body, along with the relaxation of blood vessels, heart action, and proper bowel function.

It's estimated that as many as 80 percent of Americans are deficient in this essential nutrient. This is due in part to the food choices we make – junk food and fast food do not have much magnesium – and to the food itself. Our cropland has been depleted of magnesium over the years, and conventional fertilizers typically only replace nitrogen, potassium, and phosphorous. Organically grown food is better since the faming practices and fertilizers used are more complete.

Children are not immune to a magnesium deficiencies either, especially considering that many of the foods they eat like hot dogs, pizza, and soda are all magnesium deficient. Dr. Leo Galland, author of *Superimmunity for Kids*, believes that hyperactive children need extra magnesium due to their high adrenal activity. He recommends 6 mg per pound of weight per day in these cases in the form of magnesium citrate or 1½ teaspoons of milk of magnesium a day.(23)

You have probably heard about how important obtaining enough calcium is. This is true, but most people don't realize that the calcium must be balanced with magnesium for optimal results. In fact, if you get too much calcium and not enough magnesium, bad things can occur. A high calcium-to-magnesium ratio in the diet can lead to a heart attack. Finland has the highest rate of heart attacks in the world, and the Ca:Mg ratio there is 4.0:1.0. In the U.S., the Ca:Mg is around 3.5:1.0 to as high as 6.0:1.0. The recommended ratio is 2.0:1.0. So is it any wonder that the U.S. ranks so high in heart attacks? Considering this, taking extra calcium (without balancing it with magnesium) in hopes of keeping your bones strong may actually be setting you up for a heart attack.

Experts say that our bodies evolved in prehistoric times on a Ca/Mg ratio of 1.0:1.0, and this is what we should try to get in our diet. In the early 1900's, dietary magnesium in the U.S. was 500 mg/day whereas now it's barely 200 mg/day. The RDA for magnesium is 6 mg/kg of body weight or 6 mg per 2.2 lbs of body weight. So if you weigh 150 lbs., you should get at least 400 mg of magnesium a day. Growing children need more magnesium – from 7-10 mg/kg/day, and pregnant women should get up to 15 mg/kg/day. As you get older, the amount of magnesium you absorb goes down. By age 70, magnesium absorption is only two-thirds of what it was at age thirty. And experiments show that chronic marginal magnesium deficiency reduces life span in test animals.

Consider that sugar uses up magnesium. Coffee, and alcohol cause it to be excreted, and carbonated beverages and processed foods (luncheon meats, hot dogs) contain phosphorus which binds to magnesium making it insoluble and unable for the body to absorb. Drugs can also cause a magnesium deficiency. In fact, a lot of side effects of some medications are actually magnesium deficiency symptoms. Birth control pills, diuretics, digitalis, cardiac glycosides, tetracycline, cortisone, and even insulin can create a magnesium deficiency. So if you're on any kind of medication, you need to be sure you're getting enough magnesium.(24) If not, you may be looking at heart problems.

Diabetes can be caused by a number of factors ranging from our lifestyle of bad food, deficiencies, and no exercise, to our exposure to water, food, and air that has been contaminated with a myriad of chemicals, many of which mimic or interfere with our hormones. There are also theories that vaccines could cause diabetes in children. (See chapter on vaccines.)

The telltale signs of diabetes are excessive thirst, frequent and copious urination, a highly acid system, rapid weight loss, constant hunger, severe itching, weakness, fatigue, and high sugar levels in the blood and urine.

If you've been determined to need insulin, it's best to take it. However, by adopting a better, cleaner and more natural lifestyle, the symptoms and severity of your disease can be handled and alleviated. I have heard of many people who have changed their diet and exercise patterns and decreased their need for insulin. In rare cases, some have even been able to go off it completely.

A most important thing to do is to change your diet and the diet of your child – whether you are diabetic or not. The typical American diet of fast food hamburgers, pizza, coke, and chips is certainly not conducive to the health of your pancreas. In fact, if you keep eating like that, diabetes is probably just around the corner. Fresh fruits, vegetables, whole grains, good organically grown meats, nuts, seeds, greens, fresh vegetable juices, raw milk, and spring water are what the pancreas and the body needs to function correctly. Remember, it's the repeated spike of sugar in the blood that causes the pancreas to work too hard. Over time, it wears out, and blood sugar problems arise.

Killing Us Softly

What substance do you think the following paragraph describes?

> It removes rust spots from chrome car bumpers; cleans corrosion from car battery terminals; removes grease from clothes: just put some into your washer and run through a regular cycle. It's great to clean a stained toilet: put some in and let it sit for one hour, then flush clean. It has a pH of 3.4, which is very acidic. (Car battery acid is around 2.0. The pH of human blood is normally 7.4. And if the pH of your blood dips below 7.2, you die.) It will dissolve a tooth or human bone: put a tooth in this stuff and in ten days it will be gone. It will also dissolve a common metal nail and loosen a rusted bolt in minutes because it is extremely corrosive.

Did you guess a household cleaner, disinfectant or maybe even a industrial chemical? Sorry. The substance I'm referring to is the all-American cola drink. That's right. Soda pop.

Back in 1942, the average consumption of soft drinks per person per year was just 60 12-ounce cans. Now children drink almost 900 cans a year. Between 1942 and 1998, production of soft drinks increased nine fold. The biggest consumers are 12- to 19-year-old males, drinking an average of almost 2½ 12 ounce sodas (28.5 ounces) per day. That's 868 cans of soda pop a year. Teenage girls drink about 1.7 12-ounce sodas per day. Twenty years ago, the average consumption for boys was just three quarters a can per day. One fifth of one- and two-year-old children also consume soft drinks, averaging seven ounces (almost a cup) per day.[25,26] The elderly are drinking more soft drinks too. Those aged 40 - 59 increased consumption from 2 percent to 5 percent between 1977 and 2001 and for those over 60, consumption went up from 1 percent to 3 percent.[27]

One reason for the increase in consumption, aside from the ubiquitous advertising, is that over the past 40 years, bottles and cans have grown in size from 6½ ounces to 12-ounces to the present 20-ounce bottles. The larger the container, the more beverage people are likely to drink, especially when they assume they are buying single-serving containers. In 1998, Americans spent over $54 billion to buy 14 billion gallons of soft drinks. That's an average of 56 gallons of soft drinks for every man, woman, and child in America. In 2000, sales were even higher, topping $57 million.(28)

Although soft drinks are now commonplace, they are a very recent addition to the human diet. We survived and thrived for millions of years without them. Now they are connected to a host of health problems: obesity; diabetes and other blood sugar disorders; heart disease; osteoporosis and bone fractures; nutritional deficiencies; eating disorders and food addictions; neurotransmitter dysfunction; and neurological and adrenal disorders.(29) To say, as a National Soft Drink Association's poster (intended for teachers) proclaims, that soft drinks are a "positive addition to a well-balanced diet" is positively untrue. The poster goes on to say: "As refreshing sources of needed liquids and energy, soft drinks represent a positive addition to a well-balanced diet. . .These same three sugars also occur naturally, for example in fruits. . . In your body it makes no difference whether the sugar is from a soft drink or a peach."(30)

First, it's true that the body needs liquids. Although a soft drink does contain about 90 percent water, it also generally contains caffeine (six of the seven top-selling soft drinks contain caffeine). Caffeine is a known diuretic, a substance that causes increased urine and water excretion. It's estimated that for every can of soda a person consumes, the body requires about two glasses of water to replenish what was lost due to the caffeine's diuretic action. That holds true for any caffeinated beverage, coffee and tea included. You may think you're replenishing water in your body when you drink that soda, but in reality, you're actually contributing to dehydration.

Second, the sugars in the soft drink may, on paper, look like the sugars found in fruits, but they are not. A manufactured, synthetic or processed sugar does *not* have the same effect on the human body as a sugar found in its natural state.

Many soft drinks now contain artificial sweeteners to cut down on calories from sugar. Two of the major ones used are saccharin and aspartame, and both have been linked to urinary-bladder cancer. Now Congress has required products made with saccharin to have a warning label – but this has done little to curtail consumption. Acesulfame-K, another artificial sweetener approved in 1998, is considered suspect by some cancer experts.(31) Now *Splenda* is the number one artificial sweetener in America and in many sodas. But it has been linked to liver and kidney problems, thymus gland shrinkage, and reduced growth rates.

Soft drinks are Americans' single biggest source of refined sugar. Twelve- to 19-year-old boys get about 44 percent of their 34 teaspoons of sugar a day from soft drinks. Girls get a little less – only 40 percent. That translates to about 15 teaspoons of sugar a day for boys and 10 teaspoons a day for girls. One thing to keep in mind here is that these are averages for all children. Considering that some kids don't drink any pop at all, the children who do drink it are really taking in more than that average.

As teens have doubled or tripled their consumption of soft drinks, they now drink 40 percent less milk. Twenty years ago, boys consumed twice as much milk as soda and girls consumed 50 percent more milk than soda. Now, boys and girls consume twice as much soda pop as milk. Michael Jacobson, executive director of the nonprofit Center for Science in the Public Interest (CSPI) says, "Many teens are drowning in soda pop. It's become their main beverage, providing many with 15 percent to 20 percent of all their calories and squeezing out more nutritious foods and beverages from their diets. It's time that parents limited their children's soft-drink consumption and demanded that local schools get rid of their soft-drink vending machines, just as they have banished smoking."[32]

Marianne Manilov, the executive director of the Center for Commercialism-Free Public Education, castigated schools "for sacrificing their students' health by selling out to *Coca-Cola*. The marketing agreements virtually ensure that more kids will be drinking more soda – while their health classes are discouraging consumption. Taxpayers must provide schools systems with adequate funds so schools don't become reliant on junk-food companies."[33] Since the adult market is essentially stagnant, the soft-drink companies are going after the young and the innocent. An article in *Beverage* magazine stated: "Influencing elementary school students is very important to soft-drink marketers."[34] So important they spend billions of dollars each year on advertising aimed at children. They run ads on *Channel One* – the classroom TV network seen by eight million junior and high school students every day. *Coca-Cola* paid one Colorado school district $11 million over more than 10 years to advertise in the hallways and sides of busses. Amazingly, the schools have quotas, so consumption, even in the classroom, is encouraged by the administration.[35]

If that's not bad enough, get this: At a press conference, CSPI displayed baby bottles with *Pepsi*, *Seven-Up*, and *Dr Pepper* logos. Those companies have licensed their logos to a major maker of bottles, Munchkin Bottling, Inc. One study found that parents are four times more likely to feed their children soda pop when their children use those logo bottles than when they don't.[36]

Let's look more closely at the documented health impacts of soft drinks. When you consider soft drinks in the context of obesity and overweight, it's interesting to note that obesity rates have risen in tandem with soft-drink consumption. Heavy consumers of soda pop have been shown to have higher calorie intakes. Michael F. Jacobsen, Ph.D., writes, "While those observations do not prove that sugary soft drinks cause obesity. . .Heavy consumption is likely to contribute to weight gain in many consumers."[37]

The National Institutes of Health recommends that people wanting to lose weight cut back on consuming soft drinks and drink water instead. Nutritionists and weight-loss experts routinely advise overweight people to consume fewer calories, especially "empty-caloric foods" such as soft drinks. Soft drinks now account for about 25 percent of sugar consumption and sugar is an empty-calorie food.

They are called "empty-calorie foods" because they have no nutritional value besides calories. A soft drink contains no vitamins, minerals, enzymes, or fiber that gives a food its nutritional value. All you get when you drink a can of soda is calories (and caffeine, artificial flavoring, and acid), which can be used for energy production or stored as fat. Since we're exercising less, guess where most of it goes?

Several additives used in soft drinks can cause occasional allergic reactions. Yellow No. 5 dye causes runny noses, hives, and asthma as well as lymphoma, thyroid tumors, and chromosomal damage.[38] Cochineal, a red coloring agent, can cause life-threatening allergic reactions, and other dyes have been shown to cause hyperactivity in sensitive children.[39]

Soft Drinks and Osteoporosis

It's a well-recognized fact that low calcium intake contributes to osteoporosis, a disease that leads to fragile and broken bones. It's estimated that teenage girls in the U.S. are getting only 60 percent of the recommended amount of calcium, with soft-drink drinkers consuming almost one fifth less than non soft-drink drinkers.[40] This means these girls are replacing healthier beverages such as milk (although super-market milk is not so healthy these days as you'll find out later).

Not only that, but the very nature of soft drinks is that they deplete calcium in the body. It's all a matter of simple chemistry. The pH of most soft drinks is around 3.4. That's highly acidic. Neutral pH is 7. The pH of healthy blood is slightly alkaline, being 7.4. It's fatal if your blood pH drops to 7.2. When you ingest acidic food or drinks (such as a soft drink), the body must neutralize the acid. It does so by drawing on its stores of calcium (and some magnesium) from the bones, teeth, and muscles.

I'm sure you've heard of the calcium in heartburn medicine; some antacid brands even go so far as to promote their product as "bone-building" (which they are not). It's there to neutralize the acid in your stomach that causes gas and heartburn. Not unlike a farmer liming his field. Lime is calcium carbonate, and he spreads it on the field to raise the pH to a more neutral condition, which promotes better plant life. That's what our bodies do naturally when we consume a substance so high in acid (low pH). We have to neutralize it by robbing calcium out of our bones, muscles, and teeth. The end result? Osteoporosis, weak and brittle bones, and cavities.

Do soft drinks cause this? In a study published in *Pediatrics & Adolescent Medicine* in June 2000, the researchers concluded that cola beverages were "highly associated with bone fractures." They expressed ". . .concern and alarm about the health impact of carbonated beverage consumption on teenaged girls."(41) Another study reported in the *Journal of Adolescent Health* also found a "Strong association between cola beverage consumption and bone fractures in girls. . . The high consumption of carbonated beverages and the declining consumption of milk are of great public health significance for girls and women because of their proneness to osteoporosis in later life."(42)

To drive this important point home one more time, Dr. Bess Dawson-Hughes, a bone-disease expert at the Jean Mayer USDA Human Nutrition Research Center on Aging at Tufts University in Boston, says, "I'm particularly concerned about teenage girls. Most girls have inadequate calcium intakes, which makes them candidates for osteoporosis when they're older and may increase their risk for broken bones today. High soda consumption is a concern because it may displace milk from the diet in this vulnerable population."(43)

Caffeine is one of the ingredients in soft drinks that contribute to calcium loss. Linda Massey, Ph.D., a bone researcher at Washington State University in Spokane, says that caffeine can indeed be hard on your bones. "The more regular coffee a woman drinks, the more calcium is excreted in her urine," she says. Janet Barger-Lux of Creighton University's Osteoporosis Research Unit in Omaha, Nebraska, goes further, "This loss amounts to about 5 milligrams of calcium for every 6 ounces of coffee or two cans of cola."(44) Yes, soft drinks also increase the excretion of calcium the urine. Drinking 12 ounces of a caffeine-containing soft drink can cause the loss of about 120 milligrams of calcium (roughly 2 percent of the U.S. Recommended Daily Allowance).(45)

It's a simple equation: Soft Drinks + Human = Soft Bones (and Rotting Teeth, as we shall see). If things keep going the way they have been, it may not be long before you start seeing hip replacement surgery on teenagers.

Soft Drinks and Tooth Decay

Drinking soft drinks regularly bathes the teeth in and acidic sugar-water for long periods of time. Refined sugars promote tooth decay. So it's not a surprise that a study between 1971 and 1974 found a strong correlation between the frequency of between-meal consumption of soda pop and cavities.(46)

The phosphoric acid in soft drinks also plays havoc on teeth. As this acid lingers in the mouth after a sip of soda, the body must pull calcium ions from the teeth in an attempt to normalize the saliva's pH (which should be around 7.4). As the calcium is stripped away, so is the enamel. This explains why dentists are noticing a condition in teenagers that was previously found only in the elderly – a complete loss of enamel on the teeth, resulting in yellow teeth.(47)

Food for Thought

When dentists do cosmetic bonding, they first roughen up the enamel by removing some of it with a chemical compound. That chemical is none other than phosphoric acid – the same found in soft drinks.

Soft Drinks and Upset Stomach

There's another risk from phosphoric acid (and other acids in sodas such as acetic, fumaric, gluconic) and caffeine: stomach aches. These acids and caffeine upset the fragile acid-alkaline balance of the stomach, creating a continuous acid environment that leads to inflammation.(48) Oftentimes the lament of "Mommy, I have a tummy ache" can be prevented by keeping the child away from sodas or other acidic and caffeinated beverages.

Soft Drinks and Heart Disease

In some people, a diet high in sugar may promote heart disease, some researchers contend. An estimated one quarter of adults has high levels of triglycerides and low levels of HDL cholesterol (the "good" cholesterol – HDL stands for High-Density Lipoprotein) in their blood. When these people eat a diet high in carbohydrates (sugar is a refined carbohydrate), their triglyceride and insulin levels rise. It's been shown that sugar has a greater effect than other carbohydrates in producing this result. No wonder excessive sugar intake also contributes to developing diabetes.

A study in Louisiana determined that overweight children were at increased risk for developing heart disease. Fifty-eight percent of the overweight kids ages five to 10 had one additional risk factor such as elevated cholesterol or high blood pressure. Twenty percent were found to have two or more additional risk factors for heart disease.(49) Since so many kids are overweight these days, there's a significant number that are close to or already have heart problems. Part of the reason is that they are getting less exercise. Another is that they are consuming more sugar, thus leading to heart problems similar to what happens in adults.

One of the most painful disorders, kidney stones affected more than one million people in 1985.(50) It's estimated by the National Institute of Diabetes and Digestive and Kidney Diseases (NIDDK) that 10 percent of all Americans will have a kidney stone during their lifetime – more in men than women. Men, incidentally, are the heaviest consumers of soft drinks. One study linked soft drink consumption with kidney stones.(51) More research is needed, but the NIDDK does include cola beverages on a list of food that patients with kidney stones should avoid.

Another thing that can contribute to kidney stones is foods rich in oxalic acid. These foods, when cooked, definitely contribute to stone formation and also calcium excretion and bone weakening. But some believe that when these foods are consumed raw (eaten or juiced), the oxalic acid is not harmful. My advice? If you do consume these foods, be sure not to cook them and only eat them or juice them occasionally. Foods high in oxalic acid include beets, soy, beet tops, black tea, chenopodium, chocolate, cocoa, dried figs, ground pepper, parsley, poppy seeds, purslane, rhubarb, sorrel, spinach, and Swiss chard.

Caffeine

Caffeine is a mildly addictive stimulant drug found in most cola and other soft drinks of all colors and tastes. An average soda pop drinker, drinking *Mountain Dew*, would have ingested 92 mg of caffeine. That's equivalent to one 6 ounce cup of coffee.

Caffeine causes nervousness, irritability, sleeplessness, and rapid heartbeat. It's been documented that children who normally do not consume much caffeine become restless and fidgety, develop headaches, and have difficulty going to sleep when they do consume it. When children age six to 12 stop consuming caffeine, they suffer withdrawal symptoms that impair their attention span and performance.(52)

Roland Griffiths, professor in the department of psychiatry and behavioral sciences at the Johns Hopkins University School of Medicine, says, "Caffeine is a mildly addictive drug, and parents might wish to limit their children's consumption of it." He goes on to say, "Americans should be mindful about their caffeine consumption. Drinking the caffeine equivalent of several cups of coffee a day can lead to insomnia, anxiety, and difficulty concentrating. Ceasing the consumption of caffeine often leads to withdrawal symptoms, such as headache and fatigue."(53) These symptoms have been reported in children as well as in adults.

Yes, caffeine is a drug. According to more than 40 scientific studies, it may cause miscarriages, insomnia, and other problems. Dr. Michael Jacobson, executive director of CSPI, says, "Caffeine is the only drug that is widely added to the food supply and consumers have a right to know how much caffeine various foods contain. Knowing the caffeine content is important to many people – especially women who are or might become pregnant – who might want to limit or avoid caffeine."(54) The Food and Drug Administration advises pregnant women to "avoid caffeine-containing foods and drugs, if possible, or consume them only sparingly." Why? Because they have been implicated in causing birth defects and underweight babies. In laboratory animals, very large amounts of caffeine seem to cause females to bear young that are malformed.(55) As far as humans are concerned, the jury on whether they in deed do cause birth defects is still out. But one report stated, "The risk for any kind of congenital abnormalities is 3.5% in individuals who consume caffeine and 1.7% in those who do not. The difference is statistically significant."(56)

Caffeine has been more strongly implicated in low-birth weight babies. Among nearly 4,000 women who gave birth in New Haven, Connecticut, in the early 1980s, those who consumed between 150 and 300 milligrams of caffeine a day during their pregnancies, had more than twice the risk of delivering under-weight babies (less than about five pounds) than those who consumed less. The risk was almost five times greater for women who consumed more than 300 milligrams a day, just three cups a day. Unfortunately, researchers haven't been able to tell if it's the caffeine, the coffee, or something else about women who consume these substances that's causing the low-birth-weight babies. A 1996 study showed more than double the risk of miscarriage in women who were consuming more than 300 mg a day of caffeine.(57)

There are also studies that show that caffeine consumption by pregnant mothers may cause decreased placental circulation, smaller brain size in off-spring, and decreased learning capacities.(58) Potential mothers, why take the chance? Just don't drink coffee and don't drink soft drinks while you're pregnant. Period. You're more likely to have a normal, healthy baby.

Food for Thought

"You know," you might say, "I understand all these things about soft drinks and coffee. But really, how bad can they be? I mean, everybody drinks them. Wouldn't the FDA or somebody ban them if they were really harmful? You're just being a worrywart." Well, people smoked for decades thinking there was nothing wrong with it. It's just a matter of time before people realize these drinks are just as bad if not worse.

Within the past couple of years, some school districts have banned the sale of soft drinks – Philadelphia, Los Angeles, Chicago and New York. This is a major step in the right direction, but it's not really a boon for our children's health since instead of soft drinks, fruit juices, and sports drinks will be sold. They are loaded with sugar, artificial sweeteners, and fluoride.

As a child's health is impaired, so is his or her enjoyment of life. That child is then more likely to get depressed or despondent or even violent. I'm not saying soda pop necessarily causes violent behavior. What I am saying once again is that the healthier a person is, the less likely he or she will have mental or emotional problems. The more a child consumes harmful substances, the less likely that child will be healthy. All these things add up. Soda pop here, food additives there, pesticides over there, TV over there. They're all straws added to the back of someone growing up – straws that can eventually break that child's back and make that child, or anyone, snap.

It's estimated that one in five kids may have some sort of mental problem. They're three times as likely to have an emotional or behavioral disorder today, as they were 20 years ago. That means that psychological disorders in kids almost tripled in the last 20 years.(59) Personally, I haven't had a soda since 1982. I stopped in graduate school when I figured that just by not buying a cola at lunch, I would save over $100 a year. ($100 was a lot of money back then.) I didn't realize the health risks associated with drinking the stuff; I quit because I needed the money. Now, when I see people who may be struggling to make ends meet drinking soda, I have to shake my head. Considering the average male teenager drinks 868 cans a year, they're spending over $500 a year on something that will cause them even more expense later – ill health.

When I worked as an environmental engineer, I inspected industrial plants to make sure all the waste and hazardous wastes were disposed of properly. It was some what of a joke among us inspectors that if we found a drum of cola on the site, it would, according to EPA regulations, be required to be disposed of at a hazardous waste disposal facility. Recently I checked with the EPA to see if that is really the case. I found that if a substance has a pH of less than 2.0, it is considered hazardous. So soft drinks don't meet this criterion because they have an average pH of 3.4. But, if a substance corrodes steel at a rate greater than 6.35 millimeters a year – roughly ¼ inch (at 65º C), it's considered hazardous.[60] I don't know if soft drinks will corrode steel at that rate, but I did discover some comments on this subject in the book *Sugar Blues* which quotes Dr. McCay, who had been in charge of nutritional research during World War II. Besides reporting to a Congressional committee that cola beverages typically contained about 10 percent sugar, he also commented that they were very corrosive. An excerpt of the committee records is interesting:

Dr. McCay: "I was amazed to learn that the beverage contained substantial amounts of phosphoric acid. At the Naval Medical Research Institute, we put human teeth in a cola beverage and found they softened and started to dissolve within a short period. . .children little realize they are drinking this strange mixture of phosphoric acid, sugar, caffeine, coloring, and flavoring matter."

A congressman asked the doctor what government bureau was in charge of passing on the contents of soft drinks.

Dr. McCay: "As far as I know, no one passes upon it or pays any attention to it."

Congressman: "No one passes on the contents of soft drinks?"

Dr. McCay: "So far as I know, no one."

Another congressman asked if the doctor had made any tests of the effect of cola beverages on metal and iron. When the doctor said he hadn't the congressman volunteered: "A friend of mine told me once that he dropped three ten-penny nails into one of the cola bottles, and in forty-eight hours the nails had completely dissolved.

Dr. McCay: "Sure. Phosphoric acid there would dissolve iron or lime-stone. You might drop it on the steps, and it would erode the steps coming up here. . . Since soft drinks are playing an increasingly important part of the American diet and tend to displace foods such as milk, they deserve very careful consideration."[61]

According to this anecdotal information about corrosion then, cola drinks and probably most other soft drinks would indeed be classified as a hazardous waste according to EPA guidelines.

Sugar

In 1975, the book *Sugar Blues* by journalist William Dufty was published. It is a shocking exposé of sugar, its history and the health problems that arise from its continued use. Before going into its possible health effects, a brief discussion about just what sugar is and how it evolved is in order so that you will better understand just what we're dealing with here.

Sugar is refined sucrose, often called simple sugar. It's produced by a number of chemical processing steps from the juice of the sugar cane or sugar beet. In processing, all fiber, protein, and minerals (which comprise about 90 percent of the plant itself) are removed.

Simple sugars (monosaccharides and disaccharides) are sometimes called *rapid sugars* because they don't need digestion and are rapidly absorbed into our bloodstream. Most sweeteners, natural or otherwise, are composed of simple sugars. When they are absorbed into the bloodstream, they cause a rise in blood glucose levels that are unnaturally high. Glucose is a single sugar molecule. It results from the breakdown of disaccharides and is the only sugar used by the cells in the body. In fact, it is the only thing the body ever uses as fuel. When the blood glucose level in the blood rises, it results in a condition called hyperglycemia, and is one of the symptoms of diabetes. When the pancreas functions as it should, it will produce and release enough insulin to remove the excess glucose from the bloodstream. If the pancreas is impaired, it cannot keep up and hyperglycemia results.

As the body senses the increased glucose in the blood, insulin production increases, but when the intake of sugar is stopped, the pancreas does not recognize this right away, there's a time lag. So as the insulin keeps pouring into the bloodstream, there's less and less sugar to go around. The result is that the glucose level in the blood falls too much. Low blood sugar, or hypoglycemia, is the result. Symptoms of hypoglycemia include depression, dizziness, crying spells, aggression, insomnia, weakness, and in extreme cases loss of consciousness.

When the blood glucose level falls too low, the adrenal glands kick in to mobilize the body's stores of glycogen (a carbohydrate found in the liver and muscles – the storage form of glucose) to bring the sugar level up to normal. Glucose is also synthesized from proteins and other substances when the blood level of glucose falls too low.

So, when too much sugar is ingested, there's a seesaw effect of the metabolism. The pancreas reacts to produce insulin. This results in hypoglycemia. Then the adrenals react and glycogen is released from the liver to bring the blood sugar up to normal. Not only is the sugar level of the blood going up and down in extremes, but also the pancreas, adrenals, and liver are being overworked.

When the pancreas wears out, diabetes manifests. But there are other effects. As the sugars are absorbed, the body turns them into excessive amounts of saturated fatty acids and cholesterol. If these are not burned off through activity, they accumulate under the skin, in our liver, kidneys, arteries, and other organs. That's why so many diabetics have weight problems and cardiovascular complications. If they don't exercise (and they are less likely to not to want to since their blood sugar levels are so inconsistent), they get fat.

Since sugars increase our body's production of adrenaline by fourfold, two major things happen. One is that the body goes into a state of stress – the fight or flight response. This stress reaction increases the production of cholesterol and cortisone. Cortisone is known to inhibit the immune system – so allergies and infections are more likely. Also, as insulin levels rise, the release of growth hormone is decreased. Growth hormone is known to activate the immune system. So, the more sugar, the more insulin, the less growth hormone, the weaker the immune system.

The second thing is that along with the pancreas, the adrenals simply get tired and wear out. Eventually they cannot produce the necessary hormones for proper cellular function. Stress cannot be handled as well.

Another reason that sugar is so bad is that it does not contain the vitamins, minerals, and cofactors necessary for its own metabolism in the body. So the body must draw on its stores of these nutrients in order to metabolize it. Sugar leaches out vitamins B, C, and D, and minerals like calcium, magnesium, iron, zinc, chromium, and phosphorous. The more sugar you eat, the more minerals and vitamins you need, and the fewer minerals remain in your body.

Sugar not only robs the teeth, bones, muscles, and blood of a great percentage of their minerals, but also causes irritation and weakens mucous membranes. This irritation and inflammation can result in breathing problems (asthma and emphysema) and digestive problems such as heartburn.

As vitamins and mineral stores in our body decrease, the body is less able to carry out other functions that require them. It cannot metabolize fats and cholesterol as efficiently or convert cholesterol into bile acids. So cholesterol levels rise, the metabolic rate goes down, fats burn more slowly and gall stones are formed. As all this is happening, the person certainly feels less and less like exercising, so body weight increases even more: A vicious cycle.

William Coda Martin, Ph.D., believes that sugar is a poison because it depletes the body of its life forces, vitamins, and minerals. He says,

> What is left consists of pure, refined carbohydrates. The body cannot utilize this refined starch and carbohydrate unless the depleted proteins, vitamins and minerals are present. Nature supplies these elements in each plant in quantities sufficient to metabolize the carbohydrate in that particular plant. There is no excess for other added carbohydrates. Incomplete carbohydrate metabolism results in the formation of toxic metabolites such as pyruvic acid and abnormal sugars containing five carbon atoms. Pyruvic acid accumulates in the brain and nervous system and the abnormal sugars in the red blood cells. These toxic metabolites interfere with the respiration of the cells. They cannot get

sufficient oxygen to survive and function normally. In time, some of the cells die. This interferes with the function of a part of the body and is the beginning of degenerative disease.(62)

Essentially, eating sugar is worse than eating nothing at all since it robs the body of minerals and vitamins, along with the energy demands of detoxification and elimination from the body. You can survive for quite some time on nothing but water, but eating sugar and water can kill you sooner. In fact, in 1816 the French physiologist F. Magendie published his results of a series of experiments with dogs in which he fed them nothing but sugar or olive oil and water. All the animals died in a shorter time than if they consumed nothing but water.(63)

If you eat sugar every day, a continuously over-acid condition results and more and more minerals are required from deep in the body in the attempt to rectify the imbalance. Finally, in order to protect the blood and keep it in a slightly alkaline condition (since sugar creates an acid condition), so much calcium is taken from the bones and teeth that osteoporosis and decay, respectively, result.

Excess sugar eventually affects every organ in the body. Initially, it is stored in the liver, as already mentioned, in the form of glycogen. Since the liver's capacity is limited, it will soon expand like a balloon. When the liver is filled to its maximum, the excess glycogen is returned to the blood in the form of fatty acids. These are taken to every part of the body and stored in the most inactive areas – the belly, buttocks, breasts, and thighs.

When these places are filled, the fatty acids are then distributed to the active organs such as the heart and kidneys. This causes their activities to slow down and tissues to degenerate and turn to fat. The whole body is affected by their reduced ability, and abnormal blood pressure is created. The circulatory and lymphatic systems are taxed, the red corpuscles are altered, an overabundance of white blood cells is created, and tissue regeneration and repair are slowed. The parasympathetic nervous system is affected and the organs governed by it (such as parts of the brain) become inactive and paralyzed.

As you can see, it's not just the body that suffers, but the mind also. Dr. E. M. Abrahamson and A.W. Pezet, in *Body, Mind, and Sugar,* say "since the cells of the brain are those that depend wholly upon the moment-to-moment blood sugar level for nourishment, they are perhaps the most susceptible to damage. The disturbingly large and ever-increasing number of neurotics in our population makes this clearly evident."(64)

The late endocrinologist John W. Tintera said, "It is quite possible to improve your disposition, increase your efficiency, and change your personality for the better. The way to do it is to avoid cane and beet sugar in all forms and guises."(65)

Nobel Prize winner Linus Pauling, M.D., and other prominent doctors believe that mental illness is a myth and that emotional disturbances are the first symptom of a person's inability to handle sugar. In *Orthomolencular Psychiatry,*

Dr. Pauling writes, "A deficiency of [vitamin B_{12}] whatever its cause, leads to mental illness, often even more pronounced than the physical consequences. Other investigators have also reported a higher incidence of low B_{12} concentrations in the serums of mental patients than in the population as a whole and have suggested that B_{12} deficiency, whatever its origin, may lead to mental illness."[66]

Remember that sugar is stripped of its vitamins when it is processed. The B vitamins are leached from the body to help metabolize the sugar when we eat it. Thus, this could lead to a vitamin B_{12} deficiency. The B vitamins play a major role in brain function, so their presence in our body is of utmost importance. They are not only supplied to us from the food we eat (provided it's unprocessed), but also a significant amount of them are normally produced in our intestines by bacteria. However, refined sugar actually kills these bacteria, and in so doing our stock of B vitamins can get depleted.

In *Megavitamin B_3 Therapy for Schizophrenia*, A. Hoffner, M.D., advised patients to follow a good nutritional program with the restriction of sucrose and sucrose-rich foods. An inquiry into the dietary history of patients diagnosed as schizophrenic showed that their choice of foods was rich in sweets, candy, cakes, coffee, caffeinated beverages, and foods prepared with sugar. These foods stimulate the adrenals as noted earlier and can cause adrenal exhaustion.[67]

In the 1940s, John Tintera, Ph.D., found that the symptoms of hypoadreno-corticism (the lack of adequate adrenal cortical hormone caused by adrenal exhaustion) were similar to those found in people whose systems were unable to handle sugar. These symptoms were fatigue, nervousness, depression, apprehension, craving for sweets, inability to handle alcohol, inability to concentrate, allergies, and low blood pressure. He started using a simple glucose tolerance test (GTT) to find out if a person could handle sugar. He said,

> A glucose tolerance test. . .could alert parents and physicians and could save innumerable hours and small fortunes spent in looking into the child's psyche and home environment for maladjustments of questionable significance in the emotional development of the average child. The negativism, hyperactivity, and obstinate resentment of discipline are absolute indications for at least the minimum laboratory tests: urinalysis, complete blood count, and the five-hour glucose tolerance test. . .[68]

Dr. Tintera stressed that improvement was "dependent upon the restoration of the total organism. . .the importance of diet cannot be overemphasized."

Obviously, if a child or adult is consuming large amounts of sugar his or her metabolism and brain function is being compromised. This not only affects his or her resistance to diseases like diabetes, but also impacts their mental health as well. Sugar can undermine just about every area of the body. Dr. Joseph Mercola, director of the Optimal Wellness Center, has listed 78 ways sugar can destroy your health. He compiled this list in conjunction with Nancy Appleton,

Ph.D. (You can see the list at his website www.mercola.com/sugar.) Along with the list are 78 different scientific references concerning the hazards of sugar from a number of doctors and researchers. Evidence enough of the hazardous nature of this white powder.

Patricia Hardman, Ph.D., Director of Woodland Hall Academy, a school for children with hyperactivity and learning disabilities in Maitland, Florida, says,

> We can change a child's behavior dramatically by lowering his or her intake of sugar. If a child comes to school extremely depressed or complains that nothing is going right, or if he flies off the handle and can't be controlled, we ask him what he's been eating. It's almost always the case that the night before he had ice cream or soda or some other food with a lot of sugar. We had one child who was tested for his IQ and scored 140. Three days later he was tested and scored 100! It turned out that grandma had come for a visit and, that morning had made the child pancakes for breakfast. Of course, they were smothered in store-bought sugary syrup. We waited another three days without sugar and tested him again. Sure enough, he scored 140. There's no doubt about it. Sugar makes children poor learners. At Woodland Hall, sugar is eliminated from the diet of every child."[69]

It's not just disposition and intelligence that is affected by sugar. The very survival of your child may depend on avoiding it. In his book, *Type A Type B Weight Loss Book*, H.L. Newbold writes,

> The teenage suicide rate has doubled since 1968, largely because mothers demonstrate their love by keeping the refrigerators stocked with sugary soda drinks and feed them cereals for breakfast and spaghetti for dinner. [Remember, white flour products quickly turn into sugar in the stomach and have essentially the same effect on metabolism as sugar does.] Why do we insist upon rotting the brains of a whole generation of children, turning them into scholastic failures, delinquents, dropouts and welfare recipients? Why do we drive more and more of them to suicide by feeding them ever more processed foods? I'll tell you why: Many people are getting rich at their expense. We look askance at African tribes when they cut faces and rub dyes into the wounds and when they circumcise women. That's child's play compared to what we do to our children. In our society, it's perfectly all right to maim and kill – so long as we do it in a socially acceptable way."[70]

Food for Thought

I have gone to pro-sugar web sites to see if there was any documentation on the benefits of sugar consumption. Although I found comments like "sugar represents a positive addition to the diet" and "sugar is a good, pure food that supplies much needed energy," I found nothing to the effect that there has been any research done to prove it. On the other hand, *Time* magazine reported back in 1958 that a Harvard biochemist and his assistants had worked with mice for more than 10 years – bankrolled by the Sugar Research Foundation Inc. – to find out how sugar causes dental cavities and how to prevent this. In the 10 years of research, they discovered that there was simply no way to prevent sugar from causing dental decay. When the researchers reported their findings in the *Dental Association Journal*, the Sugar Research Foundation Inc. withdrew their support.(71)

I like to think of myself as an open-minded person. I try to look at all sides of a situation and then come to a decision on what the truth is. But try as I might, I cannot find one good or even harmless reason to eat sugar or sugar products (like high fructose corn syrup). Little do people realize that sugar is so bad for their health and well-being.

William Dufty quoted one author as saying, "It is a rule of thumb. The more you see a product advertised, the more of a rip-off it is." I would add, "and bad for your health." Do you ever see fruit and vegetables advertised? But they have to brainwash you into drinking sodas and eating junk food. I remember the first cola I drank when I was about four years old. I threw it up all over the refrigerator door. (It's one of my first memories.) My body naturally rejected it – literally – because as we now know, it's a toxic waste. My body knew better, but my mind kept forcing it on me until I built up a tolerance, and then a craving. Just like alcohol, cigarettes, junk food, and drugs. You first reject these poisons, then grow to need them. That's the way addictions are. I don't mean to be a hardnosed, but if you need that coke, pastry, candy bar, or coffee, you have a food addiction. The best way to beat an addiction, is to replace it with something healthy. Go buy a juicer with all the money you're going to save by not drinking sodas, and distract yourself from your addiction or craving by getting busy juicing!

There are plenty of books on juicing, so I won't get into recipes here except to tell you the one I use as my standard: a couple carrots, two big bunches celery, bunch of cilantro, thumb-sized piece of ginger, maybe some parsley, spinach, dandelion, or arugula, maybe some pineapple. Mix the juice up and pour into a Mason jar. Add a dollop of raw honey that will help keep the juice fresh, seal, and store in refrigerator. Drink at least a pint of this a day, in between meals. I don't drink straight fruit juices because there's too much concentrated sweetness, even though it's wholesome and raw.

History of Sugar

Much of the colonization of the Western world has resulted because of the sugar trade and the fight to control it. From the early settlers of the West Indies to the American Revolution to the slave trade, sugar has played a major role. At first it was a very expensive commodity, used only by kings, royalty, and the very rich. They used to snort it like cocaine, and it was taken precisely because it gave people a high. (People now are so used to this high that it's a normal state of being. Kind of like a drug addict needing more and more drugs to feel an effect and not being able to feel normal without at least some in his system.) Certain diseases were associated only with the rich, and the poor, sugarless farmers seemed to be immune. But as the industry grew and processing methods improved, the price came down more and more people could afford this high. The diseases started to spread to the common folks. Natural healers were seen as witches, burned at the stake, and hanged, because they admonished people to abstain from sugar. "The great confinement of the insane," as one historian called it, began in the late 17th century, after sugar consumption in Britain had escalated for 200 years from a pinch or two in a barrel of beer, here and there, to more than two million pounds per year. Sailors suffered when sugar was introduced as rations, and scurvy became rampant. Sir Frederick Banting, the co-discoverer of insulin, noticed in 1929 in Panama that among sugar plantation owners who ate large amounts of their refined stuff, diabetes was common. Among the native cane-cutters, who only got to chew the raw cane (replete with vitamins and minerals), he saw no diabetes.

Some researchers believe that sugar was the cause of or instrumental in causing the bubonic plague. "By 1662, sugar consumption in England had zoomed from 0 to some 16 million pounds a year. . .Then, in 1665, London was swept by a plague. More than 30,000 people died that September. . .People who lived in the country virtually without sugar seemed to escape the plague. Had anyone called it the sugar plague, they might have been denounced as menaces to commerce and crown and strung to a gibbet."[72]

Could it be the cause of tuberculosis too? "In relation to consumption, now called tuberculosis and blamed on a bacillus, evidence suggests that a sugar-rich diet may create the necessary conditions in our bodies [for the disease to take hold]. . .Three hundred years ago, in the 1700s, deaths from tuberculosis. . .increased dramatically. The highest incidence occurred among workers in sugar factories and refineries. . .In 1910, when Japan acquired a source of cheap and abundant sugar in Formosa, the incidence of tuberculosis rose dramatically."[73]

Dr. Weston Price traveled the world examining the dietary habits of primitive tribes and cultures. He noticed without exception that when these peoples were exposed to the white-man's food (white flour and white sugar), they invariably contracted tuberculosis and the amount of dental caries (cavities) increased dramatically.

Why don't we see tuberculosis now? When the human body is first exposed to a harmful substance, it is very sensitive to it, and the reactions can be very severe. Over time and through the generations, the body builds up resistance and adapts to some degree to overcome the toxicity. This is not to say that it is no longer toxic, but the manifestations of symptoms may take longer and change characteristics. Instead of tuberculosis, we may see diabetes or cancer instead. But a poison is still a poison that eventually takes its toll on the body.

Now sugar is in just about everything. It's not required to be listed on food labels if it's used in certain ways in the product. In addition, the labeling is often misleading or difficult to understand. "Made from natural ingredients" on the label means nothing these days. Heck, plastic is made from petroleum, which is a natural product. The label may call sugar corn syrup, dextrose, or a carbohydrate. Oftentimes people don't realize they are still buying a product with sugar in it. You'll be hard-pressed to find things with absolutely no sugar added. Finding a product with a label that specifically states *No Sugar Added* is the safest bet.

A press release from the Center for Science in the Public Interest titled, "America: Drowning in Sugar," states that a petition was made to the Food and Drug Administration to require food labels to declare how much sugar is added to soft drinks, ice cream, and other foods. The petition was filed in 1999 by 72 health experts and organizations and spearheaded by the Center for Science in the Public Interest (CSPI). Michael Jacobson, executive director of CSPI, says, "Sugar consumption has been going through the roof. It has increased by 28 percent since 1983, fueling soaring obesity rates and other health problems. It's vital that the FDA require labels that would enable consumers to monitor – and reduce – their sugar intake." As of the date of the publication of this book, the change to the "Nutrition Facts" label has yet to occur.[74]

"Listing added sugars on labels would alert consumers as to how much added sugars are in a serving of food," Jacobson says, "It's vital that food labels give consumers the information they need to reduce their consumption of added sugars." Another press release from CSPI in June 2000 said:

> The USDA advises people who eat a 2,000-calorie healthful diet to limit themselves to about 10 teaspoons of added sugars. However, USDA surveys find that the average American consumes 20 teaspoons a day, twice the recommendation. . .Just one month ago, the federal government's new edition of *Dietary Guidelines for Americans* recognized that many consumers are eating too many sugar-rich foods. The document urges consumers to "Choose sensibly to limit your intake of beverages and foods that are high in added sugars."[75]

However, if the added sugars are not listed on the label, there is no way consumers can know just how much sugar they are consuming. Many typical American foods provide a large fraction of the USDA's recommended 10-tea-spoon-a-day sugar limit in just one serving. A typical cup of flavored yogurt provides 70 percent of a day's worth of added sugar (seven teaspoons). A cup of regular ice cream has six teaspoons, a 12-ounce *Pepsi* has just over 10 teaspoons, as does a quarter-cup of pancake syrup.

As you can see, if you eat like a typical American, you're going to get your dose of sugar because it's hidden in many products. The average American will eat about 140 pounds of sugar every year. The best way to go is to shop at a health food store, buy mostly unprocessed, fresh food, and maybe even grow a garden. If you do go off sugar, or at least eat less of it, you may experience withdrawal symptoms, so be prepared. The same holds true for your kids. They may temporarily complain, but the long-term benefits greatly outweigh the inconvenience.

Avoiding & Dealing with Diabetes

The best way to avoid and deal with diabetes is to adopt a lifestyle that will support your body such that your organs and blood can function correctly. That means you should stop consuming sugar, artificial sweeteners, refined carbohydrates, and even excess fruit. Be sure to eat the proper fats, protein, get adequate magnesium, and adequate iodine. Making garlic, celery, apple cider vinegar, and bee pollen a part of your daily diet may help heal and maintain your pancreas and thus your blood sugar. Remember, as I mentioned in the Obesity chapter, unheated honey is not harmful to the pancreas and actually helps heal it.

Carol Johnson, Ph.D., professor of nutrition at Arizona State University, did a study with people with Type II diabetes which showed that people who took 2 tablespoons of vinegar before a high-carbohydrate meal cut their blood-glucose rise in the first hour after a meal by about half [76] She said, "Scientific studies over the past 10 years show benefits from vinegar consumption. It's inexpensive and can be easily incorporated into the diet. Used in combination with diet and exercise, it can help many people with Type II diabetes."[77] Another study in Sweden showed that those who ate pickles (cucumbers preserved in vinegar) after a high carbohydrate meal had smaller blood-sugar spikes afterwards.[78] So having a Total Health Drink (see Obesity chapter) not only can help you lose weight, but help your blood sugar too.

Garlic has also been shown to help blood glucose levels in test animals [79] One study using garlic extract for 14 days "significantly decreased serum glucose, total cholesterol, triglycerides, urea, uric acid. . .while increased serum insulin in diabetic rats. . ."[80,81]

Cinnamon has now been clinically shown to improve glucose levels in people with Type II Diabetes as reported in *Diabetes Care*.[82] People who took as little as one gram a day (about a quarter of a teaspoon) cinnamon showed an 18 percent to 29 percent reduction in blood sugar levels than those who didn't take the cinnamon. The cinnamon takers also had reduced cholesterol levels (from 12 percent to 26 percent decrease over the 40 day trial period) and lower triglycerides (23 percent to 30 percent decrease). In test animals, skeletal muscle of cinnamon takers was able to absorb 17 percent more blood sugar per minute compared to those not taking the cinnamon. A study at the USDA Human

Nutrition Research Center reported that taking cinnamon increases the body's insulin-dependent ability to use glucose roughly 20-fold.[83]

Cinnamon is especially effective in lessening the impact on your blood sugar if high-carbohydrate foods are eaten. Adding cinnamon to the meal slows the rate the stomach empties, which decreases the rise in blood sugar levels.[84] Test animals on a high-fructose (carbohydrate) diet that were fed cinnamon had the same ability to respond to and utilize blood sugar as the test animals on a normal diet.[85]

Cinnamon appears to help Type II diabetics improve their ability to respond to insulin by not only stimulating insulin receptors, but also inhibiting an enzyme that inactivates them. Cinnamon is also a powerful antioxidant.[86]

An easy way to get cinnamon in your diet is by adding a couple sticks of it to the Total Health Drink after you've blended the other ingredients together. You can get the powdered kind (organic, please) and sprinkle it on food or add it to beverages. Remember, the less you tamper with something, the more effective it will be, so using the sticks of cinnamon in a drink is probably best.

Simple additions to your diet, and avoiding things that cause blood sugar spikes is the only true way to avoid and even reverse diabetes.

CHAPTER VI

Asthma

Throughout the United States, asthma is on the rise and becoming a serious health risk, especially to our children. Asthma is a chronic inflammatory disorder of the airways characterized by variable airflow obstruction and airway hyperresponsiveness in which prominent clinical manifestations include wheezing and shortness of breath.[1]

Asthma (16.1 million adults and 6.8 million children in U.S. have it) is one of three pulmonary (lung) diseases grouped under the umbrella term of Chronic Obstructive Pulmonary Disease (COPD), the other two being emphysema (4.1 million in U.S. have it) and chronic bronchitis (9.5 million in U.S. have it).[2] According to the World Health Organization, almost three million patients die of COPD-related complications each year. But this figure is probably higher since many COPD deaths are inaccurately attributed to pneumonia and other causes.[3] COPD affects about 37 million people in the U.S. And is the fourth leading cause of death (131,000 per year) behind cancer, heart disease and stroke. COPD typically affects people over 45, and 90 percent of people who get it smoke or have smoked. Symptoms include chronic cough, shortness of breath, wheezing, not being able to take a deep breath and excess sputum production. Surprisingly, almost 80 percent of people in a recent survey of smokers didn't recognized that smoking puts them at greater risk of COPD.[4]

COPD can be diagnosed with a simple breathing test called spirometry that is non-invasive and can be performed in the doctor's office in just a few minutes. Of course, typical treatment of COPD is with drugs, but recent research reveals that the commonly used drugs called inhaled *anticholinergic* (IAC) drugs, maybe causing more harm than good. A study published in the *Journal of the American Medical Association* examined 20 different trials using IAC medication and showed that using them increased the risk of heart attack by more than 50 percent and increased the risk of cardiovascular death by 80 percent.[5] The risk of having a stroke was increased markedly as well. Another class of drugs called inhaled corticosteroids (ICS) has been shown to increase the risk of COPD patients getting pneumonia by 34 percent.[6] COPD sufferers who get pneumonia are much more likely to die because their lungs are too weak and damages to overcome the excess mucus.

There's a strong connection between the three COPD diseases, as evidence by the fact that sufferers are prescribed the same medications (*Ventolin, Bricanyl, Serevent, Prednizone* etc.). So as you read the following discussion on asthma, most of the recommendations apply to any form of COPD.

A U.S. Public Health Service pamphlet says, "There are irritants in the environment such as cigarette smoke, cooking odors, and aerosol sprays that can adversely affect a person with asthma. These should be avoided as much as possible. An asthmatic should not smoke nor be active outdoors for prolonged periods of time during air pollution alerts."[7] Asthma expert Dr. R. Michael Sly says, "Air pollution is an established cause of increased morbidity (illness) from asthma, and intense air pollution has caused increased mortality (death)."[8]

The prevalence rate for asthma increased 75 percent from 1980 to 1994. By 1993-1994, an estimated 13.7 million people reported asthma during the preceding 12 months. This increasing trend in rates was evident among all races, both sexes, and all age groups. Estimates in 2005 are that about 20 million Americans have asthma, and 9 million of these people are children under the age of 18. The most substantial rate increase in asthma occurred among children ages 0 to four years (160 percent from 22.2 per 1,000 to 57.8 per 1,000), and children aged five to 14 years (up 74 percent from 42.8 per 1,000 to 74.4 per 1,000). It appears that asthma is affecting children at younger and younger ages. If someone has asthma, they probably suffer from allergies too. Seventy percent of people with asthma have common allergies.[9,10,11]

From 1975 to 1993-1995, the estimated annual number of office visits for asthma more than doubled from 4.6 million to 10.4 million. By 2004, physician office visits due to asthma reached 13.6 million.[12] Between 1979 and 1994, the estimated national number of asthma-related hospitalizations increased from 386,000 to 466,000. Asthma is not just an inconvenience – it can be deadly. Asthma attacks kill about 5,000 people a year.[13]

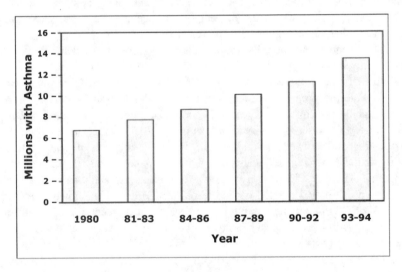

Figure 4.
Estimated average annual number of people with self-reported asthma during the preceding 12 months, 1980-1994.

According to the report "Action against Asthma" from the Department of Health and Human Services:

> We are facing an asthma epidemic. . . From 1980 to 1996, the number of Americans with asthma more than doubled, to almost 15 million, with children under five years old experiencing the highest rate of increase. Reasons for these increasing rates are unclear. Yet even if rates were to stop increasing, asthma would remain an enormous public health problem. Not only does it keep children in fear and pain – it keeps them out of school. In every classroom with 30 children, there are likely to be at least two with asthma. That adds up to over 10 million school days lost to asthma each year. And the problem is not limited to children. Asthma is the leading work-related lung disease. Moreover, the disease kills over 5,000 Americans and results in half a million hospitalizations every year. As serious as asthma is, it doesn't strike evenly. Minorities and the poor are hit especially hard.
>
> The steady rise in the prevalence of asthma constitutes an epidemic, which by all indications is continuing. Even if rates were to stabilize, asthma would continue to be a profound public health problem, responsible for 9 million visits to health care providers per year, over 1.8 million emergency room visits per year, and over 460,000 hospitalizations per year. . .Asthma is a common chronic disease of childhood, affecting an estimated 4.4 million children. . .Taking care of asthma is expensive and imposes financial burdens on patients and their families, including lost workdays and income, as well as lost job opportunity. A 1998 analysis. . .estimated the cost of asthma in 1996 to be over $11 billion per year.[14] Health care provider visits were up to 12.7 million a year, school days lost up to 12.8 million and the cost of asthma was $16.1 billion by 2003.[15]

The traditional medical community says the causes of asthma are not known and sites an interaction between environmental and genetic factors as the most likely culprits. Some studies suggest that indoor allergen exposure is a risk factor of the initial onset of asthma.

There is also widespread agreement among physicians that one outdoor air pollutant, sulfur dioxide (SO_2), causes asthma attacks in susceptible individuals. The 24-hour atmospheric legal limit for SO_2 is not to exceed 0.14 parts per million (ppm). One article about asthma (published in 1991) made note that during the Reagan administration the limit was 0.4 ppm and that the "EPA opposed the tighter regulation, saying that asthma is a 'transient and reversible' condition (even though it kills more than 5,000 Americans each year) and it's simply not worth it to force reductions in SO_2 to benefit asthmatics. The electric power industry applauded."[16]

Sulfites added to food to prevent discoloration can also trigger asthma attacks. Manufacturers put sulfites in all sorts of foods without having to clear it with the U.S. Food and Drug Administration (FDA), which regulates most food additives. Sulfites are one of the food additives that have been around for so long that they were placed on the list known as *Generally Recognized As Safe* (the GRAS list) in 1958 when food additive regulations began.

In 1986, the FDA banned the use of sulfites on fresh fruits and vegetables, largely because of the hazard to asthmatics. Health advocates wanted the FDA to ban all uses of sulfites on food, period. The FDA said in a memo (which was leaked to the press in 1988) that they knew that a million asthmatics were endangered by sulfites in other food, but that the FDA had decided, after much thought, not to do anything about the problem. This time, the food industry applauded.

The official position of the U.S. EPA is that either asthma isn't related to pollution or that asthmatics are such a small fraction of the population that setting pollution standards to protect them isn't worth the effort. Considering the fact that now many believe that asthma is an epidemic, it's hard to believe it isn't worth the trouble.

In a recent review of the current scientific literature, the Institute of Medicine (IOM) drew several conclusions about the role of numerous indoor air exposures and the initial development of asthma. The IOM found that exposure to house dust mite allergen can cause the development of asthma in susceptible children. They also determined that exposure to environmental tobacco smoke is associated with the development of asthma in younger children. Maternal smoking during pregnancy was suggested to have a stronger adverse affect than exposure after birth.[17]

Reducing exposure to certain allergens has been shown not only to reduce asthma symptoms and the need for medication, but also, in some studies, to improve lung function. The IOM committee found that exposure to allergens produced by cats, cockroaches, house dust mites, and environmental tobacco smoke causes exacerbations of asthma in sensitized individuals. Common air pollutants such as ozone, sulfur dioxide, and particulate matter are known to be respiratory irritants and can also worsen asthma symptoms. Any of these pollutants or irritants can combine synergistically, thus exacerbating the problem.

The report from the Department of Health and Human Service concludes: "In summary, we have made progress but we are not yet close to understanding the causes of the asthma epidemic nor to providing optimal care. . ."

The typical treatment for asthma is drugs. But they have serious, sometimes life-threatening side effects such as high blood pressure, worsening ulcers, osteoporosis, diabetes, glaucoma, cataracts, increased growth of body hair, irregular heart beat, personality changes, hyperactivity, nausea, vomiting, liver damage, triggering another asthma attack, and death. Sudden deaths among asthmatics still clutching their inhalers are not uncommon. Two federal drug officials have concluded that asthma sufferers risk death if they continue to use four hugely popular asthma drugs – *Advair, Symbicort, Serevent* and *Foradil*. But these views are not shared by everyone in the government, and the money involved is so huge (*Advair* sales in 2007 were $6.9 billion and may approach $8 billion in 2008) that I doubt you'll see much happen to stop their sales. Of course, drug company spokespeople say the evidence is inconclusive. These drugs are especially hard on children, and one of the officials who spoke out against these drugs thinks they should no longer be used by people under the age of 17.(18)

Food for Thought

The increase in asthma in the U.S. is no real mystery. As we saw with cancer, obesity, and diabetes, and as we shall see with other degenerative diseases, the increases can be correlated with the degeneration and pollution of our environment and food supply. While the medical community tries to point the finger at genetics and luck as the evil spirits, the truth of the matter is that as our environment (internal as well as external) degenerates, so do we. Throwing another drug at it is not the answer, as has been proven so often in the past.

Drugs do not solve any medical problem – they just delay the inevitable and suppress symptoms. This is what drugs – the kind from the drug store or the kind on the streets – do to the body: Drugs interrupt, interfere with, delay, or stop the normal transmission of nerve impulses or other cellular communications and transport mechanisms in the central nervous system (brain and spinal cord) or peripheral nervous system (everything else). That's it. They do nothing to build up or repair the body. They simply alter the transmission of information. Sometimes this will change the expression of a disease – the acne, cancer, herpes, or whatever, may go away, but the underlying source of the problem is still there and then manifests in another part of the body with different symptoms. People with one disease usually have multiple problems. If someone gets "cured" of cancer with radiation, chemotherapy, or drugs, you can bet that there's something else still wrong with them.

Why does it seem that drugs help or cure some conditions? Most problems in the body are really some form of inflammation. Asthma, fever, arthritis, sinusitis, psoriasis, congestion, skin eruptions, liver, heart, brain problems. . .they all (especially in their early stages) are simply a form or inflammation. From the modern medical perspective, inflammation is bad and needs to be treated – so drugs are prescribed to stop it. But from the natural health and healing perspective, inflammation is an indication that the body or the specific part of the body is speeding up its metabolism to cleanse itself of toxicity.

If you let the fever or inflammation run its course, the toxicity will be purged and the metabolic rate will return to normal. The tissues will be cleaner and healthier and the body better off because of the cleansing. Making sure you don't contribute more toxicity during the inflammatory event or after it will help it subside quicker and will prevent it from returning. Most inflammation events the body initiates last between three days to a week or so provided more toxins are not added during the event and adequate nutrients are available for repair. That's why there's a saying that goes, "Treat a cold with drugs, and it'll last a week. Leave it alone, and it'll last seven days."

The drugs you take to stop the inflammation and thus the symptoms are actually poisonous to the body. The body reacts in order to get rid of the poison of the drug by increasing the actions of the elimination organs of the body such as the liver and kidneys. This response requires energy, so the body shunts its energy of repair of the inflamed area to that of getting rid of the more toxic poison (the drug). The inflammation, and thus the symptom, stops because the body was doing something more important – saving itself from the systemic poisoning of the drug.

Medical research – as performed in medical schools and universities all around the world – focuses on how a disease or illness can be ameliorated (lessened) by administering a substance into or onto the human body. I spent a year in medical school studying for a Ph.D. in anatomy and physiology and saw what goes on there first-hand. The professors were concerned with two things: teaching the medical students and doing research. The research was *always* aimed at finding a way to alter the biological system by administrating a new drug or combination of drugs or performing a destructive procedure such as radiation. I repeat – these do nothing to nourish or cleanse the body. They simply stop the symptoms from appearing.

The best analogy is that of the oil gauge on your car. If the oil gets low, the oil gauge light will go on. It's a warning signal that something is wrong. The sensor in the engine detects the absence of oil, transmits its message through a wire to the light on the dashboard, which alerts you of the problem. You may not like to see the light go on, and it may be an inconvenience or even discomfort to have to stop and add oil – but you'd better stop and do it or your engine will burn up.

But what if when you saw the light go on, you simply cut the wire to the gauge and kept on driving? Would this be smart? Would you be able to drive very long? That's what drugs do. They stop you from sensing something is wrong, or they alter the transmission of the nerves so the problem may seem to be gone, but is just rerouted to another part of the body.

In some instances, a drug will actually increase the activity of nerves. The best example of this is to watch how pesticides work. If you've ever watched a bug after you sprayed it with a pesticide, you probably noticed how it twitches violently until it dies. The pesticide gets inside the bug and floods the synapses of the nerves (the gap between the nerve cells – kind of like the gap on a spark plug) with the appropriate neurochemical (the spark that jumps the gap). The nerve cells fire and fire like crazy until the bug's little body is totally exhausted and depleted and then it dies.

If you have a pain or other aberration in your body, it's a signal that something is wrong. The receptors in your body have detected something is out of whack and send messages to your brain and you sense pain. But what if you just cut the nerves between the problem and your head? The pain stops, and you think everything is back to normal. This is exactly what aspirin and all other pain - relievers, alcohol, and recreational drugs do. The nervous transmission is interrupted, and you "feel no pain."

In the case of heart medication, oftentimes the intricate actions of the cells in the heart are altered to affect a change that is perceived as beneficial. I distinctly remember my physiology professor saying in reference to one heart medicine: "You see, in this case we had to effectively poison a part of the heart cells to modulate the contractions."

Yes, I agree that perhaps in some extreme emergency cases drug intervention may be necessary. But even so, the underlying cause of the problem is not corrected at all. And as the body is poisoned over a long period, other problems will manifest. Any drug – from the innocent-looking aspirin to chemotherapy drugs, from caffeine to illegal street drugs such as crack cocaine and heroin, and from something as seemingly harmless as sugar to the over prescribed *Ritalin* – *any* drug injures some part of the body in order to make another part function differently.

It's not just manmade drugs that do this. Many pharmaceuticals were derived originally from plants. The classic case is *Valium*. Its active substance is valerian, which comes from the valerian plant. This has been known for centuries to decrease pain and put a person in a calmer state. But does that justify its use? Not everything natural is suited for the human body. Cocaine is from coca leaves of the South American shrub *Erythroxylon coca*. Eating some plants may actually kill you. So just because something grows and is not processed in a chemical plant does not necessarily make it good. The way to overcome, and I mean truly conquer a disease, is to get the body back to functioning correctly. This is done by: 1. Supplying the body the proper building blocks for repair, regeneration, and maintenance; and 2. Eliminating and/or removing any interfering substances like toxins or normal cellular waste products. That's all you have to do. The basic fundamentals to health are really not that complicated, although specific problems may require special remedial solutions to speed the healing up. The underlying solution to any health problem is to treat the body in accordance with natural laws and in harmony with our biology and physiology.

Asthma and allergies are both inflammatory events. They indicate a body that is overwhelmed with toxicity. When the body encounters an impurity such as an allergen, it reacts by releasing histamine, which stimulates the secretion of mucus. The mucus grabs on to the allergen or impurity and tries to eliminate it through sneezing, coughing, and watery eyes.

A side effect of too much histamine is tightening of the bronchial tubes, which may go into spasm causing wheezing, coughing, shortness of breath, rapid breathing, difficulty exhaling, anxiety, and dehydration – a typical asthma event.

Asthma can also be caused by being sensitive to carbohydrates. Nutritionist David Getoff says he's seen this sensitivity go away by eliminating all grains, sugars, artificial sweeteners or alcohols in as little as 45 days. You can check out his website www.Naturopath4you.com for a complete description of this diet. And remember, shortness of breath can be a symptom of congestive heart failure.

Asthma patients were shown to have significantly lower levels of cellular magnesium. The researchers concluded that increasing the concentration of magnesium helped stop bronchial spasms by dilating the bronchial tubes. They also stated that the lack of magnesium was probably a major cause of the bronchial spasms.[19]

Magnesium is a calcium antagonist, so it relaxes airways and smooth muscles and dilates the lungs. Another study involving 2,633 adults showed that a diet low in magnesium may cause the development of asthma and chronic obstructive airway disease.[20]

The drug treatment of asthma involves drugs that are "magnesium wasters" such as *Prednisone* (cortisone), *Theophylline* (Aminophylline), and beta blockers. These actually cause the body to get rid of magnesium and other vital nutrients such as vitamin C, zinc, and vitamin K. Prolonged treatment with these drugs can cause a severe magnesium deficiency that can result in arrhythmia and sudden death.[21]

Food for Thought

Supplementation with magnesium will undoubtedly help asthma and allergies. But you should do this under supervision of a qualified health care professional. I in no way advocate going off your asthma medication cold-turkey and haphazardly. Add the right foods to your diet that contain a lot of magnesium, and maybe take a magnesium supplement or use magnesium oil. With time, your levels of magnesium in your blood with climb, and the chance of a bronchial spasm will decline.

Considering the symptoms of asthma, emphysema or chronic bronchitis – the shortness of breath and the feeling of the need for more air – one would think that those who suffer from these would benefit from increasing their breathing and the amount of oxygen they take into their lungs. However, this is not true. In fact, just the opposite is now believed to occur.

To explain this we need to look at the functions of the two main blood gases – oxygen (O_2) and carbon dioxide (CO_2). Oxygen is often thought of as the good gas. It's needed for respiration to take place in your cells. You can think of respiration the same as the process of combustion in an automobile engine. You breathe oxygen into your lungs (the carburetor) so the heart (fuel pump) can deliver the oxygen to the tissues and cells. Oxygen is removed from the blood stream (fuel line) and combines with fuels (fats and carbohydrates) to burn and produce useable energy. One of the by-products (exhaust) of this energy production is carbon dioxide, often thought of as the bad gas. You breathe in oxygen, you breathe out carbon dioxide. Simple, right? On the surface it is. But it's a bit more complicated.

Carbon dioxide has a much more important role in this process and in the overall functioning of the body than we've been led to believe. It is not just a waste gas and we don't exhale just to get rid of it. We exhale in large part to *regulate* the concentration of carbon dioxide in the blood stream and in the body. Incredibly, the concentration of carbon dioxide in the blood stream is actually crucial to how well the cells can utilize oxygen and how well the body functions overall.

"In fact, carbon dioxide is the regulator of all bodily functions either directly or indirectly, making it the fourth requirement of survival" (behind oxygen, water and food).(22) Carbon dioxide is involved in countless chemical reactions throughout the body, largely determines the amount of tension in smooth muscles, and is critical for the transfer of oxygen out of the blood and into the tissues.

When you breathe, oxygen gets attached to the hemoglobin in your red blood cells. It is then circulated through the blood stream to other parts of the body. The oxygen must then detach from the hemoglobin before it can enter another cell. This is accomplished by exchanging it with carbon dioxide. In fact, oxygen cannot come off of hemoglobin unless carbon dioxide takes its place.

If the level of carbon dioxide in the body is too low, there's not enough of it to take the place of oxygen on the hemoglobin, so the oxygen stays there and is not released into your tissues. Your tissues become oxygen deprived, your muscles may spasm, the blood pH may rise, and a long list of symptoms may result.

If you breathe too deeply and too often, you exhale too much carbon dioxide, not enough oxygen is released from the hemoglobin, and you feel like you need to breathe more. The more you breathe, the more breathless you feel. Your blood may be nice and red and full of oxygen, but that does your tissues no good. The oxygen is not in the blood for the blood's sake, it's there to be delivered to the cells where it's used in respiration. So too much and too heavy breathing (hyperventilation) results in oxygen deprivation to your cells!

Here's a simply way to prove this: Breathe as fast as you can for the next minute or so. You'll find you'll get dizzy, your fingers and lips will tingle and you might feel like passing out. If your brain was receiving more oxygen, you wouldn't feel ill – you would feel relaxed and invigorated. When you deep breathe, you end up feeling ill because your brain isn't getting more oxygen, it's actually receiving less oxygen because the amount of carbon dioxide has gone down and less oxygen is coming out of the bloodstream and into the brain tissues. Fainting happens when your brain doesn't get enough oxygen; either from not getting any (like when you hold your breath too long), or not getting enough (like when you hyperventilate and not enough is released off of the hemoglobin).

Here's why over-breathing leads to asthma: Hyperventilation (breathing too much) causes not enough oxygen to be released from the hemoglobin which leads to decreased oxygen in the tissues which leads to biochemical disturbances which leads to inflammation and constriction of the airways (and other tissues).

The amount of oxygen in the atmosphere is about 21 percent, while that of carbon dioxide is negligible. It's easy to get enough oxygen into the blood and most of the oxygen inhaled into the lungs is eventually exhaled. Even when you do deep breathing, the concentration of oxygen in your blood does not rise significantly. Using mouth-to-mouth resuscitation to revive someone shows that it's possible to revive seriously ill people with less oxygen than is normally inhaled. In fact, recovery rates for seriously ill people have been shown to be faster when carbon dioxide pressure increases in the bloodstream.[23,24] It's interesting to note that the womb has a higher concentration of carbon dioxide than the outside atmosphere, and that a fetus grows and develops in this carbon dioxide rich environment.[25]

You may have heard from some companies that sell air purifiers that ozone (O_3) is healthy and will help increase the amount of oxygen in your bloodstream. But consider that ozone is a strong oxidizing agent and can be very damaging to the body. Perhaps in low concentrations (as found in nature), it's OK and even beneficial. But to use it to increase cellular oxygen is actually a moot point, since if there isn't enough carbon dioxide in the body, you can have all the oxygen in the world in the bloodstream and it still won't be delivered to the tissues.

Although these facts about carbon dioxide and respiration have been known for over a century, practical and useful application of them didn't occur until late in the 20th century. A Russian doctor named Konstantin Buteyko noticed that his healthy patients' breathing was slow and shallow, while those with serious illnesses and those close to death breathed very often and deeply.

Dr. Buteyko himself suffered from high blood pressure, a rapid heart beat, and frequent headaches. So he began forcing himself to breath as if he were healthy – slow and shallow. He soon discovered that his illnesses disappeared. When he went back to breathing faster and deeper, his symptoms returned.[26]

As a result of his research and experiments, he deduced that hyperventilation has the potential to create a wide variety of health problems. Some of the diseases that may manifest due to chronic hyperventilation are:

asthma	sleep apnea	migraines	frequent urination	angina
diabetes	hypertension	bronchitis	chronic fatigue	epilepsy
eczema	palpitations	hypoglycemia	depression	Alzheimer's
snoring	rhinitis	arthritis	panic attacks	stroke

Proper breathing doesn't just affect the respiratory system; it affects every system in the body. Which symptom appears in an individual depends on their genetic make-up, their strengths, and weaknesses. One person may exhibit asthma if they have weak lungs, while someone else may exhibit arthritis if they have weak joints.(27)

Chronic hyperventilation is all too easy a state to fall into. One reason for this is the constant unfounded rhetoric that deep breathing is good for you. Now you see why that's not true and actually harmful. It's not that a lot of oxygen is bad – it isn't, and those on supplemental oxygen should not discontinue its use. But how oxygen gets out of the bloodstream and into the cells is just as important as how much oxygen is in the blood.

Dr. Buteyko isn't the only one to observe that increasing the concentration of CO_2 in the blood is a good thing. In the excellent book *The Einstein Factor*, author Win Wenger, Ph.D., tells of how over the course of a summer he went from the bottom to the top of his class because he increased his CO_2 concentration. His story is worth repeating:

> In the summer of 1959, I attended summer school in an attempt to make up for some serious deficits in my grades. Because my afternoons were free and the school had a pool, I spent several hours each afternoon swimming. I found that, for some reason, swimming underwater felt better to me than normal swimming. An unusually large amount of my time was therefore spent each day holding my breath for extended periods, as much as 4½ minutes at a time. A remarkable thing occurred. Despite my lackluster academic record, my poor study habits, and the demanding course load I had taken on, my grades suddenly shot through the roof. On test after test, I found myself scoring 100. By the end of the summer I had literally gone from the very bottom of my class to the top.(28)

Dr. Wenger goes on to explain that he learned why this happened years later when he met Dr. Glenn Doman, medical director of Philadelphia's Institutes for the Achievement of Human Potential, who explained to him how CO_2 affects blood supply: Whenever the CO_2 content of the blood increases, our bodies interpret it to mean that our oxygen supply is being cut off. In response, the carotid arteries (that carry blood to our brains) open wide to allow more blood to the brain, thus drenching it with oxygen.

Getting more oxygen to the brain not only activates areas that are usually dormant, but slows down the constant die-off of brain cells (take note, Alzheimer's patients). Dr. Dorman even developed a technique he called *masking*, where the person breathes into a constricted space for a few minutes. Each exhalation contains a little less oxygen and a little more CO_2 thus increasing the blood supply to the brain. He says that doing this regularly for 30 second intervals every 30 minutes for two to three weeks will improve brain function.

But masking is tricky, requires a specially designed mask, and is really unnecessary if you do the breathing exercises Dr. Buteyko recommends (see below). One comment on Dr. Dorman's explanation is necessary here – that it's not only the carotid arteries that open wide when the CO_2 level increases, but every blood vessel in your body does too. Not only does your brain get a rich supply of oxygen when the CO_2 level increases, every cell in your body does.

The cause of low tissue oxygen levels (corrected by high carbon dioxide levels) occurs when we over breathe for extended periods. Notice a baby's breath – you can hardly tell he or she is breathing at all. But when we're faced with a stressful situation, our body goes into the fight or flight mode, certain hormones are released, our metabolism increases, and we breathe harder. Being repeatedly stressed, be it emotional, mental, or physiological (bad food, toxins), causes us to over breathe as a habit, resulting in chronic hyperventilation. This causes decreased CO_2 and decreased oxygen delivery to all our tissues.

Dr. Buteyko developed a way to retrain the body to breathe so carbon dioxide in the body returns to normal. When this happens, oxygen utilization returns to normal, tissues and cells start functioning properly, and better health ensues. This new method of breathing is rightly called The Buteyko Method after its founder. It's not well known in the U.S. at this time, but is taught in medical school in Russia and is covered by insurance in Australia. In fact, over 250,000 people in Russia have taken the workshops to learn the method. A recent article was published in the *NY Times* in November, 2009 says it is effective for asthma.[29]

The Buteyko Method is taught by only a few practitioners in the U.S. and their main focus on helping people with asthma. The classes last a couple hours a day and are given for 5 days straight. There are many reports of asthmatics or emphysema sufferers never needing to use medications again after just the first day's class. Even if you don't have asthma or COPD but are suffering from other physical, mental, or emotional problems, or just want to get healthier and fee better, doing the Buteyko Method would probably help you immensely.

Food for Thought

I took the Buteyko Method classes a couple years ago. I can tell you without a doubt that it was one of the best things for my health I've ever done. I took the classes out of curiosity and because I had sleep apnea and snored so loud the windows rattle. (Not really, but it was *loud*.) The Buteyko Method is starting to get some recognition here in the states. Julian Whitaker, M.D., a practicing physician who also sends out one of the nation's most popular natural health newsletters, says of the Buteyko Method,

"This theory makes a lot of sense to me. . .People with asthma tend to breathe rapidly, deeply, and through the mouth. As a result, their CO_2

levels are low. To prevent further CO_2 losses, the smooth muscles of the airways constrict and spasm, bringing on shortness of breath and other signs of asthma. . . To counter all of this, Dr. Buteyko created a series of exercises designed to restore normal breathing, raise CO_2 levels, and dilate the airways. These breathing exercises have been shown to dramatically improve symptoms and reduce drug use. . .I've read scores of testimonials from people who have used this breathing technique to overcome asthma."[30]

The method is very simple and it's best if you learn it from a licensed Buteyko practitioner. You can find a list of them at their website www.Buteyko-usa.com. (By the way, Dr. Whitaker also recommends magnesium to help with asthma.) Although I'm going to give you a real short introduction to one of the breathing exercises taught in the Buteyko class, please note that Dr. Buteyko was against people learning his method by themselves without proper professional guidance. He even did studies showing that those who tried to do it alone had a very low success rate while those being taught by a licensed practitioner did very well indeed. That being said, I feel obliged to give you an introduction to it so you can feel the benefits. Hopefully, this will encourage you to go take the classes.

If you do this exercise right now, I guarantee you'll feel more relaxed and calmer afterwards. You may also experience a runny nose, yawning, or sighing. That's because your muscles are relaxing (they are finally getting more oxygen). You may even feel sleepy. In fact, it's a great thing to do before bed or if you're having trouble sleeping.

Sit upright on the edge of a regular chair with your feet flat on the floor and your hands on your thighs. Your back should be straight. Breathe in through the nose (never through the mouth) slow and shallow. Breathe as little as you can without making yourself gulp for air.

Slow and shallow. . .slow and shallow. You should breathe so your diaphragm goes down on the inhale and up naturally and with no effort on the exhale. Do that for five to ten minutes. If you feel like yawning or sighing, fight it. Don't take a deep breath ever.

After five to ten minutes, stop and breathe normally. After about a minute of normal breathing, exhale normally and hold your nose like you're about to jump in a swimming pool. Hold your nose and don't breathe. This is after you exhale (with little air in your lungs), not after you inhale (with a lot of air in your lungs). Keep holding your nose until you feel a fairly strong urge to inhale. Don't hold it until you *have* to inhale, just until you *kind of* have to. Then do another set of the shallow breathing.

Do as many of these cycles as you want. If you do this every day, you'll see that you'll be able to hold your breath for longer and longer periods (the recommendation is to do this for 30 minutes, 3 times a day during the first week). This means you're retraining your breathing and more and more oxygen is getting into your cells. As that happens, you'll see big improvements in your health. You'll also notice, surprisingly so, your chest wants to expand and your posture will improve. That's because again, your muscles and tissues are relaxing with the increased supply of oxygen, and your muscles are lengthening to their rightful length. Here are a few other pointers to get you going in a "better breathing" direction:

1. Do not do deep breathing exercises – ever. They make you light headed for a reason. . .they deprive your brain of oxygen!

2. Breathe as shallow and slow as you can during the day.

3. Always breathe through your nose. never through your mouth – your mouth takes in too much air. (Even during exercise – if you have to breathe through your mouth, slow down the exercising until you no longer have to.)

4. If you snore or have sleep apnea, take some one-inch wide masking tape and tape your mouth shut before you go to sleep. Yes, that's right – tape your mouth shut! I do it every night now and sleep much better. They sell a special kind of tape just for this purpose – so check out the Buteyko website. (Your spouse may want you to leave the tape on your mouth all day, but just having it on at night is enough!)

5. Sleep on your side or on your stomach.* Sleeping on your back allows too much oxygen into your lungs. Babies want to sleep on their stomachs. No one has "educated' them yet. I know that sleeping on your stomach may not be ideal for your neck, but if you don't have neck or spine problems, I would give it a try. Personally, I put a pillow under my chest and kind of hang my head off of it, allowing a straighter spine angle and less tension in my neck.

These days, when someone is under stress, they're admonished to "Breathe, breathe, breathe. . .Take a deep breath. Relax." Well, that's really self-defeating since deep breaths actually deprive your tissues of oxygen and increase stress levels. In a few years, when people finally wake up to Buteyko breathing, you'll hear people saying instead, "Exhale and hold. Exhale and hold!" So the basketball player standing on the foul line just before taking the foul shot to win the game will no longer take a deep breath – he'll exhale and hold. And the announcer will say, "There he is, trying to calm himself down before this historic shot, exhaling and holding! Exhaling and holding! The shots up! Holy cow, I think he's gonna make it! It's GOOD! He made the shot! The home team wins! The fans go wild and storm the floor!" Exhale and hold and you'll make the shot too.

*However, there is evidence that Sudden Infant Death Syndrome (SIDS) may be caused by babies sleeping on their stomachs and new parents are advised to make sure their newborn sleeps on their back. Researchers in the U.S. say they don't know why this is. But one doctor in New Zealand thinks he's found the reason. Dr. Jim Sprott, a New Zealand scientist, says that fire retardants (that include arsenic, antimony, and phosphorus) used in the manufacturing of mattresses react with a fungus that typically grows in bedding materials to produce a toxic gas. If the baby breathes this gas at high enough levels, the central nervous system shuts down, stopping breathing and heart function.

Dr. Sprott recommends that the mattress be sealed in a high-grade polyethylene (plastic) that stops the gas from getting into the air space of the baby or using all natural, organic bedding. The New Zealand government listened to Dr. Sprott, and instituted a program of mattress wrapping seven years ago. Since then, there has not been a single SIDS death reported among the over 100,000 New Zealand babies who have slept on a wrapped mattress. During this same period, the number of crib deaths involving unwrapped mattresses was over 500.(31)

A recent study showed that if you place a fan in the baby's room that circulates the air, SIDS deaths are reduced by 72 percent. This makes sense if the true cause of death is due to the toxic gases, since they would be blown away from the baby faster than if the air is stagnant.(32) Dr. Sprott also recommends using a pure cotton under-blanket, with only cotton sheets and woolen or cotton blankets over the baby. No other bedding materials should be used, especially synthetic sheets or blankets, a duvet, sleeping bag or sheepskin. The initial research by Dr. Sprott was published in 1994, and the New Zealand mattress-wrapping program went on for seven years with a 100 percent success rate. So why hasn't the United States instituted such a program? Well, this information is being suppressed because the mattress manufacturers are required to use the fire retardants due to government regulations. They would have to change their manufacturing processes and admit that their mattresses were causing babies to die — leaving them open to major liability. In addition, crib death research has been a major source of funding for medical researchers in the U.S. They don't want their meal ticket revoked. (SIDS research has just about stopped in New Zealand.)

You can order these plastic mattress covers from www.babysnugglebugs.com. To be even safer, get an all natural, organic crib mattress from www.healthychild.com.

Carbon dioxide plays a key role in the regulation of proteins throughout the body. Proteins have what are called *amine group*. These amine groups are very sticky, and will naturally combine with carbon dioxide if it's available and this keeps them functioning normally. However, if enough carbon dioxide is not present, the amine groups will combine with sugar molecules. This renders the protein useless and toxic and can cause serious problems in many ways. Let's look at a few of these problems:

Insulin is a protein (a hormone) that the pancreas produces in order to get glucose molecules into the cell so they can be used for energy production. If insulin has sugar molecules (instead of carbon dioxide) attached to its amine groups, it won't function properly and glucose won't get into the cell, as it should. When this happens, the pancreas releases more insulin and the liver releases more sugar into the bloodstream. Not only will some of this sugar get deposited as fat, but will also combine with the additional insulin that the liver released causing it malfunction too. If this goes on long enough, the pancreas gets exhausted, can no longer produce enough insulin, and diabetes results.

Skin is made of structural proteins. If these proteins get sugar molecules attached to them instead of carbon dioxide, they can't reproduce normally. New skin won't be generated to replace the old skin, and this old skin will be filled with toxic protein-sugar molecules, which show up as age spots. These age spots are not just on the surface skin either, but can be in other places like the heart, brain, or other internal organs. They are not so much a sign of old age, but of a body that is has become toxic.

Neurotransmitters are chemicals the nervous system uses to communicate. One of them, serotonin, gives us happiness and peace of mind. Another one called dopamine gives us ambition. A third called melatonin allows us to sleep. But if these are impaired because sugar attached to them instead of carbon dioxide, they can't function properly. You may get depressed, lose interest, or have trouble sleeping.

If you have trouble sleeping because you just can't stop thinking and worrying, it may be because you don't have enough carbon dioxide in your body. Carbon dioxide lets our brain cells rest, and if there isn't enough of it, your brain cells keep going and going and they wear out prematurely. This may lead to anxiety, difficulty concentrating, and chronic fear. Enzymes malfunction if there's a lack of carbon dioxide. Digestion becomes impaired and so does the ability to absorb nutrients. (Doing Buteyko breathing is also good way to relieve gas and indigestion. Try it and see.)

Ammonia is produced by the body as a normal waste product of protein metabolism. It combines with carbon dioxide to form urea, which is naturally excreted. But is there's not enough carbon dioxide to do this, ammonia can build up to toxic levels. Symptoms may include tremors, fatigue, and the aversion to high protein foods.

One of the major benefits of carbon dioxide is that it relaxes the muscles. In fact, it's been called *nature's tranquilizer*, and if enough is available, the body relaxes. However, if adequate amounts of it are not available, muscles will become tense and overly contracted. This may be obvious with stiffness in leg, arm, and back muscles, but not so obvious in heart, lung, and muscles in internal organs.

When muscles are overly contracted (too tense), a lot of bad things can happen: If the arteries to your brain are tense, blood flow decreases and you may have headaches, bad memory, bad eyesight or hearing, fatigue or depression; if the muscles around your throat are tense, you may snore, have sleep apnea or difficulty speaking; tense lungs can lead to asthma and breathing problems; if the heart is too tense, you may get angina or even a heart attack; if the stomach is too tense, you have digestive problems or acid reflux; if the gall bladder is too tense, you get gall stones; tense bladder causes incontinence; tense uterus causes menstrual cramps; tense colon causes constipation or spastic colon; tense reproductive organs causes impotence.(33)

Food for Thought

Yes, I know, doing breathing exercises (or in this case, *lack* of breathing exercises) is a bother. I don't really like taking the time to do them either. But I always feel better afterwards and my health has greatly improved since I started. (Ladies, it is great for your complexion – you'll look years younger!) You just need to keep in mind that the time you take now to do them will help you avoid a lot of time in the doctor's office down the road. That's not to mention all the suffering and impaired functioning you'll be avoiding.

You can sneak these exercises into your daily routine. If you're waiting in line, waiting for food, or waiting for sleep, slow down your breathing. If you're watching TV, turn down the sound during the commercials and turn down your breathing. If you practice enough, your breathing pattern will reset, and you'll breathe less without thinking about it. I do the breathing a lot while I'm driving my car. I'll hold my nose for 5-10 seconds, and then breathe slow and shallow. This is very relaxing, so if you do this while driving, be careful not to get too comfortable.

A lot of this book focuses on what you put into your mouth. But what goes into your nose is also important, since we take about 20,000 breaths a day. If there's too much food going into your mouth, you'll get sick. If there's too much air going into your lungs, you'll get sick too. Changing your health can be as simple as changing your breathing, and it will never cost you a penny. In fact, it will save you money because your digestion and assimilation will improve and you won't need to eat as much. What a deal!

To summarize this chapter on asthma, you will find relief if you do a few simple things: avoid air pollution especial second hand smoke; avoid sulfites on food; get enough magnesium in your diet or take a magnesium supplement (magnesium oil), and; do the breathing exercises every day.

CHAPTER VII

Attention-Deficit and Hyperactivity Disorders

Attention disorders have been known by several names over the years. They were first documented in children in 1902 by George Still, who described 43 children with aggression, defiance, emotionality, limited sustained attention, and deficient rule-governed behavior.(1) Since then, the disorder has been given numerous names including minimal brain dysfunction, hyperkinetic reaction of childhood, attention deficit disorder (ADD), and the most current, as defined by the *Diagnostic and Statistical Manual, 4th Edition,* of *Attention-Deficit/Hyperactivity Disorder* (AD/HD). This current name reflects the importance of the inattention/distraction aspect of the disorder as well as the hyperactivity/impulsivity aspect.(2)

Symptoms of AD/HD usually arise in early childhood around the age of three unless there is some type of brain injury later in life. It is marked by behaviors that are evident for at least six months with their onset before the age of seven. There are three basic subtypes of AD/HD:

I. AD/HD – Primarily inattentive type (AD/HD-I). A person with this disorder: Fails to give close attention to details or makes careless mistakes; has difficulty sustaining attention; does not appear to listen; struggles to follow through on instructions; has difficulty with organization; avoids or dislikes talks requiring sustained mental effort; is easily distracted; is forgetful in daily activities.

II. AD/HD – Primarily hyperactive/impulsive type (AD/HD-HI). Someone with this disorder: Fidgets with hands or feet or squirms in chair; has difficulty remaining seated; runs about or climbs excessively; has difficulty engaging in activities quietly; acts as if driven by a motor; talks excessively; blurts out answers before questions have been completed; has difficulty waiting or taking turns; interrupts or intrudes upon others.

III. AD/HD – Combined type (AD/HD-C). These individuals exhibit both sets of attention and hyperactive/impulsive criteria above.(3)

For purposes of this discussion, we will be talking about the AD/HD combined type. It will be referred to as ADHD. To determine if a child has ADHD, the symptoms must be more frequent or severe than other children the same age. In adults, the symptoms must affect the ability to function in daily life and persist from childhood. And, the behaviors must create significant difficulty in at least two areas of life, such as in the home, at school, at work, in social settings, and so on

Since there is no single test to diagnose ADHD, a comprehensive evaluation is needed. This requires time and effort and is largely a subjective process. A history of the child should be taken from the parents, teachers, and child and the child's academic, social, and emotional characteristics all need to be evaluated. Often a clinician will use nothing more than a checklist for rating ADHD symptoms. It's shocking to find out that a diagnosis of such a serious problem can be made by a non-physician by simply checking eight of 14 items on a behavior checklist.(4)

Some behaviors that are prevalent in children with an attention and/or hyperactivity disorder can manifest at any time – even when the child is still in the womb. Some mothers have described their children as "punching their way out of the uterus." As infants, children may do excessive head banging or crib rocking, have long bouts of crying and screaming, be overly restless, have great thirst and large amounts of saliva and dribbling, or have fitful sleep or little need for sleep. As toddlers, these children can be easily excited, cry easily, or burst into tantrums if their demands are not instantly met. They run and climb on everything and can't sit still or concentrate for more than a few seconds. Often they will bump into furniture and walls so often that it looks as if the parents are battering them.

By the first grade, symptoms can get worse. ADHD children are easily distracted, make careless errors, don't follow-through on requests, forget to write down school assignments, or can't play games for the same amount of time as other children their age. They are not able to listen to an entire story or sit through a meal, sleep through the night, or complete a chore. They have difficulty accepting direction, discipline, and correction, and are too impulsive to think before they act. They find it hard to wait for things they want or to take turns in a game and are more likely to grab a toy from another child or hit others when upset. ADHD is not just an attention problem, but a problem of impulse control (more on that later). Their urge to act is not being inhibited, so their first reaction becomes their immediate behavior.

As these children grow older, they still have difficulty in starting and completing tasks, making transitions from one thing to another, and interacting with others. They have difficulty following through on directions and organizing multi-step tasks and have little goal orientation. New and different stimuli attract their attention and distract them easily.

Still later, other symptoms may appear such as clumsiness, fatigue, listlessness, muscle weakness, aggression, nonstop talking, increased volume of speech, body aches, poor appetite, anxiety, defiance and disobedience, nervousness, and depression, wild mood swings, bed wetting, poor hand-eye coordination, swollen neck glands and fluid behind the ear drum, ringing in the ears, excessive sweating, and self-abusive behaviors such as hair pulling.

It's important to realize that children with ADHD usually have a normal or high IQ, but because they cannot control themselves, they often fail at school. It's not that they are unintelligent; it's just that they don't have the self-discipline to learn. They have poor learning skills and underdeveloped social skills that may affect them the rest of their lives.

It's estimated that between 10 percent and 15 percent of all school children in the U.S. are affected by ADHD. That's between 1.8 million and 2.7 million children.(5). Since it is difficult to diagnose, it is believed that many cases go undetected. Up to 70 percent of children with ADHD will continue to exhibit symptoms of it in adulthood.(6) Boys are diagnosed with the disorder two to three times as often as girls.(7)

Adults who have ADHD often have difficulty concentrating for long periods, are impulsive and impatient, and may have short tempers and frequent mood swings. They can have difficulty planning ahead, be overly disorganized, and feel restless and fidgety.

It's believed that many adults with ADHD were never properly diagnosed as children. It was once widely believed that the symptoms would disappear, as one got older. However, it's now recognized that these symptoms carry through into adolescent and adult life, giving rise to job performance and interpersonal relationship problems.

Current estimate that about 4 percent to 6 percent of the U.S. population has ADHD.(8) According to one 1997 estimate, somewhere between 6.5 and 9 million adults in the U.S. have ADHD – making it as large a problem as drug abuse or clinical depression. In 1997, close to 730,000 adults in the U.S. were taking *Ritalin* by prescription for ADHD.(9) By 2004, one out of 100 adults 20 to 44 year of age were on ADHD medication, up from one out of 200 in 2000.(10) *Ritalin*, as we shall explore in depth below, is a psychoactive drug used to treat ADHD.

Food for Thought

I do not intend to exaggerate the problems of ADHD and scare you into thinking that all the possible behaviors mentioned above means your child has a disorder. Kids will be kids, and they have an amazing amount of energy and their attention span is naturally short. But some kids are showing too many of these impulsive and aggressive behaviors, and that is a problem. If something isn't done for them as soon as possible, these behaviors will become more and more ingrained and harder to change as time goes on. There are many simple and natural ways to help children with ADHD (besides using drugs), which we will explore. But please don't get hysterical if your child exhibits some of these behaviors on occasion. Most of them are part of being a child and growing up. It's my personal opinion that unless a number of these behaviors seem out of control, especially the aggressive and violent ones, there's no reason to be overly concerned. If you follow the recommendations in this book, your child will likely recover from these behaviors or never exhibit them. If you or someone you know has adult ADHD, the recommendations herein will also have a positive impact, although they may take longer to effective a permanent change in behavior and attitude.

In a medical conference in November 1999, the organizers of the conference estimated that ADHD among children in the U.S. is doubling every three to four years. The use of *Ritalin* has *quadrupled* between 1990 and 1997.[11]

The traditional medical community considers the cause of ADHD to be unknown even though it is one of the best-researched disorders in medicine. Research does suggest that it has a neurobiological basis. Stewart Mostofsky, M.D., of the Kennedy Krieger Institute and Johns Hopkins School of Medicine in Baltimore, says, "There is a lot of evidence that the brain's right hemisphere is dominant in attentional processes. Abnormalities in the brain's right frontal structure and function may be contributing to the behavioral impairments associated with ADHD."[12] It was also noted that children diagnosed with ADHD often have smaller overall brain volumes than normal children, with significantly less gray matter in their frontal brain region (especially the right frontal part). This study was funded by the National Institutes of Health, and involved 12 boys diagnosed with ADHD and 14 boys without ADHD.

It is also believed that ADHD is caused by a combination of hereditary predisposition and environmental factors. However, there have been some studies of identical twins showing that environmental factors contribute significantly to ADHD (one twin was normal, the other, exposed to environmental toxins, developed ADHD).[13] So although genetics may contribute to ADHD, it is not the only thing that may trigger it. You won't be surprised to learn that there is good evidence showing that prenatal exposure to lead, mercury, cadmium, aluminum, fluoride, cigarette byproducts, and alcohol may contribute to its manifestation.

Food for Thought

I do not mean to ignore the role that heredity and genetics play in the manifestation of ADHD because they could contribute to it. Garret Loporto, in his book *The DaVinci Method,* says that many of the characteristics of ADHD are also found in people with extraordinary talents. He calls these people *DaVincis* in honor of Leonardo DaVinci, the epitome of the *Renaissance Man.*

These people share a common genetic trait: ". . .the DRD4 exon III 7-repeat allele." He says that 'DaVinci Types' have made up to 5 percent of the world population over the course of history, and that having this genetic trait is not all bad. In fact, there's a high correlation with having this trait and one's ability to attain incredible success and genius. This gene supports risk-taking, novelty seeking, increased alpha/theta brainwave patterns, susceptibility to ADD/ADHD, propensity for genius level problem solving and creativity, and gives one what it takes to be a charismatic political leader, rock star or rebel billionaire."

DaVincis have little self-repression and "are only really content when operating at 100% threshold of their physical, mental, emotional and spiritual capacity with virtually no repression." Loporto says that sometimes the gene needs to be activated for the characteristics to manifest, and that this activation is likely done by some form of life-threatening stress. He also believes that once the gene is activated, it cannot be deactivated. The best we can do is to learn how to channel this energy into something positive. He gives ways to accomplish this – journaling, meditating, playing a musical instrument, and doing physical activities that involve short bursts of intense activity such as kick-boxing, tennis, or dancing. In fact, he says that these types of people need a lot more exercise than 90% of the population: "It's your genetic make-up that wants intense activity almost every day, and you can't escape your genetic make-up. . .The trick is to do it, to dread it, but do it, and keep doing it. Eventually it will become a habit. Dread and do. Dread and do."

Here's a list of famous people Loporto believes had or have the DaVinci gene (the ADHD genetics): Napoleon, Thomas Jefferson, Bill Clinton, Benjamin Franklin, Thomas Edison, Winston Churchill, Bono (rock star), John F. Kennedy (and most of the Kennedy's), Carl Jung, Sylvester Stallone (actor), and Robin Williams (commedian/actor), Marianne Williamson (best selling author), and of course, Leonardo DaVinci.(14)

So take heart, mom and dad. If your little one is a handful and gives you fits, he/she may just be the next DaVinci! It's best to get them exercising a lot to burn off that energy. And be sure to keep them off sugar and artificial sweeteners.

People with ADHD often do poorly in school, may drop out, have low self-esteem, and have difficulty making connections with other people. They are described as messy, disorganized, inattentive, irritable, and aggressive. Because their lives can be unrewarding and frustrating, they may become hostile and violent. In May 1999, a 15-year-old boy shot six of his schoolmates in Conyers Georgia. At the time, he was taking the prescription drug *Ritalin* for ADHD.

Peter Montague of the Environmental Research Foundation states, "At a time when Americans are searching for causes of aggression and violence among children, it would make sense to consider malnutrition, food additives, tobacco additives, toxic metals, pesticides, and other endocrine-disrupting industrial toxicants – all of which many U.S. children are exposed to from the moment of conception onward."(15) Let's consider some of these closer.

Food Additives

Food additives such as dyes and colorings have been implicated in ADHD. In 16 out of 23 studies on food additives and ADHD, it was found that these food additives exacerbated the symptoms of ADHD in some children.(16) Despite these studies (which were double-blind studies) the U.S. Food and Drug Administration has stated in one of its pamphlets "Food Color Facts" that "there is no evidence that food color additives cause hyperactivity or learning disabilities in children."(17)

Food for Thought

It's interesting to note that although the FDA published the pamphlet *Food Color Facts*, the publication was actually written by the International Food Information Council. That council is a trade association representing many makers of food additives such as *General Mills, Kraft, Pepsi-Cola, Coca-Cola, Procter and Gamble*, and others. So it's no wonder the pamphlet says there's no evidence food color additives cause hyperactive or learning disabilities in kids. Remember too that some food additives, such as the sulfites, have been known to cause death. Shame on you, FDA.

While there has been much research concerning the potential carcinogenicity of artificial colors and flavors, there have been only a few published studies examining their effects on behavioral attributes. But Ben F. Feingold, M.D., in 1970, claimed that some children showed dramatic improvements in attention deficit and hyperactivity after removing artificial ingredients from their diet. Other researchers subsequently have failed to show this consistently, according to some interpretations of their results. However, these later studies removed only one artificial item from the child's diet, when in actuality, the ADHD child is exposed to many synthetic compounds daily.

To determine if artificial colors specifically can impact a developing organism, Dr. Bennett Shaywitz of Yale University studied young rat pups exposed to a mixture of artificial colors, using amounts that would typically be consumed by American children (1 mg/kg body weight). He reported that the mixture of five dyes (blue, green, red, yellow, and orange) resulted in hyperactivity in the young rat pups. Shaywitz concluded ". . .it is apparent that food dyes affect activity levels during the first month of postnatal life."(18)

Monosodium glutamate (MSG) is a flavor enhancer used to increase the perceived taste of any item it's in. The food industry uses it to save money. Chicken soup made with MSG, for example, requires half the amount of real chicken in it to get the same taste as soup made without MSG. That's a real cost-saver for manufacturers. And it explains why world MSG production in 1976 was 262,000 metric tons.

Food for Thought

As agricultural practices have changed in the past 70 years from natural growing methods to ones that use chemicals, the nutritional quality of the food has concomitantly decreased. Reflective of the quality of the food is how it tastes. MSG is used in part because our food just doesn't taste like it should and needs flavor-enhancing. Grow more wholesome foods the way nature intended them to be grown, and you wouldn't need any "flavor enhancers." Taste an apple from a grocery store, and one that was grown organically – there's a big difference.

The FDA has stated that MSG is safe for most people except for those with serious asthma difficulties. But studies by L. Reif-Lehrer reported that 25 percent of a population sample who have been exposed to Chinese restaurant food (with MSG) exhibit at least some adverse symptoms.[19] MSG was routinely added to baby foods prior to the 1970s, and its use in them was halted following government suggestions.

Dr. Olney, at the department of psychiatry and pediatrics at Washington University School of Medicine, a leading expert concerning MSG, has said:

> According to a NAS [National Academy of Science] subcommittee, in considering the safety of added MSG in baby foods, one must remember that the levels added are small - not higher than 0.6 percent. . . This means that one small jar of baby food (130 g) would provide about 0.78 g of MSG or 0.13 g/kg of body weight for a human infant weighing 6 kg. Based on our finding that an oral dose of 1 g/kg in the primate or 0.5 g/kg in the mouse is sufficient to destroy hypothalamic neurons, this leaves a 4 to 8 fold margin of safety for a human infant eating 1 jar, a 2 to 4 fold margin if 2 jars are eaten and so forth. This is substantially less than the 100-fold margin generally recommended. . .in susceptibility of the mechanism of a toxic com-pound.[20]

The Food Protection Committee of the National Academy of Sciences (NAS) has declared MSG to be a safe food additive requiring no regulation. Despite evidence that MSG causes brain damage in infant rodents, the committee reasoned that the primate infant (humans are primates) was not likely at risk because it has a more mature central nervous system and more highly developed blood-brain barrier at birth.

Subsequent to this ruling, Olney showed that rhesus monkeys (a primate also) exposed to a single dose of MSG developed brain damage (in the hypothalamus). He says, ". . .it seems unrealistic to deny primate susceptibility to the MSG effect."

Another study using 75 infant mice was done to determine at what level MSG and aspartate could cause brain lesions. All but the very lowest level administered to the mice had harmful observable effects on brain cells. It was found that MSG and aspartate can combine their damage potential when fed tithe animals together.(21)

Another Olney study was performed to investigate the possibility of long-term effects from MSG ingestion. Olney examined 38 originally healthy Swiss albino mice from birth to nine months of age. Twenty of these animals received injections of MSG daily. The MSG-treated animals appeared stunted in growth and shorter than the controls after 30 days. The average weights of five-month-old animals were significantly less if they did not consume MSG than if they did. It's of particular interest to note that the MSG-treated mice actually consumed less food than their thinner control counterparts. This implies damage to the brain area responsible for controlling body weight.(22)

Food for Thought

Could this in part explain the growing obesity pattern in our youth and even our population at large? Have you ever heard someone complain that they continued to gain weight even though they ate practically nothing? I'm sure there are a number of factors responsible for weight gain in children and adults, but could MSG, that's in a lot of snack foods (check out the *Doritos* label) , be partly responsible?

Olney also reported that the MSG animals were quite lethargic when they were adults, and they lacked the sleekness of body coat seen in the controls. The reproductive capacity of the MSG females was also modified in that they repeatedly failed to conceive. Olney concludes:

> These observations, linking MSG treatment of the neonatal (the first four weeks after birth) mouse with a syndrome of manifestations, including skeletal stunting, marked adiposity, and sterility of the female, coupled with histopathological findings in several organs associated with endocrine function, suggest a complex endocrine disturbance. . .The assumption that MSG is an entirely innocuous substance for human consumption has been questioned. . .the finding that neuronal necrosis can be induced in the immature mouse brain. . . raises the more specific question whether there is any risk to the developing human nervous system by maternal use of MSG during pregnancy. . .(23)

One child who was experiencing "innumerable seizures" (100 or more a day) showed dramatic improvements after MSG was removed from his diet. This was reported by Dr. L. Reif-Lehrer of Harvard Medical School in the journal *Federal Proceedings*. The child did not respond to dilantin (a common drug for epilepsy), but had symptoms "Completely alleviated by a diet that excluded exogenously added glutamate." When the child is fed an MSG meal, the seizures return. Dr. Reif-Lehrer says, "In some individuals, glutamate may be getting through the blood-brain barrier, or to certain areas of the hypothalamus, and may result in undesirable effects. . ."[24]

It's clearly evident that MSG can have subtle as well as devastating effects on children and adults alike. It's best to avoid it. If you consume nutritious foods, you won't need any flavor enhancers.

Chemicals and Pesticides

Most recently, research has implicated pesticides and exposure to low levels of industrial chemicals to cognitive problems such as ADHD. Undoubtedly, combinations of environmental pollutants may contribute to the problem.

A report entitled *In Harm's Way*, by a team of physicians in Cambridge, Massachusetts, says that millions of children in the U.S. exhibit learning disabilities, reduced IQ and destructive, aggressive behavior because of exposures to toxic chemicals. Drs. Ted Schettler and Jill Stein et al. link toxic exposures during early childhood and even before birth, to lifelong disabilities including attention disorders and poorly controlled aggression. As of June 2000, estimates indicate that ADHD, dyslexia, and uncontrollable aggression affect about 12 million children under 18 in the U.S. (almost one in five). The number of children classified with learning disabilities and placed in special education programs increased 191 percent between 1977 and 1994. Experts estimate that autism rates rose from around four per 10,000 in the early 1980s to between 12 and 210 per 10,000 in the 1990s, and now it's about one in 150.[25]

Many pesticides kill insects by killing cells in the nervous system. These pesticides can also disrupt the development and functioning of the human's nervous system too. Studies show that children in communities that use pesticides a lot score lower on memory, physical stamina and coordination tests, and display more aggressive behavior than children in relatively pesticide-free areas.

Government "safe" exposure levels are based on individual chemicals. But children can be exposed to many chemicals at the same time, which can be far more damaging. One study found that certain combinations of pesticides produce changes in thyroid levels that are not observed when the chemicals are tested individually. Proper thyroid levels are essential for brain development. Other studies show that exposure to a combination of mercury and PCBs, two pollutants that accumulate in fish, can produce even greater effects on neurological development than either pollutant alone.[26]

Of 890 pesticide active ingredients, the EPA says 140 are neurotoxins and some 20 million U.S. children under age five eat an average of eight different pesticides on their food every day. In addition, there are between 2,400 and 4,000 industrial chemicals now on the market that are neurotoxic. The EPA estimates that nearly a billion pounds of known neurotoxins were released directly into the air and water in 1997. The authors of *In Harm's Way* write:

We should not need to identify with certainty exactly how much and through what mechanism a neurotoxic pesticide impairs brain development before coming to the conclusion that public health is not protected when the urine of virtually every child in this country contains residues of these chemicals. . .We do not need to exhaustively understand the mechanism by which methyl mercury interferes with normal fetal brain development before concluding that it is not acceptable for freshwater and many ocean fish to be sufficiently contaminated with mercury to threaten developing brains. We know how to reduce the environmental releases of mercury so that fish are once again safe to eat regularly. We can modify manufacturing practices so that lead use in products goes steadily down instead of up. We can eliminate or modify outmoded technologies that produce the dioxin that contaminates fetuses and breast milk. We know how to do these things. . .In sum, our current regulatory system is like a trial in which the criminal defendant gets to serve on the jury. If we want to have children who can play, think and learn normally, we will have to change corporations and our government so that protecting brain development comes ahead of protecting profits.(27)

Lead

The *American Journal of Public Health* called lead poisoning an epidemic among American children. The U.S. Department of Health and Human Services referred to it as "the most important environmental health problem facing young children."(28) The EPA report *Lead in Your Home: A Parent's Reference Guide* (a free government publication) says, "In the United States, about 900,000 children ages one to five have a blood-lead level above the level of concern." The report goes on to discuss the health effects of lead:

Lead is poisonous because it interferes with some of the body's basic functions. A human body cannot tell the difference between lead and calcium, which is a mineral that strengthens bones. Like calcium, lead remains in the bloodstream for a few weeks, then it's absorbed into the bones, where it can collect for a lifetime. Although children are especially susceptible to lead exposure, lead can be dangerous for adults too. In adults, high lead levels can cause:

- Increased chance of illness during pregnancy.
- Harm to a fetus, including brain damage or death.
- Fertility problems (in men and women).
- High blood pressure.

- Digestive problems.
- Nerve disorders.
- Memory and concentration problems.
- Muscle and joint pain.

Lead can affect anyone, but children ages six and younger face special hazards. In part, this is because the bodies of children in this age group develop rapidly. It is also because young children tend to put things in their mouths. . . It is important to know that even exposure to low levels of lead can permanently affect children. In low levels, lead can cause:

- Nervous system and kidney damage.
- Learning disabilities, attention deficit disorder, and decreased intelligence.
- Speech, language, and behavior problems.
- Poor muscle coordination.
- Decreased muscle and bone growth.
- Hearing damage.

While low-level exposure is most common, exposure to high levels of lead can have devastating effects on children, including seizures, unconsciousness, and in some cases, death.

Lead poisoning is not easy to detect. Sometimes no symptoms occur, and sometimes the symptoms are the same as those of more common illnesses. Some of the early signs and symptoms of lead poisoning in children are:

- Persistent tiredness or hyperactivity.
- Irritability.
- Loss of appetite.
- Weight loss.
- Reduced attention span.
- Difficulty sleeping.
- Constipation.(29)

The report goes on to say, "The only way to know if you have lead poisoning is to get a blood test from your doctor. Many people mistake the symptoms of lead poisoning for other common illnesses. . .Sometimes there are no symptoms at all." This applies to adults and children alike.

Food for Thought

Would it surprise you to learn that the symptoms of lead poisoning in children and adults are all classic signs of ADHD? I have two comments about this: One is that I wonder how many doctors prescribe a lead blood test for the hyperactive children they see before they prescribe *Ritalin*? I think every pediatrician in the country should be mailed the above referenced publication and be required to read it. Philip Landrigan, chair of the department of community and preventive medicine at Mount Sinai School of Medicine in New York City, says that any evaluation of a child suspected to have ADHD should start with screening for lead. My other comment is that since lead stays in the blood only a couple weeks or so, before it is absorbed into the bones, a blood test may not catch the fact that the child (or adult) was previously exposed to lead. A better test would be a tissue mineral analysis, which tests hair or fingernail samples. It is a long-term picture of a person's exposure, not just a snapshot of a blood test that might miss something. Really, both should be done.

Are there ways to get the lead out? Yes. The diet recommended in this book will help. Other things include: eating cilantro or its juice; taking special clay baths that pull out toxins; ensuring there's adequate magnesium and iodine in the blood and diet so the body can expel the lead or other heavy metals and taking *Epsom* salt or magnesium oil baths or foot soaks; exercise; small detox pads that are taped to the bottom of your feet that have been shown to pull toxins out of the body.

Here's a recipe that will help chelate (grab hold of and remove) heavy metals from the body. It's called *Chelation Pesto*: 4 cloves garlic;, 1/3 cup Brazil nuts; 1/3 cup sunflower seeds; 1/3 cup pumpkin seeds;, 2 cups packed fresh cilantro; 2/3 cup flaxseed oil; 4 tablespoons lemon juice; 2 teaspoons dulse powder; Bragg's Liquid Aminos (kind of like soy sauce, but healthier – at health food stores). Blend all the ingredients (except flaxseed oil and Bragg's) in a blender or food processor (you may have to add some water) until it's pasty. Then add the oil and a squirt or two of Bragg's to taste. Store in a dark glass jar. This freezes well, so you can make a lot and store it. Eat two teaspoons a day. If you start experiencing detoxification reactions, stop. Resume once symptoms are gone, and eat this several times a week for maintenance.

According to the American Academy of Pediatrics, between two million and four million American children have sufficient lead in their blood to reduce their physical stature, damage their hearing, decrease hand-eye coordination, and shorten their attention span enough to impair their ability to learn in school and diminish their IQ. Sad thing is, this damage is thought to be permanent.[30,31]

About 400,000 babies are delivered each year with toxic levels of lead already in their blood. Interestingly, the fetus acts as a "sink" for lead (and cooper, aluminum, cadmium, and other toxic metals) that is difficult for the mother to eliminate. Of the children living below the poverty level, some 55 percent have toxic levels of lead and one child in six is exposed to toxic levels of lead from the environment. Even low levels of lead are associated with hyperactivity, attention deficit/hyperactivity disorder (ADHD), and developmental failures. Again, any evaluation of a child suspected to have ADHD should start with screening for lead.[32]

In fact, the American Academy of Pediatrics showed that in 18 scientific studies lead diminished a child's mental abilities. "The relationship between lead levels and IQ deficits was found to be remarkably consistent," they report. "A number of studies have found that for every 10 mcg/dL increase in blood lead levels, there was a lowering of mean (average) IQ in children by four to seven points." An average IQ loss of five points puts 50 percent more children into the IQ 80 category, which is borderline for normal intelligence.(33)

The academy says these IQ losses are permanent and they translate into reduced educational attainment, diminished job prospects, and decreased earning power, as was evident in a study in which groups of children with different blood levels of lead were tracked through high school. The high-lead children had higher absenteeism in school, lower class rank, poorer vocabulary, and longer reaction times with poorer hand-eye coordination. The high-lead group also was seven times less likely to graduate from high school and had reading scores two grades below expected.

As for adults, as many as 4 percent to 5 percent of U.S. Adults have ADHD and only about 20 percent of them know it. Oftentimes an adult who has ADHD is characterized as being lazy, stupid, disorganized, unable to finish tasks, or a trouble maker. These people are usually as smart as the next person, but just have trouble with attention and self-control.(34) Since as many as 67 percent of children diagnosed with ADHD continue to have symptoms of the disorder into adulthood, it's important that we address its probable causes as early as possible.

It's interesting to note just what is considered excessively high levels of lead. In 1960, it was said that it was safe for a child to have 60 micrograms of lead in each deciliter (a tenth of a liter) of blood (60 mcg/dL). In 1975 the medical community determined that this in fact was too high, and lowered it to 30 mcg/dL. By 1985, it was determined that 25 mcg/dL was the safe limit. But that was found to be too high too. In 1991, the safe limit was lowered again to 10 mcg/dL. Now, the National Research Council believes this level is still too high.

For adults, the CDC says that elevated blood levels are those above 25 mcg/dL. Adult exposure to lead can cause anemia, nervous system dysfunction, kidney problems, hypertension, decreased fertility, and increased miscarriages.(35)

The Centers for Disease Control (CDC) says, "Blood lead levels at least as low as 10 mcd/dL can adversely affect the behavior and development of children." What this means is that the federal government has set an "acceptable" level of lead in blood (10 mcd/dL) that it acknowledges does not protect children. Damage to children has been documented at blood-lead levels considerably below 10 mcg/dL. The federal Agency for Toxic Substances and Disease Registry cites studies showing that children's growth, hearing, and IQ can be diminished by blood-lead levels as low as 5 mcg/dL.(36)

Between 1991 and 1994, the CDC tested the blood of a representative sample of the U.S. population for lead poisoning. They report that 4.4 percent of children ages one to five have at least 10 mcd/dL. That 4.4 percent represents about 890,000 children in the U.S. In some cities of the northeastern United States, it's estimated that 35 percent of preschool children have 10 mcg/dL or more of lead in their blood.[37]

Yet both the federal Department of Housing and Urban Development (HUD) and the U.S. EPA have set standards for lead in dust that, if met, essentially guarantee that childhood lead poisoning at the level of 10 mcg/dL will continue. Even if the current government standard for lead in dust were reduced to one tenth its present level, it would still allow children to be poisoned by lead in dust.[38]

It seems the whole philosophy behind all these safety standards is not one of "How do we prevent lead poisoning?" but more of "How much lead is safe for us to put into our children?" This even though there is convincing evidence that lead is a poison even at extremely low levels and that it has been poisoning people for many thousands of years.

Food for Thought

Ancient Greeks and Romans mined lead, and its toxicity was well established, even back then, long before the birth of Christ. Roman miners sometimes died from what the medical literature of the time called *lead colic*. One of the reasons the Roman Empire fell, according to some historians, was that they used lead pipes for water (they abandoned their stone aqueducts) and had lead in their pottery. The accumulation of lead in their tissues would have led to mental problems. Could the crazy act of Nero playing a fiddle on the balcony as Rome burned below him have been because he had lead poisoning?

In 1989, the EPA reported that more than one million elementary schools, high schools, and colleges were still using lead-lined water storage tanks or lead-containing components in their drinking fountains. The EPA estimates that 20 percent of human exposure (including children) is attributed to lead in drinking water.[39]

Lead has also been implicated in aggressive behavior (in addition to delinquency and attention disorders) in boys between the ages of seven and 11. In the *Journal of the American Medical Association*, Herbert Neeleman examined 301 boys in public schools in Pittsburgh, Pennsylvania, measuring the lead in their bones and relating it to their behaviors as reported by the boys' teachers and parents and by the boys themselves. Boys with more lead in their bones consistently had more reports of aggressive and delinquent behavior and problems paying attention. The boys' behavior was measured at age seven and again at age 11. The behavior of the boys with more lead in their bones got worse as they grew older. On the other hand, behavior did not change among boys with less lead in their bones. The study also examined nine other variables in addition to lead (parents' socioeconomic status, mother's age, presence or absence of a father in the home, etc.) But even with all those variables taken into account, the relationship between lead and behavior was still statistically significant.[40]

Other studies have made the correlation between lead and aggressive behavior as well. In 1975 in Virginia, researchers compared 67 lead-exposed 11-year-olds to 70 non-exposed children to see if lead exposure was related to behavior problems. Nineteen of the lead-exposed children were described as "hyperactive, impulsive, and explosive, and as having frequent temper tantrums." Only five among the nonexposed group were described that way.[41] One year later, the group was reevaluated. Fourteen of the lead-exposed children were described as having problems with lying, stealing, running away, and setting fires. Six of the non-exposed children were described this way.

In a study in 1994 in Boston, 1,782 children were examined for the amount of lead in their teeth and whether they had behavioral problems. Problem behaviors increased as lead levels in the children's teeth increased.[42] In 1982 in Tennessee, a study was done examining the level of lead in children's hair. The lead levels in hair of 26 "problem children" were nearly twice as high as a control group of 29 students who had no behavioral problems.[43]

One scientific paper observed that as the concentration of lead in children increases, so does the incidences of violent crimes approximately 20 years later, when the children are grown. Bernard Weiss said in an article in the *International Journal of Mental Health* that the connections between brain-damaging lead and destructive behavior at least partially explained the increases in crime.[44]

As early as 1943, the correlation between levels of lead in children and behavioral problems was documented. In a study by Randolph Byers and Elizabeth Lord, 20 children who had recovered from "mild lead poisoning in infancy" were examined. Although none of the children had exhibited overt signs of lead poisoning, the growth and development of their nervous systems had been seriously impaired. Of the 20 children examined, only one had progressed normally in school. Many of the children were emotionally impaired. Byers and Lord said many of the children had "unreliable impulsive behavior, cruel impulsive behavior, short attention span, and the like." Three of the children were expelled from school – one for setting fires, one for repeatedly dancing on the desks, and the third for sticking a fork into another student's face. One of these lead-exposed children was reported to have attacked teachers with knives and scissors.[45]

Roger D. Masters, Ph.D., and his coworkers at Dartmouth College say that pollution causes people to commit violent crimes (homicide, aggravated assault, sexual assault, and robbery). Masters has developed what he calls the neurotoxicity hypothesis of violent crime, which holds that the toxic metals lead and manganese cause learning disabilities and increase in aggressive behavior and the loss of control over impulsive behavior. These traits combined with poverty, social stress, alcohol, and drug abuse, individual character, and other social factors can produce individuals who commit violent crimes.(46) In the largest study of its kind, of 1,000 black children in Philadelphia, showed that both lead levels and anemia were predictors of the number of juvenile offenses, the seriousness of juvenile offense, and the number of adult offenses for males.

Environmental sources of lead are everywhere. The main source of lead for children is house dust from paint that is disintegrating. Aside from remnants of the paint laced with lead in our homes, house dust also contains lead tracked into homes from soil outside. Forty-two million families live in housing that contains an estimated three million tons of lead in the paint. That's equivalent to about 140 pounds of lead per household. As that paint slowly disintegrates into house dust, it becomes available for a child to get on his hands and into his mouth and lungs. If a child ingests just 150 micrograms per day, the National Research Council says, the child is poisoned.

Manufacturers used to put lead pigments in paint because the pigments made the paint last longer and cling to surfaces better. They no longer do so, but some significant risks remain since as the paint breaks down with age, the dust it sheds contains significant amounts of lead. In 1978 the Consumer Product Safety Commission (CPSC) banned its use in paints for use in residences, on children's toys, or on household furniture.(47)

Food for Thought

If you think that the United States is on the cutting edge of health care, consider this: Australia passed a law curbing lead in paint in 1920. But they were *behind* the times. France and Austria had banned the use of lead in interior paint all the way back in 1909. I guess they thought centuries of known health problems from lead were enough proof of its toxicity. But the U.S.? We banned it in 1978. Maybe we're just plain old dumb from all the lead we've been ingesting all these years.

Drinking water is another source: the EPA estimates that over 800 municipal water systems serving some 30 million people have lead levels that exceed federal guidelines. The FDA estimates that a significant amount of lead exposure comes from food that's been in contact with ceramic hollowware, including coffee mugs with a ceramic glaze. Frequent use of them can contribute to elevated lead levels. Lead poisoning was often referred to as *the potter's disease* because those who made pottery with lead glazes often contracted it.

Should you worry about this with your everyday dishes? Probably not. Modern ceramics made by commercial firms are usually harmless. And major importers of pottery such as *Pier One* and *William-Sonoma* voluntarily prohibit the sale of lead-glazed items in their stores. The FDA has also mandated those imported items not safe for food-use must have a permanent stamp stating so. But you do need to be wary of pottery made by artisans or folk-potters in other countries that are brought into the U.S., or old heirlooms that have been in the family for years and passed on from generation to generation. There is concern that using a glazed mug for coffee or other acidic beverages may leach lead out of the glaze. If you don't know where you got a piece of ceramic ware, don't use it with anything you would consume.

Oil companies used to add lead to gasoline to stop engine knocking, but dangerous lead particles escaped into the air through auto exhaust systems. In 1978, the EPA reduced the amount of lead allowed in gasoline, hence the term *unleaded*. Lead was also used in fixtures, pipes, and pipe soldering, and can leach into water that flows through the pipes. In 1986, and again in 1988, Congress changed the Safe Drinking Water Act to restrict the use of lead in pipes, solder, and other components used in public water systems and residential and nonresidential plumbing. However, lead may still be found in pipes manufactured prior to 1986 that are still in use today.

In 1995, the United States banned the use of lead solder in food cans. It was found that the lead solder used to seal the food cans leaches into the food. Although it has been banned in the U.S. for this use, lead solder may still be found in cans imported here from other countries.

Most people would think that since lead has been eliminated from some products, it's no longer a problem. It's true that changes in the law have greatly reduced the amount of lead released into our homes, air, and environment. And the average blood level in U.S. children has gone down from 16 mcg/dl to 5 mcg/dL during the last 15 years. But remember, lead does not go away. It persists in the soil, gets into our food chain, and gets tracked into our houses. There is still an estimated 30 million tons of lead in our soils as a result of using lead in gasoline and industry. The lead problem will be with us for many years. That's why the Academy of Pediatrics says, there are still many children at high risk of exposure. The National Research Council, in its 1993 book on lead, states:

> Once lead is mined and introduced into the environment, it persists. Over time, lead in various forms becomes available to the body as small particles. Most of the 300 million metric tons of lead ever produced remains in the environment, largely in soil and dust. That explains, in part, why background concentrations of lead in modern North Americans are higher by a factor of 100 to 1,000 than they were in pre-Columbian Americans. Today's production levels turn into tomorrow's background exposure, and despite reductions in the use of lead for gasoline, overall lead production continues to grow and federal agencies have not addressed the impact of future increases of lead in the environment.[48]

The National Research Council says modern humans are estimated to have total body burdens of lead approximately 300 to 500 times those of our prehistoric ancestors who had blood lead level of only 0.016 mcg/dL (micrograms per deciliter) (determined from measurements of human bones). This, if considered the background level, is 625 times lower than the 10 mcg/dL now considered safe for our children.[49]

Lead in the brain damages glia cells, a special kind of cell associated with inhibition (impulse control) and detoxification (eliminating poisons from the body). Manganese, another potential toxin, has the effect of lowering levels of serotonin and dopamine, which are neurotransmitters associated with impulse control and planning. Masters notes that low levels of serotonin in the brain are known to cause mood disturbances such as depression, poor impulse control, and increases in aggressive behavior.

Let's take a closer look at manganese. Children who are raised from birth on infant formula and who are not breastfed will absorb five times as much manganese as breastfed infants, Masters reports, and the absorption of manganese is increased when there is a calcium deficiency.

Food for Thought

Soft drinks increase the amount of calcium excreted in the urine, possibly leading to a calcium deficiency, possibly leading to higher blood levels of manganese, possibly leading to a loss of impulse control, possibly leading to. . .?

Because of the increased manganese absorption by babies who drink infant formula and who are not breastfed, Masters considers infant formula toxic. Surprisingly, impoverished mothers are less likely to breastfeed their babies. Seventy-3 percent of infants born to mothers with more than 12 years of education were breast fed, compared with 31 percent of infants born to mothers with less than 12 years of education. "The effects of manganese toxicity associated with infant formula are thus greatest for the poor, for ethnic minorities and for those with little education," Masters says. Masters also says that toxic metals affect an individual in complicated ways. For example, because lead diminishes a person's normal ability to detoxify poisons, lead may heighten the effects of alcohol and drugs.

He also points to studies showing a synergistic effect between toxic metals and poor diet. It's been thoroughly documented that the uptake of lead is greatly increased in individuals who have a diet low in calcium, zinc, and essential vitamins. The amounts of lead and manganese that wouldn't harm a well-nourished individual may poison undernourished children.[50] Federal studies of nutrition make the point that black teenage males consume, on average, only about 65 percent as much calcium as whites; it follows that their risk of metals toxicity would be higher.

To explore the link between metals toxicity and the propensity to violence, Masters acquired data from the FBI for violent crimes in all counties of the

United States. He correlated those with data on industrial releases of lead and manganese, and on alcohol consumption, which has been shown to increase the uptake of toxic metals. He found that counties having all three measures of neurotoxicity – lead, manganese, and high alcohol consumption – had rates of violent crime three times the national average. He says that the highest levels of lead uptake are reported in precisely the demographic groups most likely to commit violent crimes (inner-city minority youths).

Masters notes that neurotoxicity is only one of many factors contributing to violence, but adds that he believes it may be especially important in explaining why violent crime rates differ so widely among geographic areas and by ethnic group. He says that traditional sociological approaches to crime cannot explain why the availability of handguns or drugs triggers violent behavior in only a small proportion of the population, a proportion that varies greatly from place to place. Part of the explanation may be the way the physical environment affects brain chemistry and behavior. "The presence of pollution is as big a factor as poverty," Masters says in an interview in the *New Scientist* magazine. "It's the breakdown of the inhibition mechanism that's the key to violent behavior." When our brain chemistry is altered by exposure to toxins, he believes, we lose the natural restraint that holds our violent tendencies in check.(51)

It is well established that lead poisoning occurs mainly in poor neighborhoods. In 1998, 13.5 million children (about 18.9 percent of all children in the U.S.) lived in poverty. Children living in low-income families are eight times as likely to be lead-poisoned as children who are not poor. Black children are five times as likely to be lead-poisoned as white children. One researcher said, "the homes of black children [in the study] had higher levels of lead-contaminated dust and their interior surfaces were in poorer condition."(52)

The General Accounting Office (an investigative branch of Congress) stated in 1999 that "hundreds of thousands of children exposed to dangerously high levels of lead are neither tested nor treated" because state governments are refusing to comply with the law.(53) That law was passed in 1989 and requires all infants (12 months old) and toddlers (two years old) in the Medicaid program to be tested for lead poisoning. (Medicaid is a federally funded medical insurance program for economically disadvantaged people.) But this guideline is not being followed and it is it not being enforced. In summary, the Environmental Research Foundation states:

> . . .we have a federally mandated blood-lead standard (10 mcg/dL) that permanently dumbs down any children who meet it, which is nearly a million children at any moment, and roughly 200,000 new dumbing-downs are occurring each year. Medical authorities agree that the only real solution is primary prevention – keeping lead contaminated dust away from children. Credible estimates show that the federal government could make a profit of $1.08 billion by undertaking primary prevention in federally owned or assisted housing, but instead the government requires

the dead-canary approach, blood-lead testing, which the states then refuse to carry out. We know. . .that public policies that put the onus on the private sector can make a big difference – but most states have failed to adopt such policies.(54)

Food for Thought

How could the federal government make a profit on lead abatement? It's estimated that the first-year cost of reducing lead hazards in federally owned and federally assisted housing would be $458 million. However, the calculated benefits from lead – abatement, such as reduced costs for medical care and for special education, plus increased salaries and resulting economic boost that go with higher IQs, would be $1.538 billion – a net benefit of $1.08 billion.(55) Seems that monetarily, there should be no excuse. Better to spend money doing that than on bailing out banks that don't know how to make a simple loan. Maybe the halls of Congress and the White House are painted with lead paint!

Mercury

Mercury contamination may also be responsible for behavioral problems, learning disabilities, and ADHD. As early as the 1860s, a clinical disorder from mercury exposure was identified among *felters* (people who made the felt linings of hats and clothes). The term *mad as a hatter* was even coined to denote the strange behavior of people who did this kind of work. In the 19th century, mercury was known to be a deadly poison and back then it was known as Quick Silver (taken from the German phrase *Quak Silber*). People who put mercury, or Quak Silber, into other people's mouths were known as *quacks* – a term now used to denote a person who practices questionable medical procedures. Some believe it's no great surprise that dentists have a high rate of suicide. Mad Hatter's Disease may have become Mad Dentist's Disease.

Mercury exposure can come from seafood intake, environmental exposures at work and home (especially from mercury fungicides used in farming), and yes, from the silver fillings in a person's mouth. These "silver" fillings contain approximately 52 percent mercury. In a study reported in the *Journal of Dental Restoration*, those people in the study (including children) who had amalgam fillings had significantly greater levels of mercury in their blood. The authors concluded, "These examinations show that amalgam restorations contribute. . . to the origins of mercury in the organism [in children as well as adults]."(56) Another study, reported in the same journal, confirmed that blood concentrations of mercury are higher in people with amalgam fillings, and that the ". . .blood mercury concentrations were positively correlated to the number and surface area amalgam restorations and were significantly lower in the group without dental amalgams."(57)

Levels of mercury in the brain are directly proportional to the number of amalgam fillings in the mouth. While 78 percent of Americans have dental filling, 95 percent of people with disorders of the central nervous system such as multiple sclerosis, epilepsy, paralysis, and migraines also have silver dental fillings.[58]

But other sources of mercury abound. Prior to the 1990s household latex paints routinely contained mercury as an antifungal agent. Other possible sources include batteries, dyes, electronics, fluorescent lights, plastics, and many others.

Another major source of mercury contamination comes from incinerating garbage. Approximately 187 incinerators nationwide emit almost 70,000 pounds of mercury each year. Originally, incinerators were thought to be a solution to keep mercury out of landfills and hence away from ground water. But studies have shown that the scrubber and filter technology that cleans smoke of toxic gasses fails to work on mercury. One of the biggest sources of contamination of mercury in some parts of the country is from coal-burning energy plants. There are no plans to limit mercury from these plants. Gary Glass, an EPA mercury researcher in Duluth, Minnesota, said, "In the past, we would take our mercury wastes and bury them so they would contaminate the ground water in just one place. Now we've gotten smarter – we're blowing it into the air so it can go everywhere."[59]

Although safety standards for mercury exposure are based on clearly visible signs of neurological problems, researchers point out that this is outdated thinking that doesn't take into account possible behavioral, biochemical, carcinogenic or other subtle effects such as lowered intelligence and premature senility. It accumulates in fish in its most toxic form, methyl mercury. The EPA estimates that 1.16 million women of childbearing age "eat sufficient amounts of mercury-contaminated fish to pose a risk of harm to their future children."[60] Joan M. Spyker and colleagues at the Minnesota Medical School and Johns Hopkins School of Public Health also reports, ". . .attention should be directed to the fetus since the unborn organism is much more susceptible to the toxic effects of methyl mercury than the adult.

Methyl mercury easily crosses the placental barrier and is concentrated in fetal tissues; it has a greater affinity for the embryonic central nervous system than for that of the adult."[61] Methyl mercury arises (especially in the mouth) when it combines with a methyl molecule, which is nothing more than carbon and hydrogen. Mercury is very reactive chemically and this reaction is likely to occur. Methyl mercury is 100 times more toxic than plain, elemental mercury and "is especially toxic to the brain and nerve tissue, which may explain amalgam's relationship to multiple sclerosis, epilepsy, and emotional disturbances."[62]

Children with attention deficit disorder are shown to have altered dopamine levels in their brain (dopamine is a neurotransmitter in the central nervous system). One study at Duke University Medical School has shown that even very low levels of methyl mercury result in dopamine and norepinephrine (a hormone) brain neurotransmitter changes. The researchers conclude that mercury exposure could produce both short-term and long-term effects on behavior and the growth of the organism exposed.(63)

Workers chronically exposed to mercury are shown to consistently have behavioral weaknesses along with short-term memory problems and mood-state problems. In a study in Singapore, 94 dentists and 54 people who were not dentists were evaluated. The dentists who had elevated mercury concentrations in the air in their office were found to have poorer scores in mood, finger tapping (reaction skills), logical memory, and visual reproduction.(64)

In a landmark study at the Rocky Mountain Research Institute, it was shown that amalgam mercury (from fillings) affects the neurotransmitters' uptake of dopamine, serotonin, acetylcholine, and norepinephrine. This points to a bio-chemical basis for why people who have silver amalgam dental fillings experience significantly higher levels of depression, excessive anger, and anxiety than those without such fillings. Low levels of serotonin are implicated in a lack of control, which may manifest as irritability, loss of temper, and explosive rage. The leader of the study, Robert L. Siblerud, suggests that in using amalgam, dentistry unwittingly may be contributing to this country's growing epidemic of depression, anger, anxiety, violence, alcoholism, the need to smoke, and other impulse disorders.(65)

Food for Thought

Dentists, although allowed to put silver amalgams into people's mouths, must dispose of scrap amalgam as a toxic waste following strict governmental guidelines and alert their dental hygienists of its toxicity. It's illegal to put it in the garbage, sewer or down the drain, but it's okay to fill our cavities with it. If you want to get on your dentist's bad side, ask him what he has to do with his scrap mercury fillings. Then ask him why.

Just to show you how far-reaching the effects of amalgams can be, consider the case of one woman who had hers removed: "With time, everything improved. Her complexion cleared, the bloating decreased, and she felt connected to her body again. Her thyroid became normal, she no longer felt pain in menstruation, her heart didn't hurt, and the schizophrenia was gone."(66)

At low doses, mercury exposure can produce impairments in language ability, attention, and memory; at high doses it can cause mental retardation, vision problems, and problems walking.

Hal Huggins, D.D.S., is a world-renowned expert on mercury, its use in dentistry and its effects on biological systems. He discovered many of the problems with mercury while working as a dentist himself. Although the American Dental Association says that silver amalgam fillings are safe, Huggins vehemently disagrees: "Does mercury pose a health problem? I can give you an unequivocal 'yes'. . ." He goes on to say that it's been proven that as mercury comes out of fillings, it forms a toxic compound in the mouth, methyl mercury, which is mercury's most poisonous form. Enough of this compound can cause illnesses. Those illnesses have been reduced or eliminated by amalgam removal.

An article in the *Journal of Orthomolecular Medicine* echoes his conclusions:

> The findings presented here suggest a correlation between many health complaints and mercury amalgam fillings. Removal of amalgam fillings results in significant improvement of these symptoms. These same symptoms which are improved or eliminated in amalgam-removal patients are present but undiagnosed in the general population.[67]

Of particular note is a section on mercury and how it can affect the unborn fetus, which may result in birth defects:

> It's bad enough that methyl mercury destroys our adult tissues, but it can also cross the placental barrier and do chromosomal damage early in life. The mechanism is simple. Mercury is attracted to what are called active sites on genetic code molecules called deoxyribonucleic acid (DNA). Chemicals react with other chemicals in the body by coming together in a docking mechanism, similar to a spacecraft at a space station. When mercury is in the vicinity, it can twist a molecule a few thousandths of a degree. Now when the molecule tries to dock with another molecule, it can't because the docking points no longer match. . .This defect can also prevent molecular reactions from taking place. The mercury sits on a spot where other specific molecules are supposed to park. It is impossible for two things to occupy the same space at the same time, so interference in molecular reactions occurs, causing a birth defect.[68]

Mercury stops the normal cellular division in mitosis of the developing fetus, causing an abnormal cell. If this new, abnormal cell is capable of reproduction, the abnormality may show up as a birth defect. Chromosomes can also be altered by mercury, since mercury is good at cleaving off segments of chromosomes so they don't contain the appropriate number of genes. If the chromosomal damage is in the heart or brain, a spontaneous abortion is probable.[69]

Dr. Huggins says:

> Just what could be the source of this mercury? The first three months of pregnancy is the time a baby is most susceptible to mercury-produced birth defects. Mercury from the mother's fillings can cross the placental barrier and do its damage within

seconds. Enough animal research has been done over the years to indicate on exactly which day of pregnancy an exposure to mercury will produce a cleft palate in test cases. Why not share this information with pregnant women? While you should check with your obstetrician before you have any dental work done, I recommend having mercury fillings removed as soon as possible.(70)

Mercury in a filling not only gets into the bloodstream directly, but mercury vapor emitted from the filling can penetrate the mucousal lining of the mouth. A number of scientific studies indicate that from 20 mcg/m^3 to 150 mcg/m^3 (micro-grams per cubic meter of air) may be found in the mouth of a person with amalgam fillings. One hundred mcg of mercury vapor is 500 times greater than the level the EPA says is safe and 3,300 times greater than the level regarded as an acute exposure by the Agency for Toxic Substances and Disease Registry (the ATSDR). In 1991, the World Health Organization stated that there is no known "no-observable-effect level" (NOEL) for mercury vapor. That means that any and all levels of mercury vapor are considered harmful. The ATSDR lists mercury as one of the top 20 most hazardous substances known to man.(71) Yet, we fill our teeth and our children's teeth with it.

Huggins says it takes but a few atoms of mercury to create a birth defect and only one microgram to create other disturbances. One 16-year-old boy was chronically fatigued and could barely function. The removal of one small filling resulted in full teenage activity. One 11-year-old girl was having seizures every 15 minutes. Neurologists were baffled as to why. She had her amalgams removed, and within five days, her seizures stopped.

He also points out that mercury can deactivate zinc, which cannot only contribute to birth defects, but also affect the development of children. Zinc is important for intelligence, bone growth and healing and, along with magnesium, is vital in the healing process. Zinc is also a key element in the insulin molecule, and a deficiency of it may contribute to diabetes (in children as well as adults). Zinc levels can also be decreased by the consumption of caffeine and alcohol.

Other symptoms of suspected reactions to dental materials include unexplained irritability, constant or very frequent periods of depression, unexplained chronic fatigue, difficulty with short-term memory, sudden unexplained or unprovoked anger, jumpiness, jitteriness, and nervousness, constant death wish or suicidal intent, frequent insomnia, and other behavioral and physiological problems.(72)

Food for Thought

On November 15, 2000, the judge of the Superior Court of California in San Francisco signed a consent decree that states there's a link between birth defects and silver-mercury dental fillings. A new law says this will have to be disclosed to California dental patients. This is a 180-degree turn around from the American Dental Association's policy – still current – that silver mercury amalgams are safe and that any dentist who suggests otherwise to his patients can have his license revoked. In California, dentists with more than 10 employees must post this warning starting February 15, 2001:

WARNING:
Amalgam Fillings Contain a Chemical Element Known to the State of California to Cause Birth Defects or Other Reproductive Harm

Interestingly, the California Dental Association refused to allow the word "mercury" to be used in this warning sign or while informing their patients of the risks.(73) Let's hope this awareness will spread across the country and new laws will be enacted in each state requiring similar warnings. Considering there are about 250,000 mercury fillings put into our mouths per day (down from one million per day in the 1970s due to the controversy over mercury toxicity), it's important not just for our own health, but the health of future generations. We need to promote awareness of this problem and how to avoid it. Sweden no longer allows mercury amalgams, and Germany has stated that no mercury should be placed in pregnant women or even in women who could become pregnant. It's a shame to think that a baby may be born deformed simply because some company wants to maintain its profit margin. I have had my fair share of work on my teeth, and I can tell you without hesitation that what goes on in your mouth has a big impact on your total health. My suggestion is to not have amalgams put into your teeth or the teeth of your child. There are many new materials that can be used instead that are just as effective and a lot less toxic. Find a dentist who understands the hazards of amalgams – these informed professionals are growing in number every day and it should not take you long to find one. If your child has amalgams already, have them removed by a dentist who is experienced and knows how to do it correctly. Some insurance companies will pay for this if you can justify it. Remember, mercury is an accumulative poison, and is not easily excreted from the body. Every bit of exposure to it builds up in your child's tissues and will have long-term effects.

Women are oftentimes encouraged to have their cavities filled (usually with mercury fillings) when they are pregnant. This is so they will be less likely to have the discomfort of an abscessed tooth during the final weeks just prior to delivery. This is tantamount to encouraging women to expose their fetus to mercury, which as we now know can cause birth defects. See the Resource Guide on finding an informed dentist.

Mercury is also used in the preservative *thimerosal* in many vaccines. Huggins comments: "Thimerosal is the preservative in immunization shots, so anytime you get an immunization shot you are undergoing the same procedure that in the University Lab that we used to give animals auto-immune disease – give a little tiny injection of mercury. When you get an immunization shot you are getting a little tiny dose of mercury there."(74) (Thimerosal is covered in more detail in the chapter on vaccines.)

Aluminum

High levels of aluminum affect the central nervous system, and are believed to play a role in Alzheimer's disease in the elderly and hyperactivity in children. Aluminum can be ingested from food and water contaminated when cooked in aluminum pans or stored in aluminum foil. Most soft drinks come in aluminum cans and aluminum can be in these beverages. It's also found in coffee, bleached flour (all white flour products and pastas, but not the whole grain kinds), and drinking water. Municipal drinking water plants typically use a chemical called Alum, which contains aluminum, which ends up in the tap water. If someone has a deficiency of magnesium and calcium, the toxic effects of aluminum are increased, so it's necessary to have a diet with sufficient amounts of these two nutrients.(75)

Cadmium

Cadmium is the most toxic heavy metal on the planet (with mercury being the second) and is a highly toxic neurotoxin. It concentrates in the kidneys, liver, and blood and is harmful from the time of conception onward. The half-life of cadmium in the body is from 17 to 30 years, so it's very difficult to remove it from tissues. Once in, it interferes with the absorption of zinc, which is a vital nutrient necessary for many biochemical reactions in the body. Conversely, adequate levels of zinc in the diet may protect against the adverse effects of cadmium.

Zinc is involved in more than 60 enzymes in the body including those regulating digestion, protein synthesis, vision, the immune system, and prostate health. It's been shown to prevent some birth defects and acts to calm the nervous system (zinc is sometimes called a *sedative* mineral that stabilizes emotions). Our soils are depleted of zinc so getting enough zinc in the diet is sometimes difficult, especially if one is a vegetarian. Zinc is found mainly in animal products, so someone on a vegetarian diet may lead to a zinc deficiency. Also, zinc will compete with copper, so if zinc is inadequate, copper toxicity may occur.(76)

Zinc and copper smelters and refiners release more than two million pounds of cadmium into our air every year. Cigarette smoke is a major source of cadmium, coffee is the second largest source, and refined white flour products also contain high amounts. A study of over 150 children showed that those with a high intake of refined carbohydrates (white flour) had the highest levels of cadmium in their tissues. Since most of the junk foods like pretzels, tortilla chips, pizza, etc. contains mostly white flour, it's no surprise that children can accumulate higher than normal levels of cadmium, which may contribute to behavioral and learning problems. If the pregnant mother consumes large quantities of these type foods, some of the cadmium may be passed on to the fetus.(77) Whatever the source of cadmium, studies show that many children with learning disabilities have significantly higher levels of cadmium and lower zinc levels than normal children.

Copper

Like cadmium, excessive copper in the body displaces zinc and contributes to emotional sensitivity, mood swings, and erratic behavior. Other signs of copper toxicity include fatigue, depression, headaches, premenstrual tension, and skin problems. Again, since toxic metals can pass through the placenta, copper toxicity can be passed from mother to child. Junk foods, soda pop, and other non-nutritious foods can lead to copper toxicity.(78) Vegetarian diets are typically high in copper (whereas meats contain more zinc and less copper), so vegetarian diets can also lead to copper toxicity. As the prevalence of vegetarian diets has increased, so have the incidences of copper imbalances.(79)

It's important to realize that toxic metals compete with the beneficial minerals in many biological reactions. Lead will replace calcium, and cadmium can replace zinc. Avoidance of toxic metals and sufficient intake of the good minerals helps to keep these biological reactions functioning normally.

Diet

Poor diet undoubtedly contributes to ADHD, and it's been reported that malnutrition can trigger ADHD.(80) Simply put, if a child does not eat well or has certain food allergies, chances of behavioral and learning problems are increased not to mention compromised overall health.

Certain deficiencies should be watched for, especially zinc deficiencies and essential fatty acid deficiencies. Both have been shown to occur frequently in children with ADHD. Donald Rudin, Ph.D., co-author of *The Omega-3 Phenomenon,* believes that deficiencies of omega-3 oils (an essential fatty acid) are partly responsible for the increase in emotional and behavioral disorders and wide-spread illnesses.(81)

Foods at a typical supermarket may look good, but modern chemical fertilizers supply only three basic nutrients (N, P, K – nitrogen, phosphorus, potassium), and the soils our crops are grown on are no longer rich in all the minerals needed to produce healthy, nutritious plants. Instead what we get are exhausted crops not healthy enough to survive natural growing conditions making the heavy use of pesticides and herbicides necessary to grow them. In addition, the chemicals used on crops oftentimes kill the important soil microorganisms that help the plant roots absorb the minerals.

It's not just the plants that have been affected by depleted soils and modern agricultural methods. The animals we eat are now raised in lots and pens and not allowed to roam freely. Their feed is contaminated with metals, hormones and antibiotics, dyes, and additives. Plus, their feed comes from the same fields we grow food for people and has the same depletion of minerals. So it's important you and your children eat as much organically raised food as possible and as much meat from free-roaming, naturally raised animals.

Even though you hear a lot of talk about how bad fat is in the diet, the fact is that we need a fairly good amount of good fats to be healthy. These good fats include the essential fatty acids (EFAs), which are building blocks in the membranes of every cell.

If you're worried about gaining weight by eating fat, you don't need to be if you're eating the right kind of fat. Mary Van Elswyk, Ph.D., a leading authority on fat, explains:

> Obesity results when the body is unable to process nutrients. You've got all this stored fat unable to convert to energy, and you're not able to make proper use of it. The cells are literally starving. Then it becomes a vicious cycle: Your body is looking for more energy; you eat more to provide it, but cells don't have access to it and your body holds onto it. If you improve the nutritional status throughout the body with the correct vitamins, minerals and essential fatty acids, cells will function better and be able to access the fat.[82]

So eating the right kinds of fat and avoiding the bad kinds can actually help you lose weight because your body will function better. Although the body needs about twenty different fatty acids to be healthy, it can make all of them except two – omega-3 (linolenic acid) and omega-6 (linoleic acid), which must be obtained from the diet.

Unfortunately, modern food processing destroys the essential fatty acid content of many foods. Even the fish, chicken, and meat produced have lower levels of EFAs because the feed for these animals is not as nutritious as the food the animal would eat in the wild or as a free-range animal. Further, many of the items in our diet such as drugs, sugar, caffeine, and refined carbohydrates tend to block EFA absorption and metabolism. A zinc deficiency that may result from metal toxicity also adversely affects the functioning of EFAs.[83]

Some research has shown that children with ADHD oftentimes cannot absorb or metabolize EFAs normally, resulting in an EFA deficiency. The requirements for EFAs are thus higher in these children. Hyperactive male children outnumber female children by about three to one. These boys need two to three times more EFAs than the girls, reportedly because they have more difficulty converting EFAs to prostaglandins. (Prostaglandins are tissue-like hormones that control body functioning at the cellular level). Asthma, eczema, and other skin problems are also more prevalent in hyperactive children because of prostaglandin insufficiency. Children with EFA deficiencies usually have abnormally high thirst. Since wheat and pasteurized, commercial milk can block the biochemical conversion of EFAs in the body, these products should be avoided by all children, and especially those with signs of ADHD. (Raw milk is acceptable to feed to children.)

Other things that interfere with EFAs and their metabolism are diets high in hydrogenated oils and food colorings (especially yellow dye), low zinc in the diet, low vitamin E, C, B$_3$ (niacin), and B$_6$ (pyridoxine).[84]

Children especially need a diet high in fat. Their nervous system is developing and fat supplies a fair amount of energy production and slows the metabolic rate. Calcium and some vitamins need fat in order to be absorbed, and growth requires the energy of concentrated calories, like those found in fat. The sheathing around nerve fibers is called the *myelin sheath* and is nearly 100 percent fat. It's the insulator and protective cover of the nerve. If we don't have enough of the proper raw fats in our diets, these myelin sheaths will be inadequate and we'll always feel on edge. Children with ADHD oftentimes have faster than normal metabolic and oxidation rates. A diet high in carbohydrates – pasta, chips, pretzels, bread, cereal, and so on – will actually raise the metabolic rate, and fat will lower it, so replacing some of these items with a good natural fat will help the child slow down.[85]

Of course, children (and adults) need the right kind of fat (natural, unheated and uncooked as much as possible), not the fat found in fast food and chips. They also need a consistent supply of EFAs. EFAs can be found in fresh foods such as cold-water fish (salmon, sardines, cod, trout, mackerel), leafy green vegetables, nuts and seeds, flax seed oil, borage oil, evening primrose oil, avocados, and rice.[86]

Fats to avoid are those that are hydrogenated as found in margarines and shortenings – used extensively in fast foods. Hydrogenation uses chemicals and high heat, which remove most of the vitamins and minerals from the fat and changes the fat into a form that does not spoil as easily. During hydrogenation, polyunsaturated oils (*cis*-fatty acids, which are healthy) are changed into oils called *trans*-fatty acids, which are very detrimental. They alter the permeability of the cell membrane, interfere with certain enzymes and disrupt the vital functions of the EFAs in the body. Avoid products that are hydrogenated (margarine) and also partially hydrogenated oils, which have a high amount of *trans*-fatty acids. The hydrogenation process changes the oil and strips it of most or all of its beneficial EFAs. The body can't metabolize the *trans*-fatty acids because they're unnatural and they have been shown to decrease the good cholesterol (HDL) and impede liver function.

Two other fatty acids that are necessary for proper nervous system and over-all health are EPA (eicosapentaenoic acid) and DHA (docosahexaenoic acid). They are polyunsaturated fatty acids necessary for proper brain and eye development during pregnancy and proper functioning of the immune, respiratory, circulatory, and reproductive systems.[87] DHA is especially critical in brain development, so it's important for pregnant women and infants to get enough. DHA has been shown to help women carry babies to term.(88)

Although they are produced in the body from omega-3 fatty acids, it takes a long time, and children with EFA deficiencies may also develop deficiencies in DHA and EPA. A good source of EPA and DHA are fish oils – in fish tissues or cod liver oil. There is not a good vegetarian source of these two fatty acids. The best fish for these are cold-water fish such as salmon, sardines, cod, trout, and mackerel. These fish should be from the ocean or lake, not from fish farms, since farm-raised fish have less omega-3 fatty acid content.

One of the best sources of omega-3 fatty acids is krill oil. Krill is a small shrimp-like crustacean considered a delicacy and source of protein in Japan. It's abundant in EPA and DHA and has vitamins A and E. The best krill oil to get is from Antarctica and processed using the *Neptune* processing method of low heat without oxygen and is called NKOtm (Neptune Krill Oil). The phospholipids in krill oil seem to be absorbed better into the brain and work better for ADHD than conventional fish oils. Krill oil has also been shown to benefit brain, cardiovascular and vision development, and may even help joint function and the symptoms associated with PMS.

EPA and DHA are not essential (essential meaning the body must obtain them from outside sources and cannot manufacture it by itself), but are oftentimes difficult for the body to manufacture. Interestingly, people whose ancestors consumed large amounts of meat as a staple in their diets frequently cannot make DHA, EPA, or arachidonic acid (AA), and gamma-linolenic acid (GLA). So these need to be obtained from the diet. *Trans*-fatty acids, found in commercial vegetable oils and abundant in fast-food products, can interfere with the body's ability to manufacture these fatty acids as well, so obtaining them in the diet is advisable. Consuming egg yolks, liver and other organ meats, fish oils, and organically raised chickens will supply EPA and DHA. GLA can be found in borage oil and evening primrose oils and AA is found in butter and organ meats.(89)

Cod liver oil is good, but not for infants. Fish and krill oils also contain EPA, which is fine for adults, but in infants it counteracts other EFAs needed for growth. The consumption of DHA alone is best for infants.

Although some researchers might say there is not a good plant source of DHA, there is one product I have found on the market that has been shown to elevate blood levels of DHA in both infants and mothers during pregnancy and lactation. It's called *Neuromins Pro*, manufactured by MMS Pro (www.mmspro.net). This product is highly purified and is believed be less contaminated (especially in mercury) than fish oil DHA. Neuromins does not contain significant amounts of EPA.

To understand the importance of fat in the diet, when you have too many *trans*-fatty acids and too few essential fatty acids, and you have a recipe for depression. *Trans*- or hydrogenated, manmade fats were synthesized originally to extend shelf life of commercial products. The production of *trans*-fatty acids for human consumption is one of the most devastating nutritional mistakes ever made. In the effort to make foods last longer in the supermarket, all traces of essential fatty acids (such as omega-3s) are obliterated from processed foods, and *trans*-fats or partially hydrogenated oils take their place. The absence of omega-3 essential fatty acids in Western diets has contributed to an alarming increase in a number of diseases that appeared only infrequently 100 years ago. A lack of the essential fatty acids and cofactors, such as minerals and vitamins to handle fat, combined with the consumption of *trans*-fats, is more often the causal factor in obesity and cardiovascular disease than is eating cholesterol-rich foods. After all, the body needs some cholesterol – it's needed to produce crucial hormones that strongly influence mood such as pregnenolone, testosterone, progesterone, estradiol, estrone, and cortisole.(90) Too little cholesterol and you're subject to depression too.

Sugar interferes with enzymes that synthesize fatty acids, and aspirin inhibits the enzyme necessary to assimilate omega-3 fatty acids and may aggravate asthma or allergic disorders. Repeated and prolonged use of aspirin and other non-steroid anti-inflammatory drugs is not recommended.(91,92)

Food Allergies

Allergies to certain foods are another problem, not just for the overall health of children but in the development of ADHD. If a child is being bothered with allergy symptoms, he or she may appear inattentive or have other behavioral problems. It's important to identify and eliminate the offending substance to settle the child down into normal behavior.

Richard E., Layton, M.D., of the Allergy Connection says, "Children who suffer from chronic illnesses or who exhibit certain behavioral difficulties may actually be experiencing allergies. A surprising number of childhood medical conditions can be traced to food allergies. When an allergy is identified as the culprit behind a child's medical or behavioral problems, it can be controlled and even eliminated through several safe and effective treatments resulting in a happier, healthier life."(93)

Symptoms of allergies are not just a runny nose or sneezing. They can include anxiety, depression, hyperactivity, insomnia, irritability, mental confusion, personality changes, joint pain, muscle aches, acne, eczema, fatigue, digestive disturbances, ear infections, hyperglycemia, migraines, and even seizures.

A chemical produced by the body, and also found in many foods, that causes allergic reactions is histamine. It causes rashes, itchiness, and increased mucus production. Most cold, flu, and asthma medications try to block the release of histamines by the white blood cells, thereby stopping the symptoms. This does nothing to eliminate the cause of the problem, however, which, along with a general toxicity of the body, may include eating foods high in naturally occurring histamine. These include tuna, wine, preserves, sausage, sauerkraut, spinach, and tomatoes. Other foods that cause our white blood cells to release excessive histamine include milk, eggs, shellfish, strawberries, bananas, chocolate, papayas, pineapples, some nuts, and alcohol.(94)

Cheese contains high amounts of tyrosine (an amino acid), and children with ADHD have been found to have high levels of this in their blood. Other products that contain tyrosine in high amounts, and to be avoided by children with ADHD, are: chocolate; cream; coffee; citrus fruits; cheese; and yeast extracts.(95) Other foods that frequently cause allergic reactions are sugar, chocolate, peanuts, apples, carrots, tomatoes, eggs, soy, grapes, corn, oranges, red and yellow dye, and preservatives.

One topic not generally discussed when it comes to allergies is that our brain can be allergic to many things, just like our bodies. In fact, doctors have found that 90 percent of patients admitted to mental hospitals had allergies that affected the brain. When the brain is allergic, swelling and inflammation result, so it's no wonder people suffering from them may have a wide variety of mental disorders. Just about any food, but especially wheat and dairy products, can trigger a brain allergy reaction. Food additives can also be a problem.

The most common symptoms of a brain allergy in children are irritability, mood swings, sleeplessness, depression, anxiety, hyperactivity, learning disorders, lack of concentration, tantrums, fatigue, and muscle weakness. If a child is affected with a brain allergy for an extended period, his or her handwriting may deteriorate and behavior change. Certain smells can also trigger a brain allergy response. Some toxins that can do this are formaldehyde, acetone, methyl ketone, and ethyl ketone. (Check your perfume and nail polish, ladies.) A parent or teacher may jump to the conclusion there's a problem and put the child on *Ritalin* or other drug, when really it's some kind of allergic reaction. With the high amount of synthetic chemicals, additive, ingredients, and so on in our environment, an allergic reaction of some sort is almost unavoidable.

Two foods that cause many allergic reactions are *pasteurized* milk and wheat products. In fact, by taking a child suffering from allergies off pasteurized milk and wheat products, most allergic reactions usually cease.

Not only can wheat cause allergic reactions by itself, but you and your child may suffer allergic reactions because of the toxic residues in the wheat remaining from its processing. Wheat, when not grown organically, is subjected to the treatment of the wheat seed with mercury, hormone treatment to increase the size of the seed head, insecticides, fungicides, and hormone treatment to reduce the length of the stem. All these chemicals can cause allergic or toxic reactions in your child and presumably in a fetus. Oftentimes, just by using organically grown wheat products, you can ameliorate those reactions entirely.(96)

Pasteurized cow's milk is probably the food that causes the most allergic reactions in children. Although mother's milk is by far the perfect food for infants and raw cow's milk is a good second-best, pasteurized cow's milk is far from being so for children and adults. Dr. Julian Whitaker, M.D., writes in his newsletter:

> Here are three reasons kids and [pasteurized] milk doesn't mix. First, [pasteurized] milk is the leading cause of iron-deficiency anemia in infants, and in fact, the American Academy of Pediatrics now discourages giving children [pasteurized] milk before their first birthday. Second, it has been shown that [pasteurized] milk consumption in childhood contributors to the development of Type I diabetes. Certain proteins in [pasteurized] milk resemble molecules on the beta cells of the pancreas that secrete insulin. In some cases, the immune system makes antibodies to the [pasteurized] milk protein that mistakenly attacks and destroys the beta cells. . .Third, [pasteurized] milk allergies are very common in children and cause sinus problems, diarrhea, constipation, and fatigue. They are a leading cause of the chronic ear infections that plague up to 40 percent of all children under the age of six. [Pasteurized] Milk allergies are also linked to behavior problems in children and to the disturbing rise of childhood asthma (milk allergies are equally common in adults and produce similar symptoms). Even so august an authority on children as the late Dr. Benjamin Spock changed his recommendations in his later years and discouraged giving children [pasteurized] milk. . .To start with, knock off drinking [pasteurized] milk altogether. Fluid [pasteurized] milk is likely to be the most highly concentrated, easily absorbed source of growth hormones…be sure to avoid products from hormone-treated cows. A growing number of dairies offer organic or hormone-free diary products.(97)

Another problem with pasteurized milk is what's called lactose intolerance. Lactose is the sugar found in milk. At about the age of two to three years, children lose most of the enzyme called lactase, which is necessary for digesting the lactose. Most adults have about 5 percent to 10 percent of the lactase they had as in infant. If lactase is missing, the sugar does not get digested, and ends up accumulating in the intestine. This is perfect culture media for bacteria to grow on. This may cause bloating, intestinal pain, gas, and diarrhea. (Raw milk, on the other hand, contains its own lactase, which digests the lactose when you drink the milk. So this is not an issue when you drink raw milk.)

When milk is pasteurized, the lactose sugar – which is naturally absorbed slowly by the body – is transformed into beta-lactose – which is absorbed very quickly by the body. That leads to a rush of sugar into the bloodstream and a powerful insulin secretion from the pancreas. This could end up causing obesity and adult-onset, insulin-resistant Type II diabetes.

Food for Thought

If pasteurized milk is so bad for you and your child, why do they promote it as being so healthy? The dairy industry has grown, thanks to good advertising and lobbying, to be a major player in the development of dietary recommendations from nutritionists and the government alike. Again, dear friend, the bottom line is money. It's a multibillion-dollar industry.

It all started back in 1935 when a government official of a small dairy in Minnesota named George Pushing discovered he could use pasteurization to prolong the shelf life of milk. (I discuss germs in depth in the chapter on vaccines.) He said, "We can buy the milk that dairy farmers cannot sell by themselves, and by applying heat at 155 degrees Fahrenheit, even reject milk will keep for two weeks." He later admitted that pasteurization was only an economic ploy to increase profits and get control of the dairy industry since pasteurization requires expensive equipment that many small dairies cannot afford. Mr. Pushing later contracted rheumatoid arthritis, a disease that raw milk can prevent, by drinking his pasteurized milk.[98] Consider what pasteurization (cooking milk at a minimum of 155 degrees Fahrenheit for at least 15 seconds), does to milk:

Pasteurization alters and destroys the beneficial properties of proteins, vitamins, minerals, enzymes, essential fatty acids, and natural antigens. When these substances are altered through heat in this way, they become toxins the body must isolate and eliminate. The body does this by coating these toxins in mucus to transport and eliminate them.

Minerals often become glass-like and sharp, frequently lacerating liver tissue, blood, and nerve cells. If someone cannot produce enough mucus to eliminate them, they often become the cause of a myriad of allergies. Pasteurized fats become lipid oxides that are known carcinogens, and pasteurized proteins create large amounts of uric acid that can lead to muscular and glandular problems. The heat involved in pasteurization not only creates these toxic substances, but destroys almost all the nutritional value too. It is so lacking in nutrition that if calves are fed pasteurized milk, they die within sixty days. We'll see in the Ancestry Factor chapter the devastating effects of cooked milk on several generations of cats.

Pasteurization creates degenerative matter in milk on which microorganisms thrive. Many of the reports of the hazards of raw milk have really occurred because of faulty pasteurization, leading to the formation of these microbes. Nutritionist Aajonus Vonderplanitz says, "The microbes that science and medicine term 'pathogenic' are simply the symptom that degenerative matter exists. As soon as the degenerative matter is consumed, the microbes go dormant. . ."[99]

Here's more proof that pasteurization doesn't even kill all the (supposedly) disease causing microorganisms it's supposed to every time.

The *Consumer Reports* reported that one out of six milk samples bought from retail stores had a count of 130,000 bacteria per *milliliter*. In fact, the acceptable standard for pasteurized milk is about 100,000 bacteria per *teaspoon*.(100)

On the other hand, raw milk simply sours, and this microbiological activity is not pathological, as proven by tests in Europe. Conversely, there have never been any scientific studies proving that bacteria in raw milk are dangerous to health. In fact, the souring produces lactic acid and makes milk more easily digestible, especially for people with less than optimum digestion such as infants, the elderly, and infirmed. There have been countless reports of people recovering from many different ailments by consuming raw milk.(101) Dr. Bieler, a practicing physician for more than 50 years, routinely prescribed raw milk to his patients. He never saw a case of undulant fever – which is supposedly caused by unpasteurized milk.(102)

When milk was right from the farm, pure and fresh as it had been for millions of years before 1935 when some dairyman wanted to make more money, it was a good wholesome and nutritious food. It didn't contain the hormones, pesticides, antibiotics, cancer-promoting substances, and even radioactive particles it does today. All these things are done to and added to milk for one purpose – to make more money. With all this toxic material in a glass of *natures perfect food*, is it any wonder children have runny noses, ear aches, sinus infections, headaches, sour stomachs, fevers, and so on? These are the reactions of their little bodies trying to get rid of all these poisons. Gabriel Cousens, M.D., says, "I am always amazed how many have their chronic colds, sore throats, and earaches cleared up when I discover they are allergic to dairy and they stop eating diary. Even without an allergy to dairy, the tendency to colds and flu is greatly decreased when diary is eliminated."(103)

Yes, milk does contain a lot of calcium. But if the milk is pasteurized, it's mostly unavailable to the human body because it's trapped within the casein molecule, and pasteurized milk's reaction in the body is acidic. That means in order for the body to maintain the normal blood pH of 7.4, calcium, which neutralizes acid, must be mobilized from its reserves (bones and muscles) to neutralize the acidic effects of pasteurized milk. To make matters worse, modern dairy cows are now fed feed with a higher protein content than old-time grass-fed cows. This increased protein makes the milk have more protein, which makes it more acidic. This in turn makes your body more acidic when you drink it, which encourages more bone loss due to the necessity of the body to rob calcium from its bones to neutralize the acid. Although pasteurization doesn't kill all the microorganisms, it does kill some (and the healthy ones at that). Enough to make it last longer on the shelf: longer shelf life means more money.

Is it any wonder the "authorities" make you fear drinking raw milk and have made it a crime to sell it? The more control someone has over a substance, the more money will be made. But raw milk was sold in California for years, and although the health officials kept an eagle eye for problems, there weren't any. They did make raw milk illegal in California in 1990, but now is now legal again. Whereas there had been a dozen illness reports from pasteurized milk in the 1980s and 1990s (*Salmonella, Listeria*), there were none involving raw milk. On the other hand, raw milk from healthy cows is great for growing children. It's abundant in calcium, has the right kinds of fats their brain and nervous system need to develop normally, is a complete protein with minerals, vitamins C, A, E, D, B vitamins, and enzymes. All these vital nutrients are easily absorbed and assimilated by the body, which allows children to not only avoid the problems with pasteurized milk, but to grow into strong, healthy, and well balanced adults.

What's the bottom line? Stop drinking pasteurized milk and above all, don't feed it to your child. It could be causing a lot of the allergies and other problems he or she is experiencing. But raw milk and raw milk products will help bring anyone to health. Some places that will help you find raw milk are www.realmilk.com, www.rawmilk.org. But please, remember, you are buying the milk for your pets, not yourself. We all know that raw milk might kill us and is against the law because the authorities care only about what is best for us, not what's best for their wallets and corporate friends.

An Overlooked Cause of Many Allergies

There are small proteins in our bodies and in the raw food we eat called enzymes. These make biochemical reactions possible and others to proceed at a much faster rate (they are catalysts). They were first identified in the 1930's, and today over 5,000 have been discovered. If you don't have the proper enzymes or enough of them, things in your body can get sluggish. Nutrients cannot be processed (poor digestion) or transported efficiently (poor assimilation), and waste material cannot be eliminated easily (mucous buildup). This paves the way for congestion, allergies, and even more serious degenerative diseases.

In fact, Maile Pouls, Ph.D., a recognized expert in enzyme therapy, says that between 70 percent and 90 percent of allergies may be caused by the lack of enzymes.[104] The solution is very simple: eat more raw food. Each raw food has the proper enzymes included for it to be properly digested. But when food is heated as in cooking, these precious enzymes are destroyed and digestion becomes problematic.

It's interesting that all enzymes in food are deactivated at a wet-heat temperature of 118 degrees Fahrenheit. That's exactly the temperature you'll feel pain at if you stick your finger in hot water. Anything below this temperature, nature is telling you is fine to eat. Above this temperature, is harmful. (Enzymes are destroyed at a dry-heat temperature of about 150 degrees Fahrenheit.) [105]

Another way to address the lack of enzymes is to add some to your diet. They help in digestion and assimilation and thus, overall health. Dr. Pouls has seen many children with allergies, learning and behavioral disabilities, and other problems improve when they received the right enzymes. Adding enzymes to your child's diet, especially if their diet is less than optimal, can be an easy and relatively inexpensive way to help them.

There are several ways to test for allergies – the skin prick test, blood tests, and a simple one you can do at home called the *Elimination Diet*. This is where you eliminate from the diet foods that are likely to cause allergic reactions for four to seven days. These foods are milk, soybeans, eggs, wheat, peanuts, nuts, shellfish, corn, and any other your doctor may think a possible cause. More than 80 percent of people who have food allergies get relief when these foods are omitted from the diet. If the symptoms do not go away, more foods are eliminated.

Then, slowly, one food at a time is added back to the diet and you observe whether allergic reactions return. But beware: Common food allergens are hidden ingredients in hundreds of packaged or processed foods, and even as filler in some vitamins.

Another way to test if you have an allergy to a certain food is to avoid eating it for at least four days. Then eat a small amount of it on an empty stomach but before you do, test your pulse rate. Check your pulse again immediately after eating the food. If you pulse rises more than a few beats per minute, or if you have any other adverse reaction, you're probably allergic to this food. You can monitor those same reactions in your child – taking care, of course, to seek immediate medical help in the case of severe adverse reaction such as intense wheezing or extreme hives.

Food for Thought

There are certain foods that have a compound in them called *salicylates*. These are aspirin-like substances that have been shown to contribute to hyperactivity and asthma in children. These foods are tomatoes, almonds, apricots, peaches, and nectarines. Many children are also allergic to citrus fruits.

How significant can making dietary changes be? Lendon Smith, M.D., a world-renowned pediatrician, says that 80 percent of children get better from behavioral disorders just by changing their diet and taking vitamins. He believes that food sensitivity is a major factor for many children who have ADHD. William Crook, M.D., studied 182 hyperactive children. He found that most of the children's hyperactivity was definitely related to specific foods. Ninety-four percent of all hyperactive children he has seen are allergic or sensitive to some foods and food colorings. The worst food was sugar, followed by food additives.

Other foods such as milk, corn, wheat, and eggs also created problems in many kids.(106)

Dr. Alan Cott, a psychiatrist, reported in his 1977 book, *The Orthomolecular Approach to the Treatment of Children with Behavior Disorders and Learning Disabilities*, that nutritional deficiencies can have a profound effect on learning and behavior. Nutrient deficiencies can stress the body. For example, a vitamin B_{12} deficiency may cause severe psychiatric symptoms including mood disorders and paranoid behavior.

In a study performed at the California State University, children placed on vitamin and mineral supplements have been shown to exhibit significantly less violent and antisocial behavior, higher intelligence test scores, and higher academic achievements than children on placebos.(107)

However, nutritional imbalances can cause problems too. If there are excessive amounts of some B vitamins, other vitamins may not work properly. For example, mega doses of vitamin B_6 can induce folic acid deficiency. So a "shot-gun" approach of mega doses of vitamins or minerals without proper supervision can cause problems just as deficiencies can. Children who received at least 100 percent of the Recommended Daily Allowance (RDA) of nutrients did better on IQ tests than those receiving 200 percent or 50 percent of the RDA. So excesses, as well as deficiencies, of vitamins or minerals can cause problems.(108) If you do consider supplementing your or your child's diet with vitamins or minerals, it's important to proceed slowly with proper professional guidance. It's best to start with a low-dose multivitamin/mineral supplement (remember to check for fillers), but an individually tailored supplement program designed by a qualified health care professional is the ideal way to go.

Again, a diet of organically raised foods with no additives, colorings, or sugar will go far in helping you and your child remains calm and attentive. Since these foods naturally contain more vitamins and minerals than conventionally grown foods, the need for supplementation (especially if these foods are eaten raw) may be reduced or eliminated altogether. Be aware that vitamin and mineral deficiencies are more likely during growth spurts when nutrient needs are highest. If children are on drugs for ADHD, their appetite is usually suppressed due to the action of the drugs and they may not want to eat enough. Getting them off the drugs will help their normal appetite to return.

Hypoglycemia

Hypoglycemia is a deficiency of glucose, or blood sugar, in the blood. Medical research indicates that hypo, or low, blood sugar can play a significant roll in mental and emotional disorders including ADHD, antisocial behavior, criminal tendencies, drug addiction, and allergies. In one study, 76 percent of 265 children with ADHD were found to have abnormal glucose tolerance tests.(109)

The symptoms associated with impaired glucose metabolism includes the inability to concentrate, mood swings, anxiety, depression, and the tendency to be more emotional than normal. Fatigue, asthma, headaches, hyperactivity, nervousness, insomnia, irritability, restlessness, poor memory, and indecisiveness are also common with hypoglycemia.

Glucose is a kind of sugar the body uses as energy. It is not the same as sucrose, which is common cane sugar. There must be a steady supply of glucose in the bloodstream for the body to function normally. The brain is especially dependent on blood glucose and glucose is its sole energy source – so constant and steady supplies of it are essential to normal brain function.

The two most significant factors that contribute to hypoglycemia are diet and emotional stress. Certain foods affect the blood sugar in different ways. For example, simple carbohydrates like white flour and sugar get absorbed very quickly from the intestines into the bloodstream. This causes insulin to be produced so that the cells of the body can absorb the glucose. If too much sugar is consumed, too much insulin is produced, and a large amount of blood sugar is absorbed in a very short period of time. This quick uptake of blood glucose then leads to a sharp drop in blood sugar – resulting in too low a blood sugar, or hypoglycemia. When this happens, many of the symptoms of hypoglycemia can occur.

As someone senses the drop in blood sugar from this quick absorption due to increased insulin production, he or she would quite naturally reach for something sweet to replenish the sugar in the blood. These sharp increases and decreases in blood sugar affect the brain and nervous system and the endocrine system as well. Since the pancreas is being over stimulated to produce too much insulin, it is being overworked. Repeated events like this can eventually exhaust the pancreas causing insulin production to be permanently impaired – leading to diabetes. In the short term, the person is on a roller coaster of blood sugar peaks and valleys and experiences emotional and mental instability.

It's important to realize once again that the child thought to have ADHD may simply be suffering from a physiological problem brought on by environmental stressors – in this case, hypoglycemia. Any child experiencing emotional or learning problems should have their blood sugar checked. Simple adjustments in diet could eliminate the cause and preclude the need for any other type of intervention such as drugs.

The modern western diet is probably the best one in the history of the world to promote and cause hypoglycemia. Foods like white bread, sugar, soda pop, sugared cereals, and all other refined carbohydrates are absorbed too quickly into the bloodstream since they require little to no digestion. Even natural products like honey, dried fruit, fruit, and fruit juice can exacerbate the problem. What's the solution?

First off, eliminate or severely restrict all sugar. No more soda, no more sugar-filled snacks, no more sugared fruit drinks, or *Kool-Aid*. Although sugar in fruit is a good food, even too much of it can cause problems – so keep fruit consumption low to moderate and be sure to eat the whole fruit by itself along with no other foods (this improves digestion). You should also eliminate or restrict all kinds of refined carbohydrates such as white bread, pasta, pizza, crackers, and so forth. Replace these with their whole-grain counterpart.

Whole grains and vegetables provide slow-release energy: No more peaks and valleys and no more exhaustion of the pancreas. A steady blood glucose level will go far in helping maintain concentration, calmness, and emotional stability. Remember, grains like rice should be soaked before cooking to make them more digestible.

A diet with adequate amounts of protein is also necessary. Cold water fish, chicken, turkey, lamb, and beef – organically raised if possible – are good sources of protein. Other good sources are eggs, leafy green vegetables, sunflower seeds, pumpkin seeds, and almonds. Most dietitians now recommend a diet high in complex carbohydrates like pasta and rice, and little protein and fat. Is this healthy? Historical evidence does not support it. Healthy, primitive cultures ate large quantities of meat, fish, and fat along with vegetables, nuts, and seeds.

A person with a fast metabolism will require more protein and fat in the diet. This needs to be kept in mind for children since their metabolism is naturally faster than adults. They undoubtedly need more protein and fat in their diets. Small frequent meals are also advised for those with blood sugar problems. Five or six small meals are better than three large ones. Between meal-snacks when hungry are also advised, even when overweight is an issue. Just choose carefully. As long as you provide good, fresh, wholesome, and organically raised foods with no sugar or other additives, letting children eat all they want when they want is fine. Since they are getting nutritious foods, and not addictive foods, their body will operate correctly and natural hunger will arise when food is really needed.

Food for Thought

When I was a kid, I was a hot dog freak. Anytime our family went out to dinner, it's all I would eat and any time I could choose a food, it was hot dogs. I think my body was trying to tell me something. I needed the protein and the fat that was in the meat. Of course, I didn't need the nitrates, additives, and preservatives. But kids need high protein and fat in their diets. Fats will calm them down, and protein is necessary for growth. Of course it should be high-quality protein and fat from organic sources if possible.

Another thing that causes or exacerbates low blood sugar is stress. When stress is encountered, the adrenal glands are activated to mobilize the body's energy reserves of glycogen in the liver and muscles. This in turn causes an increase in blood sugar, which eventually peters out, creating a low blood sugar situation. High stress levels strip the adrenals of vitamin C and the B-vitamins, which will cause them to eventually become exhausted. Caffeine also over stimulates the adrenals leading to blood sugar problems.

Good foods to help deal with sugar cravings are bananas, walnuts, and fresh pineapple. A mineral supplement high in magnesium and trace minerals can also help with sugar cravings. After about a week off refined sugar, the cravings will go away. Getting your child off refined sugar and all the products it's in is one of the best things you can do, not just for your child's health, but your sanity as well.

Food for Thought

As you are discovering, it is my belief that abnormal behavior, be it attention deficits, hyperactivity or aggression is caused by something tangible – that's to say physical/chemical/biological. Although sociologic/psychological conditions may contribute to problems, these sociologic/psychological conditions had to have first arisen themselves out of some sort of biological aberration. Out of this aberration springs forth behaviors inconsistent with a healthy organism.

This is not to say that sociologic/psychological programs or strategies are not helpful or necessary – I believe they are. But they are more of a form of damage control and are not getting to the true cause of the problem – that being the degeneration of the human organism physically, chemically, and biologically. Our environment – what we are exposed to, what we eat, and how we exercise are the major determinants to health be it physically, mentally, or emotionally. If we nurture ourselves with the natural things that bring health, we will become more understanding, more loving, and more mentally and emotionally equipped to handle the stresses of life.

Single-Parent Households

One article suggests that the rise in ADHD, and other mental problems in children, are in part due to more single-parent households (up from 15 percent in 1979 to 22 percent in 1996).[110] Divorce is one cause of single-parent households, but also the fact that many women are having children out of wedlock and are forced to raise them largely by themselves. Even when the parents stay together, our fast-paced world, the need for both parents to work to make ends meet, and the resulting lack of attention paid to our children undoubtedly take their toll.

A study of more than 21,000 children between four and 15 years old showed that in 1979, doctors reported psychological problems in 6.8 percent of the children and in 1996, 18.7 percent.[111] Children are almost three times as likely to have an emotional or behavioral disorder today as they were 20 years ago. Emotional problems (other than behavioral problems like ADHD), which include depression and psychosomatic illnesses, went up from 0.2 percent in

1979 to 3.6 percent in 1996. The researchers concluded that living in poverty or in a family with only one-parent increases the likelihood of a child having psychological problems. Children growing up with only one parent were almost twice as likely to be diagnosed with a psychological disorder. However, Alan Hilfer, a child psychologist, feels that it's a complex problem and that there are other factors that contribute to children's problems such as the tremendous availability of drugs and weapons. "I see children at younger ages being pulled to the dark side," he said.(112)

Another study released by the National Institute of Mental Health says that up to 2.5 percent of children and 8.3 percent of adolescents in the U.S. suffer from depression.(113) Depression onset is occurring earlier in life today than in past decades, and depression in youth may predict more severe mental or physical illness in adult life. Depression in young people often occurs along with other mental disorders such as anxiety, disruptive behavior, substance abuse disorders, and even physical illnesses such as diabetes.

Depression is associated with an increased risk of suicidal behaviors. In 1997, suicide was the third leading cause of death in 10-to 24-year-olds. In adolescents who have major depressive disorders, as many as 7 percent may commit suicide when they are young adults. This risk is higher in adolescent boys than girls.(114)

In childhood, both boys and girls are at equal risk to develop depression disorders. During adolescence, however, girls are twice as likely as boys to develop depression.(115)

Another disorder that warrants mention is called Bipolar Disorder. It's rare in young children, but can appear in older children and adolescents. It involves unusual shifts in mood, energy, and functioning and may begin with either manic and/or depressive symptoms. Symptoms include severe changes in mood – either extremely irritable or overly silly and elated, inflated self-esteem, increased energy and sexual thoughts and feelings, disregard of risk, decreased need for sleep, increased talking, being easily distracted with attention moving constantly from one thing to another. Children who are severely depressed and exhibited ADHD-like symptoms with excessive temper outbursts and mood changes may have Bipolar Disorder. Traditional treatment is usually with drugs – mood-stabilizing medications. One thing to be aware of is if your child is taking drugs for ADHD and has Bipolar Disorder, the drugs may trigger or worsen manic symptoms – perhaps the very symptoms you were hoping to control.(116) I talk about other psychological problems in the chapter on depression.

Food for Thought

A sound body, a sound mind. It's no coincidence that people with emotional problems also have some physical problem as well. You know that you're more likely to snap when you've had a tough day or not enough sleep or have a headache or whatever. The easiest and surest way to improve one's mental disposition and decrease the likelihood of depression or behavioral problems is to be physically healthy and fit. Our young people are becoming emotional casualties. They are also out of shape and overweight. It's vitally important that we get them outside, away from the TV and computer games, and get them physically active. When one exercises, the body produces natural painkillers – substances called endorphins. They are very close chemically to drugs such as morphine and opiates. That's why you feel better after a good workout. The bloodstream is flooded with these endorphins, and you can actually get kind of high – called *runner's high*. People can get addicted to this natural high and literally *have* to get out and run or work out. It's the body's natural mechanism to ensure you want to exercise. You simply feel better. Now, our lazy and pampered youngsters get high by using drugs, when really that feeling was meant to ensure that one go out and exercise. Exercise increases oxygenation to the brain, allowing it to function better and be more relaxed. It results in clearer thinking, less stress, less anxiety, better sleep, better digestion, and a better disposition.

Touching and Moving

Recent studies show that the absence of touching, cuddling, and movement for a baby can lead to learning and behavior disorders. In a study of 49 cultures, there was shown to be a direct correlation between the lack of physical affection, especially touching and movement during infancy and childhood, and the amount of adult crimes. The National Institute of Child Health says that early deprivation of touching, contact, and movement results in abnormal social and emotional behaviors later in life. These abnormalities include hyperactivity and depression.(117)

The role of movements such as rocking in a cradle, touching things, crawling, walking upright, running, swinging arms, skipping, and other activities help the brain to develop coordination and balance. Since learning is a sensory process that must be reinforced by proper motor functioning of the brain, it's important for babies and children to learn how to move. Movement stimulates the brain cells and helps regulate other brain functions that control physical, mental, psychological, and social development. Not enough movement can cause poor sensory integration, which may cause difficulties in learning to read, write, and do arithmetic. Touching and movement in infancy and childhood is important to help the brain develop normally.

If a child did not get enough touching and movement, it is not too late to help him or her develop the areas of the brain that were adversely affected. One therapy is called sensory integration therapy, which involves increased stimulation in six sensory and motor areas: visual, auditory, touching, mobility, language, and manual skills. Other therapies include writing, and *Brain Gym,* discussed a bit later.

Food for Thought

As our society becomes more technological, many old-fashioned traditions fall by the wayside. It used to be that babies were kept in cradles and were rocked back and forth throughout the day. Now, children are kept in bassinets, which are stationary and immobile cribs. The fetus gets rocked and moved continually while in the womb and needs to be moved and touched as an infant. But now mothers don't hold their babies as much and carry them around in plastic carriers with no direct physical contact. Touching is as much a nutrient as food. Those who do not get enough develop behavioral and physical deficiencies.

I remember in my college psychology textbook there was a discussion on the importance of touch in early life. There were pictures showing three cages with a baby monkey in each. The first cage was totally empty. The baby monkey died within a day or so. The second cage had a figure of a mother monkey made out of wire. The baby monkey in this cage tried to cuddle, even on this cold wire. It died within a few days. The last cage had the same kind of wire figure covered with soft cloth. The baby monkey in this cage cuddled on this surrogate mother, lived the longest, and survived the experiment. It's important to touch and cuddle your baby and child. Do it as much as possible and the chances your child will develop normally mentally, physically, emotionally, and socially are greatly increased.

A more recent study showed that newborn rats who received repeated touching from their mothers received a number of benefits that helped negate stress later in life. These Harvard researchers also examined orphans who had been left alone in their cribs as babies. It turns out that the lack of touching and caressing sets up a hormonal response that continues well past infancy. Many of these orphans developed into distant, highly-stressed, lonely children who had difficulty coping with normal human interaction and touch.(118)

Diagnosis of ADHD

The diagnosis of ADHD is not a simple task. As you can see from the list of possible symptoms listed earlier, the determination of ADHD is purely a subjective task. What one person sees as a problem significant enough to classify it as ADHD, another person may not.(119)

There is no positive medical or scientific test such as a blood test or a brain scan that can be used to help determine if someone has the problem. The diagnosis today, as a decade ago, relies totally on behavioral criteria, which are evaluated subjectively. According to the *Diagnostic and Statistical Manual (DSM-IV),* which establishes the official criteria for testing ADHD, there are 14 activities (such as fidgeting, blurting out answers, interrupting, etc.) that must be evaluated before a diagnosis can be made. Each one depends on the evaluators' perspective, which may not be the same as someone else's. That makes diagnosis particularly difficult and open to debate in each case. And how many evaluators inquire about food sensitivity or heavy metal exposure?

Lawrence H. Diller, M.D., author of *Running on Ritalin: A Physician Reflects on Children, Society, and Performance in a Pill* is a highly recognized expert on ADHD. He says, "What often strikes those encountering DSM criteria for the first time is how common these symptoms are among children generally." He adds that diagnosis of ADHD is "very much in the eye of the beholder."[120] In *Driven to Distraction* by Hallowell and Ratey, the authors said, "There is no clear line of demarcation between ADD and normal behavior."[121]

Mary Eberstadt, in her article "Why *Ritalin* Rules," recounts performing a nonscientific test on adults using a questionnaire commonly used to help diagnose ADHD. The questionnaire was given to 20 people, all of whom were successful, mostly professional adults. She found that "Apart from the exceedingly anomalous two scores. . . All the rest of the subjects reported answering 'yes' to at least a quarter of the questions – surely enough to trigger the possibility of an ADD diagnosis. . ."[122]

Diane McGuinness goes a step further. "The past 25 years has led to a phenomenon almost unique in history. Methodologically rigorous research. . . indicates that ADD and Hyperactivity as 'syndromes' simply do not exist. We have invented a disease, given it medical sanction, and now must disown it. The major question is how we go about destroying the monster we have created. It is not easy to do this and still save face. . ."[123] Richard E. Vatz says, "Attention-deficit disorder is no more a disease than is 'excitability.' It is a psychiatric, pseudo-medical term."[124]

In 1998, the National Institutes of Health convened a conference on ADHD with the panel consisting of 13 doctors and educators. Part of the reason for the conference was to help nail down the criteria and evaluations for diagnosing ADHD. As one of the panelists put it, "The diagnosis is a mess."[125]

Considering what's at stake here, that being the health and future of our children, it's simply amazing that the medical community and the public at large are so quick to label a child as having an attention deficit disorder. Especially considering that the diagnosis is "in the eye of the beholder."

The question has arisen whether ADHD is a result of some biological, physical abnormality. Some research has suggested that this is not the case. G.S. Golden, an expert on brain function, says, "Attempts to define a biological basis for ADHD have been consistently unsuccessful. The neuroanatomy of the brain as demonstrated by neuroimaging studies, is normal. No neuropathologic substrate has been demonstrated."[126]

Keep in mind, however, that although there is evidence that strictly biological or anatomical conditions may not cause ADHD, biochemical imbalances may, so the overall health of the child (or adult) needs to be considered. A medical exam by a physician should be conducted when there is a question whether a child is affected. This should include hearing and vision tests to rule out other medical problems that may be causing symptoms similar to ADHD.

There has also been research that shows that a small number of people with ADHD may have a thyroid dysfunction.(127) Stephen E. Langer, M.D., points out that hypothyroidism can manifest itself in poor short-term memory and difficulty in concentrating. A study at Georgetown University showed that these two symptoms occurred in more than half of 109 cases of hypothyroidism.(128) Nathan Masor reports that in hypothyroidism thinking is slow and memory impaired, which often compounds emotional conditions such as listlessness, restlessness, irritability, and miscellaneous body pains. He says that oftentimes these symptoms go away with daily thyroid therapy indicating that in most cases, they were due to hypothyroidism.(129) Besides supplementation with thyroid hormone (which can only be done under a Medical Doctor's prescription and supervision), the diet needs to include all essential nutrients, especially the B vitamins. The lack of thiamin (B_1) and cyanocobalamin (B_{12}) can slow thinking, cause irritability, and cause memory lapses.

An interesting double-blind study by Dr. Ruth Flinn Herrell was performed where she added just 2 mg of vitamin B_1 to the daily diet of one group of children and a placebo to a second group. The first group's mental and physical abilities rose from 7 percent to 87 percent, while the second group's remained almost the same.(130)

J. MacDonald Holmes, Ph.D., reported in the *British Medical Journal* that a vitamin B_{12} deficiency brought on mental and emotional symptoms such as mood disorders, agitated depression, difficulty in thinking and remembering, confusion, visual and auditory hallucinations, epilepsy, and delusions.(131)

In addition to good nutrition, aerobic exercise is important in encouraging brain and memory function, according to Professor Robert Rivera, a memory expert at Valley College in Van Nuys, California. He has found that better blood and oxygen circulation to the brain can cause an increase in a person's IQ as much as thirty points.

This is understandable considering that the gray matter of the brain, where thinking is done, uses 25 percent of our oxygen intake. The blood going to the brain must have an oxygen saturation of 90 percent for us to think efficiently. If it's reduced to 85 percent, the ability of fine concentration and fine muscular coordination decreases. Rivera thinks that oxygen deprivation may also lead to emotional instability. Hypothyroidism can cause oxygen deprivation in the brain because it is usually associated with decreased blood circulation and a general decrease in the rate of metabolism.(132)

Treating ADHD

In a 1995 article in the *Journal of College Student Psychotherapy*, Peter R.

Breggin, M.D. and Ginger Ross Breggin discuss how to handle children with ADHD:

> The symptoms or manifestations of ADHD often disappear when the children have something interesting to do or when they are given a minimal amount of adult attention. . .When a small child, perhaps five or six years old, is persistently disrespectful or angry, there is always a stressor in that child's life – something over which the child has little or no control. Sometimes, the child is not being respected because children learn more by example than by anything else. When treated with respect, they tend to respond respectfully. When loved, they tend to be loving. . . Children do not, on their own, create severe emotional conflict within themselves and with the adults around them.(133)

Breggin says that most so-called ADHD children are not receiving enough attention from their fathers in particular, who may be separated from the family or too preoccupied with work and other things. The treatment that has shown to be most successful is more rational and loving attention from the young person's father. And since many young people are so hungry for the attention of a father-figure, the attention can come from any male adult. He notes that seemingly impulsive, hostile groups of children calm down when a caring, relaxed, yet firm adult male is around.

Studies show that children who receive good and adequate treatment for ADHD in the form of increased attention and caring from adults respond in a very positive manner. Many professionals note that ADHD tends to go away during summer vacation, when the child is in a less structured environment and free to pursue things that interest him.

Smaller schools with smaller class sizes have a dramatic effect on children and their emotions. The teachers can get to know their students better and understand their basic needs. A smaller, more child-oriented school setting can make behavioral problems virtually disappear.(134)

In July 1993, the *New York Times* reported, "students in schools limited to about 400 students have fewer behavior problems, better attendance and graduation rates, and sometimes higher grades and scores. At a time when more children have less support from their families, students in small schools can form close relationships with teachers." Teachers in these schools, said the article, have the opportunity for "building bonds that are particularly vital during the troubled years of adolescence."(135)

When an already troubled student is put into a smaller school, she tends to respond positively. "They are shining stars you thought were dull," said New York City teacher Gregg Staples. Breggin and Breggin say that, "Children respond so quickly to improvements in the way that adults relate to them that most children can be helped without being seen by a professional person." Oftentimes, psychotherapists can help a child without ever seeing the child himself, but rather, working with their parents to help them become more loving or more disciplined, which can indirectly transform the child.

Berggin and Berggin go on to say, "Children can benefit from guidance in learning to be responsible for their own conduct; but they do not gain from being blamed for the trauma and stress that they are exposed to in the environment around them. They need empowerment, not humiliating diagnoses and mind-disabling drugs. Most of all, they thrive when adults show concern and attention to their basic needs as children"(136)

Ritalin

Some drugs that act as stimulants or "speed" in most adults can have a calming effect in children and even in some adults. When a child is diagnosed with ADHD, he or she may be given a drug to keep them under control. The most widely used drug is methylphenidate hydrochloride, or *Ritalin* – a powerful stimulant, especially to the central nervous system that usually takes effect in 30 minutes and peters out in three to four hours. The use of stimulant drugs such as *Ritalin* and amphetamines to treat ADHD began in the 1960s.(137) *Ritalin* is classified as a Schedule II controlled substance in the same category as cocaine, methadone, and methamphetamine.(138)

Close to four million children in the U.S. are currently prescribed *Ritalin*.(139) The number of children taking *Ritalin* for ADHD has approximately doubled every four to seven years since 1971. It's estimated that its use quadrupled between 1990 and 1997, and the *New York Times* reported on January 18, 1999, that the production of *Ritalin* has increased 700 percent since 1990. Just how much *Ritalin* is going into our kids? In 1997 U.S children ingested more than 10 tons of *Ritalin* to control ADHD.(140,141) The use of the drug is spreading to younger and younger children; in 1995 almost half a million prescriptions were written for children between ages three and six.(142)

The percentage of children with behavioral problems being prescribed the drug has increased also. In 1989, 55 percent of children diagnosed as ADHD left the doctor's office with a prescription for *Ritalin*, and in 1996, that percentage had climbed to 75 percent. Meanwhile, the number receiving psychotherapy fell from 40 percent in 1989 to 25 percent in 1996. Jeff Goodwin, a former pediatrician commented:

> It is easier for physicians to prescribe a drug and categorize a disorder as hyperactivity than it is to deal with the problem. Health services are being cut back, so you have doctors saying, "Take this and live happily ever after.". . .The reason *Ritalin* use has gone up is that we are in an era when psychiatric services are devalued and therapy is not paid for by insurance companies.(143)

It's not just children who are on it. In 1997, between 6.5 million and 9 million adults in the U.S. had been diagnosed with ADHD, and about 730,000 of them were taking *Ritalin* by prescription. Most of these adults were children diagnosed with ADHD who have continued treatment.

In November 1998, *Time* magazine ran a feature story on *Ritalin*, which reported:

> For years *Ritalin* has been a godsend for children who were so hot-wired they were simply unreachable, and unteachable. In severe cases, the benefits of *Ritalin* (and the family of related drugs) on these children's ability to function and learn and cope are so direct that advocates say withholding the pills is a form of neglect. . .Some doctors find themselves battling anxious parents who, worried that their child will daydream his future away, demand the drug, and if refused, go off to find a more cooperative physician. Some parents feel pressured to medicate their child just so that his behavior will conform a bit more to other children's, even if they are quite content with their child's conduct – quirks, tantrums, and all.(144)

"It's a fixed, stable, low-dose drug," according to Philip Berent, M.D., a consulting psychiatrist. He says that critics who claim diet, exercise or other treatments work just as well as *Ritalin* are kidding themselves. "The quickest way to end that criticism is to spend a week with a hyperactive child. We aren't talking about kids who ODed on Halloween candy."(145)

However, Lawrence Diller, M.D., author of *Running on Ritalin,* makes an interesting point. "What if Tom Sawyer or Huckleberry Finn were to walk into my office tomorrow? Tom's indifference to schooling and Huck's 'oppositional' behavior would surely have been cause for concern. Would I prescribe *Ritalin* for them too?" The disorder is surprisingly ill defined – no one is sure whether it's truly a neurochemical imbalance or not.

"Let's not deny *Ritalin* works," said J. Zink, Ph.D., a Manhattan Beach, Calif., family therapist who has written several books on raising children and who lectures extensively around the country. "But why does it work, and what are the consequences of over prescribing? The reality is we don't know."

Scientists don't know why *Ritalin* seems to help kids with ADHD, but they have some clues: they know which parts of the brain are involved in impulse control and which chemicals in the brain respond to *Ritalin*. How these two pieces of the puzzle fit together, however, is still unclear.(146)

We do know that amphetamine drugs like *Ritalin* help the body to produce adrenaline, or they mimic its effects. Low adrenaline levels in children causes the same hyperactive symptoms of ADHD – restlessness, poor attention, and difficulty understanding and solving problems. Consequently, the child cannot filter out all the incoming stimuli to his or her nervous system, which results in excessive activity in the parts of the brain that regulate attention and sleep. If adrenaline is increased, the child will calm down. *Ritalin* relaxes these low-adrenaline children by helping them produce more adrenaline.(147)

The amount of adrenaline the body produces must be in specific amounts, neither too high nor too low. If too low, the child will have difficulty concentrating and be restless. If too high, the child may become hyperactive. Timothy Jones, M.D., of Yale University found that when children were given the sugar equivalent of two 12-ounce colas, their adrenaline levels were twice as high as adults given the same amount. He suggests that in increase in adrenaline could be why some children become hyperactive after eating sweets and recommends they not eat sweets on an empty stomach.(148)

Ritalin is what is a psychotropic (mood altering) or psycho stimulant drug. It is pharmacologically classified with amphetamines ("speed") and is very similar chemically to cocaine. In 1995 the Drug Enforcement Administration (DEA) published a report on the drug that said, "Methylphenidate (*Ritalin*) is a central nervous system (CNS) stimulant and shares many of the pharmacological effects of amphetamine, methamphetamine, and cocaine. . .It produces behavioral, psychological, subjective, and reinforcing effects similar to those of d-amphetamine including increases in rating of euphoria…"(149)

Author Richard DeGrandpre in *Ritalin Nation,* quotes a 1995 report in the *Archives of General Psychiatry:* "Cocaine, which is one of the most reinforcing and addicting of the abused drugs, has pharmacological actions that are very similar to those of methylphenidate (*Ritalin*), which is now the most commonly prescribed psychotropic medicine for children in the U.S."(99) The American Psychiatric Association says that cocaine, amphetamines, and methylphenidate (*Ritalin*) are "neuropharmacologically alike," that abuse patterns are the same for the three drugs, and that people can't tell their clinical effects apart in laboratory tests.(150) Further, they can substitute for each other and cause similar behavior in addicted animals. The FDA classifies methylphenidate in the high addiction category (Schedule II), which also includes amphetamines, morphine, opium, and barbiturates.(151) How many parents are told this before the prescription is written for their child?

In the 1980s, methylphenidate (*Ritalin*) was one of the most commonly used street drugs; youngsters sell their prescribed methylphenidate to classmates who take it for a "high." John Merrow, executive producer of a PBS documentary on ADHD, reported that *Ritalin* is so plentiful that a black market has developed on the school playground. *Ritalin* can be crushed and snorted for a cheap and modest buzz, and it has become a "gateway drug" in junior high school, frequently being the first drug a child experiments with.(152,153) The Drug Enforcement Administration reports that as early as 1994 *Ritalin* was the fastest-growing amphetamine being used "nonmedically" by high school seniors in Texas. DeGrandpre says that in 1991 there were about 25 emergency room visits of children ages 10 to 14 connected with *Ritalin* abuse. By 1995, the number had climbed to more than 400 visits – about the same number of visits as for cocaine.(154)

Richard DeGrandpre goes on to report that "lab animals given the choice to self-administer comparative doses of cocaine and *Ritalin* do not favor one over another. . .a similar study showed monkeys would work in the same fashion for *Ritalin* as they would for cocaine."

Newsweek, in 1995, reported, "The prescription drug *Ritalin* is now a popular high on campus. . ." In *Running on Ritalin,* Diller quotes several undercover narcotics agents who say, "*Ritalin* is cheaper and easier to purchase at playgrounds than on the street." The 1995 *Time* feature article says that, "more teenagers try *Ritalin* by grinding it up and snorting it for $5 a pill than get it by prescription." Many teenagers do not consider *Ritalin* to be anywhere near as dangerous as heroine or cocaine because they think that since their younger brother takes it by prescription, it must be safe.(155) They don't realize it is addictive.

Hallowell and Ratey, in *Driven to Distraction* say that, "people with ADD feel focused when they take cocaine, just as they do when they take *Ritalin.*"(156) *Ritalin* works on children the same way cocaine or related stimulants work on adults: It sharpens short-term attention span. This "peak" is followed by a "valley," when the child "rebounds", from its effects. (Similar to, as they say on the streets, "coming down" off a drug). One mother comments about her daughter's *Ritalin* rebound: "She'd hold herself together all day, but the minute she got home she'd have this breakdown. You'd be asking the impossible to have my child come home, have a snack, and do her homework right away."(157)

Withdrawal symptoms can include inattention, hyperactivity, and aggression – the very things the drug is supposed to prevent – along with appetite suppression and insomnia (the drug adversely effects children the same way adults are affected by such drugs).(158) That's why handbooks on ADHD given to parents advise them to see their doctor if they feel their child is losing too much weight, and why some children who take *Ritalin* are also prescribed sedatives to help them sleep. A catch-22.

Methylphenidate can cause permanent disfiguring tics and suppress growth (height and weight). Much of the brain's development takes place during the years in which children are given this drug, and thus the brain's size could be reduced. Although there have been no consistent brain abnormalities found in children with ADHD, one study found brain shrinkage in adults labeled ADHD who have been taking methylphenidate for years. The authors of this study suggest, "cortical atrophy may be a long-term adverse effect of this [methylphenidate] treatment."(159) Michael F. Jacobson and David Schardt in *Diet, ADHD & Behavior - A Quarter-Century Review,* found that *Ritalin* causes liver cancer in mice (although not in rats).(160) The DEA also says:

> Most of the ADHD literature prepared for public consumption
> and available to parents does not address the abuse liability or
> actual abuse of methylphenidate. Instead, methylphenidate is
> routinely portrayed as a benign, mild stimulant that is not
> associated with abuse or serious effects. In reality, however, there
> is an abundance of scientific literature which indicates that
> methylphenidate shares the same abuse potential as other Schedule

II stimulants. . . Abuse data indicate a growing problem among school-age children. . . ADHD adults have a high incidence of substance disorders, and that with 3 to 5 percent of today's youth being administered methylphenidate on a chronic basis, these issues are of great concern.(161)

Doctors do not always warn of these dangers. And they do not tell parents that there are virtually guaranteed non-drug methods to improve the conduct of nearly all so-called ADHD children through more interesting and engaging schools and a more loving, attentive family, let alone changes to diet and physical health. Nor do they discuss what diagnosis and treatment might do to a child's self-esteem. Once labeled with ADHD, a child is viewed differently, and even normal behavior could be interpreted as problem behavior requiring drugging. This diagnosis can follow the child through his school years and even throughout life. Side effects (both short-term and long-term) of taking prescription drugs can wreak havoc on the child's mental as well as physical health.

Our children are not only getting attention disorders and learning disabilities, they're getting depressed too. It's estimated that 3.4 million Americans under 18 are said to be "seriously" depressed. In 1997, approximately 800,000 antidepressant prescriptions were written for drugs such as *Prozac*, *Zoloft*, and *Paxil*, for children, some as young as 5 years old. Many of these kids were also taking *Ritalin* – not surprisingly since depression can be a by-product of the drug and ADHD. Antidepressants can lead to agitation and nervousness in anyone, but in children they can trigger full-blown manic episodes. Doctors are not sure how these drugs affect a young, still elastic brain.(162)

It's interesting to note that healthy adults respond in the same way children do to these drugs (methylphenidate and other stimulants such as cocaine and amphetamines), regardless of whether they are diagnosed with ADHD or hyper-activity. Diller says that methylphenidate "potentially improves the performance of anyone – child or not, ADD-diagnosed or not." And, psychologist Ken Livingston says, "studies conducted during the mid-seventies to early eighties by Judith Rapaport of the National Institute of Mental Health. . .clearly showed that stimulant drugs improve the performance of most people, regardless of whether they have a diagnosis of ADHD, on tasks requiring good attention. Indeed, this probably explains the high levels of "self-medicating around the world" with "stimulants like caffeine and nicotine."(163)

One of the brand name drugs used to treat ADHD is *Concerta*. In 2004 there were 7.8 million prescriptions of *Concerta* filled. (This is just one of several ADHD drugs remember.) It contains methylphenidate, the same active ingredient in *Ritalin* as do most of the other ADHD drugs on the market. The bottle's label warns of possible psychiatric side effects. But other side effects that are not listed have also been reported such as hallucinations, suicidal thoughts, aggression, high blood pressure, arrhythmia, and racing heartbeats.(164) Even if the label showed these other side effects, it would have little to no effect on the rates of prescription. It's been shown numerous times that warnings have no effect on prescription rates.(165) (This goes for all prescription medicine such as heart medications, cholesterol-lowering medication, erectile dysfunction medications, and so on.)

The latest in ADHD medicine is a skin patch that also contains methylphenidate called *Daytrana*. It lasts for 9 hours, versus 4 hours for a pill of *Ritalin*. It's more convenient in some ways, and can be removed if it causes side effects. But it's just another way to numb children's minds into complacency without addressing the underlying cause of the disorder (if in fact, the child *has* a disorder).(166)

Food for Thought

So what has taken place is this: A "disease" – ADHD – is "created" with such a nebulous, subjective, broad scope of symptoms that almost anyone can be diagnosed as having it – especially kids who are naturally full of energy and have short attention spans. Then, a drug is called upon that will "improve the performance of most people" (can't-miss prognosis!) to get the child into "compliance," settle down and not be a threat or bother to anyone. It's very clever, don't you think? So clever that more than 10 tons of *Ritalin* are ingested by kids all across the country every year. Just think of the profits! I think we're on to something!

How could such a potentially harmful substance be foisted upon our children with the consent and even encouragement of the parents? Here's something to consider:

In 1991, the U.S. Department of Education formally recognized ADHD as a handicap (under the Individuals with Disabilities Education Act and Section 504 of the 1973 Rehabilitation Act). The department then directed all state education officers to make sure that local school districts establish procedures to screen and identify ADHD children. Those children would then be given special educational and psychological services. New funding to the schools was then possible.

The U.S Department of Education told school superintendents that there are "three ways in which children labeled ADHD could qualify for special education services in public school under existing laws." In 1990, the Individuals with Disabilities Education Act mandated that "Eligible children receive access to special education and/or related services, and that this education be designed to meet each child's unique educational needs" through an individualized program.

So, ADHD children are now entitled by law to a long list of services including separate special-education classrooms, learning specialists, special equipment, tailored homework assignments, social services, mental health care, speech therapy, counseling, and psychological services. So, it's in the interest of the school to have children with ADHD because it will get better funding for services they think are necessary in areas directly related to ADHD and also other areas not necessarily related to ADHD. And what school doesn't want more free money?(167)

Children are regularly tested by teachers for emotional, social, mental, and physical disorders (especially ADHD) inside public schools. As stated earlier, the diagnosis of ADHD can be made by a non-physician. Once a child is diagnosed and labeled with ADHD, school health officials have the authority to treat them by prescribing and administering *Ritalin* (a Schedule II drug, remember). Other drugs that may be used are *Valium, Lorazepam*, and *Prozac*.

CHAAD (Children and Adults with Attention-Deficit/Hyperactivity Disorder), a nationwide ADHD support group, mounted a campaign in 1995 to have *Ritalin* changed from a Schedule II drug to a Schedule III drug, which would have made it far easier to obtain. CHADD considers itself the leading information center for ADHD.

CHADD's petition to the DEA to reclassify *Ritalin* as a Schedule III drug was cosigned by the American Academy of Neurology and was supported by other distinguished medical bodies including the American Academy of Pediatrics, the American Psychological Association, and the American Academy of Child and Adolescent Psychiatry. However, it was uncovered that Novartis (then called Ciba-Geigy – the pharmaceutical giant that manufactures *Ritalin*) had contributed nearly $900,000 to CHADD over five years and that CHADD had failed to disclose this.

The DEA stated it had concerns over "the depth of the financial relationship between CHADD and Ciba-Geigy." They said that Ciba-Geigy "stands to benefit from a change in scheduling of methylphenidate." They expressed concerns over the use of methylphenidate and that nongovernmental organizations and that parental association in the U.S. were actively lobbying for the medical use of methylphenidate, not to mention that "Methylphenidate shares the same abuse potential as other Schedule II stimulants." When it learned of the DEA's concerns, CHADD withdrew its petition to decontrol *Ritalin*.(168)

Food for Thought

When an individual or organization with credentials says something, people tend to listen and believe. If a group like the American Academy of Pediatrics wanted *Ritalin* decontrolled, it's easy for someone not informed to take it for granted that they must know what they're talking about and that the substance is not that dangerous or harmful. But, as evidenced, there were perhaps less than noble reasons these associations wanted it

> decontrolled – and an open checkbook could easily sway them to agree with their pharmaceutical friends.

Approximately 90 percent of *Ritalin* production is consumed in the U.S., but not every nation sees it as a godsend. Sweden, for example, withdrew methylphenidate from the market in 1968 after a number of abuse cases, and has not reintroduced it since.

Alternative Ways of Treating ADHD

Remember, ADHD is a very loosely diagnosed problem; what one person may see as ADHD, another may not. Oftentimes the diagnosis is made simply so that an unruly but "normal" child can be silenced and easier to handle. Remember, children are bundles of energy, and their attention span is naturally short. But in our fast-paced, "both-parents-working-let's-put-the-child-in-day-care" world, it's easy to understand why parents don't have the patience with their little Tom Sawyer and why a more easily controlled child is an attractive alternative – even if drugged. But is a little peace and quiet now worth the possible nightmare later?

Food for Thought

It's a good thing that *Ritalin* wasn't around when I was a kid. I surely would have been put on it. I drove my mother crazy. Although I could sit quietly for a while in a chair if I was given a reward, I usually ran around and never stopped until I worked myself into a state of near exhaustion. When I was about three years old, I would somehow unlock the front door early in the morning before my parents were up, and bolt out of the house with no clothes on whatsoever. I'd scoot around the neighborhood in my little push-pedal Chevy car going 100 kiddie miles an hour buck naked. My parents were awakened many times by the neighbor down the street knocking on the door with naked little Bobby in his arms. This was in Queens, New York, in the late 1950s. Try that today and see what happens. I also remember going Trick-or-Treating when I was seven, past dark, accompanied by only a friend. My, have things changed!

The first thing a parent should do if a child is difficult to handle is to pay him more attention and give him as loving an atmosphere as possible. Give your child a hug a few times a day. A prominent male figure is important. Ask the child questions, pay attention to him, take an interest. If at all possible, move the child into a school with smaller class sizes.

Improve the child's diet. Eliminate or minimize processed foods, foods with additives, colorings, and foods containing sugar or sugar like ingredients (high fructose corn syrup and artificial sweeteners). Buy organic foods as much as possible since they are free of pesticides and their nutritional value is greater. Also, encourage your child to eat as much raw, uncooked food as possible.

Reduce or eliminate all white flour products. That includes pizza, breads, pastas, Twinkies, and so on. Find a source of raw milk, and have your child drink that instead of soda pop or fruit juices. Try supplementing your child's diet with a good source of omega-3 fatty acids such as fish oil or krill oil. Don't be afraid to feed your child fatty foods (the less cooked, the better) since his/her developing brain and nervous system needs that fat desperately. Making these dietary changes alone will probably make a huge difference in you child's behavior and may eliminate his or her learning disability.

Since our water supply is greatly compromised, either buy good bottled water or get a water purification system. The fewer pollutants going into your little loved ones, the better their brains will be able to function.

Limit your child's exposure to television. Leonard Shalin, M.D., says that since TV is *image based* only, it puts the brain into an alpha brainwave pattern, fostering right-brain dominance, whereas reading a book requires the left-brain's beta brainwave functioning. Shalin says that the detrimental influence of TV is from its passive influence as it precludes interactive neural stimulation. When a child is at play, this neural stimulation is present, and thus the brain develops as it should.(169)

Russell Barkley, author of *ADHD and the Nature of Self Control* says that ADHD is now considered a "developmental issue of self-control." Lack of impulse control is the inability to regulate the emotional energy flow, which is required to focus. It causes an "act now, think later" behavior that results in increased emotional agitation and a feeling of being like a "cat on a hot tin roof" – agitated and restless.(170)

While *Ritalin* may control the symptoms of ADHD, it does nothing to change the underlying condition. That condition, no matter the cause, is one of lack of impulse control and the inability to focus – which leads to agitation and frustration.

Jeanette Farmer has an interesting perspective on ADHD and impulse control. She is a certified handwriting movement specialist, and contends that the lack of impulse control is in large part due to a lack of proper brain and neural development. She says that this can be corrected or avoided by teaching children correct penmanship – which helps develop the neural pathways that lead to learning and impulse control. Impulse control, reading, and learning are inextricably, linked, and they depend on the proper balanced development of the two hemispheres of the brain.(171)

The brain is divided into two hemispheres – left and right. Each has its own unique and specific function. The left hemisphere does what is called "hard thinking" and is mostly concerned with conscious awareness. It uses logic, reason, thinks in words, plans, is ordered, controlled, and structured, and its focus is external and narrow. The right hemisphere does what is called "soft thinking" and is mostly concerned with unconscious awareness. It uses emotions, intuition and creativity, thinks in pictures, is spontaneous, is unstructured, has an internal focus, is holistic, diffuse, and unfocused (covering a wide area). Impulse control is tied to the emotionally influenced right-brain, while the ability to focus and stay on task is tied to the left-brain. Farmer says,

> The child is born in a natural right-brain state, a state primarily motivated by the intertwined factors of instant gratification and lack of impulse control. Normally, the child gradually matures out of that state by gaining some degree of impulse control, influencing a gradual shift in dominance to the left-brain for the vast majority of the population. That is, when all goes well – but any number of environmental, nutritional, medical, educational, parental influences or conditions may preclude that normal and natural transition. Due to the increased stimulation in multi-sensory handwriting training, it can play a powerful role in aiding that transition.(172)

Handwriting with the right hand activates the left hemisphere, since the nerves from the body cross over to the opposite side (the *contralateral* side) of the brain and stimulates the left hemisphere's language capacities. (Where this nerve crossover takes place is called the *pyramidal decussation* or *motor decussation*, in the lower part of the brainstem called the *medulla oblongata*. This is near the second vertebra in the neck [also called the *axis*], or just below the base of the skull. That's your anatomy lesson for the day.) By activating and using the left hemisphere, it becomes increasingly less submissive and more dominant in the over-all functioning of the brain. That is to say that as the left-brain is used, the impulsiveness of the right-brain is subdued. It is brought under control and the child or person can function more out of a thinking than reacting way. Leonard Shalin, M.D., in his book *The Alphabet versus the Goddess*, says that any form of writing influences left-brain dominance. Farmer continues:

> Impulses are the essence of the emotional life force that drives behaviors. Learning to control impulses has profound implications for future success in life. No psychological skill is more valuable than the ability to resist impulses, the root of self-control. Lack of impulse control and instant gratification are linked. Research in 1960 nearly 40 years ago with four-year-olds and marshmallows deliver a telling message about impulse control as a predictor of future success.
>
> A group of four-year-olds was gathered around a table with some marshmallows on it. The researcher told them that he had to go do an errand and if they could wait until he got back they could have two marshmallows. If not, they could have one right then. This proved to be a dramatic telling test. These students were tracked down when they graduated from high school. Those who

could delay gratification and endure frustration were more socially competent, personally effective, self assertive and better able to cope with frustration of life. They could better direct their energies to achieve functional productivity. Moreover, it predicted a 210-point advantage in SAT scores some 17 years later. Clearly impulse control should be a major educational concern. . .

I have found that when the right-brain dominant child is thrown into a left-brain system and expected to perform using processing skill not yet in place, it immediately sets up stress and anxiety in trying to meet expectations. Stress has such a negative impact on the brain that it can easily shut down the learning process and the ability to lock information into the working memory. . .A neurophysiologist and well experience teacher, Hannaford believes that movement is essential for learning and thought. . .My personal experience leads me to believe that learning disabilities are made, not born. I believe it is learning styles and a dominance issue, which should be rightly called "learning differently." While research clearly supports handwriting's role in helping establish dominance, failure to sufficiently stress the process is an underlying factor that has subtly influenced achieving the educational crisis. . . Obviously, if I can use handwriting, as a fine motor process, to "retrain the brain," (a shift in dominance pattern) then it must have the inherent capacity to "train the brain" (develop impulse control and cause a shift in dominance) in the first place. . .Fine motor control (as needed in writing) and emotional control are deeply intertwined - it capitalizes on the left-brain-right hand connection. . . Intentional movement taps the unconscious (emotional) mind. As impulse control is an "act first and think later" factor, training the brain impacts behavior. It can't be gained by just wanting it, simply "trying harder" or by straining, willing it, or coercing the mind to function. A specific game plan is necessary to develop that innate potential – it comes from repetitive actions that imprint the brain.(173)

Carla Hannaford, Ph.D., says that hemispheric dominance is an educational issue that is vastly ignored. In Hannaford's book *Smart Moves - Why Learning is Not All in Your Head* she contends that learning disabilities are a brain dominance issue. Hannaford says that "up to 80 percent of all American school children could be diagnosed as learning-disabled." She found that 78 percent of left-brain dominant children were considered gifted and talented while 78 percent of right-brain dominant children were in special education (dyslexia, learning disabled, etc.). This underscores the importance of activating the left hemisphere. Not only does the left hemisphere deal with concepts that are largely factual and logical (which would show up on test scores), but its activity and activation subdues the right hemisphere's tendency to be impulsive, disorderly and out of control.(174)

Food for Thought

Often creative people are seen as a little "loose in the head." The "absent- minded professor" types. These creative people are often not very well organized or neat and have a difficult time completing tasks.

I contacted certified handwriting movement specialist Jeannette Farmer to see if her handwriting exercises could help adults, and if these symptoms had to do with a brain dominance imbalance. She told me that yes, by consistently activating the left hemisphere, the right hemisphere's impulsiveness can be subdued even in adults. She said,

"Adults with unremediated ADD create a number of life changing problems such as difficulties in maintaining long term relationships or even holding a job. Self-defeating behaviors require 'retraining the brain.' Current research finds that humans operate out of a 'comfort zone' by sheer habit and automatic responses over 90 percent of the time. Without changing automatic responses, it's as the old saying goes, 'if you continue to do what you've always done, you will get what you have always got.' To make positive behavioral changes, one must get out of that well established 'comfort zone.' Handwriting movement exercises provide a fast track to creating change by 'retraining the brain' due to increased neural stimulation, offering potential for new habits and responses."

Interesting, I thought. So I started to do the handwriting exercise she recommends in her manual *Training the Brain to Pay Attention the Write Way*. In this manual she also recommends doing the writing movements to music (which she supplies) with a beat of 60 beats per minute, which also has the capacity to *entrain* the brain and make learning more efficient. Upon doing the exercise, I felt an immediate difference. I seemed to calm down, although I hadn't noticed I was anxious, and I felt more at peace. The rest of my day, when I do these exercises, is easier, flows more smoothly and I'm not as prone to getting upset. I personally have not seen the results of these exercise with children, but Farmer assures me that children who do them consistently not only make tremendous leaps in their learning abilities, but are calmer, more centered and have greater self-esteem. You can order the manual and tape on line at www.retrainthebrain.com.

Another way to address brain integration to encourage better learning and impulse control is through a method called *Brain Gym* developed by Paul E. Dennison, Ph.D., and his wife, Gail. (www.braingym.com). *Brain Gym* uses easy and simple exercises to *switch on* the brain that allows it to take in and process information more effectively. The end result is increased awareness, increased focus without being over focused, better learning, easier recall, longer memory, and better decision making. I took the *Brain Gym* class several years ago, and believe it is not only good for those with learning disabilities or behavior problems, but everyone, no matter what their age or current health condition. Dr. Dennison says,

"Doing *Brain Gym* movements not only builds and reinforces effective neural connections and pathways; it relaxes us and activates centralization and focus. . . It also opens the heart, inviting us to interact. When the mind, body, and heart are active and integrated, people blossom. They learn easily, they become creative, they are compassionate and friendly, and most importantly they find meaning in their lives and are happy. I'll always remember the young woman who approached me in a workshop and said, 'Dr. Dennison, thank you for teaching me this work. I use it with my husband and children. It's helped us come together as a family. For us, *Brain Gym* is another way to say, 'I love you.' "

Over the years, I've taken just about every self-help/development class you can think of. Most try to help you get past problems using pretty much the mind alone. These methods might relieve some mental anguish and it might feel good to have someone understand your problems, but the relief is usually short-lived. Soon you're back to making the same mistakes and creating similar problems in your life. *Brain Gym* goes about change in a totally different way. It essentially reorganizes your brain and creates new, more effective neural pathways that are more efficient. Since the brain is actually functioning and thinking differently, you make different, more efficient decisions, and your life gets smoother. All without necessarily confronting the "baggage" that got you stuck in your self-defeating ruts in the first place.

I like to think I'm giving you some rare gems of advice. This is definitely one of them. Whether you have a child with a learning disability or just want to improve your life and the lives of loved ones, please check out *Brain Gym*. www.braingym.com. (888) 388-9898.

The bottom line of all this is that perhaps one of the reasons so many children are fidgety and have learning and self-control problems is that they are not practicing their writing or moving around enough. I know it sounds simple, but by activating the brain in the way movement does, it most definitely changes not only its function, but also its physiology – that being it creates new neural pathways and actually can grow new neurons. After Albert Einstein died, researchers removed his brain and examined it to see if they could determine if there were any distinct differences in his brain compared to a person of normal intellect. What they found was that his brain was no larger than normal (it was even a little smaller), and it did not weigh more. But, it had an amazing number of neural pathways in it – many more than a normal person's. Research has shown that these neural pathways develop as the brain is used. That is, the more you flex your noggin', the stronger it gets – and the smarter you are.

Experiments in rats bear this out too. A rat that is in a rich and diverse environment will develop more neurons than a rat in a sterile, boring environment. The less our children are encouraged to learn, the easier we make it for them, the lower the standards become – the dumber they will be and the more impulsive they will be. As our school systems have become more lackadaisical, so has the insistence on good handwriting skills, and so has the intellect of our children declined and their impulsiveness increased.

Literacy in America

Forty two million American adults can't read at all and 50 million are unable to read at a higher level that is expected of a fourth or fifth grader. The number of adults that are classified as functionally illiterate increases by about 2.25 million each year and 20 percent of high school seniors can be classified as being functionally illiterate at the time they graduate.[175]

In 20 years, from 1972 to 1992, the literacy rate in America fell from 13th worldwide to 49th. In 1992, according to government statistics: 2.5 million young adults graduated from high school with one million of them being functionally illiterate; 22 percent, or 42 million adults are functionally illiterate; only 5 percent of 17-year-olds can read at an advanced level; 57 percent of California's 4th graders, 58 percent of Hawaii's and 75 percent of Washington, D.C.'s read below basic grade level – and several other states were not far behind. Only 13 percent of today's 16- to 25-year-olds read at Level 4 or 5, the highest proficiency levels. During the 1990s, there's been a 30 percent increase in the need for special education services.[176]

Food for Thought

The *Princeton Review* analyzed the transcripts of famous debates of politicians and found something unexpected happening: the vocabulary and complexity of the language is getting lower and lower.

In the Abraham Lincoln/Stephen A. Douglas debate in 1858, the candidates spoke in language expected to be used by 11th and 12th graders. In the John F. Kennedy/Richard Nixon debate in 1960, the grade level of the language used was what would be expected to be used by 10th graders. In 1992, Bill Clinton spoke at a 7th grade level while George H.W. Bush spoke at a 6th grade level. In 2000, Al Gore spoke at a 7th grade level and George W. Bush spoke at a 6th grade level. The article said, "In short, today's political rhetoric is designed to be comprehensible to a 10-year-old child or an adult with a sixth-grade reading level. It is fitted to this level of comprehension because most Americans speak, think, and are entertained at this level. This is why serious film and theater and other serious artistic expression, as well as newspapers and books, are being pushed to the margins of American society. Voltaire was the most famous man of the 18th century. Today, the most famous 'person' is Mickey Mouse. . . Many eat at fast food restaurants not only because it is cheap, but because they can order from pictures rather than menus."(177)

Diane McGinnis, Ph.D., in her book, *Why Our Children Can't Read and What We Can Do About It*, points out that illiteracy correlates with school dropout rates. A large percentage of adolescent criminal offenders are functionally illiterate. She sums up her research by saying, "The truth provided by these statistics is that children's reading problems, and ultimately adults' reading problems, are caused by the school system, and not because there is something wrong with poor readers. It is impossible that 30 percent to 60 percent of all schoolchildren have an inherent or 'brain-based' deficit leading to reading failure."(178)

McGinnis's research identified four essential principles of successful reading. Neither the *whole language* approach nor the *phonics* approach are based on any of these principles. Rather, she says, "that when the sequence of reading and spelling instruction is compatible with the logic of the alphabet code and the child's linguistic and logical development, learning to read and spell proceeds rapidly and smoothly for all children and is equally effective for poor readers of all ages."

In short, the good old-fashioned way of learning to spell and read is the way that works best in the long run. It is the sequential, step-by-step processing style of this form of learning that activates the left hemisphere of the brain, forcing it to develop. As the left hemisphere develops, so does impulse control, since the right hemisphere's spontaneity is subdued.

Neuropsychologist R. Joseph suggests that repetition is the essence of learning. Children thrive on repetition since it promotes self-mastery, which is closely tied to developing the powers of self-control. He says that physiologically, repetitive movement hones the neural pathways, where nerve cells in a particular experience become more complex, more sensitive, and more easily activated. In short, repetition is necessary in learning. In fact, it's been determined that for a child to learn something new, it needs to be repeated an average of eight times. And, to unlearn an old behavior, and replace it with a new one, the action needs to be repeated an average of 28 times – 20 times to eliminate the old behavior and eight to learn the new one. Repetition ensures that an action becomes a habit. Once it is, doing the action requires less energy and can be performed with less effort.(179)

Repetitive exercises by-pass the "thinking" brain (the cortex) and influence the deeper levels of our emotional brain. The "conditioning process" stimulates neural pathways, which in turn create new dendrites (a part of a nerve cell), and synapses (gap between nerve cells). Remember Einstein's brain – extremely rich in neurons and neural pathways. Repetitive movement allows a better balance between the "thinking" brain and "feeling" or emotional brain, which promotes the integration of the right and left hemisphere. This process is called sensory-motor integration. Repetitive movements, like those in Jeanette Farmer's writing manual or the exercises of *Brain Gym*, stabilize and regulate the emotional energy flow, and the dynamics of emotional release, while honing the neural pathways no matter what your age.

Handwriting has the power to tap the emotions. James Pennebaker, M.D., did research at SMU, which found that just 20 minutes a day for one week spent writing to ventilate emotional issues produced a measurable influence on the immune system. And rhythmic movement gives us a sense of well being.(180) Multi-sensory experiences greatly enrich the learning process. By combining music with movement, more of the brain is stimulated and the brain functions in a more balanced and powerful way.

Sound in itself can have a dramatic effect on us. Alfred Tomatis, a French physician, has done pioneering research on sound and the human body. He found that hearing and touch are closely related and that every neural process passes through or relates to the inner-ear cochlea's system as the principle congregating point for all our senses. He contends that every cell in our body registers sound (it "feels" the sound) and passes the information on to higher centers for processing. (No wonder people like to dance.)

Don Campbell of the Mozart Effect Resource Center says that music impacts the mind, body, and spirit simultaneously. Heart patients derive the same benefits from listening to 30 minutes of classical music as they did from taking *Valium*. The right music can lower heart rate and blood pressure because the heart tends to speed up and slow down to match the pace of the music.(181) No wonder "rock & roll" can incite riots!

Food for Thought

Since sound and touch are closely linked – that is, sound has an actual physical impact – extremes of loud rock music could be sought after just as much if not more for this physical-impact stimulation than for the music itself. In our "touch-starved" society, could this be why loud, raucous music is so popular among children and teenagers? Maybe it's a substitute for the touch they didn't get at day care or because mom and dad were too busy working or they were put in a plastic carrier as babies.

The rhythm of the music can alter brainwaves and breathing patterns and music can affect intelligence and productivity. Students who listened to 10 minutes of Mozart prior to taking SATs generally scored higher than those students who were not exposed to the music.

Rhythm and movement stimulate the frontal lobes of the brain and enrich language and motor development. Young children especially need this stimulation that movement and rhythm provide to establish a pattern of recognition for learning in the future. Exercise along with calm music can do wonders for children who have emotional problems and learning disabilities. As these movements are repeated, the brain creates new neural pathways and the child's mind improves. As this occurs, the left and right hemisphere's activities become more balanced and the child learns, at the root level, self-control. Since the movements and music will calm the child, their stress level goes down.

High stress levels tend to impair reason and logical thinking. As reason and logic are reduced, so are the choices a person can make confronting a given situation. One who cannot think clearly cannot see the solution, or the choice of taking a specific action, which could logically lead to a solution. Thus, as choices decrease, brain function goes down to the lower levels – more along the lines of the fight or flight reaction. As a person thinks on this lower level of awareness, the chances of a reactive, aggressive reaction increases. Simply put, as stress increases (environmental or physiological), judgment, reason, and choice are reduced, leading to reactive, possibly aggressive behavior.

Cheryl Beckett, Ph.D., in her book *Growing Up Inside Out*, reveals that children's stress levels (in elementary and junior high school) were found to be as high as those for top executives. Stress overload is a major problem for those with ADHD. They struggle to cope with educational demands that require specific information processing that is not yet in place (possibly because they have not learned to write and read correctly).[182]

The child then gets anxious, feels like he's dumb, with a resultant increase in stress and anxiety. As this stress level increases, the child is more likely to rebel and be aggressive because they are now operating not out of reason, logic, and impulse control, but from an imbalance, right-brain dominated, fight or flight mode. Try as he might, the learning just won't sink in simply because the brain is not trained to process the information yet. So he is labeled ADHD or learning disabled. If he finds out he has such a label, he get even more stressed out because now he is "different." More stress leads to more reaction without thinking. Another vicious cycle. If the child practices movement-learning and handwriting, along with making the proper nutritional changes, the brain will function better, learning will increase and stress will go down. All without taking drugs akin to cocaine.

CHAPTER VIII

Depression

Depression is a serious medical condition that affects thoughts, feelings, and the ability to function in everyday life. Depression can occur at any age. According to the National Institute of Mental Health (NIMH), there are three different mood disorders: major depressive disorder; dysthymic disorder (chronic, mild depression), and; bipolar disorder. As of 2006, 20.9 million American adults, or 9.5 percent (that's almost one in ten) of American adults experience one or more of these mood disorders.[1]

Major depressive disorder is the leading cause of disability in the U.S. for ages 15 - 44, and affects about 14.8 million American adults (about 6.7 percent of the U.S. population age 18 and older). Dysthymic disorder affects about 1.5 percent of the U.S. population age 18 and older – or about 3.3 million adults. Bipolar disorder affects about 5.7 million American adults, or about 2.6 percent of the U.S. population age 18 and older.[2]

The World Health Organization cites depression as the fourth leading cause of disease worldwide, causing more disability than heart attacks or strokes. It's expected to be the second leading cause of disability for people of all ages by 2020.[3]

Depression results from abnormal functioning of the brain. An interaction between genetic predisposition and life history appear to determine a person's level of risk. Episodes of depression may be triggered by stress, difficult life events, side effects of drugs or other environmental factors.

Major depressive disorder brings a halt to one's ability to function in everyday life. Dysthymic disorder is less severe, but may still involve long-lasting symptoms that persist for at least two years (one year in children). Bipolar disorder is characterized by cycling mood changes: severe highs (mania) and lows (depression), often with periods of normal mood in between.

When in the mania cycle, the person may be overactive and have a great deal of energy. Thinking and judgment may be impaired. The person may feel elated and full of grand schemes that might range from unwise business decisions to romantic sprees, have abnormally high self-esteem, decreased need for sleep, increased talkativeness and the propensity to take unnecessary risks. When in the depressed cycle, the person may exhibit any or all of the symptoms of depression. The generally accepted symptoms of depression are:

- Persistent sad, anxious, or "empty" mood, or no feelings of any kind
- Feelings of hopelessness, pessimism, guilt, worthlessness, helplessness
- Loss of interest or pleasure in activities once enjoyed, including sex

- Decreased energy, increased fatigue
- Difficulty concentrating, remembering, making decisions
- Trouble sleeping, awakening in the morning, or oversleeping
- Appetite and/or weight changes
- Thoughts of death or suicide, or suicide attempts
- Restlessness, irritability
- Persistent physical symptoms, such as headaches, digestive disorders, and chronic pain (4)

The NIMH fact sheet I got these statistics from covers all sorts of mental disorders, not just depression as shown below. Although I won't cover all of these in detail, a look at the numbers is telling. . .

- Suicide: 31,655 died in 2002 due to suicide. The highest rate of suicide occurs in white men over 85 years of age. Four times as many men as women die by suicide, yet women attempt suicide two to three times as often as men.
- Schizophrenia: 2.4 million American adults 18 and older (1.1% of adults)
- Anxiety disorders: 40 million (18.1%). These include obsessive-compulsive disorder, phobias, post-traumatic stress disorder, and panic disorder.
  - Panic disorder: 6 million (2.7%)
    - Agoraphobia: 1.8 million (0.8%)
    - Other specific phobias: 19.2 million (8.7%)
  - Obsessive-compulsive disorder: 2.2 million (1.0%)
  - Post-traumatic stress disorder: 7.7 million (3.5%)
  - Generalized anxiety disorder: 6.8 million (3.1%)
- Eating disorders
  - Anorexia nervosa: 0.5% to 3.7% of females will suffer from anorexia
  - Bulimia: 1.1% to 4.2% females will suffer from bulimia
  - Binge eating: 2-5% of Americans experience binge-eating disorder in a 6 month period
- Attention Deficit Hyperactivity Disorder (ADHD): 4.1% of adults
- Alzheimer's disease: 4.5 million Americans (more than doubled since 1980)

The most common symptom of depression is fatigue. Waking up at 2 to 4 a.m. on a regular basis is another common indicator of depression leading to early morning mood problems. If you lose interest in most of your daily activities, "just don't care" anymore and find that nothing in life gives you pleasure, chances are you're depressed. If someone has a lot of guilt, blames themselves for everything, expects the worst, and is generally pessimistic or hopeless, they are exhibiting signs they may be depressed. If someone complains incessantly about money, their job, housing, wants to run away and can't make up their mind anymore, doesn't talk, stays in bed, has no sense of humor, and has poor personal grooming habits, they may also be depressed.

All of us at one time exhibit many of these traits, and that's normal. But when someone is mired in this kind of attitude and behavior, it's probably a problem that needs to be addressed.

Depression is responsible for about 66 percent of all suicides. Although the medical community recognizes what the symptoms of depression are, there is no universally accepted diagnosis for it.(5) But one commonly used diagnostic criteria is known as SIGECAPS – sleep, interest, guilt, energy, concentration, appetite, psychomotor and suicide. If four or more of these traits are shown to be abnormal, it indicates major depression. Even with all these descriptions, about two-thirds of people with depression are not diagnosed as such, and only one-third of patients receive adequate treatment.(6)

Women are twice as likely to experience depression as men, and depression is the leading cause of disability in women. Women are 2½ times more likely to be depressed during the transition to menopause than when premenopausal.(7) Only one in three women with depression will seek professional help. It occurs most frequently in women between the ages of 25 and 44 years of age, and about 10 percent of women will experience postpartum depression in the months after the birth of a child.

Food for Thought

A study published in the *Archives of Pediatrics and Adolescent Medicine* reported that if a young female is depressed, there's about a 25 percent greater chance that she will be physically abused by her male partner.(8) So someone's attitude can directly effect how she/he is treated? Interesting concept. But don't think, "she brought this on herself," since depression is not something someone can really control -- at least directly. It's a result of the body (of which the mind is part) no longer being able to take stress, and that stress is most often from environmental sources. But, the good news is, once we know about these outside stresses, we can indeed control them and improve or avoid depression (and thus, abuse).

Although women experience depression more often than men, men are more likely to commit suicide because of it -- especially if they are separated, widowed, or divorced. Men who have recently become unemployed and retired men are more likely to become depressed, and depression increases their risk of cardiovascular problems.

The average age of the onset of depression has continued to drop over the last 100 years and it's estimated that now there are 20 times more incidences of depression than in 1945. People are getting depressed more often and at younger ages.(9,10) Nearly 3 percent of children and over 8 percent of adolescents are considered depressed with pubescent girls twice as likely to experience it as pubescent boys. Suicide is the third leading cause of death for people between the ages of 15 and 24, and the sixth leading cause of death for children between the ages of 5 and 14.

Depression affects about 6 million elderly people in the U.S. As many as 20 percent of older adults and as many as 50 percent of those in nursing homes suffer from depression. This age group has the highest suicide rate.[11,12] Chronic illnesses (an illness that lasts for a long time and cannot be cured completely) predisposes a person towards depression. Up to one-third of individuals with chronic illnesses experience depression. Forty to 65 percent of people who have had a heart attack experience depression as do 40 percent of those with Parkinson's disease, 40 percent of those with multiple sclerosis, 25 percent of those with cancer or diabetes, and 25 percent of those who have had a stroke.[13]

The general treatment by the current medical community includes anti-depression drugs and psychotherapy. There are other, natural ways to get out of depression and we'll examine these in a minute. But first, let's look at the mainstream treatments and their problems.

Mild and less severe depression has responded to cognitive-behavioral therapy (CBT) (designed to modify thought patterns) and interpersonal therapy (IPT) (which focuses on the roles a person plays). These give support to the patient and a new way of looking at their situation. A psychologist or psychiatrist can help in this regard.

For more severe forms of depression, the doctor would typically prescribe an antidepressive drug. These include the newer selective serotonin reuptake inhibitors (SSRIs), the older tricyclic antidepressants (TCAs) and monoamine oxidase inhibitors (MAOIs).[14] Some people may respond to one class of drug, and not the others, and there's really no way of telling before hand which one that will be. So any prescription is just a guess by the doctor. Usually about 60 percent of patients are helped with the first drug prescription and 80 percent with the second. The patient is put on the drug for at least 4 - 6 months until recovery is noted and then another 6 months to prevent a relapse. But once off the drugs, recurrence of depression occurs more than 70 percent of the time, and many psychiatrists put patients on the pills for life – called "maintenance therapy."[15]

Drugs may alleviate the symptoms of depression, but they don't come without problems. One study showed that the SSRIs *Prozac* and *Paxil* can cause acute gastrointestinal bleeding.[16] Another study in 2004 showed that those taking *Prozac*, *Paxil*, *Zoloft*, and *Anafranil* had a three times greater risk of hospitalization for gastrointestinal bleeding or ulcers.[17] In very severe forms of depression, electroconvulsive therapy (ECT) may be used.

Food for Thought

Speaking of gastrointestinal bleeding, it also occurs from taking non-steroidal anti-inflammatory drugs (NSAIDs) such as aspirin, ibuprofen, and naproxen. In fact, gastrointestinal bleeding from these drugs is responsible for an estimated 16,500 deaths in the U.S. each year. So if you're on any of these for pain management or are taking an aspirin a day to keep your blood thin because you have heart disease, think again. You can get the same benefits from taking all natural foods like fish oil or krill oil – without the nasty side effects. I discuss NSAIDs more in the Arthritis chapter.

Adverse reactions to SSRI antidepressants, according to the Physician Desk Reference (PDR) include (the list below is the specific list for the antidepressant *Luvox* - others are similar):

Frequent: amnesia, apathy, hyperkinesis, hypokinesis, manic reaction, myoclonus, psychotic reaction; Infrequent: agoraphobia, akathisis, CNS depression, convulsion, delirium, delusion, depersonalization, drug dependence, emotional liability, euphoria, hallucinations, hostility, hysteria, incoordination, increased salivation, increased libido, paralysis, paranoid reaction, phobia, psychosis, sleep disorder, stupor, twitching, vertigo.[18]

These reactions are not just theory, either. They are based on clinical trials on the drugs in real people. I wonder how many doctors go over these possible adverse reactions with their patients before they prescribe them.

Amazingly, the prescription of antidepressant drugs for adolescents and children has increased dramatically – a 500 percent increase since 1998 – and now it's estimated that 10 million children in the U.S. are taking them. Soon these drugs will be used in youngsters as often as adults.[19,20]

Psychiatric drugs are even being prescribed to kids two to four years old for reasons such as bed-wetting, pain relief, anxiety, and ADHD. In 1991, 100,000 preschoolers were on these drugs, and by 1995, the number had jumped to 150,000 – a 50 percent increase.[21] This despite the fact that there is little evidence that these drugs work on children (that is, in the positive sense), that their use in children and not approved by the FDA, and that these antidepressants have been shown to cause suicides.

A scientist at the FDA reviewed 20 clinical trials of different antidepressants involving more than 4,100 children. He concluded that there was a definite link between kids who took antidepressants and suicidal behavior. But the FDA wouldn't let him publish his report. Instead, they substituted a report from doctors and professionals which avoided the suicide issue.[22] Even though the research shows that antidepressants can actually worsen depression and cause thoughts of suicide, and even though the FDA was forced to change the package insert for 10 of these antidepressants to reflect this, the sale of them keeps climbing. The use of these drugs by children is now growing by about 10 percent a year. (This class of drugs even outsell drugs that treat the heart, arteries, and blood pressure combined by $9 billion more in 2003 – $37 billion for antidepressants vs. $28 billion for heart medication).[23] Further proof that there's a problem is indicated by the fact that in early 2004, the United Kingdom banned nearly all antidepressants for kids due to the increase risk of suicide.(24)

It's not just suicide that happens more often when kids are put on these SSRIs. Violence happens too. Evelyn J. Pringle is an investigative journalist who has researched and written numerous articles about the U.S. drug policies for children. Below is a lengthy excerpt from one of her excellent articles concerning antidepressants and kids:

> Dr. Ann Blake Tracy is the Director of the International Coalition for Drug Awareness, holds a doctorate in biological psychology, and is a specialist in the adverse reactions to SSRI medications. . . Dr. Tracy can recite hundreds of horror stories involving violence by people taking the same drugs that TeenScreen is marketing to more children. "The professor on *Prozac* who bit her mother to death; the Stanford graduate on *Paxil* who stabbed herself in the kitchen while her parents slept; the mother who bludgeoned her son and then drank a can of *Drano*; and the 12-year-old girl who strangled herself with a bungee cord she attached to a plant hanger on the wall."
>
> "Most of these drugs are not approved for children, but it doesn't stop doctors from prescribing them," Tracy points out. Besides causing suicide, enough evidence now exists to prove that psychotropic drugs have played a major role in the senseless acts of violence by school-age children in the country in recent years... On April 15, 2001 16-year-old Cory Baadsgaard took a rifle to his high school in Washington State and held 23 classmates and a teacher hostage. Cory sat in jail for 14 months before finally being released based on expert testimony by psychiatrists that his behavior was an adverse reaction to the drugs he was prescribed. Cory has no memory of his actions at the school that day. Twenty-one days before the event, he had been taken off *Paxil* and prescribed a high dose of the drug *Effexor*. . . Cory's father Jay told *Insight News*. . . "The morning that Cory went to school and did what he did, my wife and I just knew that it had to be something with the drugs. . .One of Cory's friends described the incident to Jay, "Cory was yelling and then he just stopped, looked down and saw the gun in his hand and woke up. . ."
>
> It has never been revealed if Dylan Klebold [he and Eric Harris were the two teenagers who opened fire on their classmates at Columbine High School in April 1999] was on any legal drugs at the time of the shootings, but an autopsy revealed that Harris was on the psychotropic drug *Luvox*. . . Dr. Tracy says, "All you have to do is read the *Luvox* package insert to see that Eric's actions were due to an adverse reaction to this drug. . .Show me a drug anywhere that has listed mania and psychosis as frequent

adverse reactions. That is what the insert says for *Luvox*. There is no doubt in my mind that *Luvox* caused Eric Harris to commit these acts. . ."

A little known fact is that a few days before the Columbine Tragedy, Eric Harris had been rejected by the Marine Corps specifically because he was taking the drug *Luvox*.

In 2001, 18-year-old Jason Hoffman, shot five students and teachers at a California High School while on the drugs *Celexa* and *Effexor*, and he too was rejected by the Navy one day before he went on his rampage, according to the *San Diego Union-Tribune*.

In a letter to his mother, Hoffman said, "I want people to know that what happened was not the real me, I was just angry, maybe my medication. It was a fluke of the moment. The person was not the true Jason Hoffman," he wrote. On Oct. 29, 2001 Jason Hoffman killed himself by hanging from a vent screen in his jail cell, the *Tribune* reported.

Kip Kinkel was 15 on May 21, 1998, when he murdered his parents and then went to Thurston High School in Springfield, OR where he shot and killed two students and injured 22 more. Kinkel was on *Ritalin* and *Prozac* at the time of the killings even though *Prozac* was not approved for pediatric use. . . Seven years after the senseless killings by Kinkel, on December 18, 2003, Eli Lilly sent letter to British healthcare providers warning that *Prozac* was not recommended for any use in children.

Twelve-year-old Christopher Pittman was on *Zoloft* when he shot his grandparents and set their house on fire, and says his violence was caused by the drug he was on. Before *Zoloft*, he had been on *Paxil*.

Dr. Tracy explains how this happens. SSRIs suppress "the REM state or dream state (of sleep). . . These drugs allow a person to be awake but at any time they can slip into the REM state. This is why people often discuss how they couldn't tell the difference between the dream and reality. These drugs are horribly damaging to the entire system. . ."

Dr. Tracy has consulted on many cases where children engaged in violent behavior including one 15-year-old boy on *Zoloft* who shot and killed a woman and is serving life in prison; a 17-year-old boy on *Paxil* for three months who jumped off an overpass into the path of a trailer truck; a 14-year-old girl prescribed *Paxil* to deal with the suicide of her father (who was on *Paxil* before killing himself) drank Drano in a suicide attempt; and a 16-year-old boy on *Paxil* who stabbed a woman over 60 times, drove his car into a cement abutment in a failed suicide attempt and is now serving life in prison.

"In each of these cases," Tracy told *Insight News*, "individuals close to them were shocked at the violent and destructive behavior because it was so out of character for them."

Drug companies are finally starting to be held responsible for violent behavior associated with these drugs. A jury in Cheyenne, Wyoming recently determined that *Paxil* "can cause some individuals to commit suicide and/or homicide." The jury decided *Paxil* caused Donald Schell to shoot his wife, daughter, and granddaughter before killing himself after being on the drug only two days. The jury allocated 80% of the fault on *Paxil* drug maker GlaxoSmithKline and awarded the surviving family members $8 million in damages.

On June 18, 2003, GlaxSmithKline issued a warning to British physicians against the use of *Paxil* in children, acknowledging failure of clinical trials "to demonstrate efficacy in major depressive disorders and doubling the rate of reported adverse events – including suicidal thought and suicide attempts – compared to placebo."

In Bismarck, ND, 10 days after Ryan Ehlis began taking *Adderall*, he shot and killed his 5-week-old baby and then turned the gun on himself. He survived and was tried for the murder but was acquitted after the Judge agreed with psychiatrists who testified that the murder resulted solely from a psychotic state caused by the drug.

In February 2005, Canadian regulators ordered *Adderall* off the market after the drug was linked to 20 sudden deaths and a dozen strokes. Of the 20 deaths, 14 were children.

There has been a lot written about the increase in teen violence and school shootings but no one has identified a common denominator in the lives of these kids with one exception – the drugs. . ."We've got a nightmare on our hands with these drugs, an absolute nightmare," Tracy warns. "We've got kids on these drugs that are ticking time bombs in every school in America. When all this is over and we count up the dead, we're going to be in shock," she adds.(25)

Food for Thought

I marvel at the drug ads that are on TV these days – people running though the flowers happy as can be, or playing with their children and having the time of their lives. All thanks to that little pill they get from their friendly drug dealer. . . uh, excuse me. . . physician. How wonderful. "Side effects may include, drowsiness, lack of motivation, jumping off a cliff, stabbing yourself, shooting up your school, drowning your kids in the bathtub, or killing your wife and kids. Ask your doctor if _____ is right for you!!!"

Isn't it amazing that commercials like these actually work? A 1999 study by *Pharmaceutical Research* said that the TV ads got 24.7 million consumers to talk to their doctors about a medical condition they had never discussed before seeing the ads.(26) This kind of advertising is not allowed in Europe.

Then there are the prescription drugs for high cholesterol, prostatitis, incontinence, erectile dysfunction, attention deficit, high blood pressure, insomnia, and diabetes testing equipment. We never had all these commercials years ago. Back then all you saw were ads for *Alka-seltzer* and *Doans* pills. Ever wonder why?

In 1977 the FDA significantly relaxed guidelines for direct-to-consumer ads so that the volumes of side effects of the drugs need not be reported in the ad. A GaxoSmithKline spokesperson said the ads for *Paxil* "are critical. They do a lot. . .in encouraging people who may have the symptoms to come in and seek treatment." "[The advertising] really influences their sales dramatically. Patients are going into their doctors' offices and, before they have a diagnosis, they are saying, I want that *Paxil.*"(27) And 71 percent of patients who ask for a drug they had seen advertised leave the doctor's office with prescription for it.(28)

Then you see on the evening news how people get arrested for selling or smoking marijuana. People smoke it because it makes them feel better, so why don't they just make it legal? I've never heard of anyone committing suicide or shooting their classmates while high on pot. In fact, from what I've gathered, people become more agreeable and mellow. Although there are health risks associated with its use, they don't seem to be any worse than the risks of using antidepressants. In fact, they appear to me to be minor in comparison. But it's a plant that anyone can grow in their own backyard, and you can't get a patent on it, so that leaves the drug companies grasping at control. The guy selling pot on the street corner is a criminal and can go to jail, and the doctor, pharmacist, or drug company CEO pushing *Prozac,* which causes suicides and homicides, is considered an upstanding citizen and gets rich. Crazy world, isn't it? (I in no way advocate marijuana usage and in fact condemn any kind of drug, man-made or natural. I am only pointing out the hypocrisy and insanity of our current system.)

Looking over the literature, there's so many problems with these antidepressants it's hard to discuss them all, but I will mention a few more, without going into much detail. *Paxil* has been show to be ineffective in treating depression in people under the age of 18, and children taking it are twice as likely to have suicidal or self-harm thoughts. The British government therefore no longer allows *Paxil* to be prescribed to anyone less than 18 years of age.(29)

Prozac has been linked to an increase in certain kinds of brain tumors.(30) If a pregnant woman is on *Prozac*, her baby is more likely to have respiratory problems and be born lighter and sleepier than normal.(31)

Antidepressants are likely to cause a decrease in sex drive for both men and women. Up to 70 percent of those on antidepressants report sexual side effects.(32) Further, the drugs may impair the ability for someone to experience romance. Dr. Helen E. Fisher of Rutgers University and author of the book *Why We Love: The Nature and Chemistry of Romantic Love*, says, "We know that there are real sexual problems associated with serotonin-enhancing medications. But when you cripple a person's sexual desire and arousal, you're also jeopardizing their ability to fall in love and to stay in love. . . people should be aware that these drugs dull the emotions, including the positive ones that are central components of romantic love."(33)

Food for Thought

If all this isn't depressing enough, consider this: On April 29, 2002, U.S. President George W. Bush issued Executive Order 13263 establishing the New Freedoms Commission on Mental Health (NFC). It recommends screening all children for mental illness, and along with the TeenScreen program, will ensure that every student receives a mental health check-up before finishing high school. That's a potential 52 million school children being screened, and if determined a little "off," they will be recommended to be put on drugs. (Already, 10 million children in the U.S are now taking these mind-altering drugs even though, as we've seen, they can cause suicide, mania, psychosis, and homicide.) Further, eventually every person in America will be screened for mental illness. And once screened and determined to have a mental problem, will be recommended treatment. And what do you think that treatment might consist of? Drugs, perhaps?

The NFC used the Texas Medication Algorithm Project (TMAP) as its model, which also screens people for mental health problems and prescribed high-profit prescription drugs to them. (Wasn't George Bush governor of Texas?)

An article by columnist Mike Adams says the NFC is. . .

". . .poised to consolidate the TMAP into a comprehensive national policy to treat mental illness with expensive patented medications of questionable benefits and deadly side effects. So, at first glance, it certainly appears that this is no more than a good old boy strategy for boosting the profits of pharmaceutical companies through political influence – it's the same old game. . . Just how much support has come from these companies? The Bush administration has very close financial ties to the pharmaceutical industry. . .George Bush, Sr. was also a member of Eli

Lilly's board of directors, and George Bush, Jr. Appointed Eli Lilly's Chief Executive Officer to a seat on the Homeland Security Council. . .Eli Lilly made $1.6 million in political contributions in 2000. Four-fifths of that went to the Republican Party and presidential candidate Bush. It is, in fact the same company that started up the Texas project. And now, many members of the New Freedom Commission have also been found to have ties with pharmaceutical companies and have served on their advisory boards. . .Under the Bush administration, the pharmaceutical industry has done extremely well in terms of boosting sales and generating profits. And it looks like the Bush administration is determined to continue the drugging of America, no matter what the cost to American taxpayers. They won't stop, it seems, until every American is dosed up on a dozen simultaneous prescriptions that generate tens of billions of dollars in profits for the pharmaceutical industry each year. People don't need mandatory screening for mental health disorders. They don't need to be put on multiple prescription drugs that turn them into zombies and may, in fact, cause them to commit suicide or engage in violent acts. . .We don't need more bombs, more drugs and more government-mandated health initiatives that masquerade as good science while in reality only offer another financial trap that will push Americans even further into household debt and poverty. . .If there's any mandatory mental health screening that should be taking place, it should start with the officials running the Bush administration, and then continue on to take a look at the people running the FDA, and those in charge of the pharmaceutical companies. Because from all the available evidence, it appears to me that these people have lost their minds in a mad attempt to generate obscene profits regardless of the cost to human life, individual privacy, and human rights. . .Above all, to call this new plan the 'New Freedom Commission' is perhaps the ultimate insult to the intelligence of the American people. . .Dosing people up with prescription drugs that alter their brain chemistry and take away their normal healthy brain function is not freedom. In fact, it is chemical enslavement, and the perpetrators behind this diabolical plan are truly the enemies of freedom, democracy, and the ideals that America historically stands for."(34)

I don't care what your politics are. With all the money that's being and can be made pushing drugs on people (antidepressants accounted for $11.2 billion in sales worldwide in 2004 – up from just $240 million in 1986 – and if you include antipsychotic drugs, sales were nearly $20 billion in 2004)(35), any reasonable person has to at least consider that something other than the people's best interests may be determining public policies. If that is in fact the case, it's "just plain wrong." And here's just how wrong it may be? The government is using your tax dollars to fund programs that will push people into using drugs. In effect, the pharmaceuticals are getting governmental assistance to sell more drugs, with our government paying the bills.

Evelyn Pringle, in her article *Big Pharma Bankrupting U.S. Health Car System,* says that the pharmaceutical industry ". . . is bankrupting the nation's health care system by convincing prescribing doctors to over-medicate patients with expensive psychiatric drugs and then send the bills to government programs like Medicaid and Medicare. . .Medicaid alone spends an estimated $3 billion a year for these antipsychotic medications."(36)

This over-drugging is happening to children and the elderly alike. The mass drugging of children on Medicaid is happening all over the country. In 2001, psychiatrist Dr. Stefan Kruszewski, was hired to review psychiatric care provided by government-funded agencies in Pennsylvania to identify fraud, waste, and abuse, and found cases of what he refers to as "insane polypharmacy," where children were placed in state-run treatment facilities and over-medicated with the new antipsychotic and anticonvulsants sometimes for years.

Two years ago, Brian Flood, the Texas Health and Human Services' Inspector General, and Texas Comptroller Carole Deeton Strayhorn, began reviewing information on how doctors were prescribing stimulants, antidepressants and antipsychotic to children on Medicaid. The studies revealed that children were being prescribed multiple psychiatric drugs and some children as young as 3 were taking the mood-altering medications. Ms. Strayhorn's study found a case where one child had 14 prescriptions for 11 different mediations, at a cost of $1,088 a month. Mr. Flood's review of a two-month period of Medicaid records determined that 63,118 children were on stimulants, antidepressants or antipsychotic, with nearly one-third of the kids taking drugs from more than one of the 3 classes of drugs at the same time. The review of records found that doctors had filed 114,315 claims amounting to more than $17 million for the children. Drug makers have found ways to influence prescribers who tend to the elderly in nursing homes to funnel Medicare funds to Big Pharma through senior citizens. In one 2003 study published in the *Archives of Internal Medicine*, researchers found that 75 percent of long-term care elderly residents were receiving psychotropic medications.

Another study published in August 2004 *Archives of Internal Medicine*, noted that 41 percent of prescriptions, for 765,423 people over age 65, were for psychotropic medications. A more recent June 13, 2005, study in the *Archives* examined the quality of antipsychotic prescriptions in nursing homes for approximately 2.5 million Medicaid beneficiaries and found that "over half (58.2%)," received drugs that exceeded the maximum recommended dosage, received duplicate therapy, or under the guidelines, had inappropriate conditions for the medications to begin with. The study determined that more than 200,000 residents received antipsychotic therapy but had "no appropriate indications for use." On May 1, 2006, the *London Free Press* reported a study by Toronto's Institute for Clinical Evaluative Sciences that showed seniors who were prescribed the new SSRIs such as *Prozac, Paxil,* and *Zoloft* were nearly 5 times more likely to commit suicide during the first month on the drugs than those patients given the older class of medications used to treat depression.

Pediatrician Dr. Lawrence Diller, Author of the book, *Should I Medicate My Child,* testified before an FDA advisory committee in September 2004 on the rampant off-label prescribing of SSRI drugs to children after learning about eight previously undisclosed studies that proved the drug makers knew all along that SSRIs were linked to suicide in children but kept the findings hidden from doctors who were prescribing the drugs. Dr. Diller said the final blow was learning of these eight studies and that the loss of credibility within the medical profession extended beyond psychiatry into all of medicine and ended his testimony by stating: "The blame is clear: The money, power and influence of the pharmaceutical industry corrupts all. The pervasive control that the drug companies have over medical research, publications, professional organizations, doctors' practices, Congress, and yes, even agencies like the FDA, is the American equivalent of a drug cartel."(37)

To show you just how far this corruption can reach, parents can be charged with child abuse or neglect crimes if they take their child off of their prescription psychiatric drugs.(38)

It's estimated that every day between 3,000 and 5,000 North Americans begin taking *Paxil.*(That's just one of a dozen or so SSRIs) There were 25 million new prescriptions written for the drug in 2001 alone.(39) There's another estimate that as many as 10 percent of Americans have at one time taken a serotonin booster kind of drug.(40)

Although according to the Association of American Physicians and Surgeons, psychiatric drugs are no more effective or safer in treating mental disorders than non-drug treatments or older, less expensive drugs, children in foster care are put on them all too often: 60 percent of foster care kids in Texas; 66 percent in Massachusetts; and 55 percent in Florida take psychiatric drugs. That's simply astounding again considering that these drugs were designed to treat adults, and no real studies have been done on their effects in children.(41) To boggle the mind even more, if a parent of a child on the drugs, or an adult who is taking the drugs, complains of an adverse reaction, it is commonly dismissed as anecdotal or unscientific. This when the drugs have no scientific studies supporting their claims.

As far as helping someone feel better, antidepressant drugs don't work much better than taking a placebo. In fact, one analysis of published clinical trials showed that 75 percent of the response to antidepressants can be duplicated by a placebo – and that just 18 percent of the drug response is in fact due to the actual drug itself.(42) Dr. Michael Browne is a psychologist in Minneapolis and in private practice for 25 years and on the University of Minnesota faculty. He's done his own research on antidepressants. He said, "I was just completely astounded by what I found. The claims for the effectiveness of antidepressants were greatly exaggerated. I looked closely at the evidence, and it's not there. . .And I found that the evidence was exaggerated not just for antidepressants, but for virtually every single psychiatric medication." Dr. Browne says more. . .

> You know where psychiatrists get their information? They get their information from the drug companies. . .Twenty years ago people thought of depression as an emotion – depression meant you were sad. . .The drug companies have done an exceedingly good job of convincing us all that depression is a medical disease. . .And it's not really so surprising that these medications don't work. If a person is very seriously unhappy, and it goes on for months and months, what does that mean? That means there's something very seriously wrong in that person's life. It's not for trivial reasons. And common sense tells us it's not likely to be easy to change that.(43)

Food for Thought

Even a senior executive with GlaxoSmithKline pharmaceuticals admits that their drugs don't work that often. Allen Roses, the worldwide vice-president of genetics at GlaxoSmithKline, said, "The vast majority of drugs – more than 90 percent – only work in 30 or 50 percent of the people. I wouldn't say that most drugs don't work. I would say that most drugs work in 30 to 50 percent of people."

Here's an overview of drugs for specific illnesses and the percentages that they help someone (e.g. 30 percent means it helps 30 out of 100 people who take the drug):

Alzheimer's - 30%	Asthma - 60%
Depression (SSRI) - 62%	Diabetes - 57%
Incontinence - 40%	Migraine - 52%
Cancer - 25%	Rheumatoid arthritis - 50%
Schizophrenia - 60%	Hepatitis C - 47% (44)

So most drugs work *as intended* only about half the time – and 75 percent of this response could be from the placebo effect. But I believe that any drug in any dose for any condition has a negative impact on the human body – visible or not – insofar as it's an unnatural substance the body must deal with.

If you take an antidepressant, watch out if you ever try to quit. Not only is it next to impossible for some people to go off the drugs, some people suffer terrible and debilitating withdrawal symptoms if they try. In Europe, patients are warned that coming off *Paxil* could trigger severe withdrawal symptoms; while in America, it's advertised as non habit-forming.(45) Although the drug companies say that these symptoms rarely occur, there have been numerous law suits involving thousands of people against the drug companies because they weren't warned about the addictive nature of the drugs and the problems of going off of them.

Food for Thought

When *Valium* was introduced years ago, it was hailed as a breakthrough because, as the manufacturer drug giant Roche claimed, it was not addictive. A few years later, it was the number one cause of addiction in the U.S.

Then came *Xanax*, made by another big pharmaceutical company Upjohn. They said *Xanax* was better than *Valium* because it wasn't addictive. Then *Xanax* became the number one cause of prescription drug addiction.(46)

Now all the "experts" tell you that SSRI's are not addictive. Many drug company sponsored studies "prove" this. (Remember, as Mark Twain said, "There are lies, there are damn lies, and then there are statistics.")

What's that saying? "Fool me once, shame on you. Fool me twice, shame on me." *Valium*, then *Xanax*. They fooled us even more than once – they fooled us twice (so shame on us). And now they're trying to fool us again.

Withdrawal symptoms may include dizziness, sensory disturbances, anxiety, nausea, sweating, panic attacks, crying spells, problems with balance, shock-like electrical sensations, gastrointestinal problems, and sleep disturbances. Symptoms start within 24 to 72 hours after discontinuing the drug and may persist for weeks. The incidence of withdrawal symptoms are highest with *Paxil*, followed by *Luvox* and *Zoloft*, followed by *Celexa* and *Prozac*.(47) The drug industry doesn't call it "withdrawal" (like someone on the street would call it), they have to make it sound scientific, so they call it *Antidepressant Discontinuation Syndrome*.

Whatever you name it, coming off these drugs can be a nightmare. Dr. Joseph Glenmullen, a clinical instructor in psychiatry at Harvard Medical School says, "We see withdrawal symptoms that can be so severe that patients feel held hostage to the antidepressant."(48) Dr. Glenmullen is also author of the book *Prozac Backlash*, a good book to read if you're taking an antidepressant. Another good book is *Prozac: Panacea or Pandora?* by Ann Blake Tracy, Ph.D.

Dr. David Healy, a renowned psycho pharmacologist, had this to say in a Federal Court case about whether ads for *Paxil* were misleading the public saying that *Paxil* was non habit-forming (which would incorrectly indicate there would be no withdrawal symptoms).

> . . .Between 5,000 and 7,000 people start on *Paxil* daily. Of these, approximately 70% are in North America (between 3,000 to 5,000 people). Of these patients, at least one-third will have difficulties with withdrawal symptoms. That is, at least 1,000 to 2,000 Americans per day enter the risk pool. Of these, 1,000 to 2,000, at least 10% will have severe problems either in terms of the duration of withdrawal or in terms of the severity of the medical complications. Accordingly, approximately 200 Americans per day are entering the risk pool for serious problems as a result of the *Paxil*, and this rate of flow of patients is being increased due to the direct-to consumer advertising stating that *Paxil* is not addictive, non-dependence producing, and non habit-forming.[49]

The judge fortunately ruled that the ads were misleading and forced GlaxoSmithKline to discontinue showing them, saying, "Indeed, the *Paxil* labeling in other countries warns of withdrawal reactions following discontinuation of *Paxil*."

Food for Thought

Why do you think there are warnings of withdrawal reactions with *Paxil* in other countries? Do you think it's because the pharmaceutical company is doing it on their own? I don't think so! It's because the other countries' health departments forced them to say it. Just another piece of evidence showing who *really* determines public policy in the U.S.

Just in case you're wondering and as an example of the complexity and toxicity of an SSRI, here's the chemical formula of *Paxil*:

$C_{19}H_{20}FNO_3$-HCL- ½ H_2O (the F is fluoride). Each tablet also contains dibasic calcium phosphate dihydrate, hydroxypropyl methylcellulose, magnesium stearate, polyethylene glycols, polysorbate 80, sodium starch glycolate, titanium dioxide, and one or more of the following: D&C Red No. 30, D&C Yellow No 10, FD&C Blue No 2, FD&C Yellow No 6.[50]

I don't know why they would care what color the pills are – I guess they want it to look appealing. . . "Look, honey, the pill is orange! Don't you want to eat an orange pill?"

If someone does decide to go off these drugs, they should do it very, very slowly under a doctor's supervision. Quitting "cold turkey" can be more dangerous than staying on the drugs. This is VERY IMPORTANT! Do NOT try to go off of these drugs without medical supervision!

My advice is to avoid these ineffective, habit forming, expensive pills altogether. If you or someone you know is on them, start as soon as you can to go off them – again, with medical supervision. There's a lot of natural ways to address depression and other psychological issues that and most of the time will do the job, without disastrous side effects.

Food for Thought

There's a new device that was recently approved by the FDA to treat depression, so you may start hearing about it. It's a device that's surgically implanted in the upper chest that stimulates a nerve leading to the brain. In the one clinical trial run on the device, it was shown to be totally ineffective in helping those with depression and had a number of nasty side effects. In fact, the scientific staff at the FDA itself rejected it. One member of the FDA even said, "As an M.D. interested in science, it seems to me that such an approval would be akin to approving an experimental product." However, the director of the Center for Devices and Radiological Health at the FDA, Dr. Daniel G Schultz, approved it anyway.(51) The manufacturer contends that it's the only option for those with chronic, treatment-resistant depression, even though the clinical results show otherwise. But I'm sure there's big money at stake here, so this ineffective, potentially harmful device gets approved by the man in charge. Who's he working for, anyway?

Here's some more juicy tidbits about our all caring FDA: More than half of the money the FDA spends reviewing drugs comes from the drug industry itself; 80 percent of the FDA's resources are geared towards approving new drugs; only 5 percent of the FDA's resources go into ensuring drug safety. The following was taken from an interview with Dr. David Graham, the senior drug safety researcher at the FDA who has worked there for 20 years. He said,

"As currently configured, the FDA is not able to adequately protect the American public. It's more interested in protecting the interests of industry. It views industry as its client, and the client is someone whose interest you represent. Unfortunately, that is the way the FDA is currently structured. Within the Center for Drug Evaluation and Research about 80 percent of the resources are geared towards the approval of new drugs and 20 percent is for everything else. Drug safety is about 5 percent. The 'gorilla in the living room' is new drugs and approval. Congress has not only created that structure, they have also worsened that structure through the PDUFA, the Prescription Drug User Fee Act, by which drug companies pay money to the FDA so they will review and approve its drug. So you have that conflict as well. . .Death from adverse drug reactions is one of the leading causes of death in the United States. It turns out that most of these adverse reactions are actually what are expected in the sense that they are an extension of the drug's action. For example, we know that drugs for diabetes can lower your blood sugar. If you're more sensitive to the drug than the normal person, it lowers your blood sugar too much, causing you to have a seizure while driving your car, and you get killed, well, you died from an adverse drug reaction, but it wasn't something unexpected.

"The blood thinner *Coumadin* is another example. That drug provides a benefit, but it is also responsible for probably more deaths than any single drug currently marketed. But it has a recognized benefit and there aren't other drugs to do what it does or to do what it does well. So physicians accept that there are patients who are in a serious situation and who might die without the drug, so they take it.

"Yes, drugs cause a lot of harm. Unfortunately, we haven't quantified the benefits. For most of these drugs it's more belief. It's faith. We have faith that they'll confer a benefit, but the FDA hasn't demonstrated that they confer a benefit. We're getting much better at quantifying the risks. In the future what we need to do is just take the risks and look hard and dispassionately at what the real benefits are. If the benefits aren't there we shouldn't be having discussions about labeling the drug. You need to weed the garden patch of drugs that aren't doing what they're supposed to do. The FDA has not been very good about that; it likes to cultivate all these weeds."(52)

For more on the corruption at the FDA, check out Dr. Gary Null's *Prescription for Disaster* video documentary available at his website, garynull.com.

Natural Ways to Beat Depression

An obvious way to beat depression is counseling. Most of the time people get depressed not because of a chemical imbalance (as the drug companies want you to believe), but because there's something wrong in their life. Cognitive Behavioral Treatment (CBT) can help people handle their emotions better and provide tools for dealing with future issues. Research has shown that oftentimes psychotherapy is superior to medication in the long run.

Just talking things out can be a big help to most. Personal communication – a relationship with a therapist, friend, or family member – can do wonders. It's a necessary part of life, whether someone has mental problems or not. Dr. Browne says,

> Whether it's a child's mental health problems or an adult's, no mental health problem grows out of a vacuum. They grow out of the contest of the relationships that they exist in. The way I understand it, bears spend a lot of time alone in the woods. That's just how the biology of bears is. Their biology suits them to spend

months at a time in the woods eating nuts and berries. That's not true for human beings. For the millions of years of our biological history, we are beings that can only live in relationships. That's a fundamental fact of human nature, that we have to have relationships. And whatever the mental health problem is – whether it's depression, or anxiety, or schizophrenia – you have to look at the network of relationships within which that person has lived their life. And if you ignore that, you've missed the boat.(53)

So if you're feeling blue, don't be afraid to open the lines of communication with a loved one. If that's not possible or realistic, then go to a counselor and pay someone to listen to you. (They *have* to be interested in your problems then!) If you can't afford that, then get on the internet and search for free counseling or suicide prevention hot lines. At least you can get things off your chest, and a counselor may have different perspectives on your problems that will help you deal with them. Whether it's a family issue, chronic pain issues, fear, obsession, compulsion or whatever, talking about it is usually therapeutic.

There are also some self-help methods that can do wonders. I've experimented with quite a few myself to deal with stresses, and they can oftentimes make life go a lot smoother. I already mentioned *Brain Gym* (www.braingym.com) in the chapter on ADHD. Although the *Brain Gym* exercises may not seem like they will solve your problems directly, they help your mind function better, which will help you handle the stress and keep you from making more bad decisions that compound your problems.

Other self-help methods are the Sedona Method (www.sedonapress.com) and, the Emotional Freedom Technique (or EFT, www.emofree.com)

EFT is easier to use and can be done easily on yourself with little mental effort, and on children, adults, or the elderly without them even knowing it. The best way to describe it is that it's psychological acupressure. You probably know what acupuncture is – where they stick needles into your body in certain areas to stimulate certain nerve pathways. Well, with EFT, you tap on certain places of your body while talking or thinking about your problems. This tapping stimulates your nervous system to eliminate the "hang-ups" you have about that particular problem, allowing your nervous system and mind to relax. It's proven to work wonders with many people who are depressed.

There have also been great results with EFT for dealing with all sorts of phobias, anxieties, and habits. The originator of EFT, Gary Craig, has treated hundreds of veterans with post-traumatic stress disorder. These men have had nightmares, insomnia, cold sweats, and other symptoms from remembering what they went through in battle. Often time, after just a session or two, their symptoms are eliminated and never come back. The vets say that they still remember the events, but they simply don't trigger the emotional response any longer. Parents who learn EFT can tap on their child when he or she is upset and it calms them down. There are many reports of a child yelling and screaming and making a scene, and after a couple minutes of tapping, they calm down and behave. There are numerous M.D.s, Ph.D.s, and therapists who use EFT as part of their practice. Using EFT can help you deal with just about any issue you may have, including how to handle coming off antidepressant drugs. So give it a look. I think you'll be pleasantly surprised at how much it can help you and your family. A very good EFT practitioner is Dale Paula Teplitz at www.daleteplitz.com.

Psychological issues like being abused as a child, getting divorced, losing a loved one, being raped, etc., naturally can have devastating impacts on our lives. That's where counseling or EFT can help. But how well a person handles these problems and can come to some kind of peace with them can also be affected by how balanced the person is physiologically and biochemically. Someone with normal nerves and neurotransmitters will naturally be able to deal with a difficult time in their lives easier than someone who is imbalanced.

These days, I believe many people who are depressed have some biochemical imbalance that makes it difficult for them to be happy or content, and these imbalances lead to poor decisions that lead to upsets in our lives. We've already looked at some toxins that cause people to behave abnormally such as like lead, mercury, pesticides, fluoride, and others. I show in the section on fluoride (in the chapter on osteoporosis) that the primary active ingredient in *Prozac* (as in other SSRIs) is a fluoride compound – specifically fluorine. Fluorine is also the active ingredient in rat poison and many pesticides and sodium fluoride is added to public water supplies (which then ends up in our food).

Food for Thought

One of the first occurrences of fluoridated drinking water was found in Germany's Nazi prison camps. In the book *The Crime and Punishment of I.G. Farben*, author Joseph Borkin relates that the Gestapo had little concern about fluoride's supposed effect on teeth; their alleged reason for mass-medicating water with sodium fluoride was to sterilize humans and force the people in their concentration camps into calm submission.

As you will see in a future chapter, sterility is fast becoming a major problem in this country. Part of the reason for it, I believe, is because of the use of fluoride in our drinking water, medications, toothpaste, and food.

The other thing to be concerned about is how fluoride tends to make us calm and submissive. It appears to me that the general public in America just doesn't care about things like they used to. Everyone seems to be giving up. In the sixties and seventies, there were protests about the war in Vietnam, black power, and women's rights. Recently, not so much. People are more concerned whether they have enough chips to munch on while watching their big-screen TV, if they have enough minutes on their cell-phone, or what the celebrities are up to. I don't know if this is what the government and industries are intending or not. It sure doesn't look like they're doing anything to slow it down or stop it, however. All the research and data I am revealing in this book is just as available to them as it is to me and you – so you would think they would consider it when making public policy or designing a drug or product. I guess the question to ask is, "Does submissive behavior bring more profits?" If so, then they're probably all for it.

Consider that in August 2006, the FDA approved the fumigating of fruits and vegetables with a concentrated fluoride gas that will leave, according to some studies, a residue of at least 70 ppm. Fluoridated drinking water has about 4 ppm fluoride.(54)

Another ingredient in antidepressants is chlorine. Chlorine causes birth defects. A Swedish study showed that women who take *Paxil* are twice as likely to have a baby with cardiovascular malformations.(55) In February 2006, the FDA approved revisions to the drugs safety label to indicate the increased risk of birth defects. How many doctors are aware of this, and how many would tell their patients? Low birth weight is more likely if the mother was taking *Paxil*, and infants who were breastfed by mothers taking *Prozac* grow significantly slower than normal.(56,57) Women are more likely to get depressed. What's this say about future generations?

Fluoride is also known to suppress thyroid function; and low thyroid function can cause depression. So a person on antidepressants gets in a vicious cycle: They're depressed and then take a pill that causes more depression.

Low thyroid function, or hypothyroidism, is in fact a major cause of depression. Up to 20 percent of all chronically depressed people may be depressed because of an under active thyroid.(58) I would say that it's even a higher percentage than that, because there's an estimated 13 million Americans who have a thyroid problem and don't realize it (undiagnosed cases). So the first thing you should do if you think you might have a medical reason for being depressed, is to check and see if you have a thyroid problem. If you're going to a doctor because of depression (and low blood sugar), ask him/her about this (Don't be surprised if they dismiss your suggestion, however; and if they refuse to consider it, I would get a different doctor.) This goes for children too. As we're learning, diseases are showing up in people earlier and earlier in life, so although hypothyroidism usually manifests in middle age or later, it could still occur in children and teenagers. We'll find out how to self-check for hypothyroidism a little later.

The thyroid can be overactive too, and this is called hyperthyroidism. But the vast majority of thyroid problems are an under-active, hypothyroid and that's what we will focus on here. Other diseases of the thyroid include goiter (enlarged thyroid and usually under-active), thyroiditis or Hashimotos disease (inflammation causing either hyper or hypothyroidism), Graves disease (hyperthyroidism) and, lumps or nodules, which may be cancerous.

It's estimated that about 27 million Americans have some form of thyroid disease – half of them being undiagnosed as having it. It's the most common glandular disorder after the pancreas (diabetes). Women are four times as likely as men to develop thyroid problems – one out of eight women has a thyroid condition, and women are even more likely to have an impaired thyroid soon after giving birth.(59)

The thyroid gland is a small, butterfly-shaped gland at the base of the neck over the trachea, or windpipe. Its job is to extract iodine from blood to produce two hormones – thyroxine (T_4), and triiodothyronine (T_3) – that regulate the energy usage of every cell and organ in the body. If there are not enough of these two hormones, everything in your body tends to slow down. Symptoms include chronic fatigue, feeling cold, diminished concentration, and memory and weight gain. In time, the symptoms get worse and may include dry skin and brittle nails, constipation, muscle aches, or cramps, PMS, slow heart rate and longer menstrual periods with heavier flow, erectile dysfunction, and hair loss (especially on the outer part of the eyebrow). Since the disease brings about irregular ovulation, untreated women may have trouble conceiving and they also have a higher-than-normal rate of miscarriages and premature delivery.(60)

The standard way a doctor will test for thyroid disease is to perform a blood test to determine the level of Thyroid Stimulating Hormone (TSH). TSH is a hormone that's secreted by the pituitary gland. High levels of TSH mean you have an under active thyroid. Low levels mean you have an overactive one. Although this test has been the benchmark used by the medical profession, researchers are now learning that previously considered "normal" TSH levels could still cause hypothyroidism. One doctor reports that 90 percent of his patients he diagnoses with hypothyroidism have completely normal TSH levels.(61) Because of this, millions of people who are currently on thyroid medications are not getting the proper kinds and amounts of medicine to totally alleviate symptoms.(62) Other ways to check for hypothyroidism can be done at home. One is called the Barnes basal body temperature (BBT) test. Here's how you do it:

Get an oral thermometer (don't use a digital one) and shake it down before you go to bed at night and put it on your nightstand. In the morning, before getting up or moving around, place it under your arm in your armpit and hold it there for 10 minutes. While you're lying there, take your pulse rate too. Simply put your forefinger and middle finger from one hand over the wrist of the other arm where the veins are and feel around for the pulse. Count the number of heartbeats for 15 seconds, and then multiply by four to get the beats per minute. When the 10 minutes are up, take the temperature reading, and write it down. Do this every morning for at least four days straight. The normal basal temperature is 97.8 degrees F to 98.2 degrees F. If your average temperature for the four days is from 97.6 to 98 degrees F, then you could have hypothyroidism. If your average is below 97.6, you probably do have hypothyroidism. If your pulse rate is below 65, then you may have a lower functioning thyroid also. For women, you want to do the test starting the second day of menses so your hormones released at other times of your cycle don't increase your body temperature.

The traditional medical answer to hypothyroidism is to replace the hormones the under active thyroid is not producing with the synthetic drug levothyroxine, trade name *Synthroid* (other trade names include *Levothroid* and *Levoxyl*). It's one of the top selling drugs in the U.S., so it just goes to show you how prevalent hypothyroidism is.

But getting the right dose of *Synthroid* – which is strictly T_4 – can be tricky, and some researchers believe that some people would be better off taking a drug that included T_3 as well. Some doctors prescribe a natural product that is the desiccated thyroid gland of pigs (trade name *Armour Thyroid*), thinking it's superior to the synthetic drugs since it contains all the thyroid hormones. Personally, I believe taking the desiccated thyroid would be better for you than taking isolated synthetic hormone. An article in the *New England Journal of Medicine* reported that natural hormones are far superior, especially with respect to brain function and mood.[63] Undoubtedly, taking these products can help someone feel better. But there is a reason someone's thyroid gland goes bad, so let's see if we can improve the situation by working on the causes instead of the symptoms.

A cause of thyroid disease may be the lack of sufficient iodine in the diet. That's why common table salt is fortified with iodine. But that form of iodine is not ideal, and many people are on salt restricted diets these days, so just getting iodine in salt may not be enough.

Fish is a good source of iodine, but it's also contaminated and a lot of people don't eat that much of it these days. So if you think you may be hypothyroid, check to see if you have enough iodine in your system with the iodine patch test described below. If you are iodine deficient, consider eating foods rich in iodine such as beef liver, turkey, asparagus, white onions, broccoli, fish, kelp and other seaweeds.

Conversely, there are foods that rob the body of iodine. These are called goitrogenic foods because they promote goiters and the development of hypothyroidism. These foods are cabbage, kale, soy products, horseradish, mustard, corn, broccoli, turnips, carrots, peaches, strawberries, peanuts, Brussels sprouts, rutabaga, turnips kohlrabi, radishes, cauliflower, millet, spinach, watercress, mustard greens, and walnuts. If you have or suspect you have a under active thyroid, you should limit the consumption of these foods. Cooking tends to lessen the severity of the thyroid-suppressing effects of most of these. I go into much more detail on iodine and just how important it is in the chapter on breast cancer. Everyone is encouraged to read it.

Check for an iodine deficiency by doing the iodine patch test or have an iodine-loading test done (see breast cancer chapter). Women on estrogen replacement therapy (ERT) need to be careful when it comes to their thyroid, since ERT can make thyroid hormones less available in the bloodstream, possibly causing hypothyroid symptoms.

If you are deficient in iodine, the best way to correct it is to eat foods rich in iodine, but the right supplement is OK. Seaweeds are the richest source of iodine. They include kelp (kombu in Japanese), nori, wakame, and dulse. You can find dried versions of all of these at any health food store. Kelp and dulse come in flakes in shaker-bottles so you can use them like salt from a saltshaker. It's best to get seaweeds that have been harvested by hand and dried naturally without any additives. There are iodine supplements, the best being *Nascent Iodine* (see Resource Guide), and sometimes I feel supplementation is warranted. But it's always best to get your nutrition from food as much as possible.

Food for Thought

I went into detail on iodine in the chapter on breast cancer, but here's more: Potassium iodide (SSKI) is recommended by public health authorities (usually in tablet form) as a way to protect the thyroid gland if a nuclear bomb goes off or a nuclear power plant melts down. It's also used in hospitals to prepare someone for thyroid surgery. But there are other uses of SSKI. Johathan V. Wright, M.D. And medical director of the Tahoma Clinic says that SSKI can be added to water that may be contaminated with microorganisms to avoid infections – just add a few drops to a glass of water. It's also useful in eliminating bladder infections and if applied to open acne pimples, clears them up in a day or two.

Dr. Wright reports that "6 to 8 drops of SSKI taken in a few ounces of water daily will frequently reduce fibrocystic breast disease to insignificance within three to six months."(64) He continues, "at least thirty other women I've worked with in nearly 30 years have helped ovarian cysts disappear within two to three months with the same quantity of SSKI. Again, make sure to monitor your thyroid function!" (Note: A new product called *Nascent Iodine* is even more effective than SSKI. See the Resource Guide.)

Thick scars (called Keloids), fistulas, and sebaceous cysts can be lessened or healed by rubbing SSKI on them a couple times a day. Sebaceous cysts are cysts that contain oily, fatty material that usually appear on the face, groin, or labia. The iodine dissolves the fatty, oily material allowing your body to slowly reabsorb and dispose of it. In fact, iodine makes fats, oils, and waxes (cholesterol is a wax) more soluble in water. One study showed that taking iodine for several months actually reversed atherosclerotic clogging of arteries. Dr. Wright said, "I recommend 4 to 6 drops of SSKI and niacin-containing B-complex daily. . .for anyone with significant cholesterol-related atherosclerotic clogging. Thyroid function must be monitored!" Is it any wonder, then, that cultures that eat diets rich in seafood, which is high in iodine, have less cardiovascular disease?

Since SSKI can soften and sometimes eliminate scars, it's useful in the treatment of Peyronie's disease, a thickening along the shaft of the penis, making erections curved and painful. Rubbing SSKI into the thickened tissue twice daily softens and lessens the fibrotic area over a period of several months, allowing for more normal function.

SSKI can also help: bronchitis or emphysema (COPD); swollen glands in the throat or groin areas; fungus under toenails; infected hangnails; vaginal infections; and, if you soak beans in water with SSKI for an hour or so before cooking, you won't get nearly as much intestinal gas! (That's true, but I don't recommend you ever eat beans since they are so difficult to digest.)

Lugol's Solution is another medically useful iodine product, but I am not sure if it can be used the same as SSKI. Potassium iodide can have interactions with other prescription medications, so be sure to check with your doctor before using it.

Oftentimes people get hypothyroidism because their adrenal glands are worn out, upsetting the body's hormonal balance. The thyroid fights to compensate, but eventually wears out. Adrenal exhaustion is common in people that have to handle a lot of stress. So keep this in mind and try to relax. You don't always need to "sweat the small stuff."

Eating soy products can also lead to hypothyroidism. I devote a whole section to the problems with soy later in the book. Suffice it to say here that soy is a terrible food, and should always be avoided (except naturally fermented soy). Remember, fluoride suppresses thyroid function. So it's important to drink water that doesn't have it. This includes most municipal water supplies. Commercial products like orange juice, other fruit juices, baby formula, soft drinks, and sport drinks all have significant amounts of fluoride. Use toothpaste that doesn't contain fluoride.

One thing to avoid for good thyroid health is smoking. Smoking contains the heavy metal cadmium, which directly suppresses thyroidal function and indirectly suppresses it by inhibiting the action of zinc, which stimulates the thyroid. So although smoking may seem to give you a lift, in the long run it's running you and your thyroid down. Ladies, smoking is also believed to trigger early menopause and affect fertility.

Taking care of your thyroid is one of the best things you can do to avoid or get out of depression but there are other things that will help too. The brain is mostly fat, and half of that fat is DHA (one of the omega-3 fats). If the brain is not fed correctly, it won't operate correctly. So getting enough of the right kind of fats is critically important to how your brain functions, including whether you're depressed or not.

A lot of research in the past few years has shown this to be true. Specifically, the getting enough omega-3 fatty acids have been shown to help prevent and reverse depression. Low omega-3 levels in the blood are linked to major depression, bipolar disorder, schizophrenia, substance abuse, and attention deficit disorder. One study of 106 people found that those with higher blood levels of omega-3s were found to be more agreeable and less impulsive, while those with lower blood levels were more likely to report mild or moderate symptoms of depression, and a more negative outlook on life.[65] Other studies support this finding.[66,67,68] This has been found to be true not only for the general population, but also for the elderly – low omega-3 levels were associated with depression.[69] Considering all the elderly on anti-depression drugs, this is significant.

Another study showed that subjects on the omega-3 fatty acids who were already on antidepressant medication had improvements in sleep and libido and decreases in depression, anxiety, lassitude, and suicidal thoughts.[70] This study also showed that large amounts of omega-3s were not necessary to notice improvement and that just 1 gram a day of EPA (one of the omega-3s) let to the most significant improvements. Bipolar disorder is helped when omega-3s are in adequate supply [71], as well as the depressive symptoms in women suffering from premenstrual syndrome.[72]

A study published in *The Lancet* showed that people who rarely ate fish (including shellfish) are more likely to suffer depression than those who consumed it often [73], and post-partum depression is more likely in women who seldom ate fish [74]. An old wives-tale was that eating fish made you smart. Seems like it makes you happier, too.

Flax seeds and walnuts have omega-3s as well as fish, but the vegetable sources contain alpha-linolenic acid (ALA), which the body must convert into the omega-3s. It's estimated that only 5 percent to 15 percent of ALA is converted into the omega-3s.[75] ALA is also not as easily absorbed by the body as the omega-3s from fish. The fish with the highest content of omega-3s are sardines, anchovies, salmon, and mackerel.

Omega-3s have also been shown to increase blood flow to the brain which isn't surprising since they also provide benefits to the cardiovascular system.[76] The typical western diet is low in omega-3 fatty acids, but high in omega 6 fatty acids (which are in corn oil, safflower oil, sunflower oil, and cottonseed oils). The ratio of these omega-6s to omega-3s should be about 1:1, but in the current American diet, it's more like 6:1 or even higher. The overabundance of omega-6s and the paucity of omega-3s can lead to problems. One research article said, "Considering that highly-consumed vegetable oils have significant omega-6 to omega-3 rations, it is quite plausible that, for some individuals, inadequate intake of omega-3 fatty acids may have neuropsychiatric consequences."[77]

Consuming vegetable oils also overworks the adrenal glands. These fats tend to lower blood sugar, because they alter energy production in the mitochondria – the cells' power plants. They also suppress the production of thyroid hormone by the thyroid gland, pushing one to a slower metabolism and depression. To put it more succinctly, eating vegetable oil might make you depressed or bipolar or even worse. These oils are in just about everything these days, so is it any wonder our rates of depression are 20 times greater than shortly after WWII?

Food for Thought

If you check out the bibliography for the articles I've referenced here about depression and omega-3s, you'll find that they come from some pretty prestigious journals – the *American Journal of Clinical Nutrition, British Journal of Psychiatry, Biological Psychiatry,* and others. It's not like these articles are hiding under a rock where pharmaceutical companies or even the mass media can't find them. If a drug got the kind of results that simple fish oil or krill oil does (with no notable side effects or dangers) in helping those with depression, it would be hailed as the greatest thing since sliced bread. By the way, krill oil was used in some of the studies with depression, and it's considered better and more potent than fish oil.

Some of these studies were done in the 1980s. That's a long time ago in medical terms. Certainly long enough for our leaders to realize what's going on and to steer our health ship (which is beginning to look like the *Titanic*) to more peaceful waters.

Another fat that has proven to be beneficial to the thyroid gland is coconut oil (discussed in detail in the chapter on cardiovascular disease). It does this in two important ways. One, it increases the rate of metabolism of the whole body. This is due to the fact that it takes more energy to metabolize the MCFAs (medium chain fatty acids) found in coconut oil than they provide. One study reported in the *American Journal of Clinical Nutrition* that people who ate meals containing MCFAs increased their metabolic rate about 12 percent compared to just a 4 percent increase for those eating meals with long-chain fatty acids.[78] When MCFAs are consumed, they are immediately converted into energy by the liver, not circulated in the bloodstream as lipoproteins, which then may be deposited as fat. So eating MCFAs actually helps the thyroid do its job of maintaining a sufficient rate of metabolism.

The second way MCFAs help the thyroid is due to the fact that the fats in vegetable oils are oxidized fats that actually damage the liver directly (and the thyroid). Since the conversion of T_4 to T_3 (thyroid hormones) takes place in the liver, this function is impaired if the liver is damaged. Replacing vegetable oil with coconut oil rich in MCFAs takes stress off of the liver, making it easier to function so that it can turn T_4 to T_3 more effectively.

Weight gain is often a result of hypothyroidism because of the resulting decrease in the metabolic rate. Since the long-chain fatty acids in vegetable oils depress thyroid function, and the MCFAs in coconut oil improve thyroid function, then it stands to reason that replacing vegetable oil with coconut oil will help with weight loss. And that's exactly what research studies show.(79,80)

To substitute coconut oil for vegetable oil in all your cooking is one of the best things you can do to improve your thyroid gland, control your weight, and brighten your mood. You should consume about 3 - 4 tablespoons of coconut oil per day. Real coconut every day as a snack provides tons of benefits with none of the dangers found in the popular, packaged snack foods.

If you have a thyroid or weight problem, you should avoid vegetable oils like the plague. Use extra virgin olive oil in your salad dressings, not corn oil, safflower oil, soy oil, and definitely not canola oil. Use coconut oil for all your cooking needs, and in any dish that requires oil or fat. Real, unpasturized butter is good, but it's not as stable at high temperatures as coconut oil.

Magnesium is an important mineral when it comes to depression. Not only is the production of serotonin dependant on the availability of magnesium (if you have enough magnesium, you'll manufacture enough serotonin), but magnesium also supports our adrenal glands, which help us handle stress. A magnesium deficiency can cause anxiety, fatigue, apathy, apprehension, confusion, anger, nervousness, muscle weakness, eye twitches, insomnia, and poor memory.(81)

Magnesium has already been discussed in some detail in the chapter on diabetes. Suffice it to say here, that some researchers believe that a magnesium deficiency can be the underlying cause of anxiety and depression, and that any treatment protocol for depression should begin with adequate intake of magnesium. Remember, good dietary sources of magnesium are green leafy vegetables and fresh green vegetable juice, nuts (especially almonds), coconut, figs, dates, and shrimp. You may want to supplement with magnesium oil. You can get some magnesium from mineral water.

Since acetylcholine may be lacking in your brain, it may help to eat foods rich in choline (the backbone of acetylcholine). These are eggs, beef, cauliflower, and spinach.

Besides eating the foods that help fight depression, you should also avoid the foods that can cause or trigger it. Eating sugar and grain products increases insulin resistance of the cells, and this is believed to encourage depression.(82) Truly, any food or substance that robs you of energy is pushing you towards depression. So any improvement in diet is going to improve your chances of staying happy.

The next natural thing you can do to beat depression is to exercise regularly. Exercise has been shown to greatly improve symptoms of depression, and the intensity of the workout seems to make a difference. In one study, those who did a high-intensity aerobic workout for 30 minutes, three times a week, showed a 50 percent reduction in depressive symptoms. A low-intensity, 30-minute workout three times a week showed a 30 percent decrease in symptoms, and those who did stretching exercises averaged a 20 percent decrease in symptoms.(83).

Not just that, but exercise has actually been shown to outperform antidepressant drugs in easing the symptoms of depression. Walking for 30 minutes a day has been shown to have a faster effect on depressive symptoms for certain individuals than taking drugs (84)

Dr. Mercola suggests one hour of exercise a day. But with the new way to exercise I detailed in the chapter on cardiovascular disease (short duration, high intensity) all you really need is 10-15 minutes. Consider that exercise not only increases the "feel good" chemicals naturally produced by the brain, but also actually increases your overall energy throughout the day and helps you sleep better at night. When you sleep better, you won't need as much, so you'll be saving some time there.

If you don't exercise now, start slowly. You don't need to stress yourself out any further by thinking you *have* to exercise so much a day. Do the exercises you like at a pace you can handle. When you feel up to it, increase the intensity and time. After you exercise regularly for a couple weeks, you'll actually *want* to do it. Using a rebounder is especially beneficial to the thyroid gland. Remember, the harder you exercise, the better you'll feel.

Adequate exposure to sunlight or full spectrum lighting is critical for our mental as well as overall wealth. If you don't get enough exposure to unfiltered, natural sunlight, your mood will suffer. This is nothing new. As early as 400 B.C. Hippocrates realized that lack of sunlight could cause depression. Greek and Roman doctors had patients direct sunlight towards their eyes to treat depression. Doctors of the 19th and early 20th century routinely advised patients to go south for the winter. Hospitals prior to WWII commonly had solariums, and a light bath (or heliotherapy) was popular in Europe.

This kind of depression, where one doesn't get adequate sunlight, is called Seasonal Affective Disorder (SAD). About 36 million Americans are thought to get these winter blues, and 80 percent are female. It's estimated that one million children get it too, and these kids typically withdraw from friends and sleep too much. Those who live in the north are about nine times more likely to suffer from it than those living in the south. And now, with so many people working inside all year long, people in Florida are susceptible to getting depressed too.

The symptoms of SAD are similar to depression: sufferers feel low, slow, impatient, have trouble thinking clearly and quickly, sleep more, and are withdrawn. They eat more, especially the "feel good" foods such as sweets and carbohydrates. Some will say they'd be fine if they could just be left alone.(85) Why does this happen? If there isn't adequate sunlight, serotonin levels drop.(86) Consider sunlight the same as you would a vitamin or mineral. Your body and mind need it to function normally.

Treatment for SAD involves getting adequate unfiltered sunlight (no sunscreen please) or exposure to full spectrum artificial light. Norman E. Rosenthal, author of *Winter Blues* recommends 30 minutes of exposure to high intensity light (at least 2,500 lux for 2 hours, or 10,000 lux for 30 minutes) a few times a week.(87) Benefits may take several weeks, but some people notice a difference within just a two or three treatments, and about 80 percent of patients show an improvement. "One suicidal patient turned around in three days," reported Michael R Privitera Jr., director of the Mood Disorder Clinic at the University of Rochester (N.Y.) medical school.(88).

Food for Thought

If you can't go south for the winter, you can make your own light box to get similar benefits. Just get a couple of inexpensive shop lights and full spectrum fluorescent bulbs. The price of the lights and the necessary electricity to light them for a year will be less than a couple of month's supply of *Prosac*, and a lot better for you. So if you get the winter blues – any time of the year – use your light box to brighten your mood. It works for kids too. The full spectrum bulbs are not strong enough to cause a burn – just stay 2 or 3 feet away from them. Sorry, tanning beds are not the same, and are in fact, unhealthy.

There's another way to lift your mood that's all natural and relatively inexpensive. It also does wonders for your whole body and is one of the most powerful natural healing methods there is, according to some naturopathic doctors. It does take some courage and resiliency and most people won't do it because it is quite frankly, somewhat uncomfortable, but I would be remiss if I didn't mention it. As hard as it may be to do, it's one of my personal favorite natural health methods simply because I feel so good afterwards. What is it? None other than hot and cold therapy, in the form of showers or baths.

Do some light exercise to get warmed up, or take the hot/cold shower after a workout. Take a normal shower with your normal warm water temperature. After you're nice and warm and comfortable, turn off the hot water and leave the cold water on. This will shock you and take your breath away, especially if it's winter and the water is really cold. Turn around so the cold water touches all of you, even your head and face. Keep the cold on for about a minute, and then turn the hot water back on until the water temperature is very warm to hot. Stand under the hot for a minute, then blast the cold again for a minute. Alternate hot/cold 5-7 times or more. A good thing to do before the shower is to drink some vegetable juice or the Total Health Drink or variation of it. I blend up a glass of water with garlic, ginger, fresh red pepper, honey, and cinnamon and drink some before I start the shower and sip some on every hot cycle. The healthful nutrients in these ingredients will actually be pumped into your organs and tissues during the expansion/contraction.

You'll find that the first cold blast is the hardest to take. You may want to gradually work up to total cold over the first couple cycles. But after two or three cycles, you'll find that the cold is not that hard to take, and almost feels good. Always finish with cold. By the time you've completed 6 or 7 cycles and step out of the shower, you'll feel really invigorated, and on top of the world. Really. You may even find yourself wanting more!

The reason this works to heal the body and alleviate depression is due to the effect it has on circulation. As you go back and forth from hot to cold, your blood and lymph is being pulled to the surface of the skin (when the water is hot) and then pushed away and deep into your body and organs (when the water is cold). Increased circulation improves every function in the body. In fact, any tissue that is impaired got that way because of poor circulation. That's why exercise, massage, chiropractic, and other forms of bodywork are all good. If you combine these circulation enhancers with good nutrition, you'll be able to beat just about any ailment.

You can also take hot/cold baths if you have the necessary appliances. Draw a very warm/hot bath (don't burn yourself) in one bathtub, and a totally cold bath in another tub (I've gone so far as to add bags of ice from the convenience store to the cold tub). Go from one tub to the other, staying in each for a minute or so. Immerse as much of your body as you can. Or, make the tub your cold, and then run into a hot shower.

Doing hot/cold therapy on localized areas of your body helps too. Get a showerhead with a wand attachment on the end of a hose. Spray the part of your body giving you trouble with the warm/hot for 15 seconds to a minute, then blast it with cold for the same. This can help alleviate the pain of arthritis, sprains, and congestion. It's great to help tone the skin too. If you think you have a sluggish liver (most people do), spray just under your right rib cage. If you have diabetes, spray your left abdomen where the pancreas is. If you have breast cancer, spray the area where the tumor is. For prostate problems, spray under the scrotum. Hot-cold, hot-cold, hot-cold. Circulation is good for everything.

If you're clinically depressed or are just a little down, taking the hot/cold shower once a day it will really help. If you're really determine (or desperate), do it a couple times a day. Not only will you feel better mentally and emotionally, but your body will perk up and start mending. I've read articles on Scandinavian's who plunge into lakes in the dead of winter and attribute their long lives to this seemingly crazy practice. Native American's would go in a sweat lodge and then plunge in cold water afterwards. There are some spas in Europe that specialize in this therapy, and many naturopathic doctors have used it with great success. One doctor would have his patients go sit in a snow bank, then give them a warm bath, then back into the snow bank. Recently, there are quite a few athletes – amateur and professional alike – who are using ice baths to help speed recovery and decrease muscle soreness. Special "cold tubs" are even available. Some stay in the cold water for 10 minutes or more. I have not seen any definitive research saying this helps with muscle recovery, but most athletes who do it seem to think so. Personally, I believe alternating hot/cold is best because of the increased blood and lymph circulation.

When you just sit in a tub of cold water for 10 minutes, you may be alleviating inflammation, but not necessarily increasing circulation.

I've never come down with a cold when I've done this, and always feel great afterwards. Stiff upper lip there mate! You can do it! It may be hard, but most things in life that are worth anything usually are.

To sum it up, below is a list of simple things you can do to avoid, improve, and conquer depression, not to mention greatly improve your overall health:

- Don't smoke.
- Don't drink fluoridated or any product that's been fluoridated.
- Check your thyroid with Barnes Basal Temperature test.
- Check your iodine level – eat foods high in iodine.
- Get plenty of omega 3 fatty acids.
- Get plenty of magnesium.
- Eat some coconut every day and use coconut oil instead of vegetable oil.
- Get enough sunshine or full spectrum artificial light.
- Exercise regularly – get your heart rate up.
- Don't eat sugar and cut down on grains.
- Try hot/cold therapy.

CHAPTER IX

Alzheimer's Disease

A lzheimer's Disease (AD) is degenerative brain disorder that results in the loss of memory, thinking, and language skills, and changes behavior. It is a form of dementia, which is a general term that describes a group of symptoms such as loss of memory, judgment, language, and complex motor skills. Alzheimer's is the most common form of dementia among people over age 65, representing about 60 percent of all dementias. The next most common kind of dementia is vascular dementia, caused by stroke of blockage of blood supply. Dementias are progressive diseases, affecting more and more nerve cells as time goes on, so symptoms worsen with age.[1]

Alzheimer's was first diagnosed in 1906 by a Dr. Alois Alzheimer, a German physician, who examined the brain of a woman at autopsy, who had had memory problems, confusion, and difficulty understanding questions. He discovered dense deposits outside and around the nerve cells (*Beta-amyloid plaques*), and twisted bands of fibers (*neurofibrillary tangles*) inside the nerve cells. Observing the plaques and tangles at autopsy is still the only definitive diagnosis of Alzheimer's disease.

The nerve cells affected and which die first are always in the hippocampus – the part of the brain that is considered the seat of memory. Then a cascade of cell death occurs over time, eventually spreading out to include almost every region of the cortex of the brain (except the primary visual cortex). So Alzheimer's starts with isolated memory problems, then grows to affect language, judgment, personality, and behavior as more regions of the brain are affected. Whereas cancer is runaway cell growth, Alzheimer's is runaway cell death. The early warning signs of dementia (Alzheimer's) are:

- Trouble with new memories
- Trouble finding words
- Confusion about time, place or people
- Misplacing familiar objects
- Personality changes
- Seeing or hearing things
- Depression or irritability
- Making bad decisions

Alzheimer's is diagnosed by taking a complete medical history of the patient, lab tests, physical exam, brain scans, and memory and language tests. Cognitive (intellectual) symptoms are amnesia, aphasia, apraxia, and agnosia (the four As of Alzheimer's). Amnesia is the loss of memory – short term or long term. In Alzheimer's, short term is affected first.

Aphasia is the inability to communicate effectively. The loss of the ability to speak and write is called *expressive aphasia.* If a person can't understand spoken or written words, or may be able to read but not understand a word of it, that is *receptive aphasia.* If a person pretends to understand and even nods in agreement, this is called *cover-up aphasia* (I used to do that all the time in college!)

Apraxia is the inability to do learned activities such as brushing one's teeth or getting dressed. Motor skills that require extensive learning, such as job-related skills, are the first to go. In late stages, instinctive functions like chewing, swallowing, and walking are lost. *Agnosia* is the inability to interpret signals from one's five senses. Someone may not recognize familiar people or objects, or lose the ability to recognize things like a full bladder or chest pains.

Early on, a person with Alzheimer's may show personality changes such as being depressed, apathetic, or irritable, and may withdraw from society and personal contact. Later on, one may exhibit hallucinations and delusions. The hallucinations are typically auditory or visual. These can be very upsetting to the person having them, and feelings of fear, anxiety, aggression, verbal outburst, and paranoia are common. The further the disease progresses, the more likely the patient will become depressed, aggressive, and tend to wander around.

Unfortunately, we are on the verge of an Alzheimer's epidemic. It's estimated that by the year 2050, as many as 16 million Americans will have Alzheimer's disease.[2]

Food for Thought

Sixteen million people with Alzheimer's. That averages out to 320,000 Alzheimer's victims in each of the 50 states. That's roughly the population a city like Pittsburgh, PA or Colorado Springs, CO, full of Alzheimer's victims in each state. Scary.

Between 2000 and 2030, the number of people age 65 and older will double to 70.3 million – or 20 percent of the U.S. population. Those 85 and older will rise two-fold to 8.9 million. Our country is getting older.

I get newsletters from a number of doctors and health practitioners. One doctor told of a friend he has who's a stockbroker. This stockbroker invests in a number of medical and drug companies who manufacture products or drugs for kidney disease. He does this because he says kidney disease is out of control and there's no cure in sight. One of the companies is an adult diaper manufacturer – more than 10 million American adults wear diapers. His portfolio of kidney drug, dialysis, and diaper stocks is going through the roof.

Here's a stock tip - Invest in *Depends* diapers for adults, or any other geriatric product. Invest in wheelchair companies, scooter companies, and diabetes testing equipment companies – any company that makes products for people who are incapacitated in some way. I wouldn't invest in drug companies because sooner or later people are going to wake up to the fact that drugs are killing this country, killing humanity, and are just plain evil. As the good book says, "Take no part in unfruitful works of darkness, but instead, expose them." (Eph. 5:11)

As of 2006, it's estimated that between 4.2 and 5.8 million Americans have Alzheimer's disease (or AD). That's one in ten persons over the age of 65, and nearly half of those 85 or older.[3] Worldwide, it's estimated that 18 million people suffer from Alzheimer's disease. (That means that roughly 25 percent of Alzheimer's sufferers the world over live in the U.S.) Each year about 350,000 new cases of AD are diagnosed, and 59,000 people die because of it, making it the 8th leading cause of death in the U.S.[4] Caring for individuals with AD in the U.S. costs approximately $100 billion a year. AD costs U.S. industry $60 billion due to lost productivity and absenteeism. To care for one person with AD costs between $18,500 to over $36,000 per year. Half of all nursing home residents in the U.S. suffer from some form of dementia.[5,6].

Current medical treatment for Alzheimer's disease, is with drugs. *Cognex* (Tacrine) was the first drug approved to treat AD in 1993, but is rarely used anymore because of the high risk of liver damage. Since then, others have been introduced: *Aricept* (Donepezil), *Exelon* (Rivastigmine), and *Razadyne* (Galantamine). Side effects of these drugs include vomiting, nausea, and diarrhea.

Most family members, when faced with a loved one getting AD, think that drugs are the only answer for slowing down the disease so they get a prescription. The drugs usually cost about $120-$150 a month, and over $1.2 billion are spent on AD drugs a year in the U.S. However, there is no proof that these drugs work, and some physicians and experts believe that people are wasting their money on them.[7]

The plaques and tangles of damaged cells in the brain of a person with AD are unable to produce and use the chemical messenger called acetylcholine. Since acetylcholine is involved in memory, judgment and other thought processes, people experience problems with these if it's in short supply. The drugs used to treat AD are cholinesterase inhibitors, called that since they slow the breakdown of acetylcholine. They do this by blocking the action of the enzyme that breaks it down, namely acetylcholinesterase. The more acetylcholine around, the better the brain thinks.

Food for Thought

Just as antidepressant drugs stop the uptake of serotonin so it can hang around longer, cholinesterase inhibitors stop the action of the enzyme that breaks down acetylcholine, allowing it to hang around longer too. Both drugs effectively weaken or destroy a process to compensate for a problem. They do not strengthen or support anything, but poison something to make up for a deficiency somewhere else.

This is the way all drugs work. It's why all drugs (and I mean 100 percent of drugs – synthetic or natural), have some kind of side effect (which really means that some part of the body has been poisoned), and are, in the end, deleterious to the body.

Want proof? If you notice the warnings on most prescription drugs advise people not to take the drug if they have liver problems. The liver is the main organ of detoxification. So if your liver isn't working correctly, it won't be able to handle the drug, and the drug may cause more serious problems in the liver or another part of the body. If the drug weren't toxic, it wouldn't have to be handled by the liver. Any drug puts a strain on the liver (and other organs and cells) that pollutes it and causes damage.

Conversely, a natural way to solve the problem would be to support the cells and processes that produce and use acetylcholine so that it's produced and used it the way it was intended. How do you do that? By making sure the cells are nourished adequately, and at the same time, making sure the cells can eliminate their waste easily. Doing this would likely support other bodily processes too, instead of harming them as with drugs. Or at the very least, these natural methods would do no harm. *Primum non nocere. . .* Latin for "First, do no harm." Does that sound familiar, doctors?

Dealing with Alzheimer's Disease

Family history and genetics undoubtedly play a role in Alzheimer's disease, as they do with everything. Each of us is born with certain strengths and weaknesses, and recognizing them and compensating for them is an important part of maintaining health.

To claim that someone comes down with Alzheimer's disease because it was inherited is probably far from true. Estimates are that less than 5 percent of those who get AD are from strictly inheriting it. To date, genetics testing for AD has not been found to be useful, and is not recommended. AD, just like so many other diseases, is a relatively new disease for the human race. Genetic mutations may increase the likelihood a disease manifests, but consider that mutations are rare. Consider also, why would a gene mutate? Most mutations arise due to stresses from the environment. The biggest reasons people are getting AD, and the reasons more will get it as time goes on, are because of these environmental stresses. That's the bad news. The good news is, these environmental stresses can be eliminated or lessened. The first step is to recognize them.

The traditional medical establishment says there is no cure for Alzheimer's disease. In the advanced stages, this is probably true. But if recognized early enough and natural steps are taken, its symptoms may be delayed or even reversed.

It's been shown that the level of mercury in the brain of AD sufferers is higher than normal.(8) Remember that mercury has been implicated as contributing to ADHD and autism, so it's not surprising that it would have a neurological effect on older people too. One common source of mercury is silver amalgam fillings. The level of mercury in the brain has been shown to be proportional to the number of amalgam fillings in the teeth.(9) So a good first step to avoiding AD is to refuse new amalgam fillings and to remove existing ones. I mentioned earlier that 95 percent of people with central nervous system disorders have silver amalgam fillings. You simply can't go wrong getting them out of your head.

Mercury is also found in vaccines. Is it any wonder that the most vaccinated population in the history of the world (the U.S.) is also the one with the most Alzheimer's patients? It's best for everyone to avoid vaccines completely. See the Vaccines chapter for more.

Other common sources of mercury are from fish and air pollution. Avoiding the kinds of fish that have the highest concentrations of mercury is best. The bigger the fish, the more mercury since it bioaccumulates when the big fish eat the smaller ones. Swordfish, tuna, and mackerel are big and more contaminated than shrimp, anchovies, and sardines. But fish is good for the brain (the omega-3's), so there's a bit of a trade off there. Air pollution is something hard to control. A good air purifier helps for inside air. A drastic measure would be to move to a place with good air quality.

Aluminum has also been shown to be higher in the brains of AD sufferers, especially in the beta-amyloid plaque that are so characteristic of the disease. Aluminum is known to be extremely toxic to brain neurons, so although there has been some debate of whether it causes Alzheimer's, it probably at least accelerates it progression.(10,11) Aluminum is also been associated with Parkinson's disease and amyotrophic lateral sclerosis (Lou Gehrig's disease).

People on kidney dialysis often develop a form of dementia called *dialysis encephalopathy*, characterized by speech and behavioral changes, tremors, convulsions, and psychosis. Many experts believe this occurs because there are high levels of aluminum in dialysis fluids and medications.(12)

Aluminum is found in municipal drinking water because Alum is typically used to treat the water. In fact, it has been shown that the higher the level of aluminum in drinking water, the more incidences of AD there are.(13,14) Now there's news that the fluoride added to our municipal water supplies actually increases the body's absorption of aluminum.(15) Bottled drinking water is oftentimes taken from municipal water supplies, so is no better. Steam distillation and reverse osmosis are two ways to remove aluminum from water. A good spring water (like *Perrier*) is probably your best bet in avoiding aluminum in drinking water.

Aluminum is also found in processed cheese, baking powder, antacids, buffered aspirin, anti-diarrhea products, antiperspirants, cooking utensils, foods cooked in aluminum pots, and coffee made in aluminum-containing percolators.

Aluminum cans can transfer significant amounts of aluminum into the beverages they contain, so they should be avoided. Vaccines and flu shots all have aluminum. So seniors, please think twice before getting that flu shot.

A diet low in magnesium allows aluminum to accumulate in the body easier. Malic acid (found in apple cider vinegar – see the Total Health Drink in obesity chapter) is believed to be able to pull aluminum out of tissues, even in the brain. So it may be helpful to have some apple cider vinegar daily to prevent and reverse aluminum build-up.

Cardiovascular disease, insulin resistance, and Type II diabetes increase the risk of developing AD. Cinnamon has been shown to greatly decrease insulin resistance and help keep blood glucose levels low (see Diabetes chapter). It's also good for the blood, so in these regards, adding cinnamon to your diet may be helpful in keeping your mind sharp. It's also been shown that the smell of cinnamon boosts brain activity. Dr. P. Zoladz reported that people who are exposed to the smell of cinnamon had improved scores on recognition memory, working memory and visual-motor speed.[16]

Cinnamon can be purchased in sticks (known as quill), or powdered. Of course, it's always best to buy organic. Cinnamon smells slightly sweet when it's fresh. Powdered cinnamon will stay fresh about 6 months and should be stored in the refrigerator. The sticks stay fresh about twice as long. A tea made of cinnamon and ginger has been known to help prevent and alleviate a cold or flu. (This tea is better than a flu shot, doesn't hurt, and tastes good too.) Cinnamon is also high in calcium, iron, and manganese.

A deficiency in omega-3 fatty acids, especially DHA, may be linked to the risk of developing AD and other dementias. One study showed that low levels of fish consumption was a risk factor for the development of AD in the elderly.[17,18]

Docosahexaenoic acid (DHA), is a crucial component of the brain and nervous system. Deficiencies have been linked to depression, aggression, Alzheimer's disease, schizophrenia, and multiple sclerosis in adults, and learning disabilities in children An excellent source of DHA is good old-fashioned cod liver oil, which also contains high amounts of vitamins A and D. Sally Fallon, a noted researcher and author, comments on DHA:

> Adequate DHA in the mother's diet is necessary for the proper development of the retina in the infant she carries. DHA in mother's milk helps prevent learning disabilities and vision problems. Cod liver oil and foods like liver and egg yolk supply this essential nutrient to the developing fetus, to nursing infants and to growing children Saturated fats help the body put the DHA in the tissues where it belongs.[19]

William Campbell Douglass, M.D., has some important things to say about DHA, formula, and children. The title of his article is, "A Substance Found in Breast Milk Helps Depression, Alzheimer's." I'm going to quote the entire article (with permission) because Dr. Campbell gives several recommendations and I want you to see that I am not the only one with a healthy skepticism of our government agencies.

Depression and Alzheimer's disease are reaching epidemic proportions in America, and, as a result, *Prozac* and other pharmaceuticals that supposedly treat these ailments are selling like hotcakes.

The good news, though, is that recent studies are now indicating low levels of a fatty acid called docosahexaenoic acid (DHA) contribute to the many major physical and psychological disorders in adults. These ailments include depression, aggression, Alzheimer's disease, schizophrenia, and multiple sclerosis. (To avoid any confusion, DHA is unrelated to DHEA. DHA is a fatty acid and DHEA is a hormone.)

Approximately 60 percent of the human brain is composed of fatty material, and 25 percent of that material is made up of DHA. While DHA is the primary structural fatty acid in the brain, humans cannot produce it – they must consume it.

Studies show that the DHA levels of women in America today are comparable to those women in Third-World countries. This is attributed to the trend against eating DHA-rich foods such as fish (tuna, salmon, trout, and sardines), liver, brain and other animal organs, and eggs.

Despite a growing body of evidence that DHA is the essential structural ingredient of breast milk and is lacking in infant formulas, the Food and Drug Administration continues to ban its use in the U.S. Even the National Institutes of Health have endorsed the addition of DHA to infant formula with no visible effect on the FDA.

I know you're not an infant, but it's not too late for you to benefit from the brain- and mood-boosting benefits of this wonderful supplement. It is important that you understand how this fatty acid benefits infants, though, because it directly relates to how it affects you. Hang with me on this for a little bit.

Breastfed babies have an IQ six to 10 points higher than formula-fed babies. Scientists and nutritional experts attribute this to DHA, an omega-3 fatty acid that's an essential structural component of the brain and retina. It's found naturally in mother's milk. In case it will impress you, the World Health Organization and the Food and Agricultural Organization of the United Nations also endorse the addition of DHA to infant formula.

During the last trimester of a pregnancy is when the mother transfers to her baby much of the DHA needed for the development of his or her brain and nervous system. The DHA content in the mother's diet reflects in the amount of DHA passed on to the baby. If the baby is not breastfed at all, it receives no DHA after birth and is short-changed in neurological development, thus impairing mental and visual acuity. DHA levels of premature infants are especially low, since they miss much of that last trimester and when born, haven't developed the sucking mechanism – so they are usually bottle-fed. It's a wonder they live at all, and it's a crime they aren't getting DHA in their bottle from birth.

Many European and Asian countries are producing infant formula with DHA and making recommendations of daily allowances. The American company, Wyeth Nutritional, does make infant formula that contains DHA; however, it's only available in Hong Kong, the Middle East, and Australia, since distribution is banned in the U.S.

Dr. David Kyle, chief of research at Martek Biosciences Corporation, has been involved in several studies involving DHA. He has consistently observed that formula-fed babies have far lower levels of visual and intellectual acuity than do their breastfed peers.

As I mentioned at the outset, DHA has uses beyond the newborn. Studies show that low DHA intake in infancy can lead or contribute to Attention Deficit Disorder (ADD) and Attention Deficit Hyperactivity Disorder (ADHD). We're moving up the age ladder don't give up – we'll get to you in a minute.

The government is under pressure from prominent drug companies (such as Novartis, which manufactures *Ritalin*) to keep DHA out of the information bank of the average consumer. If *Ritalin* could be replaced by a simple and safe fatty acid, Novartis would be in trouble, people might have to be laid off, and profits would tumble. Do you think a drug company could be that heartless and put profits ahead of the lives of children? Maybe you don't but I've seen it happen more than a few times.

Bill Taylor is a retired engineer who teaches elementary-aged ADD children as a volunteer and is on the forefront of the infant formula debate. He said, "There is a lot of money at stake. Scientists are dependent on drug companies for research grants." Drug companies aren't interested in a simple cure for anything and certainly not a cash cow like the ADD/*Ritalin* market.

A study done on Japanese students during the high-stress period of final exams showed that students supplemented with DHA were significantly less aggressive than students who were not supplemented with DHA. Now we get to you, my patient reader. You are no longer a baby, that's for sure, so why am I giving you all this infant-formula information? First, you probably have children – or even grandchildren – and they need to know about DHA for their children. But more relevant to you personally, consider the following:

- Studies show that symptoms of multiple sclerosis, such as muscular weakness, loss of coordination, and speech and visual disturbances, are linked to sub normal levels of omega-3 fatty acids such as DHA.
- DHA helps supply the brain with serotonin, which regulates moods, thus making one less vulnerable to stress and depression.
- Over 1,200 patients participated in an epidemiological study that showed people with high DHA levels were 45 percent less likely to develop dementia than people with low DHA levels. This suggests that proper DHA intake may reduce the risk of developing Alzheimer's disease.
- A 1997 study showed that schizophrenic patients were less likely to have been breastfed in infancy, and the lack of DHA during early brain development contributes to the development of schizophrenia.

While these last two areas need more research, science is already starting to bear witness to the desperate need of people of all ages to consume plenty of DHA. Obviously, diet plays an important part in the consumption of DHA. And while taking a gel cap of DHA is great, you've got to fix your diet, as many people are consuming foods that actually contribute to depression, Alzheimer's, and some of the other problems we've discussed.

I've preached for years about the dangers of eating margarine as a substitute for real butter. Now the devastating results are starting to hit hard. In addition to it being nutrient-free, margarine is saturated hydrogenated fat (a.k.a. *trans*-fatty acids) that causes our neuro-chemistry to go into a tailspin. You don't have to be a brain surgeon to understand the brain runs every system in the body. So when the neurochemistry is messed up, the rest of the body is messed up.

In contrast, essential fatty acids are just that, essential. The difference between *trans*-fatty acids and essential fatty acids is the exact difference between depression and a normal emotional state of mind. It's also a major factor that needs to be considered in greater detail in Alzheimer's and other brain illnesses.

Action to Take:
1) As you age, it's terribly important that you avoid any and all dairy products that aren't real or have been altered by processing. That means you can toss out any margarine, *EggBeaters*, and low-fat or no-fat dairy products. It also means

you need to get milk that's not homogenized or pasteurized. All of these fake fats and processed products accelerate the aging process and cause your brain to malfunction.

2) At the same time, you need to increase your intake of good, fatty animal meats. I know this goes against the grain of current medical dogma, but the evidence of their benefits is growing increasingly indisputable.

3) I can also recommend that you begin taking a capsule or two of DHA each day. It's not as good of a source as the fatty meats, but it's the next best thing (and essential if you're a vegetarian). You can probably find DHA at your local health food store.[20]

Remember, *Neuromins* is a good DHA supplement (See Resource Guide).

Food for Thought

Drug companies have us coming and going, since their tentacles reach deep into our government. Since the addition of DHA to infant formula is banned in the U.S., thanks to our friendly FDA, we are raising a generation of aggressive morons. After a few years of a diet insufficient in DHA and other nutrients not found in formula, the children are more likely to develop learning disabilities, attention deficits, and behavioral problems. The solution? Drug them with Substance II drugs such as *Ritalin*. First they sell the deficient formula, then they sell the drugs later. Very tricky.

Speaking of the FDA, although it may sometimes seem to be in alliance with the drug companies, it does offer some valuable information even though most of the time it doesn't know what to do with it. In an article by Isadora B. Stehlin on the FDA internet homepage, she writes, "More than half the calories in breast milk come from fat, and the same is true for today's infant formulas. This may be alarming to many American adults watching their intake of fat and cholesterol, especially when sources of saturated fats, such as coconut oil, are used in formulas. . . But the low-fat diet recommended for adults doesn't apply to infants."[21] I'll add to that that the low fat diet recommended for adults doesn't work for adults either. But you need to eat the good kinds of fat that have not been heated.

Dr. Barry Sears, in his book, the *Omega Rx Zone*, describes how in an extended care and rehabilitation center in Florida, terminal AD patients were helped by taking high doses of omega-3 fatty acids. The patients were given up to 25 grams per day of pharmaceutical grade fish oil (free of contaminants) along with modifications to their diet. Some patients went from being bed ridden and unable to care for themselves, to eating and playing normally and recognizing friends and relatives. Some were even able to go home and lead somewhat normal lives. Dr. Sears found that the amount of improvement was proportional to the dosage of omega-3's – low doses meant less improvement.(22) This was not a "scientifically based" study, but it does give hope that AD sufferers could be helped with supplemental omega-3's or changes to their diet. (I would say that high doses of clean fish oil have fewer risks than the drugs being prescribed for AD.)

The proportion of omega-6 to omega-3 fatty acids in the diet also appears to play a role in the development of AD. A high omega-6 to omega-3 ratio, as found in the current American diet, decreases the fluidity of neuronal membranes making them age faster.(23) (See the chapter on depression for more on omega-3's and omega 6's.) One study used a mixture of omega-3 and omega-6 fatty acids in the ratio of 1:4, and in a four week period, significant improvement in AD patients were seen in mood, cooperation, appetite, sleep, short term memory and the ability to navigate in the home.(24)

A study in the *American Journal of Clinical Nutrition* reported that elderly people who had low levels of vitamin D were significantly more likely to be admitted to a nursing home than those with high levels.(25) It's estimated that up to 90 percent of the elderly may suffer from a vitamin D deficiency.

Vitamin D deficiency is associated with loss of muscle strength, overall poorer physical health, depression, incontinence, cardiovascular disease, diabetes, obesity, mental impairment, and arthritis. The best way to get vitamin D is through exposure to unfiltered sunlight, so it's important that elderly people get out into the sunshine. Exposure to full spectrum indoor lighting is good too (see chapter on depression). Taking cod liver oil is the next best thing.

Other dietary considerations also appear to play a role in the likelihood of and severity of AD. Several studies have indicated that deficiencies in vitamin B_{12} and folate (vitamin B_9) are related to elevated risk of dementia or AD. One study found that people over 74 years old who had a vitamin B_{12} deficiency were twice as likely to develop Alzheimer's disease compared to those with normal levels.(26,27,28,29) Another study published in the *Journal of Neurology, Neurosurgery and Psychiatry* showed that people with a folate deficiency (and the elderly are likely to have it) have more than three times the risk of developing Alzheimer's disease.(30) Other symptoms of a folate deficiency include Parkinson's disease, birth defects, cancer, chronic fatigues, constipation, elevated homocysteine levels, hair loss, headache, heart disease, insomnia, anemia, restless legs, and paranoia.

Folate (the word *folic* comes from the word foliage, which refers to plants.) is abundant in leafy green vegetables, asparagus, peas, citrus fruits, tomatoes, beets, broccoli, cauliflower, nuts, eggs, cantaloupe, watermelon, bee pollen, and poultry and liver from organically raised animals. Folate is easily destroyed by heat, light, and oxidation, and substantial losses occur not only with cooking, but storage as well. (However, the folate in animal products is more resistant to destruction by heat than the folate in vegetables.) So it's vitally important to eat some (if not all) of these foods raw. Since the best source or folate is vegetables, it's another reason why juicing is so good for you. You can get many times the amount of folate from a glass of fresh squeezed vegetable juice than what you get from a salad or vegetable side dish.

Smoking, alcohol, and heavy coffee drinking can cause folate deficiencies, as do most drugs (aspirin and other NSAIDs, oral contraceptives, barbiturates, corticosteroids and others). It's recommended that people take no more than 1,000 mcg (micrograms) of folic acid in the form of a supplement per day, but there is no limit to the amount of natural folate one can consume. Synthetic folic acid is added to certain grain products including flour, rice, pasta, cornmeal, bread, and cereals, so consuming a lot of these could actually lead to a folic acid overload.

Food for Thought

Folate is a nutrient that is proving to be vitally important, especially due to its role in cognitive abilities and the fact that our population is getting older. The recommended daily allowance for folate is 400 mcg for adults and 800 mcg for pregnant women a day. I wish we could just go out and get a good folate supplement (folic acid is the synthetic version of folate and is what is used in supplements) and by taking it, everything would be fine and dandy. But taking supplements with as little as 0.8 mg/day of folic acid has been shown to increase the risk of dying of heart attack and stroke by 20 percent and cancer by 30 percent. Since the start of fortifying grain products with folic acid in the U.S. in 1998, the daily consumption of synthetic folic acid has climbed to over 1 mg/day/person, which is over the amount shown by this study to increase the risks of heart disease and cancer.[31] A different study reported in the *American Journal of Clinical Nutrition* stated that consuming more than 0.2 mg of folic acid daily overloads the body causing imbalances that increase the risk of heart disease and cancer.[32]

Clearly, it's best to obtain your folate from natural sources. But the question arises as to why folic acid supplementation has helped decrease the incidences of birth defects (specifically neural tube defects – see birth defect chapter). I'd explain that as follows: If the mother is woefully deficient in folate and doesn't eat properly, then supplementation is better than nothing, but not as good as making sure the diet is rich in naturally occurring folate. Since most women aren't aware of the difference in synthetic folic acid and natural folate, just giving her a pill is more expedient and probably more effective since most women wouldn't make the necessary changes to their diet to ensure adequate folate intake. Simply put, supplement if you must, eat properly if you can.

As you know, I'm a bit fan of eggs and bee pollen. One tablespoon of fresh, raw, bee pollen has about 100 mcg of folate and one raw egg has about 25 mcg of folate. Just two tablespoons of bee pollen and two raw eggs supply roughly 250 mcg of folate. Add in some of the other foods high in folate or a glass of vegetable juice, and you've got your recommended daily requirement covered (without increasing your risks of heart disease, stroke, or cancer).

Vegetarians are more likely to get a vitamin B_{12} deficiency since it's mostly in animal products. You can find vitamin B_{12} in meat, fish, poultry, eggs, milk, and spinach. Grass-fed beef and wild ocean fish have more B_{12} than grain fed beef or farm raised fish. Vitamin B_{12} is a large molecule, and taking supplements of it orally or sublingually are not very effective. The only effective form of supplementation is by injection. Medications likely decrease B_{12} absorption, and one drug, *Prilosec* (omeprazole), clearly does this.[33]

Although it is true that the body can synthesize DHA and EPA from the a-linolenic acid found in flax seeds and nuts, this ability usually declines with age. Getting omega-3's from fish oil directly explains the marked positive results they have in helping and reversing AD symptoms.

Men who ate tofu (a soy product) at least two to three times a week in mid-life, were more likely to show mental impairment in old age than those who ate little or no tofu. Another study showed the higher the tofu consumption, the worse memory became.[34,35] Smoking also reportedly doubles the normal risk for AD. Researchers believe this occurs because smoking reduces the antioxidant reserves in the body, and that perhaps smokers generally have poorer dietary habits than those who don't.[36]

Studies have reported that the risk of AD decreased substantially for those who drink a little to moderate amounts of red wine. That's up to three glasses of wine per day. The same effect was not noticed for any other kinds of alcohol. Researches believe this may be due to some antioxidants, or a substance called resveratol in the wine.[37,38] Only drink wine from organically grown grapes, since grapes grown with conventional methods are heavily sprayed with pesticides and contain sulfites.

Seniors who ate more than two servings of vegetables a day were shown to have better memory skills than those who ate few or no vegetables.[39] This is because vegetables, especially green leafy ones, contain not just folate, but vitamin E as well. Vitamin E is an antioxidant with many benefits, one of which is that it slows mental decline. Synthetic vitamin E or that found in supplements is toxic, so getting it from natural sources such as vegetables is best. Salads are fine, but it's easier to get the nutrition out of vegetables by juicing them.

Keeping your mind active also keeps it in shape and delays or even prevents Alzheimer's disease. Those over 65 who frequently took part in mentally stimulating activities were 47 percent less likely to develop AD than those who rarely did so.[40] In another study at the Byrd Alzheimer's Research Institute in Tampa, Florida, mice with the same characteristics as humans with AD, showed the same mental competency after several months of mental stimulation as mice without the disease. Project chief Huntington Potter, Ph.D., said, "The mental stimulation provided in this environment appears to stymie mental impairment. After months of mental stimulation, it was impossible to differentiate these mice from the behaviorally normal, healthy mice."(41) Activities that people can do to keep their minds sharp include: Doing crossword and other puzzles, playing cards, checkers and other games, learning a foreign language, learning to play a musical instrument, reading challenging books or articles (like this book), and using your non-dominant hand to do simple tasks (try brushing your teeth with the other hand). When you exercise your mind like this, you actually create new connections and nerve cells in your brain. It's a lot like building muscle.

Not surprisingly, physical activity also helps. "Regular exercise at least three times a week could delay the onset and reduce the risk of developing Alzheimer's, and the more frail a person is, the more he or she is going to benefit from exercise," says Dr. Eric B Larson, the director of the Group Health Cooperative's center for Health Studies in Seattle. "There's a tendency to sit down and do nothing when you start to lose function, but the opposite is probably exactly what's in order if you want to stave off Alzheimer's disease."(42,43)

Between 1994 and 2003, Larson and his team assessed the health, physical and mental function and lifestyle characteristics of 1,740 men and women over the age of 65. Those who did just 15 minutes of physical activity at least three days a week had a 32 percent lower risk of developing dementia than those exercising less than three days a week. Walking, bicycling, aerobics, calisthenics, swimming, weight training all do the trick.

Aerobic activity improves blood flow in the brain, encourages the formation of new neurons, and increases the connections between neurons. People in better shape have more activity in parts of the brain that are involved in attention. People who do just stretching or toning with no aerobic activities do not show the same improvement, so it looks like it's important to get your heart rate up.(44) It's important to realize that physical activity not just helps older people improve, but exercise in mid-life is also believed to greatly reduce the risk of developing AD later in life. Again, research shows that physical activity more than twice per week that is more intense than walking makes the difference.(45)

Proper sleep is important for memory and mental function. I don't believe you can sleep too much. If you're tired and need sleep, it's your body's signal that you need the rest. Everyone's body is different, and so are our individual sleep requirements. I believe that the more toxic a person is, the more rest and sleep he or she needs because the body detoxifies during sleep, and it rebuilds and regenerates during sleep too. One study showed that volunteers taking an hour-long nap in the afternoon had improved learning and memory skills.(46)

You may have heard of studies that say that those who only sleep seven or eight hours a night live longer than those who sleep more. I believe this is because the people who sleep less are less toxic, and therefore, don't need as much sleep. The less toxic you are, the longer you live.

The amount you sleep is an indication of your level of toxicity, not a determinant of your lifespan, and your level of toxicity is the determinant of how long you sleep. (If this last sentence made your head spin, don't worry – I did it on purpose. Ah ha! Gotcha! It made you think a little harder, didn't it? Well, don't worry, you're not stupid if you had trouble grasping it, because what I wrote is ultimately a tautology. Or to put it another way, it's a tautologous statement. What's that? I'm not going to tell you. Get up off your butt, find your dictionary, and look it up. It'll do your body and your mind some good!)

So don't deny yourself, or your elderly loved ones a nap or a long night's sleep. It's important for proper mental function. See more on sleep in the chapter on insomnia and migraines.

There are other simple and natural things that have been shown to help those with Alzheimer's disease or dementia. A hot water bottle covered with fleece has helped AD sufferers calm down and stop screaming. Putting together a memory box with items and photos of happy times activates their memories. Having a pet to hold and take care of is soothing and makes them feel needed. Sing-a-longs have a calming effect and gives AD patients a sense of belonging. Simply rocking in a rocking chair has helped those with dementia deal with depression and anxiety. Humor always helps, especially for those who are upset.(47)

Food for Thought

Speaking of humor, here's a little geriatric jocularity:

Three older gentlemen, Jack, Gary, and Lee, who played golf together, were having trouble following and finding their golf balls since their eyesight was failing. This was not just very frustrating, but expensive. One of them had an idea.

"Let's get Arnie to join us," Jack said. "He's still got 20/20 vision."

"Oh, not Arnie!" Lee complained. "He's older than any of us."

"But he can still see like a bald eagle," Gary said. "I'm with Jack. Let's get Arnie."

"Oh, all right." Lee finally agreed.

So they got Arnie to join them on their next round. Jack got up and blasted a drive, but like always, neither Jack, Gary, or Lee saw where it ended up.

"Where'd it go?" they asked Arnie. "Did you see where the ball went?"

"Sure did." Arnie replied, hitching up his pants and puffing up his chest in pride.

"So where did it go?" they demanded.

"Uhh..." Arnie thought a moment, and then mumbled, "I forgot."

CHAPTER X

Parkinson's Disease

The first reports of the symptoms describing Parkinson's disease (PD) date all the way back to 5000 BC in India, and 2,500 years ago in Chinese writings. It wasn't until the 19th century in London that a doctor named James Parkinson first described the symptoms for modern medicine.(1)

Parkinson's disease, or PD, is a brain and movement disorder that is both chronic (long term) and progressive (gets worse over time). It's characterized by tremor of the hands, arms, legs, or jaw; rigidity or stiffness of the limbs and trunk; bradykinesia (slowness of movement); postural instability; and impaired balance and coordination. Those with Parkinson's disease may exhibit a shuffled walk, muffled speech, stiff facial expressions, small, cramped handwriting, and depression. Thirty percent of Parkinson's disease victims eventually develop Alzheimer's disease or other forms of dementia.(2)

Estimates are that as many as 1.5 million Americans suffer from PD, and 60,000 more are diagnosed each year. PD usually develops after the age of 65, but 15 percent of those diagnosed are under 50, and the disease can manifest in young people. More men get PD slightly more often than women. The cost of PD in the U.S., including treatment, social security payments, and lost income is estimated to be close to $6 billion a year. Medication for an individual patient averages $2,500 a year.(3)

There is no single clinical test for Parkinson's disease (X-rays or blood tests can't detect it), but clinical tests are used to rule out other conditions. A diagnosis is usually arrived at after a neurologist's examination. Typical medical treatment includes drugs (oftentimes several at a time), with levodopa the most popular. When the drugs stop working, surgery can help some patients, but it is not a cure.

Although the actual cause of PD is not known, (genetic factors are estimated to be only around 5 percent) it occurs when a group of cells in the brain stem called the *substantia nigra* start to malfunction and die and no longer produce enough of the neurotransmitter called dopamine. Dopamine helps to regulate parts of the brain that control coordination and the initiation of movement, and when insufficient amounts are present, lack of muscle control results. In addition, the loss of dopamine production upsets the balance between dopamine and acetylcholine in the brain, which results in neural messages to muscles being scrambled. By the time symptoms appear, the patient has lost 70 percent to 80 percent of the dopamine-producing cells. Although people don't die directly from PD, it can cause other complications that could result in death.

The first drug of choice is usually some variation of levodopa (l-dopa, *Sinemet* trade name), a dopamine-precursor approved in 1970, that can cross the blood-brain barrier where it is converted into dopamine in the brain. L-dopa is now administered in combination with other drugs, which allow the l-dopa get into the brain easier and be effective for longer periods. Most PD patients can see significant improvement by taking these drugs. However, after four or five years, the drugs become less effective, and their effect can become sporadic and unpredictable leading to what's called the *on-off syndrome*. Now, many neurologists believe that l-dopa actually speeds the progression of PD.[4]

Food for Thought

Antidepressant drugs can cause depression. Alzheimer's/dementia drugs can cause impaired mental abilities. PD drugs make the tremors worse in the long run. Drugs = short-term symptom improvement (if you're lucky) with long-term systemic harm (100% of the time, no matter the drug).

Another side effect of l-dopa drugs is dyskinesia (involuntary movements and tics – sounds like PD, doesn't it?), hallucinations, mental confusion, dizziness, nausea, constipation, and dark staining of the urine.[5] It's estimated that between 15 percent and 61 percent of patients exposed to dopamine antagonists (chlorpromazine, haloperidol, thioridazine) develop drug-induced Parkinsonism [6] Of course, involuntary movements are the very thing the drugs are supposed to stop, so these drugs are far from perfect. Considering this, some doctors recommend that drug therapy be started as late as possible, to delay the inevitable loss of effectiveness of the drugs and avoid any side effects.

Results of a 15-year study reported in *Neurology*, showed that 20 percent of men and 28 percent of women in the study who had PD, had it because of poisoning by pharmaceutical drugs.[7] Drugs that have been implicated in causing PD are diuretics (reserpine), antipsychotics (chlorpromazine), heart drugs (verapamil), naproxen (*Aleve*) and other non-steroidal anti-inflammatory drugs (NSAIDs). Drug-induced Parkinsonism can oftentimes be reversed by prompt withdrawal of the offending drug. But how many doctors know this? Does anyone ever think that taking *Aleve* to relieve arthritis pain might cause PD?

Research has shown that those on *Sinemet* have an increased risk of heart attacks and strokes. One study reported that men with PD that take the drug had a 60 percent greater chance of coronary heart disease, while women had an 80 percent greater chance. The risk of a stroke was two to five times greater also.[8] This is due to elevated homocysteine levels in the blood. However, it has also been determined that supplementation with folic acid (400 - 800 micrograms per day or more) can lower the elevated homocystine levels. As noted in the chapter on Alzheimer's disease, naturally occurring folate is preferable to supplementation with folic acid due to the elevated risks of heart disease when taking the pills. Remember, foods rich in folate are leafy green vegetables, asparagus, peas, citrus fruits, tomatoes, beets, broccoli, cauliflower, nuts, eggs, cantaloupe, watermelon, bee pollen, and poultry and liver from organically raised animals.

If and when the drugs don't work, or really high doses are needed (which will eventually happen), surgery is another option. There are two different procedures: *Pallidotomy* – where a small portion of the brain called the *global pallidus* is destroyed with an electric probe; or *thalamotomy* – where a portion of the thalamus is destroyed. A pallidotomy is especially effective for reducing the dyskinesia caused by the drugs. A thalamotomy is effective for patients who have disabling tremors in the hand or arm. Another invasive technique is deep brain stimulation (DBS) where a small electrode is implanted that emits electrical pulses similar to a cardiac pacemaker. It is good at relieving tremors associated with PD. These procedures do not cure PD, but help to control the symptoms. There are other approaches such as stem cell research and human fetal tissue transplantation, but they are still experimental and unproven.

Food for Thought

Anthony Lang, M.D., a specialist in PD at the University of Toronto warns that none of the surgical procedures for PD have been exposed to rigorous, double-blind studies. "As long as there are willing neurologists and surgeons and desperate patients, this problem will persist until the professional community decides to regulate the practice of its members or until external regulations are imposed." He says that some procedures are popular for a while (such as adrenal medullary transplantation – a different procedure not related to PD), and then are later abandoned because they are truly useless and dangerous.

Pallidotomy was reintroduced in 1992, but there is still no real consensus in the medical community as to where the incision in the brain should actually be made. Neither is there total agreement as to where the electrodes used in DBS should be placed in the brain. (The original clinical trial to determine this involved only 13 patients) These facts don't really boost your confidence, do they?(9)

Then there's the study reported in the journal *Age and Ageing*, that concludes that all of the 402 patients initially diagnosed with PD (gleaned from 74 different medical practices and hospitals), only half of them, upon closer examination by specialists, actually had the disease. Of course, all of the 402 were initially put on PD medication. Some of the patients who did not have PD, actually suffered from an *essential tremor*, which requires quite different medication.(10)

So if you think you might be developing PD, be sure to have a specialist check you out before accepting any drugs. But, I'm going to show you below how you might avoid PD, and hopefully even reverse some of its symptoms.

Environmental factors and diet can be big factors in whether you develop PD, and how quickly it progresses. Medical doctors in India reported that several people developed PD immediately after exposure to organophosphate pesticides. These pesticides were common household ones such as malathion, diazanon, dursban, and chlorpyriphos. Drug treatment with l-dopa was ineffective, but most of the patients recovered fully once they were no longer exposed to the pesticide.(11)

Another major study concluded that those who use pesticides often have a 17 percent greater risk of developing Parkinson's disease than those who don't use them. Counties in California that had the heaviest pesticide usage also had the most deaths from Parkinson's disease. Rats exposed to low levels of the pesticide rotenone gradually lost their dopamine neurons and developed tremors.(12) Another study showed that part-time gardeners were 9 percent more likely to get PD, and farmers, generally considered to use a lot of pesticides, increased their chances of developing PD by 43 percent.(13) My advice is to use alternative methods of pest control, and eat organic food. You can significantly cut your risks of ever getting PD if you do.

As with dementia and Alzheimer's disease, heavy metals may also cause Parkinson's disease. High aluminum levels in drinking water causes increases in the incidences of PD. As I already discussed, aluminum can get in municipal drinking water due to water treatment methods, and fluoride (also in many drinking water supplies) multiplies the negative effects of aluminum. But aluminum can also get in ground water because acid rain leaches aluminum out of the soil.(14) Other sources of aluminum are aluminum cookware, antacids, antiperspirants, aluminum foil, baking powder, and processed foods. So get a good water filter that removes aluminum and fluoride (remember, fluoride increases aluminum absorption), or use a good spring water bottled at the source.

Other metals that have been implicated as causing PD are mercury, cadmium, copper, and manganese. Of course, you already know that amalgam dental filings are the most significant source of mercury in the body. You will also learn in the chapter on vaccines, that mercury is present in vaccines and flu shots. Copper and manganese are oftentimes found in one-a-day type vitamins, so taking these might exacerbate PD.

Not only can drugs directly cause PD, but they can also deplete magnesium, which has been shown to protect brain cells from the damaging effects of heavy metals. Magnesium competes with heavy metals for entry into brain cells, so if magnesium levels are low, the heavy metals get in and get deposited. Considering that magnesium absorption declines with age (absorption at 70 is two-thirds what it is at 30), elderly people who don't eat a diet high in magnesium and who take pharmaceutical drugs (senior citizens take on average six to eight medications regularly) are especially at risk of developing PD.(15) Millions of people also take diuretics to control high blood pressure. However, they too can cause low level of brain magnesium.

People with high levels of iron in their diets, especially when there are also high levels of manganese, are nearly two times more likely to develop PD than those with low levels. Foods that are high in iron and manganese are spinach, lima beans, peas, wheat bread, peanuts, and other nuts and seeds.(16) High levels of iron are also found in the brains of people with PD. Cooking in cast iron cookware can release significant amounts of iron, especially if you're cooking something acidic (like tomato sauce). Many elderly are lead to believe that they may develop an iron deficiency and are encouraged to take a supplement like *Geritol*, an iron-rich multivitamin. However, this may lead to an excess of iron, which can contribute to PD.

Food for Thought

The name *Geritol* is derived from the root "geri-", meaning old (as in geriatrics) with the "i" for iron. The product has been promoted from almost the beginning of the mass media era as a cure for "iron-poor tired blood." In the early 20th century, many medical doctors and other health professionals felt that much of the tiredness often associated with old age was due to iron deficiency anemia. This theory was later discredited, but *Geritol* was already well known and continued to be marketed. Now, considering excess iron can contribute to PD, there should be a warning label on good-old *Geritol*, don't you think? Interestingly, *Geritol* is now made by the pharmaceutical giant GlaxoSmithKline who also makes PD drugs. Like I say, drug companies get you coming and going.

These days, many people believe that we should take vitamins and minerals because we don't get enough from our foods. A "shotgun" approach is oftentimes used by taking a multi-vitamin loaded with everything but the kitchen sink. But what if you already had enough iron in your blood and you take a multivitamin like *Geritol* rich in iron? It's not going to do you any good, and will probably harm you in the long run.

If you're going to supplement with pills, you first need to know what nutrients you truly need. Blood tests, hair analysis, urinalysis, and other tests are all needed to determine this. Plus, most vitamins on the market are poor quality, made from inferior products and are oftentimes waste products of other food manufacturing processes. These vitamins and minerals have been so denatured that the body can hardly use them. That's not to mention the additives such as dicalcium phosphate, magnesium stearate, dyes, and others that not only directly harm your body, but render the active ingredients virtually useless. (See more on supplements in the Obesity chapter.) My advice is to save your money on all those supplements, and invest it in good quality, organic foods. You'll be getting much more nutrition, without having to worry about intake excesses and PD causing pesticides.

Those who consume a lot of sugar are three times more likely to develop PD as those with moderate intakes.[17] Any kind of processed sugar is detrimental to nerve cells and causes an overproduction of adrenaline. The nerve cells are essentially stripped of their protective layers of fat by the adrenaline, and are exposed to the harmful effects of toxins, especially heavy metals.[18]

Nerve cells are largely fat – especially the myelin sheath protecting the nerve fiber. It's essential that nerves have a good supply of the right kinds of uncooked, unprocessed fat. You won't find these in cooked meats, potato chips, and vegetable oil. Raw milk, cream, butter, coconut oil, and raw fish and meat contain the right kinds of fats that will insulate the nerves and allow them to function normally. My advice here is consistent with the findings of an experimental diet for patients with PD that was very low in protein and carbohydrates, and extremely high in fat. These patients experienced improvements in balance, tremors, and mood.[19] If the study had used only uncooked fats, I believe the results would have been even more astounding. I also believe that they would not have had to limit the protein content of the diet, since uncooked protein is good for the body too. But as far as PD is concerned, the fat is absolutely essential.

Cholesterol has already been discussed in some detail in the chapter on heart disease. As far as PD is concerned, *MSNBC* reported that men with low cholesterol levels were found to be up to six times more likely to get PD than those who had higher levels. Researchers think this may be because cholesterol helps to rid the body of environmental toxins and that it's the precursor for hormones involved in nervous system function.[20]

In another study reported in *Neurology*, it was found that middle-aged men who drink one or two glasses of pasteurized milk a day have double the risk of getting PD.[21] This is not surprising to me since pasteurized milk is difficult to digest and the calcium almost impossible to utilize. Unpasteurized milk products are fine, and good for you. But when the proteins, fats, enzymes, and minerals are cooked – as in pasteurization – they become inert. . . like glue. In fact, I imagine that drinking pasteurized milk and eating pasteurized dairy products is like taking a bottle of *Elmer's* glue (ever notice the picture of the cow on the bottle?) and squirting it into your brain. So don't drink the milk or eat the cheese (unless it's raw), and you'll be reducing the risk of getting PD.

So how can you avoid getting PD, and if you have it, is there anything you can do to stop it from getting worse or reverse it? I already mentioned that avoiding pesticides, pasteurized dairy products, aluminum, fluoride, mercury, high blood levels of iron, and sugar will help reduce your risks. Now there's a study that shows that vitamin D can help to suppress genetic weaknesses that tend to allow the disease to manifest.[22] So getting plenty of sunshine and taking your cod liver or krill oil should help you.

Some research has shown that consuming high amounts of vitamin C and E and vitamin B complex slows the progression of the disease in its early stages.(23) I believe it's best to get these vitamins from food, not supplements, and if you eat raw food, you will.

Relaxation therapy has also proven useful in treating PD, since stress aggravates it. And of course, our good old friend exercise has been shown to help. Men who are physically active in their adult life are 50 percent to 60 percent less likely to get PD later on.(24) I haven't seen any studies on what effect exercise has on people already with PD, but it can't be bad. The more circulation, the more blood to the nerves, and the quicker they can repair themselves. Short duration, high intensity exercise has shown to be better than low intensity, long duration exercise (see chapter on cardiovascular diseases for details on the best way to exercise).

I'm not a big fan of eating beans, since you have to cook them and they're difficult to digest even then. But the fava bean (*Vicia faba*), or broad bean, has an extremely good source of l-dopa, and can, in some cases, actually have the same effect on PD as the l-dopa drug. These should always be consumed whole since the pod has the highest l-dopa content.

CHAPTER XI

Arthritis, Osteoporosis, & Cavities

Arthritis is an umbrella term for more than 100 diseases and conditions that affect the joints. It is a defect in the production of collagen, the protein that is the structural part of cartilage. This causes the joint to degenerate. Arthritis is the leading cause of disability in the U.S. Currently, about 46 million Americans (22 percent) have some form of arthritis and by 2030 it's expected to affect an estimated 67 million adults in the U.S. Women, older adults, persons with little education or those who are obese, overweight or physically inactive are more likely to get arthritis.(1,2,3)

Osteoarthritis (OA) is the most common form of arthritis affecting 21 million Americans. It's characterized by the disintegration of cartilage (the part of the joint that cushions the ends of the bones). This causes stiffness, pain, loss of movement, and eventually the cartilage can wear away completely causing bone to rub on bone. This feels like a grating sensation and can produce sounds like creaking or crunching. Usually the hips, hands, knees, lower back, and neck are affected. Pain or stiffness occurs most often after overexertion or long periods of inactivity. Rheumatoid arthritis (RA) is another common form of arthritis affecting about 2.1 million people in the U.S. It's marked by the inflammation in and around joints and connective tissues (the *synovial membrane*) and strikes adults between the ages of 30 and 50, 70 percent of these being women.(4)

The risk of getting OA increases with overweight, joint injury, poor joint alignment, and aging. Diagnosis is generally made using X-rays or magnetic resonance imaging (MRI). Maintaining healthy weight is one of the most important factors in preventing OA. A study in the *Annals of Internal Medicine* found that if an overweight woman loses as few as 10 pounds, she decreases her risk of getting OA by 50 percent.(5)

Medical treatments for OA and RA are usually drugs that include corticosteriods (which are injected directly into the joint to ease inflammation), analgesics like *Tylenol* (prescription drugs being *Oxycontin, Ultram*), NSAIDs (see below), DMARDs (disease-modifying antirheumatic drugs), and BRMs (biologic response modifiers). Hyaluronic acid eases the dehydration of the cartilage and is often injected into the knees if they are affected.

Common over-the-counter NSAIDs (non-steroidal anti-inflammatory drugs) are the most popular way to ease the pain of arthritis. They include *Bayer* (an aspirin), *Advil* (an ibuprofen), and *Aleve* (a naproxen). Prescription brands or anti-inflammatory drugs include *Celebrex, Voltaren, Daypro, Lodine, Nalfon, Indocin, Toradol, Relafen, Clinoril,* and *Tolectin*. These drugs are the most widely prescribed drugs in the world with over 30 billion tablets sold annually in the U.S. alone.(6) The common side effects of these drugs are nausea and vomiting, and it's often recommended that these pills be taken along with milk or food to prevent an upset stomach.

But these drugs do a lot more harm than causing a little tummy ache. They can damage the kidneys and stomach lining, leading to ulcers and serious gastrointestinal complications. In fact, *The American Journal of Medicine* states: ". . .calculations estimate that approximately 107,000 patients are hospitalized annually for NSAID-related gastrointestinal complications and at least 16,500 NSAID-related deaths occur each year among arthritis patients alone."(7) Another report in the *New England Journal of Medicine* underscores the significance of this problem with NSAIDs no one ever hears about:

> It has been estimated conservatively that 16,500 NSAID-related deaths occur among patients with rheumatoid arthritis or osteoarthritis every year in the United States. This figure is similar to the number of deaths from the AIDS and considerably greater than the number of deaths from multiple myeloma, asthma, cervical cancer, or Hodgkin's disease. If deaths from gastrointestinal toxic effects from NSAIDs were tabulated separately in the National Vital Statistics reports, these effects would constitute the 15th most common cause of death in the United States. Yet these toxic effects remain mainly a "silent epidemic," with many physicians and most patients unaware of the magnitude of the problem. Furthermore, the mortality statistics do not include deaths ascribed to the use of over-the-counter NSAIDs.(8)

Aspirin was is a trade name of a buffered form of salicylic acid formulated by Felix Hoffman at *Bayer* industries in 1889. Since then, it has become a mainstay of over-the-counter pain relief. It's even used as a blood thinner to help decrease heart attacks and strokes. But as you can see, it can cause problems, just can all drugs.

There's another kind of painkiller that is technically a NSAID but in a subclass called *Cox-2 inhibitors*. They include *Vioxx*, which has been recalled, and *Celebrex*, which is still being sold. They were developed to be easier on the stomach. Problem is, they're hard on the heart and blood vessels. They actually increase the stickiness of blood and can significantly increase the risk of heart attacks and stroke.(9) In 2001 the FDA first became concerned when a drug company study designed to show *Vioxx* reduced gastrointestinal problems also revealed that people taking it had four times the risk of heart attack. It took until September 2004 for the drug maker to pull the drug from the market. Since then, about 50,000 people have filed lawsuits against *Merck*, and *Merck* has paid out $4.85 billion to settle tens of thousands of these lawsuits. It's estimated that anywhere from 100,000 to 200,000 people died as a result of taking this drug.

Food for Thought

Merck knew there were problems with *Vioxx* at least four years before they pulled it. Even a study in the *Journal of the American Medical Association* by a group of cardiologists in 2001 said there were problems. But did *Merck* do anything? Of course not. They just kept trying to silence the reports and kept saying the benefits outweighed the risks.(10)

And the FDA? When one doctor raised concerns about *Vioxx's* safety and was about to present it at a conference, the FDA scratched him from the program. He was also put under intense pressure and intimidation by his colleagues at the FDA because he was raising drug safety issues.(11) All this is not really surprising considering that when the Prescription Drug User Fee Act took effect in 1992, the drug companies actually started funding the FDA – a classic fox guarding the henhouse scenario. If you take drugs, don't think the FDA has done its homework, even if the drug is FDA approved.

As fall-out from this *Vioxx* debacle, The *New York Times* reported that *Merck* is trying to get the law changed that would bar most lawsuits against companies for injuries said to be caused by prescription medicines approved by the FDA.(12) Not just that, but they're trying to have the FDA, not individual juries, be responsible for evaluating the risks and benefits of a drug in future cases like the *Vioxx* case.(In case you missed it, I already discussed how many FDA officials have ties to the drug companies.)

Friends, "Of the people, by the people, and for the people," is becoming, "Of the drug companies, by the drug companies, and for the drug companies."

Oftentimes people with RA are prescribed glucocorticoids, prednisone being a popular one. These drugs are also prescribed to treat difficult skin problems. But they are known to induce osteoporosis (called glucocorticoid-induced osteoporosis) and significant bone loss, which oftentimes leads to fractures. One study published in the *Archives of Dermatology* reported that 33 percent of women being treated with glucocorticoids for RA for 5 years sustained bone fractures.(13,14)

Even *Tylenol* (acetaminophen) has been shown to cause liver damage in high doses for two weeks. "I would urge the public not to exceed four grams a day," said Dr. Neil Kaplowitz of the University of Southern California who headed the study.(15,16)

So if taking painkillers isn't safe, what's the solution then to avoiding or reversing arthritis? First – don't do things that cause it and, second – treat it with natural methods.

What causes arthritis and other bone or joint problems such as OA and RA is acid. As I talked about in the discussion about the evils of sugar, the body must maintain a certain pH (the measure of acidity) not just in order to be healthy, but to stay alive. If you continually expose yourself to foods and substances (tobacco, alcohol, drugs – whether recreational or prescription) that introduce acidity into the body, the body must find a way to neutralize it. One of the great neutralizers of acidity is calcium.

When a farmer's fields aren't producing, he'll check and see if the soil pH is right. If it's too acidic, most crops won't grow and if they do, the minerals in the soil won't come out of the soil for the plant to take up. So what does he do? He spreads lime, which is calcium carbonate. This neutralizes the acid and frees up the minerals. Well, the body, in its infinite wisdom, does the same thing when things are too acidic. It takes calcium out of bones (and muscles) to neutralize the acid. If enough is taken out, the bones and joints get weak (arthritis) brittle and porous (osteoporosis). They wear out sooner and as things start to wear away, you feel pain.

What does traditional medicine say to do? Take a drug, of course. But these drugs do nothing to rebuild the bones and joints they just mask the pain. So as time goes on, you have to take more and more painkillers to avoid the pain. The drugs themselves, as I just mentioned, increase the acidity, so in the long run, cause the joint, or bone to wear away sooner.

What you should do is allow the body to come back into pH balance. That involves eliminating the things that create acidity, and adding the things that encourage alkalinity (the opposite of acidity) and bone formation. Most of the acid comes from dietary sources: soda, coffee, tea, sugar, white bread, donuts and so on, processed foods, fast foods, alcohol, cooked meat, all pasteurized dairy, oils that are not cold processed, all soy products. Cooked and processed meat is especially bad for arthritis, gout, and rheumatism sufferers, as they are very high in acids that tend to accumulate in and around the joints. Rheumatoid arthritis of often called the *cooked food disease* for good reason. Cooking renders foods acidic, and this acid accumulates in the joints leading to pain and stiffness.

Foods that encourage alkalinity and bone formation include all raw foods (dairy, meat, fruit, vegetables), vegetable juices, and cold processed oils. One food shown to help arthritis is apple cider vinegar (see the Total Health Drink in the Obesity chapter). It's believed to dissolve the crystal deposits of uric acid that form between joints and in muscles. Dr. Angus Peters of the University of Edinburgh's Arthritis Research Institute found that drinking the honey/vinegar drink reduced the pains of arthritis 90 percent.(17)

Since arthritis and related joint problems result from excess acid, they are an indication that the acid/alkaline balance in the body is off. Iodine helps regulate the acid/alkaline balance in the blood and tissues, helps repair worn out tissues and nourishes the skeletal structure. So it's important to get enough of the right kind. See the breast cancer chapter for more on iodine.

Potatoes are very alkaline and have a high amount of potassium, minerals and vitamin C (potatoes are good to reverse scurvy). Many people have experienced tremendous relief of arthritis, rheumatism, gout and lumbago by drinking potato water first thing in the morning due to its anti-inflammatory actions and the fact it flushes the uric acid out of the joints. To make potato water, simply cut a medium-sized potato into thin slices (do not peel it, but cut out any eyes and don't use potatoes that are green or have black spots since these contain solanine – a toxic chemical), and place the slices in a large glass of water. Let this sit overnight, and drink it first think in the morning on an empty stomach. Alternatively, boil the peelings of a large potato in a cup of water for five minutes (most of the minerals are just beneath the skin), strain and drink. A poultice of raw potato peelings or cooked mashed raw potato applied directly to the joint is tremendous for pain relief. To make the wrap, boil 1 lb. of potatoes in their skins until tender. Place them in a linen sack and mash them. Apply the sack to the affected area and cover with cloth. Remove the only after it has cooled down completely. Potato juice is also said to be good for heartburn, constipation ulcers, gall bladder problems and helps cleanse the liver.

Fresh vegetable juices of green leafy vegetables, celery, red beets and a small amount of carrot, also help dissolve the acid crystals. Pineapples and its juice are exceptional in reducing swelling and inflammation in both osteo and rheumatoid arthritis. Bananas are rich in vitamin B_6, which is good for arthritis.

Garlic too is helps ease the pain of arthritis. A study at the Fyukuyama Army Hospital in Japan showed 86 percent of arthritis sufferers who received garlic extract reported improvement in their condition. It can also be used as a poultice directly to the aching areas. For this, chop up the cloves of two heads of garlic and soak for five minutes in a cup of warm olive oil. Soak a sock in warm water, then stuff the toe with the garlic mash and some of the oil. Rub into the affected area for a few minutes and feel the relief.[18]

One of the best things you can take to avoid and reverse any kind of arthritis is cod liver oil. It not only lubricates the joints, but has been shown to decrease certain chemicals that cause patients to suffer from joint pain. It's also thought that a vitamin D deficiency can cause OA, so getting sunshine and taking cod liver oil would help in that regard too.

Food for Thought

I had a bad case of arthritis or bursitis (inflammation of the bursa – a sac filled with fluid in a joint) in my shoulder years ago. It got so painful and it crackled so badly I couldn't even do pushups. Then I read about cod liver oil and started taking it two or three tablespoons a day. Within a week, my shoulder was feeling better, and in three weeks the pain and crackling were completely gone.

Not long after that, my mom had the exact same thing in her shoulder. I told her about the cod liver oil, and she too began taking it. In a few weeks, her pain and crackling were gone too. It's not surprising then to find that Great Britain's Arthritis Research Campaign found that the omega-3 fatty acids in cod liver oil reduce both pain and damage in inflamed joints.

(Don't forget the important warning about cod liver oil I made in the cancer chapter and be sure to get only the brands I recommend, since now most of them are incorrectly processed.)

In fact, cod liver oil has been shown to be practically a miracle when it comes to improving joint and bone health. But before I go into the research, I'd like to talk some about osteoporosis since joint and bone health are so closely linked.

Osteoporosis

Osteoporosis, or porous bone, is a disease marked by deterioration of bone tissue and loss of bone mass that makes the bone fragile and more susceptible to fractures. These fractures usually occur to the hip, spine and wrist, but any bone can be affected. It's estimated that 10 million people in the U.S. (8 million women and 2 million men) have it and 34 million people have low bone mass that's not yet osteoporosis.[19] Women can lose up to 20 percent of bone mass in the first five to seven years after menopause, making them the prime victims of this disease.

You can't feel your bones getting weaker so you may not know you have osteoporosis until you break a bone. The bones can get so weak that you don't even need to fall, but simple actions such as a sneeze can cause a break. Sometimes back pain might be a sign of a vertebral fracture (bone of the spine), and stooped posture or kyphosis (humpback) are usually signs that the bones have lost a lot of mass and are probably osteoporotic.

Falls are the leading cause of death and disability in old people. When a person in their eighties breaks a hip, there's a 12 to 39 percent chance they will die within a year. Thirteen percent to 50 percent of fall victims are unable to walk after their fracture, and about 20 percent of them require long-term nursing care.[20]

Food for Thought

Nobody wants to break a hip and nobody wants to melt away. So it's not surprising that the elderly are taking drugs that the drug companies say make bones denser. Most of them are in the class of drugs called bisphosphonates. *Zometa* and *Aredia* are bisphosphonates that are taken intravenously by cancer patients where the cancer has advanced into the bone, and *Fosamax* (alendronate), *Actonel* (risedronate) and *Boniva* (ibandronate) are lower dose forms taken as pills for osteoporosis. Yes, these pills do make bones denser, but at a very high price: they kill certain cells in the bone called *osteoclasts*, which are responsible for dissolving existing bone. The theory is that if these cells aren't as active, less bone will be dissolved so the bone will stay dense. This may sound OK, but bone cells are not static things. They are continually being built-up (by bone cells called *osteoblasts*) and removed (by *osteoclasts*), and this renewal of bone cells ensures they stay strong and dense. In osteoporosis, the osteoblasts slow down, but the osteoclasts don't, so you have more removal than renewal, and this makes bones less dense.

So these drugs kill off the osteoclasts and the bone stays dense. But that bone is also weaker since it has not been renewed with younger bone cells. The drugs do nothing to build bone. But they do come with serious side effects: jaw crumbling; atrial fibrillation; increased risk of ulcers; liver damage; renal failure; serious eye inflammations; and possible blindness.[21]

Jaw crumbling, or osteonecrosis of the jaw (or ONJ), is the actual melting away and crumbling of jawbone. This may occur in between one and 10 percent of *Fosamax* users.[22] Jaw crumbling has even been given a nickname by dentists and oral surgeons of *Fossy Jaw* (after the drug that causes it). Problems with these bisphonsphonates has gotten so widespread that on January 25, 2008 the Supreme Court designated all litigation by victims of *Zometa* and *Aredia* be treated as mass tort – a class action law suit against the drug manufacturer Novartis. It's ironic that a drug to stop bone loss actually dissolves the jawbone – and the existing labeling gives no warning of this possible side effect.

A study published in the *Archives of Internal Medicine* showed that women taking *Fosamax* had an 86 percent higher risk of atrial fibrillation, which can cause palpitations, fainting, fatigue or congestive heart failure, and embolic strokes.[23] Don't' let the slick ads and TV stars advertising these poisons fool you. Like all drugs, they may treat the symptom, but they don't fix the underlying problem, and in the long run cause more harm than good.

Being of small and thin frame makes osteoporosis more likely, as does having a history of broken bones. Low estrogen levels in women, low calcium intake, low vitamin D intake, excessive intake of protein, sodium and caffeine, smoking, alcohol abuse, sugar intake, soft drinks and medications all increase the likelihood of getting weak and porous bones.

By age 20, an average women has acquired about 98 percent of her skeletal mass, so building strong bones during childhood and adolescence can be the best defense against developing osteoporosis later. One study showed that girls who ate fruit and vegetables three times or more a day had, compared to girls who consumed them less than that, larger bones and improved bone density markers.[24]

I went into detail on soft drinks and osteoporosis in the chapter on diabetes, but will underscore the importance of avoiding them here. Soft drinks contain not just loads of sugar (which creates acid), put a high amount of phosphoric acid. Phosphates are especially effective in dissolving bone because in order for it to be excreted by the kidneys (phosphate is negatively charged), it must be coupled to a positively charged ion, which would be calcium.

And believe it or not, store-bought pasteurized milk, even though it's loaded with calcium, can contribute to osteoporosis. Why? The calcium in milk is in the form of calcium phosphate. Raw, unpasteurized milk contains the enzyme phosphatase that breaks the calcium away from the phosphate and allows it to be used correctly by the body. But when milk is pasteurized, this enzyme is destroyed, so the calcium remains bound to the phosphate, which is acidic and demands more calcium to be neutralized.

When people think of bones, they think of calcium. But surprisingly, calcium intake alone will not prevent fractures or osteoporosis. One 18-year study found that milk consumption and the use of calcium supplements among postmenopausal women did not decrease the risk of fractures unless there was adequate vitamin D in the diet.(25) Drinking milk fortified with vitamin D doesn't help either, since this vitamin D is the synthetic form (called ergocalciferol), and is no where near as beneficial as real vitamin D.

Vitamin K is also necessary for strong bones. It can be found in green leafy vegetables, and vegetable juicing is particularly good in this regard. It's also especially plentiful in collard greens and spinach.

And remember magnesium? I've extolled its virtues throughout this book, but need to remind you here since magnesium is extremely important to bone and joint health. Yes, the bones need calcium, but it is not absorbed and utilized correctly if there's not enough magnesium too, so just taking a calcium supplement is probably not a good idea. In fact, if you have too much calcium and not enough magnesium in your diet, the excess calcium may be deposited in soft tissues (arteries) and cause problems. The countries with the highest calcium to magnesium ratios also have the most heart attacks. Since it's difficult to get enough magnesium through diet and oral supplements due to its laxative effect, its best to apply magnesium oil to the skin or soak in it. I discussed magnesium in more detail in the chapters on cardiovascular health and diabetes.

Other minerals necessary for bone mineralization include zinc (shellfish, eggs, beef, chicken), manganese (avocados, eggs, nuts, seeds, butter), silicon (bell peppers, green leafy vegetables, whole grains, beets, brown rice) and boron (apples, carrots, grapes, raw nuts, pears, dark green leafy vegetables, whole grains).

Areas of the world with the lowest boron in the soil also have the highest rates of arthritis. Boron enhances brain function, helps prevent postmenopausal osteoporosis and can shrink prostate tumors. One study showed that women who took 3 mgs of boron a day lost 40 percent less calcium and 33 percent less magnesium within just 8 days.(26)

Silicon (silica is silicon dioxide) is necessary for the formation of collagen and connective tissue, healthy nails, skin, and hair; and for calcium absorption. It counteracts the effects of aluminum and may help prevent Alzheimer's besides being a preventative for osteoporosis. Silicon slows the aging process in tissues, but declines with age, so the elderly need larger amounts.(27)

Besides the right diet and avoiding things that cause weak bones, weight bearing exercises have also been shown to increase bone mass. I don't think children need to do these, but adults would benefit. If you already have weak bones I would not start a weight-lifting program until you have improved your diet.

Vitamin D was first recognized in preventing rickets in children. Now, researchers in Australia found that being severely deficient in vitamin D drastically increases elderly peoples' risk of fatal falls.(28) Women in the study who were given vitamin D supplements showed a 20 percent decrease in falls every time their vitamin D levels doubled. What's more, vitamin D has been found to improve bone mineral density in women, and that peripubertal girls with the highest levels of vitamin D in their blood had higher bone mineral densities.(29,30)

The researchers believe that vitamin D is not just important for strong bones, but muscles and brain function as well and that higher vitamin D levels helps in coordination and strength, which helps reduce the number of falls. Dr. Caryl Nowson of Deakin University in Melbourne said, "We're discovering that vitamin D deficiency is the deficiency of the elderly." The problems are "partly because the women were stuck in nursing homes, and partly because of the strong Australian public health message about sun and skin cancer risk." (That means, go get some sun, it's good for you!)

Two symptoms of vitamin D deficiency are bone pain and muscle pain. You may feel it in the legs with muscle weakness and difficulty climbing stars. Studies have shown improvements in muscle pain, muscle strength, and bone pain with cod liver oil supplementation.(31,32)

Robert Jay Rowen, M.D. prescribes vitamin D from cod liver oil for his osteoporosis patients. He says, ". . .in the case of osteoporosis, more vitamin D is better, and I will routinely use 1,200 to 2,000 IUs. Vitamin D is generally safe in doses up to 10,000 IUs per day. It has many other wonderful properties including lowering the risk of many cancers, blood pressure control, fluid and mineral balance and more. . .Vitamin D with calcium has been shown to reduce fractures. . ."(33)

Cod liver oil has been shown to improve health in a myriad of ways other than bone health, as I've discussed throughout the book. Some additional benefits include: It can reduce intraocular pressure suggesting a use in the prevention and treatment of glaucoma; can help with irritable bowel syndrome, colitis and Crohn's disease; is protective against childhood leukemia; applied topically, cod liver oil contributes to faster wound healing, softer skin, helps minimize wrinkles and is an excellent treatment for diaper rash and acne.(34,35,36,37,38) Cod liver oil mixed with zinc oxide ointment is better for the skin and safer than any skin cream prescription.

Cod liver oil also contains vitamin A, which can be toxic in high amounts. So limiting vitamin A to 30,000 IUs a day (about 4 tablespoons) is advisable. Two tablespoons of regular cod liver oil a day during the winter months is a good dose. In the summer you may not need as much if any depending on how much sun exposure you get. In addition, some cod liver oils are fortified with synthetic vitamin A (retinoic acid), which has been shown to cause birth defects, so make sure you're taking an all natural brand.

An interesting discovery was made concerning vitamin D and cereal consumption. Diets having high levels of cereals, especially oatmeal, were shown to cause rickets. The phytic acid in grains and legumes are to blame, making vitamin D less absorbable. So anyone, especially children, who eats cereal needs higher intakes of vitamin D.[39,40] (Yet another testimony as to the harmful effects of cooking. If you want to eat oatmeal that isn't harmful, soak it in water for several hours or overnight, warm it if you must, but not to the degree of burning your finger, and eat it. Add some raw honey and cinnamon, and you're all set. This is much more nutritious than cooked oatmeal.)

Bones and teeth are closely related to each other, so what affects the bones probably affects the teeth, and vice versa. William Hirzy, Ph.D., of the EPA said, "What's going on in the teeth is a window to what's going on in the bones."[41] He was saying that as he was discussing how fluoride, commonly added to our water supply, can cause osteoporosis. He continued, "It is well known now that fluoride produces faulty bone, more brittle, basically mimicking in the bone what is clearly visible in the teeth." Health officials and most dentists will tell you that fluoride helps prevent cavities. But does it? Let's take a closer look.

Fluoride, Bones, Teeth, & Cavities

Fluoride has been added to public water supplies since the 1940s in the belief that ingesting fluoride helps prevent cavities. It all started in 1939 when a dentist named H. Trendley Dean, working for the U.S. Public Health Service, said that high concentrations of fluoride in the water in certain areas of Texas corresponded to a high incidence of mottled teeth. (Mottled teeth are teeth with whitish flecks or spots, particularly the front teeth, or in severe cases, dark spots or stripes on the teeth.) Dean also said that there was a lower incidence of dental cavities in the communities having about 1 part per million (ppm) fluoride in their water supplies. Dean's report led to the fluoridation of drinking water at 1 ppm in order to supply the "optimal dose" of 1 mg fluoride per day if four glasses of water were drunk.

But Dean's original study suggesting fluoride ingestion was beneficial was flawed. When other scientists investigated Dean's data, they didn't reach the same conclusion. Dean was forced to state in court under oath that his data were invalid. In 1957 he admitted at an American Medical Association hearing that even waters containing a mere 0.1 ppm (0.1mg/l) could cause dental fluorosis, which is the first visible sign of fluoride overdose. And there has not been one single double-blind study indicating that fluoridation is effective in reducing cavities.(42)

Food for Thought

The EPA's Dr. William Hirzy says, "Clear back in 1934. . . the American Dental Association plainly treats the subject very matter-of-factly. It calls fluoride a general protoplasmic poison." A 1944 article in the *Journal of the American Dental Association* said, "With 1.6 to 4 ppm fluoride in the water, 50 percent or more past age 24 have false teeth because of fluoride damage to their own."(43)

These do not sound like ringing endorsements for the fluoridation of drinking water. In fact, the idea of fluoride being good for people's teeth originated with the atomic bomb's Manhattan Project – the U.S. Military program to produce the first atomic bomb (prior to World War II there was no U.S. commercial production of fluorine). The fact that fluoride was beneficial constituted the government's cardinal defense against lawsuits stemming from an environmental contamination that took place from the *DuPont* chemical factory in Deepwater, New Jersey, in 1944. The factory was then producing millions of pounds of fluoride for the Manhattan Project. And one thing left over from manufacturing nuclear weapons and nuclear power is fluoride compounds. Instead of disposing of it properly, which costs money, our beloved government saw fit to turn a profit instead by promoting its use in water supplies.

Suddenly, fluoride was proclaimed as the "wonder nutrient" that stops cavities. As more and more industries found uses for fluorides, its wastes increased. Hirzy guesses that if fluoride were required to be disposed of properly as a waste product, the administrative costs of that disposal would exceed $100 million a year – for the fertilizer industry alone. Now you know why they want it in our water instead. John R. Lee, M.D., says of fluoride, "It's a toxic waste product of many types of industry; for instance, glass production, phosphate fertilizer production, and many others. They would have no way to dispose of the tons of fluoride waste they produce unless they could find some use for it, so they made up this story about it being good for dental health. Then they can pass it through everyone's bodies and into the sewer."(44)

It's interesting how the quest for better ways to kill and maim people can be turned on their heads and used for our "benefit." The production of deadly chemicals for chemical warfare in World War I and World War II led to our chemical pesticide industry; and the production of the atomic bomb has lead to fluoridation of our drinking water. Isn't mankind resourceful? Seems to me that if it kills, we shouldn't use it. But I always have had radical ideas (and I don't work for the government).

There's evidence that suggests that fluoride in the water actually increases tooth decay. A study of 39,000 children ages five to 17 years conducted by the National Institute of Dental Research showed that children living in cities with fluoridated water had more tooth decay. When 1.0 ppm fluoride was added to the water supply there was a 5.4 percent increase in pediatric tooth decay. Another study examining 400,000 students showed that decay increased 27 percent when 1.0 ppm fluoride was increased in drinking water.(45) And it doesn't stop there as far as the health effects can go. Fluoride as sodium fluoride is another "cumulative toxin." That means it accumulates in the tissues and is not easily excreted by the body.

"Dental fluorosis" is the technical term for mottled teeth. Currently up to 80 percent of U.S. children have some degree of dental fluorosis, which has been shown to increase the likelihood of tooth decay.

Fluoride is added to toothpaste and public drinking water supplies for its supposed cavity – fighting property, but researchers have found that the ability of fluoride to prevent dental caries (cavities), if it exists at all, comes from using it topically, as in toothpaste. It has no identifiable beneficial effect when ingested. The Centers for Disease Control said in a 1999 report, ". . . laboratory and epidemiological research suggests that fluoride prevents dental caries predominately after eruption of the tooth into the mouth, and its actions primarily are topical for both adults and children." Even the CDC acknowledges that the effects of fluoride are "topical" and not "systemic," meaning that the addition of fluoride to drinking water supplies does not help prevent cavities.(46)

What exactly is fluoride and how can it affect you or your child? Its health effects can be profound and far-reaching and, as we shall see, it can contribute to ADHD, learning disabilities, lower IQs, depression, along with other health problems.

Fluoride is actually a generic term given to a wide variety of substances that contain the element fluorine. Fluoride substances are used in a wide variety of industries including agricultural, pharmaceutical, ceramic and glass manufacturers, metallurgy, breweries and wineries, aluminum manufacturing, computer chip manufacturing, petroleum products, military, drugs (especially mood-regulating drugs such as *Prozac*), and others. In agriculture, fluoride is the key ingredient in the world's most widely used insecticides and pesticides and is used as a fumigant for termites.

Sodium fluoride is registered with the EPA as a rat poison and is also a powerful roach killer. Fluoride is used in the military in the production of nuclear warheads and in certain types of nerve gas, one of which – sarin gas – is 15 hundred times more deadly than cyanide.(47) According to the *Clinical Toxicology of Commercial Products, 5th Edition,* fluoride is rated as more toxic than lead. The U.S. Agency for Toxic Substances and Disease Registry (ATSDR) ranks fluoride compounds as among the top 20 of 275 substances that pose the most significant threat to human health.(48) So toxic is the raw fluoride added to drinking water that, according to William Hirzy, Ph.D., of the EPA, if you were to take a dose of it about half the size of a 500 milligram (mg) vitamin tablet, "you'd be long dead before the sun went down."[49]

The so called "cosmetic" defect of mottled teeth predisposes the person to tooth decay. But the health effects go much further than that. Dental fluorosis is merely the first visible sign of fluoride poisoning. Since fluoride is a cumulative poison, U.S. law requires that the Surgeon General set a Maximum Contaminant Level (MCL) for fluoride in public water supplies as determined by the EPA. That MCL is 4 parts per million (ppm) or 4 mg per liter, with the consideration that the body will retain half of this amount (2 mg). They set this limit to avoid crippling skeletal fluorosis (CSF), which becomes severe when there's more than 4 mg/l in the water. A daily dose of 2 mg to 8 mg of fluoride is known to cause severe CSF.[50,51] But did the EPA know this when they set the (too high) MCL?

Yes, they did. In 1998 EPA scientists declared that this 4 ppm level was fraudulently set in a decision that omitted 90 percent of the data showing the mutagenic properties of fluoride.[52] Robert Carton, Ph.D., who worked for the EPA for 20 years, says that "on July 7, 1997, the EPA scientists, engineers and attorneys who assess the scientific data for the Safe Drinking Water Act standards and other EPA regulation have gone on record against the practice of adding fluoride to public drinking water."[53] Why is the EPA Maximum Contaminant Level (MCL) for fluoride 266 times greater than that of lead (4.0 parts per million for fluoride and 0.015 parts per million for lead)? Could it be that in order to add fluoride to drinking water they must make it appear less toxic?

Food for Thought

You may hear, possibly from your dentist or other proponent of fluoridation, that fluoride is found in nature and nothing to be afraid of. The ADA slogan has been, "Nature thought of it first!" It's true that fluoride is found in nature in some waters – in the form of calcium fluoride, not the sodium fluoride we're talking about here. They are totally different in their chemistry and biological effects. Calcium fluoride does not readily dissolve in water; sodium fluoride does. Calcium fluoride is not retained in the body in great amounts; sodium fluoride is. Calcium fluoride is not toxic; and sodium fluoride is very toxic. The hydrofluorosilicic acid that is the direct byproduct of pollution scrubbers in the phosphate fertilizer and aluminum industries is even more toxic – and that is what's directly added to water supplies by our government. It has never been tested for safety even though it's listed as a Class I hazardous waste by the California Code of Regulations.

Phyllis Mullenix, Ph.D., conducted a detailed study of the neurological effects of fluoride. Her results were published in the Journal *Neurotoxicology and Teratology* in 1995. She discovered a pattern of behavioral problems associated with ingestion of fluoride that ". . . matches up with the same results of administering radiation and chemotherapy [to cancer patients]. All of these really nasty treatments that are used clinically in cancer therapy are well known to cause IQ deficits in children. That's one of the best studied effects they know of. The behavioral pattern that results from the use of fluoride matches that produced by cancer treatment that causes a reduction in intelligence."(54) This was the first study to show that the central nervous system output is vulnerable to fluoride, that it accumulates in the brain and that the effects on behavior depend on the age at exposure. Consequently, IQ, learning ability, and motor function may all suffer. Mullenix's findings also showed that the developmental effects of fluoride affected the fetus as well: Doses of fluoride administered before birth produced marked hyperactivity in offspring. Postnatal administration caused the infant rats to exhibit what she calls the "couch potato syndrome" – the absence of initiative and activity.

Food for Thought

Although Mullenix's fluoride study was done on rats and not humans, they are the best testing subjects we have. Many scientific decisions are made using lab animals, particularly rats, as suitable subjects because their reactions mirror human ones. If we take this as possible in humans then, women who drink fluoridated water and ingest fluoride from other sources are more likely to have hyperactive children.

It's very interesting that many drugs used to treat brain activity have fluoride as the primary active ingredient. *Prozac* (fluoxetene) is one of these and is used to treat depression in adults. As it's doing that, however, is it also making the person less intelligent and less likely to have initiative? Is all the fluoride in our environment making us into a generation of "couch potatoes?"

A 1995 study in China found attention deficit disorders in adults developed if sublingual drops containing 100 ppm (parts per million) of sodium fluoride were administered. Toothpastes typically contain 1,000 to 1,500 ppm fluoride and mouth rinses contain 230 to 900 ppm fluoride, well above the 100 ppm shown to be a problem in the Chinese study. This study also showed that at levels of 3 ppm to 11 ppm, fluoride can affect the nervous system without first causing physical malformations.(55) So you could be suffering from this poison with no telltale teeth marks.

Fluoride has also been implicated in hypothyroidism, and in fact has been used in anti-thyroid medications prescribed when the thyroid is too active. It has an antagonistic effect on iodine and may even cause iodine deficiency. Iodine deficiency causes brain disorders, cretinism, miscarriages, and goiter, and is considered to be the world's single most important and preventable cause of mental retardation, which affects 740 million people a year.

> ### *Food for Thought*
>
> *Synthroid*, a drug to treat hypothyroidism, was, according to Scott-Levin's Source Prescription Audit in 1999, the top-selling drug in the U.S., showing that hypothyroidism is a real problem. There are thought to be many millions of people who have undiagnosed thyroid problems. Could fluoridation of our water supply and overall intake of this toxic waste be a contributing factor?

Robert Carton, the former EPA scientist, says there's research showing that a specific antibody (immunoglobulin or IgM) that is missing from patients with certain types of brain tumors is also missing from the blood of those who test as having elevated blood fluoride levels. This evidence suggests that brain tumors are much more likely among those consuming fluoride compounds.(56)

If all of the above isn't enough to convince you of the hazards of fluoride, consider that when fluorides are added to the U.S. public water systems (in the form of hydrofluosilicic acid and sodium silicofluoride), children tend to absorb more lead from the environment. This causes higher rates of diseases and behavioral problems that are associated with lead poisoning including hyperactivity, substance abuse and violent crime. Over 140 million people are served by water systems laced with fluoride with 200,000 tons of it ingested through these water supplies per year.(57)

You won't just get fluoride from your water and toothpaste. Hundreds of products on the market have significant levels of fluoride in them – partly because the water they use in processing and manufacturing is laden with fluoride, which gets into the mix. Among products with significant levels of fluoride are juices, colas, cereals, and baby juices. Most juice concentrates, including orange juice, are processed with fluoridated water. Almost every product with white grapes contains extremely high concentrations of fluoride because of the fluoride pesticide residues and processing with fluoridated water. Since many pesticides contain fluoride (because it's so deadly), it gives us another good reason to eat organic food. Eliminating all potential sources of fluoride can only do good, especially for young and developing children

As you can see, staying free from or reversing arthritis, osteoporosis and tooth decay is as much a matter of avoiding certain things as taking remedial action. Staying away from fluoride, sugar, drugs, and acid forming foods like cooked meat and dairy will go far in helping. Supplying the body with alkaline forming foods, fresh vegetable juices, vitamin D and the right fats and oils will also go far in giving you relief. Combine the two, and you're well on your way to fundamental and lasting improvement.

CHAPTER XII

Sleep Disorders & Migraine Headaches

Since sleep is when the body repairs and rejuvenates, it's important to get good quality sleep and enough of it. But these days, many people don't. Insomnia (difficulty falling asleep and/or early morning awakenings with no ability of returning to sleep) affects at least 60 million Americans and about one-third of all people in Western civilized countries report some form of difficulty falling or staying asleep, and about 10 percent of people in the U.S. have chronic insomnia. Chronic insomnia is when someone has difficulty falling asleep more than three times a week for over a month and usually involves some degree of daytime dysfunction. Accidents at home, at work and particularly on the road can often be traced back to insomnia. Recent statistics from the National Highway Traffic Safety Administration attribute fatigue to some 100,000 vehicle accidents and 1,500 deaths in the United States alone during 2004.[1,2]

Women have insomnia more often than men, and during menopause, may experience insomnia due to hormonal fluctuations. Sleep problems are also more prevalent in people over the age of 65, who generally have poorer quality sleep often due to medications, illnesses, chronic pain, depression or other health problems.[3] Although the elderly makes up only 20 percent of the U.S. population, half of all sleep medicine prescriptions are written for them.[4] Chronic insomnia may also be a precursor to, rather than a consequence of, certain psychiatric problems, especially depression.[5]

Sleep apnea affects almost 20 million people in the U.S. It's a condition in which the person stops breathing for 10 to 30 seconds during the night, and snores heavily, sometimes experiencing a choking sensation. It may cause liver problems, high blood pressure, and increase the risk of diabetes, and someone with sleep apnea is usually sleepy during the day.[6]

Food for Thought

One of the best ways to improve your sleep, and conquer sleep apnea (and snoring), is by doing the Buteyko breathing I described in the chapter on asthma. Ideally, find a practitioner and take the classes. You won't need drugs, surgery, or the *continuous positive airway pressure* (CPAP) device they sell to treat sleep apnea. The breathing exercises take some time, sure, but doing them is free, improves every aspect of your health, and you won't have to waste your time going to the doctor or trying things that don't work or may be harmful. Buteyko will change your life. I guarantee that. Children can do it too.

Sleep problems are affecting children more and more: As many as one in four children currently suffer some difficulty sleeping. And even though there isn't an approved medicine for childhood sleep problems, many doctors are prescribing them anyway. Dr. William Campbell Douglass says, besides all the sugar and carbohydrates kids eat contributing to the problem, the biggest reason for childhood insomnia is sunlight deprivation.(7)

Just a little lack of sleep can make a big difference in your health. A study at the University of Chicago showed that just six days of sleep restricted to four hours a day pushed 11 healthy young male volunteers into a prediabetic state.(8) The Institute of Medicine warns that sleep deprivation can cause an increase in hypertension, diabetes, obesity, depression, heart attack, and stroke. One study showed that those who sleep less than 4.5 hours a night have higher mortality rates than those who get seven hours. Those who sleep more than seven hours are more likely to die too, but not as likely as the ones with too little sleep.(9) People who sleep less than six hours a night were shown to have a 66 percent greater prevalence of hypertension than those who got at least six hours.(10)

Food for Thought

The study I just mentioned might lead you to think you can get too much sleep. Personally, I don't think that's true, and I'll tell you why: Your body knows best. If you're hungry, you eat. If you're tired, you rest. If you're sleepy, you sleep. The healthier you are, the more in tune you'll be with your body's needs and the easier you'll know what your body is telling you. I believe the people who got more than seven hours sleep needed it, but they needed that extra sleep because they were not as healthy as they could be. I talked about this already in the Alzheimer's chapter.

My advice is to sleep as much as you want. When your body has had enough, you'll wake up. As you heal, you may go through periods of needing a lot of sleep. Let yourself get it. You heal during sleep. Forcing yourself to get up interrupts this healing. That doesn't give you a license to be lazy, however. Get up and get moving, and you won't need as much sleep.

The treatment of choice of insomnia by most physicians is drug intervention (in 2004, $2.1 billion was spent on prescription sleeping pills), most often with drugs called benzodiazepines (*Xanax* and others) or zolpidem (*Ambien* and others). But a study done at the University of Bergen in Norway showed that the effects on insomnia using this drug were no better than using a placebo.(11) Furthermore, those taking the drug were shown to spend less time in the deeper, slower brain wave, more restful sleep than those not taking the drug.

The National Institute of Health has stated that while sleep medications may be useful for acute and situational insomnia, long-term use may cause dependency on and tolerance of the drug.(12,13)

Most sleep drugs require a prescription, but some are available without a prescription (over-the-counter, or OTC). An OTC sleep aid may be no safer than a prescription sleep aid, especially for older people. OTC sleep aids contain antihistamines, which may have side effects nervousness, agitation, falls, and confusion, especially in older people. OTC sleep aids should not be taken for more than 7 to 10 days. They are intended to manage an occasional sleepless night, not chronic insomnia, which could signal a serious underlying problem. You can get addicted to them, have withdrawal symptoms coming off of them, and have serious problems if you overdose.

Food for Thought

A lot of people might drink alcohol to help fall asleep. Although it may help you relax and fall asleep faster, it suppresses REM (Rapid Eye Movement) sleep that is necessary to wake feeling rested. So having a glass of wine or a snifter of brandy is not recommended. The over-the-counter medicine *Nyquil* is mostly alcohol as are other cold and flu medicines so they are not recommended. By the way, counting sheep is not effective in helping you drift off – Researchers at England's Oxford University found it is too boring, and that picturing a tranquil scene such as a waterfall or nice beach helped people fall asleep a full 20 minutes faster.(14)

Many other drugs interfere with sleep. A study in the *European Journal of Clinical Pharmacology* reported that some beta-blockers used to control high blood pressure interfere with sleep by reducing the sleep-inducing hormone melatonin by 80 percent to 90 percent.(15) SSRI antidepressants have also been shown to lead to trouble falling asleep or causing nighttime awakenings.

Melatonin is the hormone that sets your biological clock and tells your body when it's time to be sleepy. When melatonin levels go up, as they should later in the day, you get sleepy. James Maas, Ph.D., a researcher at Cornell University says that getting late afternoon sunshine will cause your body to produce melatonin later in the day, thus causing your biological clock to peak later, making you sleep more soundly at night. In addition, being exposed to bright light too early in the morning causes a premature peak in the cycle, causing impaired sleep.(16)

On the flip side of that is the exposure to artificial light after dark. Women who work the night shift have been shown to have a greater chance of getting breast cancer, and cancer researchers believe it's because artificial light suppresses the brain's production of melatonin, a hormone that helps regulate the sleep/wake cycles.(17) "The melatonin-rich blood collected from subjects while in total darkness severely slowed the growth of the tumors." said David Blask, M.D., Ph.D. "These results are due to a direct effect of the melatonin on the cancer cells. The melatonin is clearly suppressing tumor development and growth. In contrast, tests with the melatonin-depleted blood from light-exposed subjects stimulated tumor growth. We observed rapid growth comparable to that seen with administration of daytime blood samples, when tumor activity is particularly high," Blask said.

So it stands to reason that you should keep your bedroom as dark as possible – totally dark ideally – at night. Dr. Ott, the pioneering doctor on light research, also found that any amount of light at night disturbed the sleep cycle. If you awaken during the night, avoid light if you can, or use as little as possible to get to the bathroom and back. (Put a black-light bulb in your bathroom or use a very dim and shaded night light.)

Food for Thought

Here's a sleep-robber you probably never considered: acid reflux (heart burn or indigestion). Researchers at the Lynn Health Science Institute in Oklahoma City say that acid reflux, whether you can feel it or not, affects about one in four troubled sleepers.(18) So eating a big meal or anything that causes indigestion and gas before bedtime will throw off your sleep.

How to avoid gas (flatulence or burping)? The better you eat the less likely you'll get gas in the first place. Indigestion is just that, incomplete digestion. The gas comes from bacteria feeding off the undigested food. Why is some food not digested? A few reasons: If the food is cooked, it's harder to digest. A cooked meal may take 24 hours to digest fully, whereas the same food not cooked would take about 8 hours. Your body has to work harder to digest it, so not only do you get fewer and damaged nutrients, but it takes more work to extract them from the food.

If the foods are incorrectly combined, you may get gas. Get a book on food combining for details on this. (Beans give you gas because they are a naturally poorly combined food, which means you shouldn't eat them.) Eating to excess will also give you gas, as will eating too much of one food at a time. By eating raw foods, you'll be more able to tell when you're no longer hungry and you'll feel fuller with less food.

If you do get gas, don't run to the antacids. Try eating some celery or drinking celery juice. It's very alkaline and will put out the acid fire in your belly, and it's loaded with minerals that will help you fall asleep. Ginger can also help settle an upset stomach. Heat some in warm/hot water and add honey and lemon to make a nice tea.

The breathing method I discussed in the chapter on asthma is great for relieving gas. It relaxes all the muscles in your body, including the *cardiac sphincter* between your stomach and esophagus. This allows you to belch and eliminate the gas. Do one or two cycles of the breathing and then get up and walk around. You'll be belching in relief in seconds. Cross-crawls (a *Brain Gym* exercise), an exercise used to synchronize the left and right hemispheres of the brain, relaxes your muscles and allows belching and gas to pass. To do this, simply walk in place, and as you lift up your leg, touch it with the opposing hand: Left leg up, touch it with your right hand; right leg up, touch it with your left hand. Do this for a few minutes or until your belching stops. Doing cross-crawls and/or the breathing method before bedtime even if you don't have gas will help you relax, fall asleep faster, and sleep more soundly.

Cognitive Behavioral Therapy (CBT) is often used to help people cope with mood disorders and anxiety. It's a study all of itself, but is basically a way of training yourself to see problems differently. It's also been used to improve sleep, and one study showed that patients receiving CBT showed improvements in sleep compared with those using drug therapy three out of four times. The sleep obtained was deeper and more restful.[19] Again, those taking sleeping medication spent less time in the deeper, more restful sleep than those not taking drugs or doing CBT. The researchers concluded that CBT is far superior to drug treatment in both short-term and long-term management of insomnia. Another study using a different sleep drug (temazepam) showed the same type of results.[20]

The strategies of CBT tailored to sleep are briefly: keeping a strict schedule of bedtimes and rising times; using the bedroom and bed just for sleep (no TV or reading); addressing any fears and negative beliefs concerning sleep; learning how lifestyle and environmental factors (noise, light, temperature) affect sleep; using a progressive relaxation technique (sometimes using a prerecorded tape or CD to practice with) to release muscular tension and induce faster, more restful sleep.

The relaxation technique involves focusing on certain areas of the body and consciously releasing the muscular tension as best you can. You start with your toes, and let all the tension in them leave. You can tell yourself, "relax. . .let go" as you put your mind on them. Then focus on your whole foot and release. . .let go. Then your calves, then your thighs. . .all the way up your body to the top of your head. You'll probably fall asleep before you finish all your body parts. If not, go back down from your head to your toes.

Food for Thought

I used to have a lot of difficulty sleeping. As far back as high school I remember lying in bed and hearing *The Tonight Show with Johnny Carson* on the TV in my parent's bedroom as my anxiety grew worrying about how tired I was going to be the next day. All through college, graduate school and my engineering job, I had a hard time falling asleep, and a hard time staying awake during the day. I used to have lunch at *Burger King* or *McDonalds* and come back to work, fight like heck to keep my eyes open, just to have my head fall on the desk! I was always yawning and fighting nodding off. Embarrassing and not good for school or job performance.

After I started making healthy changes to my lifestyle, my sleep improved somewhat. I discovered some cassette tapes that put you into a slower, more restful brainwave that really helped me fall asleep. A couple companies that sell these kinds of recordings, now on CD, are www.HemiSyncForYou.com/Monroe and www.learningstrategies.com.

I no longer need these recordings and fall asleep now in about 5 or 10 minutes. But sometimes I'll wake during the night to go to the bathroom and have some trouble falling back asleep. When that happens, I use a technique called *pole-bridging* I learned from the book *The Einstein Factor*. It's a relaxation technique that involves using different areas of your brain in sequence, which causes slowing and synchronization of brain waves, and results in relaxation and sleep. It's also been shown to raise IQ levels.[21] Here's how it works:

Close your eyes and picture a pleasant scene. Perhaps you're in a meadow on a mountain top on a clear summer's day. Now describe out loud what each of your senses is experiencing. Try to really feel, hear, taste, smell, and see all these things in your imagination. Make them come to life in you. "I feel the sun on my face and a warm breeze on my skin. I hear the birds singing and the crickets chirping and I see a cloud in the clear blue sky. The taste of lunch lingers on my tongue, and I smell the honeysuckle and flowers. . ." and so on. Just keep describing what you're experiencing. It won't be long before you're asleep. This is most effective when you actually verbalize out loud, but you can also just say it in your head. You must articulate what you're sensing or it is not nearly as effective. Your mind is going to wander, and it takes some effort to bring it back, but force yourself to do so. You'll find that the sleep you have when you do this is deeper and more restful too. Here are a few other things I've found helps sleep:

1. Discontinue all drugs. Medications for arthritis, angina, prostate, depression, decongestants, cancer drugs, and so on can all disturb your sleep. As I've said and demonstrated over and over throughout this book, all drugs are poisons and have negative effects on the body. Is it any coincidence that the age-group with the most sleep problems (the elderly) is also the most drugged? I think not. Wean yourself off of drugs as you make positive changes to your lifestyle (under a doctors care), and watch your sleep improve.

2. Eat right, avoid sugar, artificial sweeteners, and caffeine.

3. Use earplugs. Even little noises upset your brainwaves and disturb sleep. Or run a fan or white-noise machine to drown-out disturbing noises.

4. Wear an eye mask or cover your eyes with a dark cloth. It's best to

sleep in complete darkness. I've covered my windows with heavy cloth, and use a dark washcloth over my eyes. As you now know, light at night upsets your biological clock. If you wake during the night as have trouble falling back asleep, you may be hungry without knowing it. Have a small snack (I have some raw eggs or a banana), go back to sleep and do the pole-bridging exercise above.

5. A warm bath with *Epsom* salts (high in magnesium) or magnesium oil (see discussion on magnesium in heart chapter) in the evening will help you relax.

6. Do the breathing exercise described in the chapter on asthma.

7. Sleep alone. Any disturbance can knock you out of restful sleep. This is especially true for men. Gerhard Kloesch of the University of Vienna who conducted a recent study said that sharing a bed "negatively impacts cognitive function and increases stress-hormone levels in men." Both men and women slept more deeply when they slept alone, but women did not suffer as badly cognitively when they slept with their husbands. Dr. Neil Stanley, a sleep expert at the University of Surrey, said,

"It's not surprising that people are disturbed by sleeping together. Historically, we have never been meant to sleep in the same bed as each other. It is a bizarre thing to do. Sleep is the most selfish thing you can do and it's vital for good physical and mental health. Sharing the bed space with someone who is making noises and who you have to fight with for the duvet is not sensible. If you are happy sleeping together that's great, but if not there is no shame in separate beds." He said there was a suggestion that women are pre-programmed to cope better with broken sleep. "A lot of life events that women have disturb sleep—bringing up children, the menopause and even the menstrual cycle," he explained. But Dr. Stanley added people did get used to sharing a bed. "If they have shared their bed with their partner for a long time they miss them and that will disturb sleep."(22)

8. Eat a good size meal before 12 noon. Fasting in the morning or going without a significant meal upsets your blood sugar and changes your biochemical rhythm. Anytime I don't eat before noon, I have a hard time sleeping that night.

9. Rub your tummy, wiggle your toes. Both will help you relax. Speaking of toes, your feet play an important role in your health for two reasons. One, they are important for balance and posture. Wearing shoes all the time restricts the foots' movement and flexibility, making correct posture and balance more difficult. Bad posture affects all of your organs and can literally cramp their function and impede proper blood flow. This can lead to health problems. Going barefoot as much as possible is a good way to relax the muscles in your feet, allowing the bones to spread out giving more stability and support. Above all, let your children (and infants) run around barefoot, even outside. A couple cuts or bruises are a small

price to pay for a child developing good posture and balance. Binding the feet with shoes all the time is almost like binding your hands – restrictive, unnatural and unhealthy. High heels are particularly bad. Two, making direct contact with the good earth discharges any electromagnetic radiation that has accumulated in the body, which is unhealthy and stress producing. Rubbing your tummy is good, deeply massaging it is better. The abdomen is the main area we harbor stress. Stress constricts not just the muscles, but blood vessels and restricts blood flow. Loosening up the tummy will improve blood flow throughout your body. Make it a nightly routine to take the tips of your fingers and firmly push down all around the abdomen for a minute or two (you can wiggle your toes at the same time). You'll find your whole body will let go, and falling asleep will become much easier. Exchanging tummy rubs with your partner is also very nice, and rubbing your child's tummy will help them too. (You can tell them how much you love them at the same time – what a wonderful feeling for a child!)

10. Get regular exercise. After 16 weeks of a moderate intensity exercise programs, subjects fell asleep about 15 minutes earlier and slept 45 minutes longer. But be sure to do your exercise at least 5 hours before bedtime.(23) Parents, let your children and babies sleep. It was shown in a study at the University of Arizona that frequent naps can boost the brain power of a growing baby.(24) This is probably true for children too, and even adults. Taking a nap or even just taking time to close your eyes and rest in the middle of the day refreshes and rejuvenates. You may not need to sleep as long at night, either.

11. Sleep grounded. Don't sleep with electric blankets, near a clock radio or other active electrical device, or with a waterbed heater on. These disturb the electromagnetic fields (EMFs) of the body. The electromagnetic fields created by these disturb the cells of our bodies 60 times per second. EMFs have been implicated in a wide variety of illnesses such as sleep disorders, stress-related and autoimmune diseases including arthritis, asthma, fibromyalgia, lupus, cardiovascular disease, and many more. Cell phones have been implicated in brain cancer and other diseases, so use them as little as possible and use a head set if you do. The problem is that our bodies take on some of the electromagnetic charges around us, and we actually act like a battery and store some of these charges. But our electrical system (our nervous system) operates on very low voltage. When we take on too much voltage from the environment, we get overcharged, which leads to stress and overproduction of adrenaline and other stress hormones. One solution is to be grounded. When we walk barefoot in the sand or on bare ground, we bring our bodies back in connection with the natural flow of electrons on the surface of the earth, which decreases stress caused by manmade electrical fields. That's one of the reasons going to the beach is so relaxing. So we sleep better, digest our food better and are happier. But most of us can't go barefoot on the beach every day,

and we all wear shoes with synthetic materials that don't allow grounding. So what can we do? A researcher named Clint Ober discovered that if you're grounded at night while you sleep, your physiology functions better. You'll get a deeper and more healing sleep, wake refreshed, and have more energy throughout the day. These discoveries led him to invent a special set of bed sheets that are actually grounded to the earth. You simply put them on your bed like regular sheets and go to sleep. The results of people sleeping on these sheets have been impressive: 85% of test subjects reported the time to fall asleep decreased; 100% woke feeling more rested; 82% had less muscle stiffness and pain; 78% reported an increase in general well being. Many subjects report improvements in back pain, arthritis, lupus, PMS, allergies, multiple sclerosis, and fibromyalgia. Not only does this technology eliminate the EMF problem, but it has been shown to help neutralize free radicals that cause pain, inflammation, and illness. He calls this grounding, *Earthing,* which also connects our bodies with the rhythmic cycles of the earth's natural frequencies. These are essential for synchronizing biological clocks, sleep cycles, and hormone production. I have these sheets and have noticed a marked improvement in my sleep, health, and performance. I highly, HIGHLY recommend you invest in this technology, not just for you and your spouse, but your children as well. In fact, with all the EMF pollution these days, I don't think it's possible to attain truly great health, or heal quickly, if you do not discharge the energy and get a fresh supply of the earth's electrons on a daily basis. Being grounded will certainly make getting healthy faster and easier. So although these sheets will cost you some money, you'll be saving money in the long run because every other healthy thing you do will no longer be interfered with or slowed due to the harmful effects of EMFs. You also won't be disconnected from the most important source of natural anti-oxidants – the earth. That's not to mention the priceless ness of simply feeling better. Many professional and college athletes including the U.S. team in the Tour de France bicycle race now use these sheets. (Now you know the secret of the man who won it 5 times in a row – wink, wink.) (25) Check it out at www.barefoothealth.com.

12. Sleep with a window open. This not only will allow fresh air in, but negative ions too, which are relaxing. In the winter, close the bedroom door, open the window a crack, and pile on the blankets or comforter. You'll sleep much better. Also, it's best to use all natural bedding materials like all cotton sheets and pillow cases. Not only are they made of non-toxic materials, but do not cause the subtle electrical disturbances (which affect the heart's electrical impulses) that polyester sheets do.

13. Remember, magnesium is needed for relaxed muscles, and fat and oils are needed for a calm nervous system. A glass of warm raw milk is nice before bedtime too. As you make healthy changes to your lifestyle, your sleep will naturally improve.

Migraine Headaches

Thirty million people in the U.S. suffer from migraine headaches, women being three times more likely than men to get them. No one is absolutely sure why some people get them and others don't, but it seems that people who get migraines have more sensitive brains. Fred Freitag, D.O of the Diamond Headache Clinic in Chicago says, "When this sensitive brain gets bombarded by outside and inside stimuli, cells in the cortex of the brain become hyper excited and start a process of electrical discharge." This causes blood vessels to dilate, which inflames surrounding tissue, leading to throbbing pain usually one side of the head, nausea, and sensitivity to light. Before the headache, about a third of people say they experience an aura – flashes of light, blind spots or zigzag line, or tingling in the face and arm. In women often hormone levels are to blame, and it seems that it's the fall of estrogen levels during ovulation that often triggers a headache.

Certain foods and substances (perfumes, food preservatives) can trigger migraines, so keeping track of what you eat may help identify these. Keeping regular hours and eating on schedule can help you avoid blood sugar fluctuations that may also cause a sensitive brain to start aching.

Regular exercise stimulates the production of endorphins, the brain's natural painkillers. Relaxation exercises (like CBT or the pole-bridging), massage and even acupuncture have helped some sufferers.

Ginger has been used for thousands of years as an anti-inflammatory and carminative (helps relieve gas and settle the stomach). It helps with morning sickness, sea sickness, motion sickness, and nausea. Drinking home-made ginger tea as you feel a headache coming on or during times when you expect to get one may help. You can find ginger root in most grocery stores. Of course, organic is best.

Ginger also has a blood-thinning effect, reducing the clumping of blood platelets. In Ayurvedic medicine, ginger is considered a heart tonic. Ginger's anti-inflammatory action can reduce pain and swelling in people with rheumatoid arthritis and osteoarthritis. Since it's easy on the stomach, it's much better than taking anti-inflammatory drugs that can cause ulcers.

To realize the benefits of ginger, you should use it at least a few times a week. I'd say if you have arthritis or a heart condition, you may want to drink ginger tea daily. It certainly won't do you any harm.

The mineral that's been shown to be of utmost importance when it comes to migraine headaches is magnesium. Studies have consistently shown that people with migraines are magnesium deficient.[26,27] One study showed that magnesium given intravenously gave rapid relief of headache pain and showed that low magnesium levels may precipitate headache symptoms.[28] People with cluster headaches are also probably magnesium deficient.[29] Oral magnesium supplementation over a four week period has been shown to help relieve migraines in 41 percent of the patients.[30] In another study a group of 3,000 patients were given 200 mg of magnesium daily, with an 80 percent reduction in migraine symptoms.(31)

It's not surprising that adequate magnesium levels will stop and prevent migraines since magnesium controls relaxation. When the blood vessels in the brain are relaxed they can dilate, reducing spasm and constrictions that can cause migraines. Magnesium also thins the blood and helps prevent lactic acid build-up that goes along with muscle tension and can worsen head pain. It also regulates the inflammatory substances that may play a role in migraines.

Women are more likely to be magnesium deficient than men, and are known to get migraines more often. Women often report having migraines just before their period, and this is the time when there's a shift of blood magnesium into bone and muscles, resulting in lower magnesium levels in the brain. Post menopausal women don't get migraines as often, so it may be that not only is magnesium shifted during menstruation, but also lost then too.

In a study in Italy, oral magnesium supplementation was successfully in relieving premenstrual mood changes.(32) Serotonin, the "feel-good" neurotransmitter depends on magnesium for its production and function, so is it any wonder that a magnesium deficiency can cause anxiety and even panic attacks? People with migraines (who are likely to be magnesium deficient), are also more likely to have anxiety disorders, obsessive-compulsive disorder, phobic disorders, neuroses, suicide attempts, and especially depression.(33,34)

Of particular concern is the research that correlates migraines with heart attack and stroke. A study at Harvard Medical School in Boston reported that people who have migraines once a month are one and a half times more likely to go on and suffer a heart attack. Those who have a migraine once a week are three times more likely to have a stroke than those who don't get them. Paul Harman at he National Hospital for Neurology in London said, "There's a stroke risk associated with migraines and it is greater the more migraines you have. But you shouldn't panic people as that stroke risk is very small compared to other risks such as smoking and high blood pressure."(35,36)

There are numerous other conditions that are related to low magnesium that are also more prevalent in women: multiple chemical sensitivity; multiple sclerosis; mitral valve prolapse; premenstrual syndrome; fibromyalgia; anxiety; depression; and temporal mandibular join (TMJ). If you have any of these, you should have your magnesium levels checked and consider supplementing your diet with magnesium.

Remember, things that rob your body of magnesium include alcohol, salt (even the smallest amount of regular table salt or salt added to processed foods), phosphoric acid (found in sodas), coffee, prolonged stress, profuse sweating, excessive menstruation, diuretics, and drugs. Everyone, especially women, be sure to eat your green leafy vegetables (or vegetable juice), nuts, seeds, and you may consider taking a good magnesium supplement and/or using magnesium oil.

Chocolate contains a substance called amines, which is thought to trigger migraines. Cheese (but not fresh milk) also contains this substance, and people susceptible to migraines should avoid both these foods. Nitrates (in hot dogs, processed meats) and MSG may also trigger migraines. Other foods that may cause these headaches included avocados, pineapples, beans, peas, lentils, pork, shrimp, alcohol, and caffeine.

Refined sugar causes a spike in blood glucose causing the release of too much insulin that causes the release of adrenaline, which is a precursor to migraines. So avoiding everything with sugar in it will help. Natural sugars like in fruits have all the vitamins, minerals and cofactors that allow a normal more gradual insulin release. Conversely, a drop in blood glucose can trigger a migraine. So eating small frequent meals (every three to four hours) of natural food keeps blood glucose steady, which may help eliminate or lessen the severity of migraines. Aspirin stimulates the pancreas much like sugar does, so it may actually cause a migraine. Other drugs also stimulate the pancreas and should be avoided.

Some other ways to ease the pain are: take a warm bath with *Epson* salts – the magnesium in the salts will help you relax; lie down to rest in a dark room; avoid bright or flashing light; put something cold on the back of your neck, such as a cold, wet cloth or ice pack; alternate hot and cold cloths where the pain is; put a cold compress on your forehead and your feet in a container of warm water; drink some fresh-squeezed vegetable juice – tomato juice is especially good; eat something even if you don't feel like it, especially something high in protein – sometimes you're hungry and don't know it when you're in such pain; massage your head and neck with magnesium oil; keep your head elevated – this will decrease pressure and help ease the pain.

Special Note:
The next four chapters are largely from my book *The Truth About Children's Health*. I'm including them here to help validate a major thesis of this book: The health of mankind in industrialized nations is declining due to unnatural conditions; and we are just a couple generations away from major health and societal problems, not being able to procreate, and massive die-off. This is discussed in more detailed in the Ancestry Factor chapter. For a detailed discussion on pregnancy and breast feeding, please see *The Truth About Children's Health*.

CHAPTER XIII

Birth Defects

A birth defect can be defined as "an abnormality of structure, function or body metabolism (inborn error of body chemistry) present at birth that results in physical or mental disability, or is fatal."[1] Simply put, a birth defect is a congenital malformation.

There are more than 4,000 known birth defects, and they are the leading cause of infant mortality in the U.S., accounting for more than 20 percent of all infant deaths. Of the 120,000 babies born each year with a birth defect, 8,000 die during their first year of life. In addition, birth defects contribute substantially to child-hood morbidity and long-term disability.[2]

Although birth defects can be caused by genetic and environmental factors, it's estimated that the causes of approximately 60 percent to 70 percent of birth defects remain unknown. The National Research Council of the National Academies reports:

> Approximately half of all pregnancies in the United States result in prenatal or postnatal death or an otherwise less than healthy baby. And major developmental defects, such as neural tube and heart deformities, occur in approximately 120,000 of the 4 million infants born here each year. Exposure to toxic chemicals, both manufactured and natural, cause about 3 percent of all developmental defects, and at least 25 percent might be the result of a combination of genetic and environmental factors.[3]

Birth defects arising from genetic causes are dependent on random variability – that is, plain old luck. (Except in instances where a mother or father has a birth defect passed on to the child. In these cases the likelihood of an offspring having a birth defect is higher.) So the percentage of birth defects caused by genetic problems should, everything else remaining equal, be about the same over generations. Given that fact, the percentages of birth defects in our population should be remaining stable. Is this happening?

Let's take a look at the National Vital Statistics reports. In 1900, there were 12.0 deaths per 100,000 live births due to congenital deformities. By 1948, the number was 13.2. But in 1997, there were 159.2 deaths per 100,000 live births.[4,5] This is over a hundred fold increase. Is this reasonable, or is something else besides genetics causing an increase in birth defects?

These statistics can be helpful, but having read this far, you should realize that there are many reasons to suspect them. For one, the reporting of birth defects over the years is less than consistent. Surveillance methods have improved since the 1960s, spurred by the serious and widespread birth defects because of the drug thalidomide given to pregnant mothers (which caused babies to be born with flippers instead of arms and legs). So the numbers have tended to go up simply because they are being reported better. Also, prenatal care has improved over the years resulting in more live births and therefore more potentially "imperfect" (rather than merely dead) babies. I could understand a slight to moderate increase in reported birth defect deaths because of these factors, but a hundredfold increase? My contention is that something other than genetics is causing this increase.

And more recent data shows a similar trend. The Centers for Disease Control started the Birth Defects Monitoring Program (BDMP) in 1973 to monitor birth defects as an early warning system of an emerging birth defects problem and to correlate the occurrences of birth defects with possible human teratogens. A teratogen (from the Greek words meaning, "monster producing") is anything that causes birth defects. From 1979 to 1987, the BDMP showed of the 38 types of birth defects monitored, 29 increased, two decreased and seven remained stable (less than 2 percent change per year). Some of the increases were dramatic – one doubled during this period, and another was estimated to be doubling every 14 years. The BDMP was discontinued during the mid-1990s and was eventually replaced by a new program comprising eight Centers for Birth Defects Research and Prevention (CBDRP).(6)

Food for Thought

I remember in my college genetics class, we did an exercise to determine if the actions the Nazis took on the Jews during the Holocaust would have a significant impact on the gene pool (the genetics of a whole population), and if those mass murders would ultimately get rid of or significantly decrease the genes of Jews in the overall population of the world (as the Nazis were intending). What we discovered was that even with this mass killing-off of the Jewish population, it was not significant in changing the gene pool, and even if the numbers were increased to the point of absurdity, the genetic pool would basically remain the same. My point is this: Under normal conditions, a change in the gene pool of a population takes many thousands, if not millions, of years. The alarming rate of birth defects in the last 50 years or so is not because of genetic probability or variability – it's because of a drastic and dramatic degeneration of the human organism that makes it more susceptible to abnormal defects. This degeneration, since genetics don't change that quickly, must then be due to environmental factors.

Although changes in human genetics cannot account for the dramatic increase in birth defects in recent years, inheritance of birth defects can certainly occur. The likelihood of a parent with a birth defect having a child with a birth defect is greater than for parents with no birth defects. A study published in *The New England Journal of Medicine* found ". . .a definite tendency for women with birth defects to also have children with birth defects." The study also found that women with birth defects were less likely to survive to adulthood, and if they did reach adulthood, they were less likely than other women to bear children.[7] Another study reported in the *Journal of the American Medical Association* showed that offspring of men with birth defects are twice as likely to have defects too. Allen J. Wilcox, M.D., Ph.D., co-author of the study, said, "What surprised us is that the children of the affected fathers had a higher risk of all kinds of defects, not just the same defect as their father." In the study, boys with birth defects had a lower-than-normal survival rate to age 20. Even if they survived to adulthood, they were 30 percent less likely to be able to father a child than other men.[8]

Food for Thought

The two studies just cited clearly show that birth defects can increase through the generations and that offspring of parents with birth defects are less likely to survive and reproduce themselves. This is most significant. In these cases what is happening is that there is a degeneration of the organisms from one generation to the next – so much so that they may not be able to reproduce. I suspect that if this study were to be continued into the third generation, we would see a further decline in reproductive capability to the point of near extinction. This, taken with the fact that birth defects are increasing in the population in general, paints a less than cheery picture. If the occurrence of birth defects continues to increase and the inability for people with birth defects to have babies (in this or subsequent generations) is true, in a short time, having to use birth control could be a thing of the past.

Birth defects will continue to increase, mainly because of the increased prevalence of teratogens. There are more than 500 new chemicals introduced into commercial use each year, added to the more than 75,000 chemicals already in commercial use. We tend to believe these chemicals are "innocent until proven guilty," so a chemical will be used until significant damage is shown to have occurred. That, along with the fact that there's not enough time or money to test all these chemicals for toxicity and teratogenicity, makes our world a very hazardous place.

In 2001 in China, there were 105 infants with birth defects per 10,000 births. By 2006, that figure had risen to 146 per 10,000 – a rapid and alarming increase. Government officials said that the increase in birth defect rates are related to environmental pollution.[9]

Besides chemicals, the environmental agents that could potentially cause birth defects are many: heavy metals such as mercury; lead; cadmium; X-rays; pesticides such as DDT; chlorine; alcohol; tobacco; recreational drugs; poor nutrition; and pharmaceutical drugs such as thalidomide.(10) Many of these agents have already been discussed. But a special mention of chlorine is in order since it is added to our water supply.

Chlorine and Other Drinking Water Contaminants

A chemical added to drinking water is chlorine, which eliminates or reduces the presence of bacteria and other microorganisms that may cause health problems if left unchecked. According to the Centers for Disease Control, about 940,000 Americans get sick and 900 die each year from waterborne microbial illness caused by contaminated tap water.(11) Another estimate by Tufts University Medical School and the EPA estimate that there are over seven million cases of waterborne diseases a year.(12) However, there is a growing concern that our water treatment methods are no longer adequate. Most treatment plants use pre-World War I technology, which employs sedimentation, filtration, coagulation, and chlorine disinfection. But the many byproducts of our modern chemical age such as synthetic organic industrial chemicals and pesticides often pass through these treatment plants unabated. A growing body of evidence indicates that a number of chemicals commonly found in tap water could be associated with cancer, reproductive effects, and developmental effects. The addition of chlorine to drinking water can also contribute to hardening of the arteries, can destroy proteins in the body, irritates the skin and sinuses, and can aggravate asthma, allergies, and respiratory problems. It's well documented that the levels of chlorine in tap water have been shown to present numerous serious health challenges.

The most common byproduct of drinking water treatment practices is the class of chemicals called *trihalomethanes* (THMs). They arise from the interaction of chlorine used to kill bacteria in the treatment plant and decomposing plant matter, naturally occurring humic and fulvic acids and other organic chemicals in the water. The federal drinking water regulations limit the total THMs in tap water to 100 parts per billion (ppb) in systems serving 10,000 people or more.(13)

Especially relevant for our discussion is that infants, children and pregnant women may be more susceptible to the effects of contaminants in drinking water than normal healthy adults. A recent study conducted in Norway indicated that byproducts in drinking water treated with chlorination may raise risks for birth defects. The report said the overall risk for birth defects rose by 14 percent in towns with both chlorinated water and water with a high amount of organic material (which would encourage the formation of THMs). Especially high were the risks for urinary tract birth defects: babies born in areas of high THMs had double the risk of urinary tract malformations. Also, there was a 26 percent rise in the risks for serious neural tube defects. (Neural tube defects are defects such as *spina bifida*, potentially paralyzing in which the spinal cord is not properly enclosed by the bone of the spine.)[14] The Agency for Toxic Substances and Disease Registry published a study in January 1998 showing that serious birth defects (neural tube defects) are associated with THM ingested from drinking water.[15] Chlorination byproducts (THMs) are also implicated strongly for causing bladder cancer and may cause colon and rectal cancer and brain tumors as well.[16]

In a study by the California Department of Health, 5,144 pregnant women were tracked and their drinking water habits studied. The outcomes of their pregnancies were compared with the amount and type of water they drank along with the total amount of THMs in the water. Sixteen percent of women drinking five or more glasses of water per day containing more than 75 ppb THMs had miscarriages. Only 9.5 percent of women who were drinking water with lower concentrations of THMs miscarried. The likelihood of spontaneous abortions was 1.8 times greater in the high-THM consumption group than the low-THM consumption group. In a similar study in central North Carolina, women were 2.8 times more likely to have a miscarriage if they had high exposure to THMs during pregnancy.[17]

Contamination by THMs can occur not only from drinking the water, but from indoor air pollution as well. Since THMs are volatile, they readily evaporate into the air. When you shower, flush the toilet, wash dishes and clothes, and so on, you can introduce these THMs into the household air. Even THMs in the *air* can contribute to neural tube defects in babies whose mothers had a high exposure.[18]

These studies looked at long-term exposures to THMs. But according to Erik Olson, a water quality expert with the Natural Resources Defense Council (NRDC), short-term exposures may be very important too and can also contribute to spontaneous abortions, fetal deaths, and serious birth defects. He says, "We may be totally overlooking the risk of short-term exposure."[19]

EPA officials admit they have no idea how many U.S. water systems exceed the federal limit of 100 ppb. But they do say that THMs increase during the summer months, sometimes to twice their normal level. So it's best not to take chances. Chlorine can be removed by a simple filtration unit on your faucet and shower. For drinking, letting the water stand for several minutes allows the THMs to evaporate.

Fluoride and chlorine byproducts are not the only thing in drinking water that may cause health problems. As already discussed, pesticides may pollute a municipal water supply or drinking water well. In addition, Volatile Organic Chemicals (VOCs) found in solvents, degreasers, adhesives, gasoline additives, and such may contain benzene, trichloroethylene (TCE), toluene and vinyl chloride, which have been shown to cause cancer, central nervous system disorders, liver and kidney damage, reproductive disorders, and birth defects.[20]

In Woburn, Massachusetts, in the 1980s, 21 children contracted leukemia (cancer of the blood) because the town's drinking water was contaminated from a shallow industrial injection well and dump, allowing VOCs to enter the reservoir. (The families' struggles were documented in the movie *A Civil Action*.) It's been shown that brain, nervous system cancers, and acute lymphocytic leukemia represent the majority of cancers attacking children – and clusters of higher than normal incidences of these diseases have been shown in areas with high VOCs in the drinking water.[21]

Philip Landrigan, chair of the department of community and preventive medicine at Mount Sinai School of Medicine in New York City, says, "I have no doubt certain VOCs in drinking water can cause cancer in children." Carolyn Poppell, program coordinator on safe drinking water for the Physicians for Social Responsibility concurs: "The concern we have is that drinking water standards are not protective of the public's health, particularly children."[22]

Oftentimes industries will get rid of their wastes by deep well injection. Sometimes they do it right, sometimes they don't. Also, ground water aquifers are very unpredictable, and leakage from one to another is possible. Dumps can also accept waste from industries, municipalities, and homes. A 1997 federal Agency for Toxic Substances and Disease Registry report noted that there are over 1,300 Superfund sites (waste dumps that are so toxic, they have to be cleaned up using masks and special clothing and equipment). The report stated that over 41 million Americans live within four miles of these toxic land dumps and are more susceptible to an increase of these toxic chemicals in their drinking water. There are over 436,000 hazardous waste sites nationwide.[23] Many dangerous chemicals can leach into the ground water from these also, not to mention pollution due to agricultural practices.

Just because you may get your water from a well does not mean it's clean. It's always best to get it checked and treat it if needed. After all, your body is more that 70 percent water. If you give it the wrong kind, you cannot get healthy, and neither can your children. Consider this: The EPA monitors 80 substances and has drinking water limits for some of these. However, there are over 75,000 chemicals produced in the U.S. Data exists for only 7 percent of the 2,700 most widely used chemicals on health effects on humans. The EPA's drinking water limits are not designed to protect children, because they are extrapolated from animal studies and based on an adult male's body weight and water consumption. As I've mentioned several times, children are more sensitive and vulnerable than adults since their enzyme systems and organs of detoxification are not fully developed. Play it safe and get a water filter or other water treatment system.

Inorganic contaminants may also be present in drinking water. They may include arsenic, barium, chromium, lead, mercury, and silver, which can cause acute poisoning, cancer, learning disabilities, and other health problems.[24] In a 1999 study by the National Academy of Sciences, arsenic in drinking water can cause bladder, lung, and skin cancer and may also cause kidney and liver cancer.

The EPA estimates that in 25 states, more than 34 million Americans drink tap water that contains arsenic levels that pose unacceptable cancer risks. The Natural Resources Defense Council (NRDC) considers it likely that in those 25 states, as many as 56 million people have been drinking water with arsenic at unsafe levels.

The current national standard for arsenic in drinking water is 50 parts per billion (ppb). That standard was set in 1942 before it was discovered that arsenic causes cancer. The National Academy of Sciences estimates that 1 person out of 100 drinking water with this amount of arsenic in it will develop cancer (based on drinking 2 liters of water a day). This is an extremely high risk considering that standards are usually set so that the risk is 1 in 10,000. And although Congress ordered the EPA to update the arsenic standard in 1974 and again in 1986, they failed to do so.[25] The new proposed arsenic standard of 10 ppb is scheduled to go into effect in 2006. Many filters can remove arsenic. Be sure the filter is certified by NSF International (800-NSF-MARK). Distillation also removes arsenic, as does reverse osmosis.

Another common contaminant in drinking water is nitrate. Nitrate (NO_3) is a naturally occurring form of nitrogen found in soil and essential for plant growth. It is very soluble and easily leaches into ground water. Nitrogen compounds are used in most fertilizers, can come from animal feedlots, municipal wastewater and sludge, and septic systems. With the intensive agricultural practices used these days, nitrates can easily contaminate drinking water supplies. The National Pesticide Survey in 1992 detected nitrates in 57 percent of domestic wells and 52 percent of community wells. It was reported that some 22,500 infants drinking domestic well water were estimated to be exposed to levels of nitrates exceeding the EPA safe drinking water limits; for community systems, the number was estimated to be 43,500 infants.[26]

Nitrate is associated with *blue baby syndrome* in infants. This syndrome was far more common in and before the 1940's, but is still possible today. Blue baby syndrome, the common name for methemoglobinemia, occurs most often in infants under six months of age whose stomach acid is not as strong as older children's and adult's. This allows a higher level of bacteria in their stomach that can easily convert nitrate to nitrite. Nitrite causes hemoglobin to be converted to methemoglobin, which does not carry oxygen well, and which babies cannot convert back to hemoglobin. This results in a reduced oxygen supply to vital tissues and organs such as the brain. When this happens, the infant will look blue (even indigo) – especially around the eyes and mouth. Methemoglobin can be changed back to hemoglobin in adults, potentially stopping this from happening, but again, not in infants. Severe cases of methemoglobinemia can cause brain damage and death.

A study in the Britain suggested that high nitrate levels also can cause juvenile diabetes. In rural areas where the nitrate levels in water were high, so were the incidences of juvenile diabetes. Nitrosamine, a breakdown product of nitrates, is known to cause diabetes in animals and has been linked to cancer, thyroid problems, and birth defects. Again, infants and young children are believed to be especially vulnerable to nitrate exposure.

There are other, less severe symptoms of methemoglobinemia: headaches, dizziness, weakness, and difficulty in breathing. The condition can be easily treated with an injection of methylene blue at a hospital emergency room.

Pregnant women, adults with reduced stomach acid and people deficient in the enzyme that converts methemoglobin back to normal hemoglobin are especially susceptible to nitrate-induced methemoglobinemia. Infants should not be allowed to consume drinking water or any other drink (including formula preparations) with a nitrate concentration above 10 mg/l NO_3-N or 45 mg/l NO_3 (these are two different ways to report nitrates, so when you have your water tested, be sure you know which value is being reported).(27)

Although infant deaths from blue baby syndrome are now quite rare (only one reported between 1960 to 1972), decreased oxygen in the blood cannot be beneficial to your baby – especially to its vulnerable, developing brain. You can remove nitrates from your water using distillation, reverse osmosis, and ion exchange methods or blending with non-contaminated water to get the concentration down to acceptable levels (use this method only in emergency situations). Charcoal filters and water softeners don't remove nitrates from water that well. Boiling the water does not make it better either, and actually *increases* the concentration of nitrates.

Since public water supplies – and many private water supplies such as wells – have become so contaminated, many people have been buying bottled water thinking it is cleaner. This is not necessarily the case, however, according to a four-year study by the NRDC. Their study included testing more than 1,000 bottles of 103 brands of bottled water. Most of the water was found to be of high quality, but about one third of the waters contained levels of contamination exceeding allowable limits. Realize bottled water products are not subject to the same rigorous testing and purity standards as those that apply to city tap water. - Here are some findings of the study:

- 25 percent to 40 percent of the bottled water produced in the U.S. comes directly from municipal water systems (even though the advertising and bottle label may claim otherwise).
- 33 percent of the bottled water tested contained bacteria (bottled water is not required to be disinfected).
- 25 percent of bottled water samples contained known carcinogens.
- 20 percent of the bottled water samples contained harmful industrial chemicals.
- Bottled water can cost between 240 and 10,000 times more per gallon than tap water.

The NRDC concluded that bottled water regulations are inadequate to assure consumers of either purity or safety, and buying bottled water is not necessarily safe.(28) It's best to buy bottled water that is bottled at the source, such as *Perrier.*

A Monster Returns

Thalidomide is a known teratogen and, according to a recent survey, two thirds of people of childbearing age are not familiar with it – a shocking fact given the tragic and widely publicized results of its use in generations past. Considering that the FDA gave approval in 1998 for thalidomide to be marketed in the U.S. Again, it's very important women know about it and understand its risks.

Thalidomide was first used in the late 1950s as a sleeping pill and to treat morning sickness during pregnancy. Of course, no one knew it caused birth defects. But in 1961 scientists discovered that the medication stunted the growth of fetal arms and legs. Taking only one dose of thalidomide early in pregnancy can severely affect the growth of fetal limbs (arms, legs, hands, feet) causing them to look like flippers instead of arms or legs. It wasn't until more than 10,000 children around the world were born with these major malformations that it was withdrawn from the market in the early 1960s.(29)

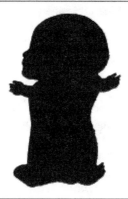

Figure 5

The dangers of thalidomide – what a baby may look like if his mother takes this medication during pregnancy.

The recent FDA approval of the drug is for the treatment of a complication of leprosy, a disfiguring skin disorder involving loss of feeling that can lead to paralysis. This disease affects only a few thousand people in the U.S. – but even so, thalidomide has been approved, giving physicians the ability to prescribe it for many more people with other conditions including women of childbearing age. It's extremely important young women realize the dangers of this drug.

Thalidomide is also sometimes used for treating some autoimmune diseases of the connective tissues including Behcet's disease and skin manifestations of dermatomyositis.

The FDA, recognizing the potential dangers of thalidomide, has taken special safeguards never before imposed with any drug. This underscores how bad it can be. Only physicians who are registered may prescribe thalidomide to patients, and those patients – both male and female – must comply with mandatory contraceptive measures, patient registration and patient surveys. That's all well and good, but the chances of someone misusing it or going off their contraceptives is there. My advice is to leave it alone all together. You can heal yourself in other ways.

You may be wondering if you can take measures to prevent birth defects. Naturally, following a wholesome lifestyle will go a long way in this regard. But there is one specific nutrient that should be mentioned here because of its importance in preventing a common form of birth defect called neural tube defect (NTD).

The neural tube is the embryonic structure that develops into the brain and spinal cord. It starts out as a tiny ribbon of tissue that normally folds inward to form a tube by the 28th day after conception. When this doesn't happen correctly and the neural tube does not close completely, defects in the brain and spinal cord can result. In the U.S., about 2,500 babies are born with NTDs each year, and many other affected pregnancies end in miscarriage or stillbirth.(30)

The most common NTDs are spina bifida and anencephaly. Spina bifida (open spine), affects the backbone and sometimes the spinal cord. Children with severe spina bifida have some degree of leg paralysis and bladder and bowel control problems. Anencephaly is a fatal condition in which a baby is born with a severely underdeveloped brain and skull. Women with diabetes or epilepsy are at increased risk of having a baby with an NTD and should consult their physician prior to pregnancy.

A certain B vitamin called folic acid, or folate, has been shown to reduce the risk of a woman having a baby with an NTD. (Other studies also suggest folic acid may help prevent cleft lip and palate malformations.) The U.S. Public Health Service, March of Dimes, CDC, and the Institute of Medicine all recommend that all women of childbearing age get at least 400 micrograms (or 0.4 mg) of folic acid every day – and no more than 1,000 micrograms per day. An adequate folate intake could prevent up to 70 percent of these types of birth defects. Women must realize that they need folic acid even before they get pregnant because by the time they realize they are pregnant, much of the neural tube formation has already occurred.(31)

Women can take a vitamin with folic acid in it to be sure they get enough. Some doctors and nutritionists actually recommend supplemental folic acid over food source folate since the body more readily absorbs folic acid from vitamin supplements than from food. But remember the research that showed that synthetic folic acid increases the chances of heart attack, stroke, and cancer.

Foods high in folate include leafy green vegetables, asparagus, peas, citrus fruits, tomatoes, beets, broccoli, cauliflower, nuts, eggs, cantaloupe, watermelon, bee pollen, and poultry and liver from organically raised animals. Synthetic folic acid is added to certain grain products including flour, rice, pasta, cornmeal, bread, and cereals, and consuming to many of these can lead to an overload in folic acid (see Alzheimer's chapter).

Considering about half of all pregnancies are not planned, it's wise for women to make sure they're getting enough folic acid every day. It could prevent a lifetime of misery. Taking this a step further, women of childbearing age should strive to lead as healthy a lifestyle as possible. Avoid smoking, drinking, street drugs, medications and over-the-counter medicines for starters. Eat as clean a diet as possible. This ideally goes for the father too. Healthy parents give rise to healthy children. Like begets like – a simple law of nature. Although the chance of having a child with a birth defect is always there just because of plain old luck, that chance can be reduced to virtually nonexistent if the parents are healthy and have healthy and vital eggs and sperm.

CHAPTER XIV

Infertility

Although fertility may not seem to directly impact your health or the health of your loved ones, the ramifications of the growing fertility problem in the United States do affect the yet-to-be-born child. With fertility problems on the rise, we have reason for concern: protecting our children assumes that there will be children to protect. If things continue to degenerate, there soon may not be.

"Infertility is defined as the inability to conceive a child despite trying for one year. The condition affects about 5.3 million Americans, or 9 percent of the reproductive age population," according to the American Society for Reproductive Medicine.(1)

A report from the National Center for Health Statistics says the percentage of infertile couples in 1995 was 18.5 percent, compared with 14.4 percent in 1965.(2) Dr. Marc Goldstein, director of the Center for Male Reproductive Medicine at New York Hospitals, said, "Infertility is definitely going up. I see it in my practice. There is a decline in fertility in men and an increase in infertility in older couples. Studies show an increase in infertility from 11 percent to 16 percent in all married couples." He believes the cause to stem in part from lifestyles that include alcohol, marijuana, and cocaine.(3)

Interestingly, there also have been numerous reports of reproductive problems in wildlife, which doesn't use drugs or alcohol. Some believe the problems are due to the presence of chlorinated chemicals that are now ubiquitous in our environment and tend to mimic estrogen. Others believe they are happening because many industrial pollutants mimic hormones, thus upsetting the delicate reproductive system. Dioxin is a chlorinated chemical that does not mimic hormones, yet Earl Gray, a senior research biologist with the EPA, testified before Congress in 1993 that, "Our studies [in rats] show that a single dose of dioxin administered during pregnancy permanently reduces sperm counts in the male [offspring in adulthood] by about 60 percent."(4) Another effect of estrogen-mimicking chemicals is that they appear to cause girls to enter puberty sooner, developing breasts and pubic hair before the age of eight – for some at as young as three years of age.(5) The authors of this study said that PCBs and DDE (a break-down product of the pesticide DDT) may indeed be associated with early sexual development in girls.

Infertility can be due to a problem with the man, women or both. It's estimated that 40 percent of couple infertility is due to the male. Not only does a lower sperm count increase the chances of having difficulty conceiving, it also increases the risk of miscarriages and birth defects.

In 1938, one half of 1 percent (that's one man in 200) of men were functionally sterile (having a sperm count below 20 million per milliliter of semen). Today, it's between 8 percent to 12 percent (between eight and 12 men in one hundred).(6) The expected sperm count of a man born in Paris in 1945 was 102 million, whereas in 1962 it was exactly half that. Pierre Jouannet, a French researcher, projects a further decline in the future. He said in 1996, "It will take 70 or 80 years before it (sperm count) goes to zero."(7) (Again, difficulty in conceiving occurs at sperm counts of 20 million or less, and sterility at five million. So effective species infertility would occur sooner than the 70 or 80 years projected for 0 sperm counts.) Not only are sperm counts going down, but cancer of the testicles has increased over threefold from 1940 to 1980.(8)

The important observation here is that infertility is increasing and increasing significantly. Some say that this is because more couples are waiting longer to try having a baby and conception rates naturally go down as we age. But in December 2005 a report from the CDC said that women under the age of 25 make up the fastest-growing segment of U.S. women with impaired fertility. In addition, the National Survey on Family Growth found that in 2002 about 12 percent of couples in the U.S. experienced impaired fecundity (the capacity to conceive and carry a child to term), which is up 20 percent from just 1995.(9,10) As I already mentioned, one estimate is that by the year 2020, people living in industrialized countries will not be able to reproduce – we will be infertile. Considering the above estimate, it may take until 2070. Still, a chilling thought.

The odds of having a miscarriage or child with birth defects rise dramatically when fathers have lower sperm counts. In a study at the University of Arkansas, it was determined that when the fathers' sperm counts were above 80 million/ml, they had only a 1 percent birth defect rate, compared with 6 percent for the general population. Miscarriages were also lower for the fathers with higher sperm counts (6 percent compared with 12 percent for the general population).(11)

Another study, in Sweden, reported in the *International Journal of Fertility*, found that married women experiencing miscarriages typically had husbands with lower sperm counts. In those men, on the average, 48 percent of their sperm appeared abnormal (two heads, two tails, etc.). Men who fathered normal pregnancies had a 25 percent higher sperm count and only 5 percent visually abnormal sperm.(12)

In a study on sperm counts and testicle abnormalities at the University of Copenhagen, Denmark, the researchers concluded that: "Recent data clearly indicate that the semen quality has markedly decreased during the period 1938 - 1990, and concomitantly the incidence of some genitourinary abnormalities including hypospadias [an abnormality of the male urinary opening], [testicle] maldescent, and cancer has increased. Such a remarkable increment in the occurrence of gonadal abnormalities over a relatively short period of time is more likely to be due to environmental rather than genetic factors. Generally, it is believed that pollution, smoking, alcohol. . .play a role."[13]

The British Medical Journal analyzed 61 previous sperm studies conducted in 20 countries. The report concluded that the average sperm counts had declined from 113 million sperm per milliliter of semen to 66 million during the past 50 years (from 1940 to 1990) – a 42 percent decline.[14] Remember, a man's fertility becomes questionable when sperm counts get down to 20 million sperm per milliliter. When the count drops to 5 million, he is considered sterile. One reference made note that the number of normally shaped sperm produced by the average man has dropped below the level of that of a hamster, which has testicles a fraction the size of a man's.[15] As early as 1981 sperm banks in the U.S. were having difficulty acquiring good-quality sperm. If the decline continued at the same rate sperm banks would soon start having great difficulty finding sperm donors whose sperm met the recommended standards. Similar observations about declining sperm quality have been noted in Denmark.[16]

It requires between 65 and 74 days for the male to make the sperm that will get his partner pregnant. Any exposure to toxins during this time can impact the health of the sperm and thus the eventual fetus and baby. Men exposed to toxic chemicals on the job or at home for two months prior to their partner's conceiving have a greater likelihood of their child's being born with health disorders including learning and behavior problems.[17]

A common misunderstanding of the process involved in producing sperm (spermatogenesis) is that the male manufactures millions of sperm daily, and that those are the sperm ejaculated that same day during sex. This is not true, however, since it takes over two months to build a sperm from start to finish. It follows that the environment it is created in determines whether it's normal or abnormal. Therefore, "all chemical exposures experienced by the man (from alcohol to pesticides) have the ability to weaken or damage this process, thereby resulting in offspring of lowered genetic potential."[18]

Food for Thought

A lower sperm count means increased chances of infertility and miscarriages and less healthy babies. Less healthy babies lead to less healthy children. The less healthy a child is, the less content he or she is. The less content, the more prone to violence, behavior problems, and substance abuse later in life. The less healthy a child, the more likely he or she will be learning-impaired, hyperactive, and unmanageable. The less healthy an adolescent is, the more likely he/she will become a disgruntled adult. My point is that some of the problems we are experiencing with today's children, adults, and violence can be traced back to conditions present even before they were conceived. It's not just the environment the fetus experiences that in large part determines the state of health of the baby, but it's the state of health of the sperm and the egg that play a large part too. If you are of reproductive age, it's vitally important to realize this because the health of your future baby in large part depends upon the health of your sperm or egg, which depends on the health of *you.*

To return to the subject of alcohol for a moment, a study at the University of Michigan showed that fathers who drank an average of two drinks a day had babies that weighed more than one third of a pound less than babies whose fathers were only "occasional" drinkers – independent of the mother's alcohol, tobacco, or marijuana use during pregnancy.[19]

At the Institute of Sterility in Vienna, Austria, physicians compared 103 consecutive couples who had sought artificial insemination with donor sperm to 103 consecutive couples who had sought help due to female fertility problems. It was found that the men in these couples who worked in the agriculture industry were more than 10 times more likely to be infertile. The researchers noted that,

> What was particularly noteworthy was that the concentrations of some environmental toxins were generally clearly higher in those semen specimens, which did not lead to fertilization as opposed to those specimens from which a pregnancy resulted. [This study] has unequivocally confirmed this observation, the number of farmers being remarkably higher in the group seeking AID (Artificial Insemination with Donor Sperm) than in the control group within the same time period. This conspicuously high prevalence can probably be explained by the increased exposure to chemical sprays. . .These toxic chemicals probably have a detrimental effect on male fertility and therefore we suggest more caution in the way they are handled.[20]

Studies in rats in Japan tested the effects that the pesticide DBCP (dibromochloropropane) and some chemically similar industrial chemicals had on fertility and sperm morphology (structure). The results showed drastic reductions in sperm counts in exposed rats compared with unexposed rats. Many sperm in the pesticide-exposed rats were missing a tail (865 per 1000), which helps explain the infertility from these chemicals.[21] No tail, no travel.

It's not too surprising that pesticides or chemicals could directly cause male infertility, but it's also been shown that the way the food itself is grown could be a factor. At the Royal Free Hospital School of Medicine in London, groups of rats were fed either a diet of totally organically raised food, food grown with chemical fertilizers or food grown with some chemical fertilizers and some manure. Of the rats fed the chemically grown food, only 11 percent had normal testicular structures. Forty-eight percent had normal structure when fed the food raised with chemicals/manure or with nothing but manure. The researchers noted, "reproductive performance was a sensitive indicator of differences between diets which had hardly shown significant differences in comparative growth tests."[22]

Essentially what they are saying is that the reproductive system is more vulnerable and more sensitive to harmful effects from chemicals than other systems in the body. Most previous studies on pesticides determine only whether lab animals die after exposure. Clearly, more research is needed to examine what effects might be realized at more subtle levels – reproductive, neurological, and immunological.

Another point to consider is that food grown organically has been shown to have higher levels of trace minerals than foods grown commercially. Organic farmers often use fertilizers such as rock powders, compost, and marine byproduct fertilizers that have higher mineral content than commercial chemical fertilizers. Chemical fertilizers typically have only nitrogen, phosphorous, and potassium (10-10-10 fertilizer) and maybe five to 10 core minerals. But medical experts are now realizing the importance of trace minerals (such as selenium, boron, chromium, etc.) in maintaining health. Therefore it is highly recommended that couples wishing to have children consume mostly if not all organically raised foods.

Food for Thought

Consuming nothing but organically raised food is a good thing for anybody. There's plenty of research backing up its advantages, and it just makes common sense. Which do YOU think is better – food raised naturally in harmony with nature, or food treated with harmful chemicals and pesticides born out of chemical warfare? If you think this is a radical suggestion, here's another: I believe that the chemical fertilizers and pesticides should be outlawed. I know it would take some time and effort and money to adjust. But remember back in the 1930s, the government had all these WPA projects it funded to help get the nation working again and out of the depression? Why couldn't our government institute a project to help farmers switch from chemicals to natural fertilizers – from chemical pesticides to natural pest deterrents? I don't know – call me a dreamer, but it could be done. If it were, America would raise future generations of super-kids and super-people, not to mention the improved health and well being of people living now. It all starts with a strong foundation. Good food = sound minds and sound bodies = good societies. Like Pulitzer Prize winner Louis Bromfield said, "'Poor land makes poor people' is a saying every American should have printed and hung over his bed."

Other environmental factors also affect sperm counts. Marilyn F. Vine, Ph.D., at the University of North Carolina reported that men who smoke had sperm counts on the average of 13 percent to 17 percent lower than nonsmokers. Three of the men in this study who smoked and then quit were found to have an increase in sperm counts from 50 percent to 800 percent. The article suggested that the toxic chemicals in the smoke are responsible for the decreased sperm counts and that by quitting the reduction in sperm count is reversible.(23) It's also not surprising that smokers have more abnormal sperm. "Male smokers have an increase in sperm abnormalities, thereby suggesting a mutagenic effect."(24) A chemical found in marijuana (THC) has been found to be directly toxic to the developing egg.(25)

The research has shown that sperm counts have decreased and infertility has increased markedly since 1940. There are a couple of reasons cited in the literature that stands out as being most significant. One is that cigarette consumption in the U.S. has increased three-to-four fold from 1940 to the early 1980s. Another is that the agricultural industry switched from natural growing methods to chemical fertilizers and pesticides in the early 1960s.

As for other chemical exposures, consider that painters are more likely to father children with defects of the central nervous system. Men who work in the aircraft industry or handle paints or chemical solvents have a higher risk of producing children with brain tumors. Paternal exposure to paints has been linked to childhood leukemias. Firemen appear to have an unusually high number of abnormal sperm and are less fertile, probably because of the toxic smoke they are

Infertility 181 exposed to (from burning carpets, paint, etc.) Dental workers (dentists and dental assistants) are more prone to spontaneous abortions, stillbirths, and congenital defects. Animal studies suggest that paternal exposure to recreational drugs and industrial chemicals can contribute to problems such as miscarriage, stillbirths, and diminished aptitude for learning in the offspring.(26)

When it comes to conceiving and giving birth to a healthy child, the environment can be a determining factor in success or failure, health or disease. In fact, Wolfram Notten, Ph.D., of the University of Wisconsin, says, "20 percent of all cases where the male is the only contributing factor to infertility can be corrected by lifestyle."(27)

Although we have focused on men to this point, women are also vulnerable to environmental stresses and toxins when it comes to infertility and reproductive problems. The most common female factor to contribute to infertility is ovulation disorders. Without ovulation, the eggs are not available for fertilization. Problems with ovulation are often signaled by irregular menstrual periods or lack of periods altogether (called amenorrhea). Stress, diet, and athletic training can affect a woman's hormonal balance, which in turn affects her ovulation. Blockages of the fallopian tubes also can cause infertility.

Oftentimes fertility drugs are prescribed to women to increase ovulation. Eighty to 90 percent of infertility cases are treated with drugs or surgery. But using those drugs does not come without risks. Multiple births occur in 10 percent to 20 percent of births resulting from fertility drug use.(28) It's believed that fertility treatments may have a direct effect on the development of ovarian cancer due to the raised concentrations of estrogens and persistent stimulation of the ovary by the drugs.(29)

In one study, John A. Collins, M.D., found that fertility treatments result in only a 6 percent improvement in achieving pregnancy over infertile couples who just kept trying. In a second study, Collins tracked the pregnancy rates of 2,000 couples; rates between the treated couples and the non-treated couples were the same. Why are treatments so staunchly advocated? Infertility treatments are a $1 billion-a-year industry.[30]

The dietary habits of the mother can play a big part in whether she gets pregnant and has a healthy child. Here's where caffeine comes in again: In a 1988 study by Allen Wilcox of the National Institute of Environmental Health Sciences in North Carolina, it was found that women who drank just one cup of regular coffee a day were half as likely to become pregnant.[31] Most other studies had this at three or more cups a day. At Johns Hopkins University a study showed that women who consumed more than 300 milligrams of caffeine a day reduced their chances of pregnancy by 17 percent in any given month. A more recent study at Yale University school of Medicine stated that the risk of not conceiving for 12 months (the usual definition of infertility), was 55 percent higher for women drinking one cup of coffee a day, 100 percent higher when they drank one and a half to three cups, and 176 percent higher for women drinking more than three cups of coffee per day.[32] Mark Klebanoff of the National Institute of Child Health and Human Development says "it's probably prudent for women who are trying to become pregnant, and especially for those having trouble, to cut back on caffeine."[33]

Coffee drinking before and during pregnancy has been associated with more than twice the risk of miscarriage when the mother drank two to three cups per day. Smoking is another impediment to conception. It's been shown that women who smoke have less chance of getting pregnant by about 10 percent. Smokers are three to four times more likely than nonsmokers to have taken greater than a year to conceive.[34]

MSG was found to cause infertility problems in test animals.[35] Other food additives such as dyes and flavorings have also been implicated in fertility problems as well as some cosmetic chemicals.

For the effects of alcohol as far as its effect on fertility, a study at the Washington University School of Medicine showed that there was a 50 percent reduction in conception in test animals after intoxicating doses of alcohol were given 24 hours prior to mating. The *Harvard Health Letter* reported in October 1992 that in the ancient cities of Carthage and Sparta, there were laws prohibiting the use of alcohol by newlyweds, due to the belief that a child conceived by intoxicated parents would be unhealthy.[36]

Your weight also can make you less fertile. In women, obesity results in an increased production of estrogen and this hormonal imbalance in turn interferes with ovulation, which of course, is the basis of successful conception. Ovulatory disorders are the leading cause of female infertility, resulting in the disruption of hormones, menstrual cycles, and conception. Approximately 15 percent of such disorders are linked to weight disorders, mainly being overweight and obese.

High estrogen levels associated with obesity can also result in pre-cancerous transformations (usually reversible) in the uterus.

Being obese also decreases a man's chances of becoming a father, even if he is otherwise health. One study in 2008 showed that obese men had lower levels of testosterone and other hormones essential for reproduction. As the body mass index (BMI) goes up, the less chance a man will become a dad.[37]

The effects of chemicals on fertility and miscarriages can be profound. Women who are consistently exposed to chemical solvents (including xylene, acetone, trichlorethylene, petroleum distillates, and others) have a more than four-fold increase in spontaneous abortions.[38] It was reported in *Time* magazine that pregnant mothers exposed to two solvent chemicals had a 33 percent miscarriage rate. (The normal miscarriage rate is 15 percent.) [39]

Birth defects occurred almost three times more often in nurse-anesthetists (nurses who help with anesthesia preparation). As far back as 1860, it was observed that wives of men who worked with lead were less likely to become pregnant, and if they did, they were more prone to miscarrying. Boguslaw Baranski, M.D., of the Institute of Occupational Medicine in Denmark observed that the "Risk of infertility increased in females who reported exposures to textile dyes, dry cleaning chemicals. . . lead, mercury and cadmium. There was a significant risk of increased time to conception among women exposed to anti-rust agents, welding, plastic manufacturing, lead, mercury, cadmium or anesthetic agents." As far as men are concerned, Baranski says, "There was also an increased risk of delay to conception following male exposure to textile dyes, plastic manufacturing, and welding. Those who unpacked or handled antibiotics had a significant association with delayed pregnancy of at least 12 months."[40]

Miscarriage risks after exposure to the following chemicals was 4.7 times greater for perchlorethylene (from dry cleaning), 3.1 times greater for trichloroethylene (from dry cleaning), 2.1 times greater for paint thinners and strippers, and 2.9 times greater for glycol ethers (found in paints). Women working in rubber, plastics or synthetics industries have an 80 percent greater chance of having a stillbirth, according to a study funded by the March of Dimes. This study also showed that women whose husbands worked in the textile industry (chemical dyes, plastics, formaldehyde etc.) had a 90 percent greater risk of stillbirth.[41]

There are many chemicals in our environment (as well as some foods such as soy) that mimic the female hormone estrogen and/or otherwise may disrupt the human hormonal system. Several currently used pesticides commonly found in food mimic the female hormone estrogen, and others clearly interfere with normal hormone function. Recent studies show that the effect of estrogenic pesticides are additive, and that exposure to estrogenic mixtures at low levels can cause the same effect produced by a single chemical when administered at a higher dose.[42] Childhood exposure to these chemicals can have harmful effects later on in life. The British medical journal the *The Lancet* said: "The various facets of declining male reproductive health seem to have a common origin in childhood, and defects that may be induced in the current birth cohort by xeno-estrogens [estrogens from sources other than the human body] or other compounds may not become apparent for a further 20 to 40 years."[43]

For all the potential risks associated with them, little is known about most chemicals – even chemicals that are produced and used in great amounts. Of the several thousand chemicals that are produced in amounts of more than 1,000 tons per year (and many at 10,000 tons per year), toxicological data of any kind exists for only a few hundred, and reproductive toxicology data exists for probably a hundred or so.

David La Roche, the secretary of the International Joint Commission, was quoted in *Esquire* magazine concerning chemicals that can harm reproduction (which number in the hundreds if not thousands), "The responsibility should not be on the people exposed to chemicals to prove they have been hurt. The responsibility should be on industry to prove that chemicals cause no harm."[44]

CHAPTER XV

Vaccines

On June 4, 2008 the *Green Our Vaccines March & Rally* occurred in Washington, D.C. It was attended by over 8,500 people, 40 autism and environmental organizations, Robert F. Kennedy Jr., Dr. Jay Gordon, Dr. Jerry Kartzinel, Dr. Boyd Hayley, and was hosted by actors Jim Carrey and Jenny McCarthy. McCarthy, whose six-year-old son became autistic immediately after a series of vaccinations, believes there is a correlation between the shots and the impairment. The American Academy of Pediatrics, on the other hand, says, "There is no valid scientific evidence that vaccines cause autism."[1]

In November 2007, the Department of Health and Human Services Division of Vaccine Injury Compensation decided to award compensation to the parents of Hannah Poling, a nine-year-old girl who became autistic within 48 hours after receiving nine routinely administered childhood vaccines in July 2000. Her parents assert that the government's decision to award them compensation vindicates that her impairment was caused by the vaccines. But the director of the CDC, Dr. Julie Gerberding, said, "The government has made absolutely no statement indicating that vaccines are a cause of autism. This does not represent anything other than a very specific situation and a very sad situation as far as the family of the affected child."[2]

Who, and what, do you believe? If you're a parent with an autistic child, you can't help but wonder if vaccines played a role or even caused it. If you just had a child, do you give them the shots, or risk having them come down with diseases the vaccines supposedly protect against?

These diseases, many believe, are caused by germs – bacteria and viruses. Bacteria are one-cell organisms that can survive and multiply on their own – in your body or on a counter top. Viruses, on the other hand, are not technically "alive," since they cannot survive on their own – they need a host organism to become part of in order to replicate. Vaccines are composed of some form of bacteria or virus that is usually injected into the person that supposedly causes the recipient to acquire immunity against a particular disease.

We're going to explore vaccines in depth in this chapter, as they relate to autism and other impairments, how they came about in the first place, and whether they help prevent disease. I must warn you that some of my comments and opinions are not just controversial, but outright revolutionary and may even be considered heretical. However, I've never been one to believe something just because an authority figure says it or popular opinion believes it, especially when it doesn't make sense to me. So tighten that seat belt and strap on a helmet, because you're in for one wild ride. . .

Here are more reports from parents who believe a vaccine affected their child:

> "Terry was a beautiful baby. . .happy, healthy, strong baby from birth. When Terry was nine weeks old, his doctor gave him his first DPT shot and oral polio vaccinations. In the 48 hours after his vaccinations, Terry started to sleep more than usual and his mother couldn't wake him up to eat. . .his skin turned grey and mottled." Terry was put on a respirator and had to be fed through a tube in his nose because he was severely paralyzed. He loves to be picked up and held close but he can't hug you back. In 1996, the U.S. Court of Claims in Washington, D.C. officially acknowledged that Terry's paralysis was a result of the polio vaccine he received as a baby.

> Within ten hours of his first DPT shot, a mother reported that her son "had a red and swollen leg and was crying a strange cry. His temperature was 105 degrees. I called the doctor and he told me to give him *Tylenol* and put him in a tepid bath. As I was putting him in the bath, his eyes rolled back in his head and he quivered all over." From that moment on, her son continued to have seizures and high-pitched screaming. Today, he is hyperactive and physically and mentally handicapped.

> After her fourth shot, an eighteen-month-old girl collapsed. Her mother said, "The day after her shot, her leg got really stiff, and she couldn't walk on it. . .The next night, she woke up screaming. It was a terrible, fearful kind of scream. My husband picked her up, and she got very silent and turned white with a purple-blue tinge around her mouth and went completely limp. We thought she was in the throes of Sudden Infant Death Syndrome."[3]

Edward Jenner, a British physician, is often credited with starting vaccinations (or inoculations) in 1796 – but the history of vaccines goes back before that, probably originating in the Orient or by the Arabs. Jenner scraped pus from the sore of a woman's hand into a cut on the arm of eight-year-old James Phipps. The boy came down with cowpox – a relatively mild disease – but later did not contract smallpox – a potentially fatal disease. There are reports the boy was sickly most of his life. He died at the age of 20 from tuberculosis (often a side effect of the smallpox vaccine). However, the same kind of inoculation failed to work with Jenner's own 18-month-old son, (who also died in his early 20s of tuberculosis), and bad reactions to inoculations in people during Jenner's day were widespread and serious. In fact, there was a serious outcry of public opinion against vaccines when they were first introduced because of their side effects and lack of effectiveness.[5,6,7]

Nevertheless, due to political and economic pressures, government mandates, bad science, and outright deception, vaccinations have become a mainstay of the traditional medical community's attempts to prevent and control infectious diseases.

The theory of how vaccines work contends that when a disease causing germ or facsimile of it is injected into a person, it stimulates the body to produce antibodies – proteins that reportedly defend it from a future invasion of similar bacteria or viruses.

The National Academy of Sciences states that the incidence of disease and death caused by vaccines is "extraordinarily low." The Centers for Disease Control says that most vaccines are 90 percent effective at preventing their target diseases. UNICEF reports that vaccines save the lives of at least 1.5 million children every year. The global eradication of smallpox during the 1970s is attributed to worldwide vaccination campaigns. Many hail the pioneering work of Salk and Sabin for developing the polio vaccine in the 1950s. Some expect polio to be eradicated as well within the next few years.

A document on vaccines by the World Health Organization prepared for parents gives general information concerning vaccines. The question is presented: "Are vaccines contrary to nature?" Their response:

> No, on the contrary, vaccines are simply utilizing the laws of nature. Science has gradually gained insight into some of the basic mechanisms utilized by nature to prevent as well as cure infectious diseases. But whereas infectious agents often cause serious disease or even death before the body can mobilize its defense, the vaccines are designed to stimulate the natural defense mechanisms in the most efficient ways, with minimal harm to the body. . .[8]

What the pro-vaccination people don't tell you is that if you go back and look at the raw data, communicable diseases have been declining at a steady rate for 150 years before large-scale vaccinations. Statistics show that there is no relationship between the decline of various diseases and the onset of immunization. Without exception, the vaccine program for each of the childhood diseases was inaugurated *after* that particular disease had begun to disappear. This includes polio. There's also evidence that vaccines have caused various childhood diseases to become adulthood diseases – with far more serious implications such as mumps in men and rubella in women.[9]

Are vaccines really hazardous to your health? Even the World Health Organization acknowledges potential dangers. It said,

> The vast majority of adverse effects following vaccination are minor, typically just a local reaction at the site of the injection. . . may occur in approximately 1 - 30 percent of the cases. . .On rare occasions, more serious adverse effects may occur, such as fever, aches or a widespread rash. . .Extremely rare cases of lasting

damage or even death have occurred. Death in association with an injection of a vaccine has mostly resulted from individual hypersensitivity to one of the components included in the vaccine. The majority of such tragedies are in principle preventable; questions concerning possible allergies are routinely explored before any immunization, and persons with a history of severe hypersensitivity reactions should be referred to relevant medical expertise.(10)

Most mothers are not aware of how many children have been killed or permanently injured due to vaccines, but the government is. They have records of thousands of children and babies who have been killed or permanently hurt by vaccines in a special database. That's just the tip of the iceberg. The FDA acknowledges that 90 percent of doctors do not report vaccine reactions at all. FDA Commissioner David Kessler stated that only one in 10 adverse events following vaccinations are reported.(11)

Even with this underreporting, every year there are thousands of reports of adverse reaction to vaccines. These reports include hospital visits, irreversible injuries, and hundreds of deaths. If you consider only 10 percent are reported, then the true figure could be as high as 120,000 adverse events annually. All this even though the Federal government set up the Vaccine Adverse Event Reporting System (VAERS) to document adverse reactions to vaccines. In 2007, nearly 25,000 adverse events were reported, including 160 deaths. In 2008, nearly 24,000 adverse events were reported including 161 deaths.(12) Clearly, there are problems with vaccines.

More proof that the government acknowledges problems with vaccines: In 1986 the National Childhood Vaccine Injury Act (Public Law 99-660) was passed. It addresses the facts that vaccines do, in fact cause injury and death. Part of this law requires doctors to inform parents of the potential risks of vaccines and to report any adverse reactions. However, as we just saw, only about 10 percent of adverse reactions are ever reported. I suspect the percentage of doctors informing parents of the potential risks of vaccines is even lower.

The National Childhood Vaccine Injury Act has a provision to give compensation to victims of vaccinations that have caused injury or death. As of January 2000, more than $1 billion has been paid out for hundreds of injuries and deaths caused by mandated vaccines, and thousands of cases are still pending.(13) Yet, this program currently dismisses 90 percent of all vaccine injury claims. The money for this fund is raised by taking a portion of the money the parents, insurance companies, or government spend on vaccines and putting it into a congressional fund. The law awards up to $250,000 if a person dies or millions to cover lifelong medical bills, pain, and suffering caused by a vaccine the government requires by law.

Food for Thought

Lest you think the government is being generous in effectively insuring manufacturers against vaccine casualties, consider how easy the program makes it for manufacturers. The bottom line is that this government-run compensation program protects vaccine manufacturers from lawsuits and the government (i.e. the taxpayers) pays out any settlement.

National Vaccine Information Center president Barbara Loe Fisher comments: "Imagine having the following business opportunity: You produce a product that the government guarantees to be free from liability and the marketplace is every child born. It certainly doesn't get much better than that. . .And the pharmaceutical industry currently has a monopoly on this 'business.' To date there has never been an independent, controlled study which proves that their vaccines are safe or even effective."[14]

There is very little control of the vaccine industry. The scientists and physicians in the pharmaceutical industry and government who are in charge of the mass vaccination system are policing themselves. There is no oversight mechanism in place to safeguard the public health.

Barbara Loe Fisher is president and cofounder of the National Vaccine Information Center (NVIC) – a consumer-led movement that monitors vaccine research, licensing, development, promotion, and policy making. She says:

> It's a dream for the pharmaceutical industry involved in making vaccines, because there's no way anybody can say no. It's a stable, ready-made market, and the enactment of the compensation law in 1986 has removed almost all liability for drug companies. . .You would think that, because vaccines are required to be used by every-one, they would be held to the very highest safety and efficacy standards, but that is not the case. What the NVIC has been pushing for is more consumer involvement in the public health decisions that are made in this country with regard to vaccination. We believe that health care consumers should have the right to choose the type of preventive health care that they want to use – including choosing whether to use one, ten or no vaccines. . .We are vaccinating in a vacuum of scientific knowledge. There have been no long-term studies set up, as has been done with heart disease and cancer, to evaluate all morbidity and mortality outcomes following vaccination in large populations of vaccinated and unvaccinated groups to see if we are paying a price for the control of infectious disease in childhood. Are we paying a larger price down the road, in terms of chronic illness?. . Today in this country, a one-year-old child can be vaccinated with ten different viral and bacterial antigens on one day. That is an incredible assault on the immune system.[15]

A vaccine is made by first acquiring the disease germ and then processing in various ways to make it suitable for the intended use. Some of the processes include adding drugs, antibiotics, diseased animal matter, aborted human fetal tissue, and toxic substances (formaldehyde, aluminum hydrochloride, streptomycin, neomycin, thimerosal [a mercury derivative]). The toxic effects of aluminum formaldehyde and mercury are well documented, and even microscopic doses of them can lead to permanent cellular damage. Vaccines containing the carcinogenic toxins formaldehyde and thimerosal are being injected into infants as young as two months old whose immune systems are not fully developed.[16]

The CDC and the National Immunization Program post a Contraindications to Vaccine Chart on their website (www.cdc.gov/nip/recs/contraindications_vacc.htm). The only official contraindication for most vaccines is if a child got a serious allergic reaction after a previous vaccine dose or exposure to a vaccine component. However, there are many health-care professionals who believe there are more reasons or situations not to give a child a vaccine. They include the child being sick or having a cold, allergy to eggs, weak immune system, and simply being too young for a particular vaccine.

The NVIC says a parent should ask the following questions before allowing their child to receive a vaccine: Is my child sick right now? Has my child had a bad reaction to a vaccination before? Does my child have a personal or family history of vaccine reactions, convulsions, neurological disorders, severe allergies, immune system disorders? Do I know if my child is at high risk of reacting? Do I have full information on the vaccine's side effects? Do I know how to identify a vaccine reaction? Do I know how to report a vaccine reaction? Do I know the vaccine manufacturer's name and lot number?[17]

DPT is a single vaccine combining diphtheria, tetanus, and pertussis vaccines into one shot. Formaldehyde is used to manufacture the vaccine and formaldehyde is known to cause cancer. The DPT vaccine contains a preservative called thimerosal – its chemical formula is $C_9H_9HgNaO_2S$ (where Hg is mercury). It also contains aluminum, which is believed to not only cause rashes soon after injection, but long-term damage to the brain. The more current vaccine DTaP, reportedly does not contain thimerosal (although the drug companies have lied about that before). Think of DPT as a triple threat: formaldehyde, mercury, and aluminum – all considered toxic.

Even the CDC admits there are more contraindications for the DPT vaccine including encephalopathy (coma, prolonged seizures, decreased level of consciousness) and progressive neurological disorder (infantile spasm and uncontrolled epilepsy). However, the CDC dismisses the following reasons not to give a baby a DPT shot: high temperature; fussiness after a previous DPT shot; family history of seizures; family history of SIDS; family history of adverse events following DPT shots; and well controlled convulsions. (Just what is a "well controlled convulsion?")

Food for Thought

Having a list of contraindications is to ensure that a person who has a high chance of being susceptible to a vaccine is determined so a serious adverse reaction can be avoided. Each box of vaccines comes with a package insert detailing the contraindications and doctors are supposed to find out if they apply to an individual before the vaccine is given. But how many doctors take the time to ask a parent if their child had an adverse reaction to their most recent vaccine, or if the child has any other characteristics that might indicate a vaccine should be avoided? As a parent, learn the contraindications and ask – even demand – to get them before letting your child get a vaccine. Do NOT assume the doctor knows everything. Remember, he or she is very busy.

One of the most frightening and suspicious things about the whole vaccination issue is that vaccines have not been adequately tested for safety or effectiveness. The proof of safety comes from the state and local officials who are just following the advice of organizations who set the policies who in turn are influenced and educated by the companies who manufacture the vaccine.

The Advisory Committee on Immunization Practices (ACIP) makes immunization recommendations that the FDA follows in licensing vaccines. Their members are appointed by the Centers for Disease Control. The Chairman of the ACIP, Dr. John Modlin, said in February 1999,

"Available data are insufficient to fully establish the safety and efficacy of Rotavirus vaccine in premature infants. . .To my knowledge we don't have data from a clinical trial specifically. . .Some bit of information from Seattle, as I recall, that had suggested that there was a slight increase in relative risk for hospitalization for premature infants. Obviously a situation where we have to make a judgment in the absence of data, and with a vaccine that has not yet been tested in the group. . ."

Modlin said that during an ACIP meeting held to determine if the Rotavirus vaccine (known to cause infant diarrhea) should be approved. Given this information, or declaration of the lack of information, the committee nonetheless voted nine to one for the Rotavirus to be given to premature infants.(18)

This story does not stop there. It turns out that Modlin did indeed have data about the safety of the vaccine from being the Chairman of the Rotavirus working group of the Vaccines and Related Biological Products Advisory Committee (VRBPAC), which decides whether vaccines are licensed (Congressional Hearings). The data showed a risk of life-threatening bowel obstructions in clinical trials of Rotavirus before the February 1999 ACIP meeting. In these clinical trials, some babies suffered obstructed bowels a week after being vaccinated – some requiring intussusception surgery to remove a portion of the intestine. The committee called these reactions statistically insignificant.[19]

Once the vaccine was introduced (1.5 million doses given to infants), bad things happened. One premature baby died and another five-month-old infant died from a bowel obstruction. In all there were 113 cases of life-threatening bowel obstructions reported because of the vaccine. Only then was the Rotavirus vaccine withdrawn from the market in October 1999.[20] In a March 1999 debate at the University of New Hampshire, Modlin defined his standard for scientific validity: "Has the information withstood the test of peer review? Has the information been published in a respected medical or scientific journal?. . .This is the standard that you should hold me to today. . .Has the information been published in a scientifically reputable Journal?" Nothing was published about the Rotavirus, and yet he voted for its approval. I guess he doesn't hold himself to his own standards. Modlin was subsequently reappointed Chairman of the ACIP.

There were trials of the Rotavirus vaccine, though never published or reviewed, showing the vaccine to have a 49 percent efficacy rate, which is low. Also, the public has no access to the actual data concerning the side effects of the Rotavirus vaccine or for the chicken pox or hepatitis B vaccines. If all these are good for us, why don't they let us see the data?

Still, if you ask your doctor about vaccines, he or she will tell you that "everyone knows" you need them, and "it is scientifically accepted" they work and are safe. However, ask him or her for proof or studies to show that, and your doctor will more than likely try to evade your questions or get angry and tell you, "It's the law."

On the other hand, if you ask someone for the data showing there are great risks associated with vaccines, and they are really not that effective (if at all), they can turn up a library full, like, I am here. Who are you more likely to trust, someone who's an open book, or someone who defiantly objects to your questions? I'm perfectly willing to consider the establishment's side of the story, but oftentimes, they don't give it out! Why not? Show me the studies and tests showing safety and effectiveness, and I'm all yours.

Another bit of history: In 1991 ACIP recommended that every new-born baby receive the hepatitis B vaccine in the hospital within hours of birth. Samuel L. Katz, M.D., was the ACIP Chairman at that time. He has stated that, ". . . there was no published peer-reviewed study" on the safety of the vaccine. Even though newborns have a negligible risk of getting hepatitis B unless the mother is infected, the vaccine was mandated for new-born babies. This was the first of its kind since no newborns were previously required to be immediately vaccinated. Not only that, but once again there was no proper safety study on the hepatitis B vaccine. Since its approval and use, there have been more than 36,000 adverse reactions and more than 440 deaths reported from it (VAERS records, which are accessible to the public through the Freedom of Information Act).

So, let me get this straight: There's little chance of a newborn getting hepatitis B, and there were no safety studies done on the vaccine, yet after they started vaccinating for it, 440 babies died and 36,000 more had adverse reactions?(21) The vaccine was originally developed to protect drug addicts who shared unsterilized needles or people who had multiple sex partners.(22) Does that sound like our babies?

Here's the extent to which the vaccine manufacturers and health officials will go to keep blame off their products: There have been cases where a child had a post-vaccine reaction resulting in seizures, coma, or death, and then the parents were charged with causing it by excessively shaking the baby (*shaken baby syndrome*). It was the parents who killed their own baby or put it into a coma, not the vaccine – so the officials say. Talk about a raw deal. First their baby dies because of a vaccine reaction, and then they get accused of murder. I bet if the defense attorney would take the time to examine the baby's vaccination record, he/she would find the baby was recently vaccinated. Wouldn't that cause an uproar in the courtroom and the news?

Encephalitis, (swelling of the brain) can be caused by a severe injury to the head, a severe burn, high fever or vaccines. Harris L. Coulter, Ph.D., a researcher and author of two books on vaccinations takes this a step further and says the childhood vaccination program is the principal cause of encephalitis in the U.S. today (and other industrialized countries). Coulter says that post-vaccinal encephalitis may be the greatest cause of developmental and learning disabilities in the country, and that "These manifestations of a vaccine reaction are identical to the symptoms of acute encephalitis from any other cause."(23) One of the most prevalent reactions to the measles vaccine – and other vaccines – is a kind of encephalitis.

Post-vaccinal encephalitis results in a loss and destruction of myelin on the brain stem and spinal cord. Remember, myelin is the fatty protective sheath around nerves that acts like insulation around an electric wire. If it's not there, all sorts of short-circuits are possible and the nerves never fully develop.

The symptoms of, "Diarrhea, vomiting, flatulence, gastroenteritis, stomach aces, enuresis, constipation, loss of sphincter control, etc., are all found in encephalitis and are frequently reported after the DPT shot. . . When the baby reacts to a DPT shot with a 'slight fever and fussiness' or 'drowsiness' for a few days, this may be, and often is, a case of encephalitis, which is capable of causing quite sever neurologic consequences." But that's not all. Severe neurologic damage can occur in a child later, even if he or she showed no acute reaction to the vaccine. In fact, "encephalitis from all other causes [fever, brain injury] is known to produce severe neurologic damage. . ."(24) So if vaccines cause encephalitis, by definition, they cause severe neurologic damage.

Coulter believes that the long-term effects of vaccines are more widespread than anyone suspected. He says that these effects are more often than not "disguised" under different names such as autism, dyslexia, learning disabilities, epilepsy, mental retardation, hyperactivity, minimal brain dysfunction. Those are the labels children are brandished with, when the cause of their problems originated with the nervous-system-attacking vaccine. These conditions then lead to violent crime, drug abuse, juvenile delinquency, and contribute to the seeming collapse of the public school system.

There have been studies showing that more violent crimes are committed by those with neurological damage than those without. Since encephalitis is neurological damage, children who have had it may exhibit cruel, abusive, and destructive behavior more often. Not just as children, but later as adolescents and adults.[25]

Hyperactivity and learning problems are another result of neurological damage and also predisposes a child to violent tendencies. An article in the *Journal of the American Medical Association* concluded that; "Adults with a history of attention-deficit hyperactivity disorder appear to be over represented in the ranks of felons."[26]

Other learning disabilities such as dyslexia are often found in convicted criminals.[27] Again, these violent tendencies may be a result of actual brain damage (from vaccine reactions?) and not necessarily from psychological or sociological problems.

Food for Thought

The number of hyperactive children has increased dramatically over the past few decades such that now more than one child in 20 is considered hyperactive.[28] Hyperactivity increases the likelihood of violent and criminal behavior, and drug and alcohol use.[29] So it's not just your imagination that crime has increased in our society. Poisons injected into babies leads to hyperactive and learning impaired children, which leads to unruly adolescents, which leads to unlawful adults.

Encephalitis (often caused by vaccines) often causes a myriad of seizure disorders including epilepsy with episodes of convulsions, petit mal, grand mal, tics, tremors, and grimaces.[30] Movements can also be impaired resulting in paralysis, cerebral palsy, weakness of arms and legs, clumsiness, and spasticity. For over a century, scientists have noticed a link between epilepsy and violent tendencies, and studies have shown that the prevalence of epileptics in prisons is significantly higher than in the general population.[32] It's an accepted fact (even by the vaccine manufacturers) that vaccines can cause convulsions, but the medical establishment denies that there's a connection between vaccines and epilepsy. Later in life, chronic encephalitis can manifest as Parkinson's disease.[31]

Another possible aberration from encephalitis is that of abnormal sexual activity and desires. These may appear as hyper-sexuality (too much sex drive usually discharged by masturbation), pornography, a casual attitude towards sex, perversions, fetishes, confused sexuality, bisexualism, and homosexualism.(33) To see a display of many of these attitudes, all one has to do is watch TV. This is what we – the most vaccinated people in the history of mankind – relate to. We relate to it because that is what we are becoming.

Hyperactive children in many cases may have some form of neurological disorder as mentioned above, and children with minimal brain dysfunction are more likely to start smoking, drinking, and using drugs as adolescents.(34)

Hyperactive children are then often prescribed drugs like *Ritalin* to control them. These drugs, harmful in their own right, then predispose the child to substance abuse and antisocial behaviors later in life. This is not to mention the increased susceptibility to other disorders such as cancer due to the poisoning effects of the vaccines.

Autism is now a well-known syndrome reaching epidemic levels. An estimated 560,000 children in the U.S. and as many as 1.5 million Americans overall have it. Experts estimate that autism rates have risen from around four per 10,000 in the early 1980s to between 12 and 20 per 10,000 in the 1990s to about 66 per 10,000 (or 1 in 150) in 2005. While the number of children with disabilities in general has increased 30 percent from 1991 – 2002, the number of cases of autism has increased a disproportionate 1700 percent. Autism costs a lot of money – in the U.S., 13.3 billion dollars a year. That's 36.5 million dollars a day.(35,36,37)

The lifetime cost of caring for a child with autism is between $3.5 and $5 million. The annual cost to the U.S. is $90 billion. Ten years ago, the disease was typically diagnosed in children at age three or four, but now it's being detected in children at age two.(38,39)

The adverse reactions to a vaccine are the same thing as the neurological complications from the disease itself. Since the introduction of the measles vaccine, the rate of autism has increased hundreds of percent. Autism has historically been called *post encephalitic syndrome* – and is essentially the same thing as measles encephalitis. Many parents report that their children were perfectly normal until the received the MMR (measles/mumps/rubella) vaccine. Then they became autistic.(40)

Robert Mendelsohn, M.D., says that the measles vaccine may cause the inability to coordinate muscle movements (ataxia), learning disabilities, paralysis, retardation, seizure disorders, aseptic meningitis, juvenile-onset diabetes, multiple sclerosis, Reye's syndrome, blood clotting disorders, and death.(41) An article in the *New England Journal of Medicine* said that giving vitamin A to children with measles reduces the likelihood of complications and their chances of dying.(42)

Regarding diabetes, the MMR vaccine has been heavily implicated in the causation of Type-I diabetes.(43) The rubella (German measles) component of the vaccine is believed to be the major suspect because rubella itself (along with mumps) is known to be a cause of diabetes. The action of the live MMR vaccine mimics that of the disease and it's believed that the rubella and mumps viruses infect pancreatic islet cells and severely reduce levels of secreted insulin.(44) Researchers believe that if measles or mumps can cause diabetes, the vaccine can too.(45)

The history of autism is particularly interesting and shows an amazing correlation to the introduction and increased use of the pertussis vaccine (and the MMR vaccine as we shall see a bit later, below). A well-known psychiatrists named Leo Kanner, while at Johns Hopkins, first described autism in 1943 in his article "Autistic Disturbances of Affective Content." He noted that the symptoms of aloneness and lack of social involvement started early and thus the syndrome was called "infantile autism."(46)

Autism is now characterized as a self-absorbed alienation where the child is detached, inaccessible, and sometimes nervously hostile. It can start very early in the child's life (*early onset autism* – 12 to 18 months), as Kanner initially observed. If symptoms are observed in a child older than three years old, it's called *late onset autism*. It was virtually unheard of before the 1970s, but now such cases outnumber early onset autism cases 5 to one.(47)

Two questions must be asked: Why did autism begin at all, and why has there been an explosion in the number of cases of autism over the past 20 years?

Many researchers have made the link between autism and government mandated vaccinations – especially the pertussis vaccine. This vaccine, to combat whooping cough, was developed in the mid 1930s and it gradually achieved widespread mandated governmental use in the 1950s. Harris L. Coulter observed, "The increase prevalence of autism in the 1950s and 1960s precisely reflected the expansion of mandated vaccination programs during these same decades."(48) This trend occurred not only in the U.S. In Japan, France, Chile, Austria, Holland, and England, the first cases of autism occurred after the introduction of the pertussis vaccine.(49)

Another reason to suspect the pertussis vaccine as being a causative agent in autism is because of the kinds of children it first affected. When autism first appeared, it did so in children of well-educated, intelligent, and affluent parents. Naturally, scientist tried to explain the outbreak of autism (unsuccessfully) as being a genetic trait. Since free vaccinations at public health clinics had not yet begun, only those who could afford private physicians and the new vaccinations they offered were having their children vaccinated. However, as free and government mandated vaccines increased across the country, so did the incidences of autism. Not just in children of affluent parents, but in children of parents of every economic, social and ethnic class as well.(50)

Food for Thought

I realize that diagnosis and terminology have advanced since the 1940s. But to not even have a name for the symptoms of autism in the medical literature of that time is telling. Dr. Yazbak says "Suggesting that a sudden and exponential increase in autistic disorders is not real, and results only from better diagnosis, amounts to denial."(51)

The agent in the vaccines believed to be largely responsible for inducing autism is mercury, which is in the thimerosal used to preserve more than 30 vaccines since the 1930s. Eli Lilly and Company assured everyone that thimerosal was safe – based on a test conducted in 1929 by a young researcher named K.C. Smithburn. Smithburn injected 22 human subjects who were already dying from meningitis with a 1 percent solution of thimerosal, and then pronounced that all the patients were reported "without ill effect." The FDA website still cites this study as evidence that thimerosal is safe, but even they concede, "Of note, this study was not specifically designed to examine toxicity; 7 of 22 subjects were observed for only one day, the specific clinical assessments were not described, and no laboratory studies were reported."(52)

This is not just bad science, but clearly unethical, and doesn't prove thimerosal is safe by any stretch of the imagination. However, based on this one ridiculous study, Eli Lilly convinced two generations of Americans that this toxic substance does no harm.

By preserving the vaccine with thimerosal, "multiple-dose vials" can be used which saves a lot of money. The World Health Organization (WHO) said, "Most vaccines could be made thimerosal-free quickly, but they would not contain a preservative. . .One solution would be to use single-dose vials, but this solution is very expensive and not always technically possible."(53)

For some vaccines, these single-dose vials are now being made, which is progress. This progress started in 1997 when, due to parental concern and the growing evidence that thimerosal was the culprit in causing the explosion in autism, the FDA, under the FDA Modernization Act (FDAMA) of 1997, carried out a comprehensive review of the use of thimerosal in childhood vaccines. Concluded in 1999, this review still proclaimed that there was no evidence of harm from the use of thimerosal as a vaccine preservative, other than local hypersensitivity reactions.

Still, on July 1, 1999, the FDA sent a letter to vaccine manufacturers requesting plans for the removal of thimerosal from vaccines – or to justify the continued use of it.(54) On July 7, 2000, the American Academy of Pediatrics (AAP) and the U.S. Public Health Service issued a statement calling for the elimination or reduction of thimerosal in vaccines for children. The FDA says on their website,

However, depending on the vaccine formulations used and the weight of the infant, some infants could have been exposed to cumulative levels of mercury during the first six months of life that exceeded EPA recommended guidelines for safe intake of methyl mercury. As a precautionary measure, the Public Health Service (including FDA, National Institutes of Health [NIH], Centers for Disease Control and Prevention [CDC] and Health Resources and Services Administration [HRSA]) and the American Academy of Pediatrics issued a Joint Statement, urging vaccine manufacturers to reduce or eliminate thimerosal in vaccines as soon as possible.(55)

Walter A. Orenstein, M.D., head of the national immunization program at the federal Centers for Disease Control and Prevention, told concerned parents that, "Thimerosal will be out by the end of the year." Spokesman for the CDC Glen Nowak said that "Our goal is to [achieve] a thimerosal-free children's immunization schedule by early 2001."(56) Remember, the FDA had previously ruled that thimerosal was totally safe.

Thimerosal is nearly 50 percent ethyl mercury.(57) Recall that the symptoms of mercury toxicity include: depression; mood swings; withdrawal; tantrums; aggression; retardation and poor attention; problems with speech, hearing and movements; vision; sleeping; eating; and allergies. It's also been noted that thimerosal completely inhibits phagocytosis in blood, which is one of most vital immune defenses.(58) Vaccinations are used to induce an immunization response, and yet one of its ingredients inhibits that very response.

According to Lars Friberg, M.D., former head of toxicology at the World Health Organization, "There is no safe level of mercury and no one has actually shown there is a safe level, and I would say mercury is a very toxic substance."(59)

Drs. Horning, Chain and Lipkin of the Department of Neurology and Pathology at Colombia University College of Physicians and Surgeons co-authored an article in the journal *Molecular Psychiatry* in 2004 that stated, "The developing brain is uniquely susceptible to the neurotoxic hazard posed by mercurials. . .Profound behavioral and neuropathiologic disturbances were observed after postnatal thimerosal [exposure]. . .The mercury [preservative] used in some vaccines can cause behavioral abnormalities in newborn mice characteristic of autism. . ." Horning et al. did their experiments with doses and timing equivalent to the pediatric immunization schedule. These findings came out just weeks after the Institute of Medicine had stated thimerosal is not connected in any way with autism. Reports are that the IOM was aware of this research, but chose to ignore it.(60)

Dr. J. C. Pendergrass and Dr. Boyd Haley say, "Pure thimerosal was toxic at the low nanomolar level – an extremely low concentration, about 10,000 times less than the thimerosal concentration found in most vaccines. These results leave little doubt about thimerosal being the toxic agent in the vaccines."(61)

Dr. David Baskin at the department of Neurosurgery at Baylor College of Medicine demonstrated "that thimerosal in micromolar concentrations rapidly induces membrane and DNA damage. . . in human neurons and fibroblasts." These concentrations were 125 nM – 250 µM concentrations of thimerosal. (That's 125 nanoMoles to 250 microMoles – much less than what's in a vaccine, even if just "trace" amounts.) (62)

Food for Thought

The most toxic element on the planet is uranium. Next is mercury. In November 2007, the U.S. House of Representative held a hearing concerning the dangers of mercury. They heard testimony from experts saying that one gram of mercury (roughly the size of a vitamin capsule) can poison 21 million gallons of water – about the volume of a good sized lake.(63)

Mercury in vaccines is bad, for sure, but let's not forget it's also part of the amalgam fillings dentists use to fill cavities. It turns out that dentists are the third largest source of mercury pollution in the country. Of course, the American Dental Association still says the fillings are safe, even though the amount of mercury in some people's mouths is enough to poison several lakes.

One concerned mother, Lyn Redwood, RN, MSN, CRNP, reviewed her son's vaccine record and found that they contained thimerosal and he had received 187.5 mcg (micrograms) of mercury – all within the first six months of life. (200 micrograms of mercury in just 23 gallons of water makes that water unsafe for human consumption according to EPA guidelines.) She said, "At each visit, two, four, and six months, he received a total of 62.5 mcg of mercury. These levels exceeded EPA's allowable daily exposure of 0.1 mcg per kilogram at two months 125-fold."(64) The EPA allowable exposure of mercury for adults is only 0.1 mcg per kilogram per day.(65)

Supposedly thimerosal has been removed from three or four childhood vaccines for influenza and one of four DTaP vaccines and has been replaced in vaccines for hepatitis B. However, many vaccines still contain thimerosal: some are still manufactured with it, some contain trace amounts, and doctors are still using up their stock of thimerosal-laden vaccines. No recalls have been issued.

Thimerosal is still in tetanus shots and many flu vaccines that have recently been introduced into the childhood immunization schedule. Each flu vaccine contains a dose of 25 micrograms of mercury, an amount the EPA considers safe only for adults weighing over 550 lbs.(66) So while the authorities are proclaiming with pride that they have eliminated thimerosal in some vaccines, they have introduced new vaccines with thimerosal in it.

Mike Wagnitz, a senior chemist at the University of Wisconsin says, "The concentration of mercury in a multi-dose flu vaccine vial is 500,000 parts per billion. To put this in perspective, drinking water cannot exceed 2 parts per billion of mercury, and waste is considered hazardous if it has only 200 parts per billion. Is it really safe then to inject pregnant women, newborns, and infants with levels of mercury 250 times higher than what is legally classified as hazardous waste?"[67]

Food for Thought

In December 2000, I went to the American Academy of Pediatrics web site to see exactly what they had to say. The press release posted was dated July 14, 1999. In it they announced new recommendations regarding the reduction and/or elimination of thimerosal in many vaccines. Although they make this recommendation, they said, "There is no evidence that vaccines containing thimerosal result in adverse reactions, and government safety guidelines for mercury exposure are still well below a dangerous level. But since very high mercury exposure from fish and other sources has caused brain damage, it is crucial to ensure that mercury levels in vaccines are as low as possible."[68]

So mercury in fish can cause brain damage, but mercury in thimerosal doesn't? Mercury is a cumulative poison. That is, it easily accumulates in our tissues and builds up over time because it is not easily excreted. Repeated vaccinations of thimerosal containing vaccines is just like eating mercury-contaminated fish repeatedly.

The kind of mercury in fish and air pollution is in the form of methyl-mercury and that in vaccines is ethyl mercury. The FDA and CDC make it sound like ethyl mercury is less toxic than methyl mercury, which it is not. Ethyl mercury is made from ethylmercuric chloride, a fungicide (which was banned). The authorities say it is excreted faster than methyl mercury, which may, in fact, be the case, but ethyl mercury crosses the blood brain barrier and accumulates in tissue more readily and stays there. Ethyl mercury has been shown to deposit twice as much inorganic mercury in the brains of primates as compared to equal doses of methyl mercury.[69]

Another study said, "By 7 days, mercury levels decreased in the blood but were unchanged in the brain. . .methyl mercury does not appear to be a good model for ethyl mercury containing compounds."[70] The concentration of mercury in the blood is of secondary importance. Its concentration in the tissues is what really counts.

What the AAP said in the 1999 press release is chicanery. They're deflecting any admission of negligence on their part by talking about mercury exposure from fish. Joel Alpert, M.D., president of AAP, said in the article, "Parents shouldn't worry about the safety of vaccines. The current levels of thimerosal will not hurt children. Reducing those levels will make safe vaccines even safer." If vaccines are already safe, then how can they become safer? If they're so safe, why take it out? Because it isn't and the growing awareness, grass-roots movement, and thousands of law suits are scaring them. All this double-talk is merely covering the AAP's, government's, and vaccine manufacturer's behind. Can you imagine the AAP, the FDA, and other health agencies saying "We've been injecting this toxic metal mercury into your children for years. It's killed thousands of your babies, and caused autism in millions more, so now we're taking it out. So sorry."

You can tell where their priorities are. Although they agreed to make thimerosal-free vaccines, they still dispensed the vaccines they had in stock that contain mercury until they run out. If thimerosal-free vaccines are "even safer," why use the "less safe" vaccines that contain thimerosal? Why not issue a recall? They do it for automobiles where there's a safety issue.

Why is it that the incidences of autism are in direct proportion to the number of mandated vaccinations given our children? Consider that in 1983 the CDC recommended 23 doses of seven vaccines for children up to age six, and the chance of a child becoming autistic was one in 10,000. In 2008, the CDC recommends 48 doses of 12 different vaccines, and the chances of a child becoming autistic is now one in 150. But according to the government and most doctors, this is not scientific proof.

On the one hand, the government and medical community speciously cite the great reduction in communicable diseases since vaccines have been used as scientific proof that they work. (This is *not* scientific proof, but anecdotal evidence. But they say it with such authority, conviction, and so often, everyone believes it's scientific.) On the other hand, they say that the explosion in autism rates have nothing to do with increased vaccination. Quite a double standard, I'd say.

If you want scientific proof, here's what you do: Take 1,000 kids from parents who want them to get the vaccines and give them the shots laden with thimerosal. There are plenty of parents who believe their children need vaccines, so that will be easy to do. Then take 1,000 kids from parents who don't want their kids to get the shots. These days, there are plenty of parents who think vaccines cause autism, so that should be easy to do too. Then see how many kids become autistic. The government balks at conducting such a study for "ethical" reasons, but they've administered vaccines that were known to be unsafe. How ethical is that?

But what if you did a study like this with 35,000 kids? Would that make the results more believable? In Chicago, there's a clinic (Homefirst Medical Services) that has catered to many children who have never been vaccinated because their parents got exemptions through Illinois's relatively permissive immunization policy. The clinic's medical director, Dr. Mayer Eisenstein, has taken care of nearly 35,000 unvaccinated children over the years. He said, "I don't think we have a single case of autism in children delivered by us who never received vaccines. We do have enough of a sample. The numbers are too large to not see it. We would absolutely know." The few autistic children he's seen were vaccinated before their families became patients.(71)

Investigative reporter Dan Olmsted, former senior editor for United Press International (UPI), whose articles appear regularly in the *Washington Times* newspaper, discovered Amish children who don't get vaccinated, don't get autism. He interviewed Dr. Frank Noonan, a family practitioner in Lancaster County, PA, who has treated thousands of Amish over a span of 25 years. Dr. Noonan said, "I have not seen autism with the Amish. . .We're right in the heart of Amish country and seeing none, and that's just the way it is."

Dr. Jeff Bradstreet, a family doctor in Florida, treats children who are home schooled who do not get vaccinated. He has actually proposed the kind of study I'm asking for, but cannot get funding. He said, "I know I can tap into this community and find you large numbers of unvaccinated home schooled children, and we can do simple prevalence and incidence studies in them, and my gut reaction is that you're going to see no autism in this group."(72)

The government has all sorts of excuses. A statement from CDC Director Dr. Julie Gerberding said, "[The Amish] have genetic connectivity that would make them different from populations that are in other sectors of the United States."(73)

Ah, the old "genetics" card. It's always easy to explain things that don't fit your paradigm with something the normal person doesn't understand plus is inherently subject to immense variability (dumb luck). Another genetics argument the authorities use is that some children have a genetic weakness that presupposes them to autism and the vaccine just exposes this weakness. (A totally ridiculous argument. That's like saying the kids who fall off a bike and break an arm had a genetically weak bone.) But if so many millions of children have this kind of weakness, wouldn't it make sense to stop using these vaccines all together? They're supposedly saving us from epidemics of "communicable" diseases, but instead, we're getting an epidemic of neurologically damaged kids. Which is worse, the disease or the cure?

Besides not getting autism, I have to wonder why Amish children aren't dying from the diseases the authorities tell us we need vaccines to prevent. Has there been a whopping cough epidemic amongst the Amish? Are they dying from measles, smallpox, or being paralyzed by polio? Are they keeling over in droves due to influenza? No, they aren't. I live in an area with a lot of Amish, and I know several families (two of them have ten children, one has seven – they are typically large families and don't seem to have the fertility problems regular Americans do). I'll tell you, these kids are the healthiest, happiest children I've ever seen, and it's a joy to be around them. They're always smiling, helpful, and well behaved. They're not dying from these dreaded diseases we're told will kill us be it not for vaccines. Although the Amish generally stay to themselves and are somewhat secretive, they do have contact with the "English" (regular white people like yours truly), and this sometimes everyday contact is surely enough to spread any disease they might have to outside people, or vise versa. How come there are no disease outbreaks because of that?

Another point about the Amish: They grow, raise, slaughter, and produce most of what they eat. They don't pasteurize their milk, butter, or eggs. They don't sterilize the equipment they use to make cream, bologna, bacon, or ribs. They don't have refrigerators. Why aren't they getting sick or dying from food-borne diseases?

Furthermore, consider why, if germs are so powerful and disease causing, we don't see outbreaks of communicable diseases in animals in the wild. When have you ever heard of mass numbers of deer, elk, wild boar, coyotes, or vultures dying from influenza or measles? Some of these animals are scavengers and eat anything they can find – like days-old road kill loaded with bacteria. Domesticated animals – which often eat processed grain products (which contain a lot of soy, antibiotics, and hormones) don't count, since they're eating less than their natural diets and may consequently become ill. Some animals like birds probably eat grain or vegetation that's been treated with pesticides, so they don't count either.

Many will blame domesticated animals' illnesses on germs, but I bet if you let these animals eat what is natural for them, they wouldn't get sick – just like the animals in the wild do not get sick. Mankind is the only living thing on the face of the earth that eats foods that have been cooked, processed, and poisoned, and we suffer immensely because of it. More on germs and "communicable" diseases by the end of this chapter, so hold on.

Back to autism. The genetics argument is no good to explain autism. For one thing, as I mentioned before, it takes many thousands if not millions of years to change a genetic component, if at all. (Some scientists question Darwinian Evolution all together. But that's another story!) It is simply impossible for our gene pool to have changed since the 1940s in any way at all, no less one that would cause a 500 percent increase in just a generation and 1,700 percent in two generations (About 60 years since autism was first diagnosed. By the way, is it a coincidence that the first cases of autism were diagnosed in the early 1940s, not long after Eli Lilly started using thimerosal in vaccines?)

Second, if a chromosome (where genetic material is) is altered, the most likely way it would be damaged would be due to some environmental pressure. Yes, there may be a weakness on the n-allel of the x-chromosome for example, but that is probably caused by a toxin (mercury, formaldehyde, aluminum – all found in vaccines), or deficiency in nutrition.

Some studies have said that autism runs in families – that a family with one autistic child is more likely to have another than a family without any autistic children and point to genetics again to explain this. I have a simpler reason: Members of the same family will tend to get the same shots. Mom, thinking she's doing her level best to keep her kids healthy, will take all her children to get the vaccines, and so more than one of her kids may get autism.

Why hasn't a study been done on comparing the number of vaccines a child receives with the incidence of autism? Actually, there was a study done in Denmark in 2002 along these lines, and the journal article proclaimed that "...neither autistic disorder nor other autistic-spectrum disorders were associated with MMR vaccination."(74) The FDA and CDC point to this study as evidence that thimerosal does NOT cause autism.

However, if the raw data of this study is reexamined, as some other researchers have done, without the statistical hocus-pocus used in the published study, the exact opposite conclusion is reached – that vaccines and the number of vaccines are directly correlated with increased number of autistic children. One non-profit anti-vaccine organization who examined the research doesn't sugar-coat it: They said, "Clearly, government and industry agreed to lie to both the medical profession and parents about the harm being done by the MMR vaccine. And of course, the other vaccines as well."(75)

So what does the AAP say now? I checked out their website again on November 10, 2008, and found "Facts for Parents about Vaccine Safety" page which says, "Valid scientific studies have shown there is no link between autism and thimerosal, a mercury-based preservative once used in several vaccines and still used in some flu vaccines." By that they mean that just because a lot of kids who were vaccinated are getting autism (anecdotal evidence) it is not scientific and does not prove there's a link. The webpage goes on to say that ". . .since thimerosal was removed from childhood vaccines in 2001, autism rates have actually increased, supplying further evidence that thimerosal does not cause autism."

Are they kidding? They say that the evidence that supports the idea that autism is caused by thimerosal is invalid because it's anecdotal (this is implied in the "valid scientific studies" comment), but in the very same paragraph, they use anecdotal evidence ("autism rates have actually increased") to try and prove thimerosal is safe! There's that double standard again. The AAP must think we're pretty stupid.

Besides, thimerosal wasn't removed from vaccines in 2001. The *LA Times* reported that Merck continued to supply infant vaccines containing a mercury-based preservative for two years after declaring it had eliminated it.(76)

Other reports are that rather than issue a recall, existing stocks that still contained high amounts of thimerosal were used as late as 2007.(77) Other vaccines, particularly the flu and tetanus vaccines, still contain it as a preservative, and still others still have it in trace amounts (which can be significant, as we'll see), and as I said, new vaccines have been introduced that have it. *That's* why autism rates have continued to climb since 2001 – *not* because "thimerosal does not cause autism."

Go to www.909shot.com find out which vaccines have thimerosal. This website also has a *Mercury Calculator* where you plug in what vaccine you're interested in and the weight of your child and it tells you how much mercury your child is receiving with each shot. It's a chilling eye-opener. This website advices parents to ask for thimerosal-free vaccines, and to demand to see not just the package insert, but the vial that's used that contains the vaccine to be sure it's in fact thimerosal-free.

Reading this "Facts for Parents about Vaccine Safety" statement on the AAP webpage makes my head spin. I know I'm going off on tangents, so please forgive me, but I think it's important you see the lies these people sink to try and cover their sins. The statement says, "At a very young age, children's immune systems are equipped to respond to many antigens at the same time, including those in vaccines as well as the ones they encounter in their daily activities such as eating, breathing and playing."

First, that is absolutely false. As I've shown several times in this book (by research from other experts and government statements), a children's biochemical sytstems 's, including the immune system are not fully developed, making them more susceptible to harm from outside agents. In fact, since children are less able to handle these onslaughts, vaccines should be the *last* thing they need. Second, even if it were true, that "a child's system is equipped to respond to many antigens at the same time," then what do they need vaccines for? They should be able to handle the germs they may be exposed to.

The webpage goes on to say, "Before a vaccine is licensed, it is studied in thousands of children and in combination with other vaccines." Who do you think those children are? Do you think they get them from some third world country or use volunteers? No – they are OUR children they are testing the vaccines on. If enough of OUR children die, they might recall the vaccine (while kicking and screaming and trying to cover it up).

A recent study showed that autism rates are higher in areas with higher rainfall. On one hand, I'd say they are really reaching on that one. On the other hand, it makes sense in some ways, since areas with higher rainfall have more pollution fall-out. It stands to reason that people in those areas would be exposed to higher levels of pollutants. (Mercury being one of them, since incinerators and coal-fired power plants emit a lot of mercury.[78] Remember the study by Roger Masters that showed that areas of higher pollution have higher crime rates.)

But if we can absorb enough pollutants from rain with microscopic amounts of pollutants to cause autism, imagine what injecting them directly into us would do! The researchers don't bring up the vaccine issue, though.

But someone is trying real hard to deflect the cause of autism away from vaccines.

I have a challenge to any adult convinced the vaccines are safe: Go and get all the vaccines on the schedule recommended by the CDC for children up to the age of 6 years with the quantity proportioned for your weight. So where a 40 pound child might get X amount of vaccine injected into them, you must have 4 times X if you weight 160 pounds. Then tell us how you feel. I suggest taking an IQ test before and afterwards so we can see if and how much the mercury and preservatives affects your brain. Since you believe these vaccines are so safe, you should have no problem taking them. In fact, if what you say is true about vaccines, germs and communicable diseases, you would be even better off afterwards.

I'll take this idea a step further: I think everyone working for the drug companies who manufacture the vaccines and the government who advocate vaccines for children (that especially includes you, Dr. Gerberding,) should do this to allay any fears parents have concerning vaccines. You could take out an ad in the *New York Times* proclaiming, "See! I just got vaccinated 48 times, and I'm doin' just fine!" That could be your slogan. . ."Forty-eight times, and I'm doin' just fine!"

But they won't do this. Just like there'd be no more wars if the politicians had to go into battle, there'd be no more vaccine carnage if the vaccinators had to be vaccinated to the same degree our kids are. Am I being unreasonable? Consider that in 1980 Russia banned thimerosal from children's vaccines and since then Denmark, Austria, Japan, Great Britain, and all the Scandinavian countries have done the same.[79] Just like banning lead-based paint way after other countries, the good old U.S. of A. is way behind the times.

Is it any wonder the U.S. is losing its place in the world as a super-power? Is it any wonder we are 49th in the world in literacy? Is it any wonder many of the decisions our leaders make sometimes appear to be totally insane?

Maybe we've all been poisoned with mercury thanks to the greedy drug companies. Remember my comment about lead poisoning and Nero fiddling away while Rome burned? Could the same kind of thing be happening in Washington D.C. due to mercury (and other neurological poisons) in vaccines, our food supply, and environment?

Boyd Haley Ph.D. echoes my feeling: "Mercury toxicity is not rocket science. Our medical establishment simply does not want to admit that a major mistake has been made. . .I know that they know, and that is what bothers me more than anything else."[80]

Dr. Mark A. Sircus said,

"It is astounding that even if a normal and healthy child goes home and dies within 24 hours after receiving multiple vaccine shots, medical authorities scratch their heads and write on the death certificate, 'This child died of unknown causes.'"(81)

Congressmen Dan Burton (R-Ind.) said,

"Despite a growing body of science linking autism to mercury and thimerosal, the protests of hundreds of thousands of concerned parents across the country, the pharmaceutical industry continues to put mercury into vaccines for both children and adults even though they know mercury is toxic to the human brain. Our Food and Drug Administration and our health agencies are asleep at the switch, and they're letting children and adults be damaged day after day by allowing mercury to continue to be put into vaccines for adults and children." (82)

Dr. Peter Mansfield comments,

"Modern medicine has backed itself into a corner, a place of refutation and rejection of basic sciences like chemistry and neuroscience, which cry out against the dangers of using mercury at any concentration in vaccines and dental fillings. The liability of the medical community for this will eventually cripple the medical establishment and investigations of the order of Watergate and the Kennedy assassination are called for. Instead of a robbery or the killing of one famous man, we have thousands of children dead and more than 20,000 new children are diagnosed with autism in the U.S. each year. . .If we are talking about mercury induced learning disabilities of a less severe nature, we get into many millions."(83)

If you don't think the government is working for the drug companies who make the vaccines, consider that over 4,200 families have filed lawsuits claiming thimerosal caused harm to their children; and besides all the legal requirements the National Childhood Vaccine act of 1986 forces these families to go through that make it virtually impossible to win their case, the CDC (a government agency) actually sold its data-base containing information (probably much of it damning) on thimerosal, mercury, and autism to a private company to make sure the family's lawyers cannot access it under the Freedom of Information Act.(84)

Stephen A Sheller, an attorney who has sued vaccine manufacturers said, "The CDC is a disgrace. It is a corrupt organization. The drug companies have them on their payroll."(85)

For the best book on autism, check out *Evidence of Harm: Mercury in Vaccines and the Autism Epidemic: A Medical Controversy* by David Kirby. It details not just the evidence that mercury is causing autism, but also the cover-ups and government's role in all this madness – including the rider on the 2002 Homeland Security Bill that would bar thimerosal litigation – making sure the vaccine-manufacturers don't lose any more or get put out of business due to all the lawsuits against them. Outrageous, a shame, a sham, a pity, and as criminal as it gets.

When thimerosal is used as a vaccine preservative, a vaccine contains 50 micrograms of thimerosal per 0.5 ml dose or approximately 25 micrograms of mercury per 0.5 mL dose. (86)

Thimerosal is not only used as a preservative in vaccines, but also during their production. Therefore, even if the vaccine does not contain thimerosal as a preservative, it may contain trace amounts ("trace" is considered 1 micrograms or less of mercury per dose by the FDA, but 0.5 micrograms per dose by the CDC. Nice, consistent government guidelines!) because not all of it is removed during manufacturing.(87) The following is straight from the CDC website:

> However, some contain only trace amounts of thimerosal and are considered by the Food and Drug Administration (FDA) to be preservative-free. Manufacturers of preservative-free flu vaccine use thimerosal early in the manufacturing process. The thimerosal gets diluted as the vaccine goes through the steps in processing. By the end of the manufacturing process there is not enough thimerosal left in the vaccine to act as a preservative and the vaccine is labeled "preservative-free."(88)

Although thimerosal is still in the product, the FDA considers it "preservative-free", even though the typical preservative in vaccines is thimerosal. This is a clever way to make the vaccine appear to have no thimerosal in it when it does. But consider that the FDA, CDC or any other agency has no substantive proof that thimerosal is safe at any dosage or concentration. The manufacturer's *Material Safety Data Sheet* for thimerosal even states that it can cause kidney and brain damage based on the fact that it contains mercury.

Food for Thought

It's shocking that one of the most toxic things on the planet is allowed, and even mandated, to be injected into harmless, defenseless, under-developed babies – while there's no proof of safety.

But I should be used to this by now.

Fluoride is put into water supplies, used as a fumigant, and put into toothpaste – with no proof of safety.

Mercury fillings are put into people's teeth – with no proof of safety.

Soft drinks are sold by the tank-full – with no proof of safety.

MSG, aspartame, and other food additives are added to countless foods – with no proof of safety.

Antidepressants are newly prescribed to 3,000 Americans a day – with no proof of safety.

Soy is added to baby formulas – with no proof of safety.

Pesticides are used on crops – with no proof of safety.

Ritalin is pumped into kids to the tune of 10 tons a year – with no proof of safety.

　If you want to stay healthy, you need to realize that the best way to decide if something is safe, is to judge for yourself.

　Jane Orient, M.D., said,

　"Educated and enlightened parents are not deceived and are quickly losing confidence in medical authority. Unfortunately, only relatively few parents are lucky enough to have access to such information and insight. Most parents around the world comply with vaccination programs unquestioningly, trusting the men of science, and having no idea that their babies are being injected with the powerful poison mercury."[89]

In 1994, the EPA revised its Reference Dose (RfD) for methyl mercury exposure, lowering its guideline for safe exposure from 0.3 to 0.1 microgram per kilogram body weight per day.[90] But even so, children and especially small children, can be inoculated with mercury levels over the recommended amounts due to trace amounts of mercury alone. But are "trace" amounts really all that's in the vaccines? Dr. Neal Halsey, who heads the Hopkins Institute for Vaccine Safety said, concerning trace amounts, "In most vaccine containers, thimerosal is listed as a mercury derivative, a hundredth of a percent. And what I believed, and what everybody else believed, was that it was truly a trace, a biologically insignificant amount. My honest belief is that if the labels had had the mercury content in micrograms, this would have been uncovered years ago. But the fact is, no one did the calculation."[91]

A vaccine with trace amounts of mercury, which the manufacturers and government consider "insignificant," can still contain 600 to 2,000 parts per billion (ppb) of mercury. Liquids with 200 ppb of mercury or more are considered hazardous waste by EPA standards. Mercury concentrations as low as 0.2 ppb have been shown to cause harm. But with just "trace amounts," the vaccine can be labeled "preservative-free," even though by definition, it's a hazardous waste.[92]

The smallest children receive approximately eight months of daily exposures of mercury in a single day if they receive all thimerosal-containing vaccines. At two months of age, children of all weight categories receive more than 30 times the recommended daily maximum exposure of mercury according to the Agency for Toxic Substances and Disease Registry guidelines.[93] The EPA guideline is 0.1 micrograms per kilogram of child per day, the Public Health Service guideline is 0.3 micrograms per kilogram of child per day and the FDA guideline is 0.4 micrograms per kilogram of child per day.[94]

Food for Thought

　Even many over-the-counter drugs recommend different dosages for different sizes and ages. Though there are guidelines for the amount of mercury a child can be exposed to, are they ever followed or even considered? Dosages are not adjusted for the size of the child – an eight-pound infant receives the same amount of vaccine that a 40-pound five-year-old receives. Did your pediatrician weigh your child last time he/she got a shot?

Boyd Haley, Ph.D., confirms this oversight along with other things I've been saying: "A single vaccine given to a six-pound newborn is the equivalent of giving a 180-pound adult 30 vaccinations on the same day. Include in this the toxic effects of high levels of aluminum and formaldehyde contained in some vaccines, and the synergist toxicity could be increased to unknown levels."(95)

Is there even one pediatrician in the country who would tell a parent: "We can't give little Johnny any more shots today because we've already injected him with the EPA recommended safety limit guideline of 0.1 micro-grams per kilogram body weight of mercury. Come back tomorrow."

Further, it is very well known that infants do not produce significant levels of bile or have adult renal [kidney] capacity for several months after birth. Bilary transport is the major biochemical route by which mercury is removed from the body (very slowly), and infants cannot do this very well. They also do not possess the renal capacity to remove aluminum, and mercury is a well-known inhibitor of kidney function.(96)

I repeat: There is NO SAFE AMOUNT of mercury (or formaldehyde or aluminum), period. Mercury accumulates in tissue every time someone is exposed. There should be NO – *absolutely zero* – amount of mercury (or other poisons) allowed to be injected into our children or anyone else. Scientists know this, the doctors who read the research like I have presented here, know this, and the law makers and vaccine manufacturers know this. For them to deny it is fraud. For them to continue administering the shots is child abuse, endangerment, and homicide.

Lifestyle can come into play as far as increased risk to thimerosal-containing vaccines. Mothers who eat more fish can have babies who are more affected since mercury is transferred to their children both prenatally and in breast milk.(97)

The EPA estimates that 7 percent of women of childbearing age in the U.S. consume at least 0.1 micrograms/kg/day of mercury from fish (above the recommended safe limit). Still, a recent study suggests that intermittent large exposures to methyl mercury pose more risk than small daily doses. Multiple vaccines on a single day can be considered an intermittent large exposure if all the vaccines contain thimerosal.

Food for Thought

It's not like everyone in our government is unaware of the problems associated with vaccines and denies the connection. We just don't hear about it in the media. The U.S. House of Representatives held a Government Reform Committee meeting on April 6, 2000, in Washington D.C. titled "Autism: Present Challenges, Future Needs – Why the Increased Rates?" The committee chairman was Representative Dan Burton, and portions of his opening statement are as follows:

"This morning we're here to talk about autism. As we learned in our August hearing, the rates of autism have escalated dramatically. What used to be considered a rare disorder has become a near epidemic. We've received hundreds of letters from parents across the country. They've shared with us their pain and their challenges. My staff tells me they cried from the heartbreak of many of these letters.

"I don't have to read a letter to experience the heartbreak. I see it in my own family. My grandson, Christian, was born healthy. He was beautiful and tall. We were already planning his NBA career. He was outgoing and talkative. He enjoyed company and going places. Then his mother took him for his routine immunizations and all of that changed. He was given what so many children were given – DTaP, OPV, Haemophilus, Hepatitis B and MMR – all at one office visit. That night Christian had a slight fever and he slept for long periods of time. When he was awake he would scream a horrible high-pitched scream. He would scream for hours. He began dragging his head on the furniture and banging it repeatedly. Over the week and a half after the vaccinations, Christian would stare into space and act like he was deaf. He would hit himself and others, which was something he had never done. He would shake his head from side to side as fast as he could. He lost all language.

"Unfortunately, what happened to Christian is not a rare isolated event. Shelly Reynolds will testify today. Her organization, Unlocking Autism, will be displaying thousands of pictures of autistic children. . .Forty-7 percent of the parents, who provided these pictures, felt that their child's autism was linked to immunizations.

"We frequently hear about children with chronic ear infections and children who became autistic after spiking a fever with their vaccinations. Liz Burt was one of the hundreds of parents who contacted us. Her five-year-old son, Matthew, has been classified autistic. He was developing normally. At age 15 months, following his MMR vaccine, he began to regress. Since the time of his vaccination, he's had chronic diarrhea. This is very prevalent in autistic children. He also didn't sleep on a regular basis for over three years. Liz took her son to numerous gastroenterologists in prominent medical facilities in the United States with no resolution. Finally, this past November, Liz took her son to London, to the Royal Free Hospital. A team of medical experts there examined Matthew. They felt that he was severely constipated. To the family, this seemed impossible since he had constant diarrhea. An X-ray indicated that Matthew had a fecal mass in his colon the size of a small cantaloupe. After the obstruction was cleared with laxatives, Matthew underwent an endoscopy and colonoscopy. The lesions in Matthew's bowel tested positive for the measles virus.

"Dr. Andrew Wakefield and Professor John O'Leary will be testifying today. Their research has uncovered a possible connection between inflammatory bowel disorder in children with autism who received the MMR vaccine and have measles virus in their small intestines. Since coming home from England and being treated for chronic Inflammatory Bowel Disorder, Matthew has finally begun to sleep through the night. I know it's a welcome relief for his family.

"Unfortunately Matthew's story is not that unusual in children with autism. . .Dr. Mary Megson of Richmond, Virginia, will testify about the correlation she has seen in children with autism and attention deficit disorder. She's seen a correlation between Vitamin A depletion and immune-suppression after receiving the MMR vaccine. . .

"There is probably a genetic component to autism. But genetics is not the only issue. Many children seem to have severe food sensitivities – particularly to gluten and casein – ingredients in the most common foods – dairy and wheat. Many of these children show signs of autism shortly after receiving their immunizations. Some of these children, as we will hear from Jeana Smith, have metal toxicities – aluminum and mercury. What is the source of these toxic substances?

"I'm very concerned about the increased number of childhood vaccines. I'm concerned about the ingredients that are put in these vaccines. I'm concerned about the way they're given. We've learned that most of the vaccines our children are given contain mercury, aluminum, and formaldehyde. Last year the Food and Drug Administration added up the amount of mercury our babies were being given to learn that in the first six months of life they received more mercury than is considered safe. Why is it that the FDA licenses vaccines that contain neurotoxins like mercury and aluminum?

"When asked about the increased rate in autism, many will immediately discount that there even is an increase. Even though the latest statistics from the Department of Education show increased rates in every state. Others will say the increase is due to better diagnostic skills. Others will say it is because the diagnostic category was expanded. California has reported a 273 percent increase in children with autism since 1988. . .

"Florida has reported a 571 percent increase in autism. Maryland has reported a 513 percent increase between 1993 and 1998. You can't attribute all of that to better diagnostic skills. . .If we want to find a cure, we must first look to the cause. We must do this now before our health and education systems are bankrupted, and before more of our nation's children are locked inside themselves with this disease. Families are forced to spend huge sums of money out-of-pocket, even when they have good insurance, because autism is often specifically excluded. California passed legislation recently to require insurance companies to cover autism. Parents spend $20,000 and $30,000 a year. What medical care is covered is often done so after extensive struggles with insurance providers. . .

"I think that as a top priority, we have to do much more research on the potential connections between vaccines and autism. We can't stick our heads in the sand and ignore this possibility. If we don't take action now, 10 years from now may be too late, not only for this generation of children, but for our taxpayer-funded health and education systems that will collapse from trying to care for these children."(98)

Another toxin that is in vaccines is aluminum, another known neurotoxin (linked to Alzheimer's disease, memory problems, liver and kidney problems, osteoporosis, seizures, coma). Although it doesn't get the attention thimerosal and mercury get, it's still bad news. Dr. Russell Blaylock said,

> Removal of thimerosal, even if complete, will not solve the problem of autism. It will help tremendously, but will not stop the epidemic of autism. . . Aluminum has a similar mode of action, though less potent. When combined with mercury, there is at least additive toxicity if not synergistic toxicity.(99)

Dr. Boyd Haley reported, "The results were unequivocal: The presence of aluminum dramatically increased the rate of neuronal death caused by thimerosal."

Dr. Gregory Ellis agrees, "I think in later years we are going to look back at aluminum the way we are looking at mercury now."(100)

So just because a vaccine may not contain thimerosal, it still can have deadly or debilitating consequences.

As we've seen, a link between hyperactivity and learning disabilities in children can be made to vaccines as well. The incidences of ADHD were already discussed in a previous chapter, but just to remind you: It became prevalent in the 1950s and by 1963 was being called minimal brain dysfunction; and the symptoms called by various names have been on the rise ever since. Nationwide, the number of children classified with learning disabilities and placed in special education programs increased 191 percent between 1977 and 1994.(101) Even with an increase in detection and reporting, that number is very high.

In her book *Endangered Minds*, Jane M. Healy, Ph.D., notes that teachers have observed that many of their students are not as bright with shorter attention spans compared with the students they had in the 1960s. Beginning in 1964 until the early 1980s, the average SAT scores (tests given to high-school students prior to graduation) in both English and math steadily declined. If that's not bad enough, Healy also shows that since the early 1960s, the tests themselves have actually been made easier. Publishers of the tests, school administrators, and teachers are all under pressure to have students look good and to show that the education system is working, when in fact, children are becoming dumber and learning impaired.(102)

The pertussis vaccine is not the only one implicated in the startling rise in autism. R. Edward Yazbak, M.D., says that the MMR (measles, mumps, rubella) vaccine, when given to women before and after conception presupposes them to having children with autism.(103) The CDC and vaccine manufacturers caution that the MMR vaccine should not be given to pregnant women. In one study by Yazbak, 18 mothers had received a live virus vaccine just before or after conception. Seventeen of the 18 women had children with early onset autism. The report goes on to say, "Several mothers who were in good health and had normal children report that after they were revaccinated with MMR or rubella vaccines they experienced health problems; they had miscarriages or delivered prematurely; they still remained rubella-susceptible; their children developed autism and other disabilities."(104)

In another study by Dr. Yazbak, 60 mothers had been revaccinated with the MMR vaccine after childbirth. Forty-five of these women now have children diagnosed with autism; another 10 have children with ADHD and four women have children with other serious health problems.(105) Yazbak, a well recognized expert in immunology, began his research when one of his grandsons, who was perfectly normal, became autistic at 15 months immediately after he received his first MMR shot. His autism worsened drastically after his second MMR shot. This boy's mother had received four MMR shots before conception, and Dr. Yazbak believes by her receiving these shots, her son became more susceptible to autism. Yazbak believes it's imperative to scientifically explore the relationship between vaccines and autism. "It is now up to them to prove that vaccines do not predispose to autism. Independent, large-scale studies should be promptly initiated," he said.(106)

The American Medical Association, The American Academy of Pediatrics, the CDC, the FDA, the U.S. Department of Health and Human Services, pharmaceutical companies and the U.S. Congress all maintain the position that there is absolutely no autism-vaccination connection and that the onset of autism around the time of an MMR or pertussis (DPT) vaccine is purely coincidence.(107)

Food for Thought

Imagine what would happen if some people or children became hopelessly deranged after taking a herb or vitamin – even if the connection of the product to the person's derangement was not scientifically established. The FDA would be on them so fast it would make your head spin. Heck, I know of one company who sold ear candles (Ear candles are long, hollow cones made of wax you stick in your ear and light on fire – the suction from the flame supposedly pulls ear wax out from deep in your ear, which supposedly helps sinuses, ear aches, headaches etc. Although I can't say how effective these candles are, I can assure you they do you no harm – as long as you don't catch your hair on fire!) who was fined and put out of business even without any complaints against them.

In spite of the large body of evidence suggesting vaccines are a causative factor in the development of autism, the government and vaccine manufacturers insist there is no correlation. It sounds very similar to the tobacco industry denying that smoking caused cancer and cardiovascular problems. There was no hard, scientific evidence to support this connection (and there still isn't!). That is, there were no scientific double-blind studies conducted under strict scientific protocols showing that this was, in fact the case. All the evidence is merely anecdotal, meaning it is hearsay and not statistically proven. But just as with the connection of the cigarettes and heart disease or alcoholism and birth defects, there is a growing number of people making the connection between their children's illnesses, injuries, and deaths to the vaccines their children were subjected to.

I predict that within the next 10 years you'll see class-action lawsuits filed against the pharmaceutical companies who make these vaccines. There have already been many lawsuits filed (and won) by individual parents claiming vaccines caused harm to their child. You just haven't heard about them because the mass media doesn't report them and the parents must file the suit in accordance with the National Childhood Vaccine Injury Act, which buffers the pharmaceutical industry from exposure. We taxpayers pay the settlements.

Are vaccines effective in preventing the disease they are designed to prevent? The first measles vaccine was given in the U.S. in 1963. But the death rate (reflective of the number of measles cases overall) had already declined almost 98 percent from its recorded high in 1900. A survey of 30 states in 1978 showed that of all the children who got measles, half of them had received the measles vaccine. Other research documents the amazing fact that someone who receives the measles vaccine is actually 15 times more likely to get the disease than someone who is not vaccinated for it.(108) There are similar statistics for other diseases that show that they too were on the decline before a vaccine was developed for them, and that the vaccine actually does little, nothing, or actually contributes to the incidences of the disease it is meant to prevent.

The pertussis vaccine is implicated in diabetes. Since the 1970s the vaccine has been known to cause over-production of insulin by the pancreas in test animals leading to exhaustion and destruction of the Islets of Langerhans cells. This prevents the cells from producing enough insulin, thus causing hypoglycemia and latter diabetes.(109) As early as 1949 it was noted that the vaccine could cause low blood sugar in children. In 1977, Gordon Stewart wrote, "More than any other vaccine in common use, pertussis vaccine is known pharmacologically to provoke. . . hypoglycemia due to increased production of insulin."(110)

J. Barthelow Classen, M.D., a former researcher at the National Institutes of Health, has done extensive studies, which support the vaccine-diabetes connection. He showed that DPT injections in lab rats caused them to have a significantly higher rate of diabetes than those not injected.(111) He also reported that in Finland there was a marked increase in the incidence of Type I diabetes following changes and increases in the childhood vaccination schedule. Dr. Classen concluded: "The net effect was the addition of three new vaccines to the 0 to four-year-old age group and a 147 percent increase in the incidence of IDDM [insulin dependent diabetes mellitus], the addition of one new vaccine to the five- to nine-year-olds and a rise in the incidence of diabetes of 40 percent, and no new vaccines added to the 10 to 14-year-olds and a rise in the incidence of IDDM by only 8 percent between the intervals 1970 – 1976 and 1990 – 1992. The rise in IDDM in the different age groups correlated with the number of vaccines given." Also, in New Zealand, the incidences of diabetes went up from 11.2 cases per 100,000 children per year to 18.2 per 100,000 children per year following a massive campaign from 1988 to 1991 to vaccinate babies six weeks of age or older with hepatitis B vaccine. That's a 60 percent increase.(112)

Children born since 1990 are the most vaccinated generation in American history and probably the world. The nation's public health "experts" currently recommend 48 vaccinations by the age of six and many people have been vaccinated their entire lives with the recommended regimen plus tetanus boosters and periodic hepatitis A and B inoculations. Never before has children's health been so in question, with numerous maladies now at epidemic proportions.

Food for Thought

Statistical analysis holds that if something changes by more than 5 percent, it's seen to be a *significant* change. If there's a change of less than 5 percent, it's seen to be *insignificant*. Many of the surveys concerning vaccines and diseases that manifest after inoculations show changes well above this 5 percent mark. This indicates a possible *causational relationship* worthy of further investigation using accepted scientifically sound protocols. But testing costs money.

More than $1 billion is appropriated by Congress to federal health agencies every year to develop, purchase, and promote mass vaccinations of American children. However, none of that money, not one penny, is used to fund independent vaccine researchers to investigate vaccine-related health problems such as diabetes and autism. The government relies solely on scientific data supplied by drug companies (who make and sell the vaccines) to approve and license the vaccines for mandated mass-vaccination programs. There is no corroboration of data with independent research. It's the fox guarding the chicken coop. The National Vaccine Information Center (NVIC) says there is a serious conflict of interest in allowing the same health officials who are responsible for researching, developing, regulating, making national policies, and promoting vaccines to also be in control of monitoring vaccine reactions and health problems associated with vaccines. We need checks and balances.

Barbara Loe Fisher, president of NVIC says,

"Health officials in federal agencies have no accountability to anyone when it comes to setting priorities for how our tax dollars are used when it comes to vaccine research. They can choose to do whatever they want to do with the money they get from Congress. And they choose to ignore the mounting evidence that vaccines are playing a role in the current epidemic of chronic disease, such as diabetes, in our society. Instead, our tax money is used to create more vaccines to add to the mandatory vaccination schedule for our children. There have never been and there are no plans to fund large independent studies to back-up the scientific validity of the government's current vaccine policies and independently confirm they are safe."(113)

Pertussis, also called whooping cough, was first described by French physician Guillaune Baillou in 1578 during an epidemic in Paris, France. There have been many other pertussis epidemics since, and most of the victims were children. Symptoms include a severe, short, dry cough, vomiting, runny nose, and later a high fever and possibly convulsions. It usually affects children between the ages of two and six years, but infants and older children are also vulnerable.(114)

Many people believe that the incidences of pertussis declined because of vaccinations. However, in America, England, and Sweden, the death rate from the disease declined by 90 percent in the 1940s before mass vaccinations.(115) Further, a study published in 1994 showed that at least 80 percent of children under the age of five-years-old who got pertussis had been vaccinated for that disease.(116)

Some reactions to the pertussis vaccine include vomiting, diarrhea, a hard swelling at the site of the injection, fever, runny nose, bronchial congestion, ear infections and possibly SIDS. However, the most distinctive symptom to the pertussis vaccine (which is part of the DPT shot) is a loud, high pitched screaming. One mother described her child's screaming after a DPT shot: "It was a blood-curdling scream like someone was stabbing him, and he never, ever cried like that. Then he became unresponsive. His arms dropped to his side, and he became flaccid. About an hour later, the same thing happened again. His arms dropped to his side, he let out this terrible scream and became flaccid."(117)

Robert Mendelsohn, M.D., the pioneer in the fight against vaccinations, has this to say about the whooping cough vaccine:

Whooping cough (pertussis) vaccine is one of the most controversial immunizations, even after all these decades of use. It is included automatically in the "triple shot" given almost all babies, the other two being diphtheria and tetanus. Yet it is the least effective of the three and the most dangerous. Most of the bad reactions, including high fever and convulsions, come from the whooping cough element, and the official recommendation is that the shot usually not be given to anyone older than six. The incidence of whooping cough in this country has certainly declined, but the disease is not that rare. Doubts persist as to whether the pertussis vaccine itself has had very much to do with the decline in the disease and whether the vaccine, if introduced today, would pass FDA standards. If you're concerned about giving the whooping cough vaccine to your child, ask your doctor if he really feels that your child should be immunized with the triple shot, or whether he believes that the duo of diphtheria and tetanus immunization is enough.(118)

Sudden Infant Death Syndrome usually happens when the infant stops breathing, most often during sleep. The medical community does not know exactly why it occurs, but the popular explanation is that the central nervous system is somehow affected so that the involuntary act of breathing is suppressed. (See Sleep Disorders chapter for more on SIDS.) Mendelsohn has his own opinion. He says,

What caused the malfunction in the central nervous system? My suspicion, which is shared by others in my profession, is that the nearly 10,000 SIDS deaths that occur in the United States each year are related to one or more of the vaccines that are routinely given children. The pertussis vaccine is the most likely villain, but it could also be one or more of the others.(119)

Mendelsohn says that breast feeding can help children avoid SIDS (along with other ailments such as allergies, respiratory disease, gastroenteritis, hypocalcaemia, obesity, and multiple sclerosis).

Food for Thought

All this bad news about the pertussis vaccine may be new to you, but it isn't to the medical community. As early as 1948 researchers from Harvard Medical School reported about children who had suffered brain damage after getting a pertussis shot. Product insert sheets from a vaccine manufacturer, the Public Health Services Immunization Practices Advisory Committee (ACIP), and the American Academy of Pediatrics all advise against further pertussis shots if a child exhibits high pitched screams or abnormal crying.(120) Isn't it comforting to know that all those experts know there are hazards with the vaccine, but the general public doesn't?

DPT shots (which include diphtheria, pertussis, and tetanus), are typically administered at two months, four months, and six months. (There is a newer version of this vaccine is called DTaP, but we will call it the DPT in this discussion). A study at the UCLA School of Medicine examined 145 SIDS victims and found a high percentage of them died soon after receiving their DPT shots: six died within 24 hours; 17 within one week; and, 27 within 28 days.(121) Another study reported in *Neurology*, the author reported that close to 70 percent of children who reportedly died of SIDS had received the DPT vaccine. The deaths were clustered around the time when the shots were given (two and four months).(122)

There have been 579 deaths adjudicated through the Federal Count of claims against vaccines since the National Vaccine Injury Compensation Program began in 1986. Two hundred twenty-seven of these were misdiagnosed as SIDS.(123) The DPT vaccine is one of the worst for causing problems. Barbara Loe Fisher of the NVIC says,

> We have been most involved in trying to inform the public about the hospitalizations, injuries, and deaths that have been associated with vaccines, particularly the DPT and DPTH vaccines. The DPT vaccine – the whole cell pertussis, or whooping cough, vaccine – is the most reactive vaccine used in the U.S. It's still on the market, even though the FDA finally licensed a less toxic, a cellular pertussis vaccine, after 15 years of pressure from NVIC and parents. Although the DTaP vaccine causes fewer reactions, it still contains pertussis toxin that is somewhat bioactive, and so has the potential of causing injury. Even though studies have shown that the DTaP vaccine is associated with far fewer severe reactions than the whole cell pertussis, or DPT, vaccine, the FDA won't take the whole cell vaccine off the market. In the compensation program that was set up under the National Childhood Vaccine Injury Act of 1986, most of the nearly 1,000 awards that have been made are for DPT vaccine injuries. There's no question that it is the most reactive vaccine that we use.(124)

So far we've addressed the problems that result from properly made vaccines. But just like in preparing anything, mistakes can be made and problems can arise in the manufacture of vaccines. Not every batch of each vaccine is as safe as the next one and some batches are more potent than others. An improperly prepared vaccine that gets past safety testing is called a *hot lot*.

Food for Thought

You would think that upon discovering a hot lot, public health officials would recall that batch of vaccines. After all, they recall peanuts, tomatoes, spinach, and such, when they are contaminated. (But those aren't made by the drug companies, just grown by poor farmers.) But hot lots of vaccines are typically not recalled.

The state of Michigan, in 1975, knowingly allowed a hot lot of DPT vaccine be given to several hundred children to see just how potent it actually was. The result? Several children suffered seizures, paralysis, and brain damage. When the parents tried to sue the state of Michigan for negligence, the case was dismissed because of the "doctrine of sovereign immunity," which protects the state from claims against it when damages are a result of services only the government can provide.(125) Just as tragically, in 1990 and 1991 in Los Angeles, approximately 1,500 minority infants were given an experimental measles vaccine. Parents were not told that it was experimental nor were they warned about immediate or long-term risks.(126)

Hot lot or not, children may have reactions to any vaccine. Most children show some kind of reaction, be it as minor as a red soreness around the site of the injection. Not all children are strong enough to handle a shot, and some react more violently than others. Some so severely they end up brain damaged or dead.

Diphtheria is an upper respiratory disease causing a sore throat, fever of 100° F to 104° F, swelling of the lymph nodes in the neck, possible heart muscle inflammation, and paralysis of the breathing muscles, which can be fatal. Robert Mendelsohn, M.D. gives us some interesting insight into the diphtheria vaccine:

". . .There is ample evidence that the incidence of diphtheria was already diminishing before a vaccine became available [as it is with all vaccines]. . .only 5 cases were reported in the United States in 1980. . .Today your child has about as much chance of contracting diphtheria as he does of being bitten by a cobra. Yet millions of children are immunized against it with repeated injections at 2, 4, 6 and 18 months and then given a booster shot when they enter school. This despite evidence over more than a dozen years from rare out-breaks of the disease that children who have been immunized fare no better than those who have not. . . Episodes such as these shatter the argument that immunization can be credited with eliminating diphtheria or any of the other once common childhood diseases. . .view of the rarity of the disease. . . the questionable effectiveness of the vaccine, the multimillion-dollar annual cost of administering it, and the ever-present potential for harmful, long-term effects from this or any other vaccine, I consider continued mass immunization against diphtheria indefensible.(127)

Polio, sometimes referred to as Infantile Paralysis, is a disease of the Central Nervous System (CNS) that plagued American children in the 1940s and 1950s. The greatest incidences of the disease are in children between the ages of five and 10 years. Early symptoms include fatigue, headache, fever, vomiting, constipation, stiffness of the neck, diarrhea, and pain in the extremities. The symptoms depend on the site of involvement of the disease in the CNS. Permanent paralysis, including fatal respiratory paralysis, may occur. However, only a small percentage of people who have the polio virus ever exhibit definitive symptoms of the disease at all.[128]

The American epidemiologist, Jonas Edward Salk, developed a vaccine for polio using inactivated or "killed" poliomyelitis viruses of three known types. The vaccine was first used in the U.S. 1954. Later, another "live" vaccine was developed by Albert Sabin and was first licensed for use in 1961.[129]

These vaccines are credited for halting the polio epidemic. However, Dr Mendelsohn reports that there is "...no credible scientific evidence exists that the vaccine caused polio to disappear."[130] In fact, polio epidemics ended in Europe around the same time as in the U.S., where the vaccines were not nearly as extensively used. What's worse is that the polio vaccine itself can cause the very disease it's meant to prevent. Even Jonas Salk stated that most of the polio cases in the U.S. since the 1970s were caused by the live virus vaccine.[131]

Besides the vaccine, is there anything else that could cause polio, or the symptoms associated with it? During one of the worst outbreaks of polio in 1948, Dr. Benjamin Sandler of North Carolina publicized findings from his research on polio showing that the disease actually resulted from the over-consumption of sugar and refined starches such as white flour products and corn meal. He showed that as sugar consumption in the U.S. increased over the years, so did the incidences of polio. In addition, countries with high amounts of sugar consumption also had high rates of polio; low consumption countries had few cases of polio. The *Asheville Times* newspaper published an article on August 4, 1948, that discussed Dr. Sandler's theory and his dietary recommendations to eliminate sweet and starchy foods. He said: "I am willing to state without reserve that such a diet, strictly observed, can build up in 24 hours time a resistance in the human body sufficiently strong to combat the disease successfully. The answer lies simply in maintaining a normal blood sugar."[132]

By the way, his dietary recommendations are consistent with those I make in this book: no sugary foods like soft drinks, candy, fruit juices, ice cream, cakes, pies, candies, etc; no cereals, breads, rolls, pancakes, etc; more protein from natural sources like eggs, fish, beef, chicken; raw milk; raw cheese. (This diet is not just good for preventing polio, but for avoiding all diseases.)

Dr. Sandler also showed that polio outbreaks occurred during the summer months when the consumption of sugary drinks and ice cream was the highest. In 1948, polio was at epidemic levels in North Carolina and its residents were desperate. So following the newspaper article and other newspaper and radio coverage, they started following his advice and sugar consumption decreased by

90 percent. The result? The number of polio victims also decreased a full 90 percent. This improvement didn't last long, however, because the manufacturers of soft drinks and ice cream made some announcements of their own discrediting Dr. Sandler's findings. By 1950, the sales of pop and ice cream were back to normal, and so were the high incidences of polio.(133)

Food for Thought

Here's a clever way to get the incidences of a disease down to make vaccinations look effective – change the definition of the disease! In 1962, Dr. Bernard Greenberg, head of the Department of Biostatistics at the University of North Carolina School of Public Health, testified in front of Congress that this was in fact the case concerning polio. He said that between 1957 and 1958, polio actually increased 50 percent, and from 1958 to 1959, it increased 80 percent (after the polio vaccine was administered). But the disease had been redefined in 1955 to mask this increase. The old definition said that the patient had to exhibit paralytic symptoms for 24 hours to have polio, but with the new definition the patient had to exhibit the symptoms for a full 60 days. Dr. Greenberg said, "This change in definition meant that in 1955, we started reporting a new disease..."(134)

In order for polio to be considered an epidemic, 20 people per 100,000 people per year had to exhibit the symptoms under the old definition and 35 people per 100,000 people per year under the new definition. Before the vaccine, cases of aseptic meningitis (similar to polio itself) were often reported as polio. After the vaccine, these cases were counted as a separate disease. No wonder the incidences of polio dropped after the vaccine: it was harder to get it, according to their new definitions.

After the polio vaccine was introduced in 1955, there were 273 cases of polio reported in Los Angeles County and 50 cases of aseptic meningitis. In 1961 there were 161 cases of polio and 65 cases of aseptic meningitis. By 1966, there were only 5 cases of polio but 256 cases of aseptic meningitis reported.(135) Numbers like that sure make it appear like the vaccine is working. But the government report that reported these numbers even stated, "Most cases reported prior to July 1, 1958 as non-paralytic poliomyelitis are now reported as viral or aseptic meningitis."(136) (Again, the symptoms of aseptic meningitis are virtually identical to those of the "old polio.")

Don't worry folks, the U.S. is not the only clever one. The same renaming charade happened in Great Britain. "After vaccination was introduced, cases of aseptic meningitis were more often reported as a separate disease from polio, but such cases were counted as polio before the vaccine was introduced. The Ministry of Health [the Great Britain version of the FDA] admitted that the vaccine status of the individual is a guiding factor in diagnosis. If a person who is vaccinated contracts the disease, the disease is simply recorded under a different name."(137)

Again in 1995, the federal government arbitrarily rewrote the definition of encephalophy (brain dysfunction) that had been used for decades. This was done in the Table of Compensable Events, used to determine what injuries, under the 1986 National Vaccine Injury Act, are eligible for compensation. Compensation for encephalophy from the DPT vaccine, with this new definition, has become virtually impossible to claim. In addition, they removed seizures from the table, although the fact that the pertussis vaccine causes them is uncontested. There's even a warning of seizures on the manufacturer's package insert! Barbara Loe Fisher comments on the changes: "The federal compensation system that we were told would be 'simple justice for children,' has become a cruel joke, a sad commentary on a national health policy that forces children to take the risk and then leaves many families to cope with the catastrophic consequences on their own when the risk turns out to be 100 percent."(138)

We've all heard the proclamations by the medical community and the mass media that smallpox was eradicated thanks to vaccinations. Maybe not. Daniel Marchini, M.D., comments: "Since (the advent of vaccines), entire whole populations and generations have been vaccinated against smallpox, and cases of fatal encephalitis and motor and mental handicaps have multiplied. . .Suddenly the World Health Organization announced (in 1978) that smallpox had disappeared and the edict to vaccinate against it in France was set aside (in 1979). . .In the following years cases of smallpox were officially reported. In truth, the illness had not disappeared, but the damage produced by the vaccine was of such importance and the legal reparations so costly (for law suits against the French State, since the vaccination was obligatory), that it became urgent to suppress this catastrophic vaccination and remove the State's accountability. . .Even though WHO recognized before 1978...that smallpox had not been beaten by vaccinations. . .the public and medical domains still believe that it was vaccination that beat smallpox."(139)

It appears the powers-that-be don't let the truth stand in their way of making billions from vaccines or deflecting blame for the harm they cause. Doctors and members of the traditional medical community, either knowingly or unknowingly, deny the existence of vaccine reactions. But it goes further than that. Rarely is a vaccine listed as the cause of death. Instead, the coroner uses the subterfuge of complicated medical language to falsify the death certificate. When in truth the death was caused by a vaccine, they say it was due to bronchial bilateral pneumonia, infantile paralysis, SIDS, shaken baby syndrome, lymphatic leukemia, tubercular meningitis, or a number of other names to ensure the real reason is not listed and thus discovered. (The suffux "itis" means inflammation or swelling. Meningitis is swelling of the meninges – the protective layer of tissue covering the brain and spinal cord.)

George Bernard Shaw was privy to these shenanigans. He wrote, "During the last considerable epidemic at the turn of the century, I was a member of the Health Committee of London Borough Council, and I learned how the credit of vaccination is kept up statistically by diagnosing all the revaccinated cases (of smallpox) as pustular eczema, varioloid or what not – except smallpox."(140)

I want to remind you that there is strong evidence that the incidences of infectious diseases were already declining when the vaccines were introduced, vaccines have actually been shown to increase the incidences of that particular disease, and the classification and diagnosis of many diseases have been changed to help reflect the "benefit to our society" of the vaccines. What could actually be happening is that the incidence of acute "infectious" diseases is really not being curbed by vaccines at all, and chronic diseases like diabetes, asthma, and autism are also increasing because of their use. The worst of both worlds.

In 1997, two highly respected magazines, *The Economist* and *Science News*, had featured articles posing the question of whether the decrease in infectious diseases in childhood through the mass use of vaccines has been replaced with an increase in chronic diseases such as diabetes and asthma. Citing data from England and New Zealand, the *Science News* article entitled "The Dark Side of Immunizations," showed that vaccinated children have a higher incidence of asthma and diabetes than do unvaccinated children.(141)

The Economist article entitled "Plagued by Cures" says that exposure to infections in childhood may prevent chronic disease later in life and that "intervening in infections may have undesirable effects on the hosts – that is, on people – as well as on the pathogens themselves." One study showed that children who had not had measles were significantly more likely to suffer from asthma, eczema, and hay fever. One theory for this is that recovery from naturally occurring childhood diseases is important so that the immune system can respond and be strengthened by viral and bacterial attacks. Depriving the immune system to naturally develop this way may cause the immune system to "eventually attack itself, which is what happens in autoimmune diseases like asthma and diabetes."(142) A study by New Zealand researchers, reported in *Epidemiology*, analyzed 1,265 people born in 1977. Twenty-three of these did not get any childhood vaccinations and none of them suffered asthma. Of the 1,242 who got polio and DPT shots, more than 23 percent later had episodes of asthma.(143)

Food for Thought

Some people do refuse vaccines and their numbers are increasing. The *American Medical News* reported on February 9, 2004 that 93 percent of pediatricians and 60 percent of family physicians reported a parent refusing a vaccine for their child.(144) Many parents are now home schooling their children to avoid subjecting them to vaccinations. (Where are the epidemics among home schooled kids?) Even some military personnel have refused to take the anthrax vaccine even though doing so could ruin their careers. But for the most part, people follow the advice of their physician. People faithfully go get their injections and subject their children to them to avoid coming down with a disease or the dreaded strain of flu making the rounds that year. But are flu shots effective, safe, and necessary?

In 1999 there were about 85 million doses of flu shots given (billions and billions of dollars worth). There are over 200 common types of influenza viruses documented (the "flu" is influenza – an infection of the respiratory tract). Which one will appear in any given year is unknown, so doctors literally guess at which strain might come around each year. Even if they guess right, there's always a chance that the virus will mutate into a new kind. Oftentimes, the flu shot leaves the person sicker than the disease itself, and there's still the chance of paralysis, seizures, allergic reactions, and death.(145)

In 1976 there were 565 cases of Guillian-Barre paralysis associated with the swine flu vaccine along with 30 unexplained deaths of elderly persons. Dr. John Seal of the National Institute of Allergy and Infections Disease says, "We have to go on the basis that any and all flu vaccines are capable of causing Guillian-Barre."(Guillian-Barre Syndrome is the inflammatory destruction of the nerve sheath causing rapid paralysis.) (146)

It's hard for me to rationalize how injecting poisons into someone can be health-promoting. Call me an extremist. Healthy things promote health. Poisons (vaccines) promote sickness and misery.

Are vaccines absolutely required by law? Most doctors and school authorities say so. However, most states provide waivers allowing parents to decline the mandated vaccines on personal, religious, or philosophical grounds. Contact your State or County Health Department and your State Board of Education and request a copy of the immunization laws in your area. Know what you are up against and learn if there's any way out of having your child vaccinated. Probably a better approach is to get a written statement from a medical doctor stating that the vaccine (or vaccines) would be harmful to the child's health. If you can find a sympathetic doctor, this would probably work. If neither of these methods works, contact the National Vaccine Information Center for help (703) 938-DPT3 or www.909shot.com.

If you try to fight the system, be prepared for resistance. Some parents have been charged with child abuse or have lost custody for not having their children vaccinated. That's why getting a doctor's statement instead of a waiver would probably be the safest and surest way to go.

Food for Thought

I just came across a letter for you to use that is not only very informative (detailing all the gross, unhealthy things that are typically in vaccines), but will give you some leverage and put the responsibility of vaccine safety back on the doctor (or school who insists your child must be vaccinated). I have no experience with this letter, but thought I should include it since it at least gives you some ammunition. If you use it, you'll probably have to find another doctor since the one you hand this letter to will probably get very angry and defensive. Watch what happens when *their* butt is on the line instead of your child's! That's a statement in itself, isn't it? I found this at: http://articles.mercola.com/sites/articles/archive/2009/03/03/A-Vaccine-Form-You-Can-Give-to-Your-Pediatrician.aspx

Physician's (or School's) Warranty of Vaccine Safety

I (Physician's name, degree (or School's Principal's name)_____, _____ am a physician licensed to practice medicine in the State of _____. My State license number is _____, and my DEA number is _____. My medical specialty is _____ (or am the Principal of _____and have told the parent or guardian of _____ that _____vaccine(s) are required for said student to be allowed to attend this school.)

I have a thorough understanding of the risks and benefits of all the medications that I prescribe for or administer (or require) to my patients (or of my students) Or . In the case of (Patient's name) _____ , age _____ , whom I have examined, I find that certain risk factors exist that justify the recommended vaccinations. The following is a list of said risk factors and the vaccinations that will protect against them:

Risk Factor _____
Vaccination _____
Risk Factor _____
Vaccination _____ (list more if necessary)

I am aware that vaccines typically contain many of the following fillers:
* aluminum hydroxide,* aluminum phosphate,* ammonium sulfate
* amphotericin B
* **animal tissues: pig blood, horse blood, rabbit brain,**
* **dog kidney, monkey kidney,**
* chick embryo, chicken egg, duck egg
* calf (bovine) serum
* betapropiolactone
* **fetal bovine serum**
* formaldehyde,* formalin
* gelatin,* glycerol,* hydrolyzed gelatin
* **human diploid cells (originating from human aborted fetal tissue)**
* mercury thimerosal (thimerosal, Merthiolate(r))
* **monosodium glutamate (MSG)**
* neomycin,* neomycin sulfate
* phenol red indicator,* **phenoxyethanol (antifreeze)**
* potassium diphosphate,* potassium monophosphate
* polymyxin B
* polysorbate 20,* polysorbate 80
*porcine (pig) pancreatic hydrolysate of casein
* residual MRC5 proteins
* sorbitol* tri(n)butylphosphate,
* VERO cells, a continuous line of monkey kidney cells, and
* washed sheep red blood

and, hereby, warrant that these ingredients are safe for injection into the body of my patient (the student). I have researched reports to the contrary, such as reports that mercury thimerosal causes severe neurological and immunological damage, and find that they are not credible. I am aware that some vaccines have been found to have been contaminated with Simian Virus 40 (SV 40) and that SV 40 is causally linked by some researchers to non-Hodgkin"s lymphoma and mesotheliomas in humans as well as in experimental animals. I hereby warrant that the vaccines I employ in my practice do not contain SV 40 or any other live viruses. (Alternately, I hereby warrant that said SV-40 virus or other viruses pose no substantive risk to my patient.)

I hereby warrant that the vaccines I am recommending for the care of (Patient's name or student's name) _____ _____ do not contain any tissue from aborted human babies (also known as "fetuses").

In order to protect my patient's well being, I have taken the following steps to guarantee that the vaccines I will use will contain no damaging contaminants. STEPS TAKEN: _____ I have personally investigated the reports made to the VAERS (Vaccine Adverse Event Reporting System) and state that it is my professional opinion that the vaccines I am recommending are safe for administration to a child under the age of 5 years. The bases for my opinion are itemized on Exhibit A , attached hereto, — "Physician's Bases for Professional Opinion of Vaccine Safety." (Please itemize each recommended vaccine separately along with the bases for arriving at the conclusion that the vaccine is safe for administration to a child under the age of 5 years.) The professional journal articles I have relied upon in the issuance of this Physician's Warranty of Vaccine Safety are itemized on Exhibit B , attached hereto, — "Scientific Articles in Support of Physician's Warranty of Vaccine Safety." The professional journal articles that I have read which contain opinions adverse to my opinion are itemized on Exhibit C , attached hereto, — "Scientific Articles Contrary to Physician's Opinion of Vaccine Safety." The reasons for my determining that the articles in Exhibit C were invalid are delineated in Attachment D , attached hereto, — "Physician's Reasons for Determining the Invalidity of Adverse Scientific Opinions." I understand that 60 percent of patients who are vaccinated for Hepatitis B will lose detectable antibodies to Hepatitis B within 12 years. I understand that in 1996 only 54 cases of Hepatitis B were reported to the CDC in the 0-1 year age group. I understand that in the VAERS, there were 1,080 total reports of adverse reactions from Hepatitis B vaccine in 1996 in the 0-1 year age group, with 47 deaths reported. I understand that 50 percent of patients who contract Hepatitis B develop no symptoms after exposure. I understand that 30 percent will develop only flu-like symptoms and will have lifetime immunity. I understand that 20 percent will develop the symptoms of the disease, but that 95 percent will fully recover and have lifetime immunity. I understand that 5 percent of the patients who are exposed to Hepatitis B will become chronic carriers of the disease. I understand that 75 percent of the chronic carriers will live with an asymptomatic infection and that only 25 percent of the chronic carriers will develop chronic liver disease or liver cancer, 10-30 years after the acute infection.

The following scientific studies have been performed to demonstrate the safety of the Hepatitis B vaccine in children_____

_____

In addition to the recommended vaccinations as protections against the above cited risk factors, I have recommended other non-vaccine measures to protect the health of my patient and have enumerated said non-vaccine measures on Exhibit D , attached hereto, "Non-vaccine Measures to Protect Against Risk Factors."

I am issuing this Physician's Warranty of Vaccine Safety in my professional capacity as the attending physician to (Patient's name)

_____.

Regardless of the legal entity under which I normally practice medicine, I am issuing this statement in both my business and individual capacities and hereby waive any statutory, Common Law, Constitutional, UCC, international treaty, and any other legal immunities from liability lawsuits in the instant case.

I issue this document of my own free will after consultation with competent legal counsel whose name is

_____, an attorney admitted to the Bar in the State of _____ .

_____ (Name of Attending Physician)

_____ L.S. (Signature of Attending Physician)

Signed on this _____ day of _____ A.D. _____

Witness: _____ Date: _____

Notary Public: _____ Date: _____

The logic behind denying someone the right to refuse a vaccine is itself flawed. If vaccines really provided immunity, then anyone who's vaccinated should be safe, even if someone who is infected is among them. If parents choose not to vaccinate their child, that child would be the only one at risk and would not endangering those who received the vaccine. But true immunity is never conferred by a vaccine – a testimony to the inexactness of the theories of immunization.

In examining 70 years of medical literature, it's apparent that scientists and doctors have long noted how vaccines can cause injury and death in lab animals and humans. So there's no guarantee they won't injure of kill your child either.

It's known and documented that substances such as mercury, aluminum, and formaldehyde are used in their manufacture. Some vaccines are even cultured from aborted human fetuses and potentially contaminated human and animal tissue cultures. (For a shocking exposé on the use of tissue from aborted human fetuses, please go to www.cogforlife.org.) But why don't the authorities and doctors tell this to the people being vaccinated? The deception goes further. Barbara Loe Fisher reports,

> Then, after the National Childhood Vaccine Injury Act was passed in 1986, when the Departments of Health and Justice worked together to rewrite the law and withhold federal compensation from three quarters of all children with vaccine associated injuries applying for help; when contraindications were narrowed and sick children started being vaccinated in emergency rooms; when each new vaccine produced was recommended for mandatory use; and when government and industry subsequently joined together to launch a mass media campaign to achieve a 100 percent vaccination rate by denying vaccine risks exist or suggesting that, if risks do exist, they are only experienced by children who are genetically compromised, there was a further erosion of trust. . . U.S. government officials continue to promote the idea that children who

die or are brain injured following vaccination have an underlying genetic disorder and that (a) either the vaccine simply triggered the inevitable; or (b) these children were predestined to die or become brain damaged even if no vaccine had ever been given. Without any empirical evidence whatsoever in most individual cases of vaccine associated death and brain damage, health officials repeat the seductive and dangerous mantra to pediatricians and parents alike when referring to children with vaccine associated health problems – underlying genetic disorder.(147)

So when parents take the state mandated vaccine risk and it turns out that the risk for their child is 100 percent, everyone has been carefully preconditioned to accept the idea that the vaccine is not responsible. The doctor is not responsible. The vaccine manufacturer is not responsible. The government is not responsible. The genetically defective child is responsible. How convenient. No need for questions to be asked. No need to report deaths and injuries following vaccination. No need to pull vaccine lots associated with high numbers of deaths and injuries off the market. No need to commit dollars or time to conduct scientific studies to find out exactly what vaccines do in the human body at the cellular and molecular biology level. No need to develop pathological profiles for vaccine injury and death or develop a genetic marker to separate out high risk children and save their lives. No need to be concerned about the immune and neurological dysfunction of these genetically defective individuals who have been legally required to sacrifice their lives on the battle-field of our nations' War on Disease.

The haunting question remains: just how many are being sacrificed? How many of the mentally retarded, epileptic, autistic, learning disabled, hyperactive, diabetic, asthmatic children in the inner cities and the suburbs and the big and small towns of America are part of that sacrifice?(148)

Food for Thought

Nobel Prize winning playwright, defender of women's rights, and one of the great minds of the 20th century, George Bernard Shaw, wrote:

"All great truths begin as blasphemies."

Please keep that in mind as you read this section, because you may think what I write here is just that – blasphemy. Be that as it may, you are about to learn of one of the great misconceptions of not just modern medicine, but of the modern world. Its a powerful health and healing concept that has been forgotten by most, ignored by some, and deliberately suppressed by others. You may think I've gone off the deep end, but I'm firmly convinced, based on scientific evidence, observation, logic, and the laws of science, that what I am about to tell you is true.

I did not invent the paradigm you are about to read – other scientists and doctors did. I am just reporting it, since I believe it correctly explains how germs really affect us and how diseases start. It shows that you are the one in control of your health and need not be dependent on drugs or vaccines. YOU have the power. Remember that. All right, here we go. . .

Not only are vaccines risky, but the understanding of how they work and of immunology in general is incomplete. The concepts of immunology are filled with assumptions and stretches of the imagination. Barbara Loe Fisher comments about the lack of understanding the medical community has when it comes to the immune system:

"I remember standing in a lab at the FDA. . .talking with Dr. Chuck Manclark, who. . .conducted pertussis vaccine research for many years at the Bureau of Biologics. . .In one conversation he pointed out to me that the problem with developing a safe and effective pertussis vaccine was that medical science still doesn't really understand precisely how the pertussis bacterium acts on the human body during the course of the natural disease and so it was difficult to develop a vaccine with the right components in it. . .If you add this basic gap in understanding to science's limited general understanding of precisely how the human immune system functions and how it interacts with the neurological system, a frontier that is being explored by the new neuroimmunologists and molecular biologists, you have a window for possible past miscalculation of the biological effects over time of repeatedly manipulating the human immune system with single and multiple antigens."[149]

Every year the vaccines for flu shots are literally shots in the dark because the manufacturers *guess* what strain of flu bug they think will be going around that year. Drugs to treat the flu, such as *Tamiflu*, are not that effective, if at all, either, and their side effects include delirium and death, especially in children. My question is, if these scientists and government officials know as much about immunology as they try to convince us they do, why can't they do a better job designing vaccines and drugs that actually work? The answer is simple: They really *don't* know what they are doing. To understand why immunology is such an incomplete, theoretical, and ultimately specious discipline, let's examine its history, and evaluate the science behind it.

In the mid 1800s, there was a debate going in the scientific community – the outcome of which would set the modern medical paradigm for the cause and prevention of disease. The principal players in the debate were Louis Pasteur and Claude Bernard. Pasteur (1822-1895) believed that disease came from preexisting microorganisms that invade the human body. He also believed that bacteria are not normally found within the body. The tissues of normal, healthy animals, he said, should be totally bacteriologically sterile. He contended that bacteria caused cells to decompose, or putrefy, thus leading to disease.

Of course, Pasteur has been proven wrong on that. Bacteriologists have since found that all animals need healthy bacteria in their bodies in order to live. Animals delivered in aseptic (germ-free) conditions, kept in sterile cages, and fed sterile food and water do not live more than a few days.

It also seems that this "contamination" by outside bacteria is essential for healthy life.(150) *ABC News* reported that there are about ten times as many symbiotic bacterial cells in our bodies than human cells, although because they're so much smaller than most body cells, they make up only about 1 – 2 percent of the body's mass. They're especially important in the digestive tract, mouth, skin, nose, and the female urogenital tract, where they perform functions like helping digestion and keeping our immune system active.(151)

Pasteur was a French chemist who first became famous for inventing a heat process that saved wine from being overtaken by mold, thus extending shelf life. This was during a time in Europe when mold was so seriously affecting the vineyards that the industry was on the brink of financial failure. His heat process, later coined *pasteurization*, gained him instant fame, and he derived his livelihood from the sale of wines and beer. He was neither a doctor nor biochemist, but was given an honorary doctorate degree which made him appear to be more than he really was.(152) In the 1870s, Pasteur experimented with inoculations similar to Edward Jenner's, and developed vaccines for anthrax and rabies. He was a prolific writer and had a vocal and flamboyant personality. He promoted his views with zest and conviction and made it his mission to preach his ideas to the world. This attitude and energy did much to get him and his ideas recognized, which further advanced his career and theories. The bottom line is, he was not just a scientist, but a good salesman. His original theories that the blood and everything else of a truly healthy person should not have one single microorganism in it have not only been proven wrong, but conveniently ignored and forgotten. Even so, the scientific community still considers him a hero.

Claude Bernard (1813-1878), on the other hand, not only had a different personality – being quiet and reserved – but different beliefs on the origin of disease as well. Bernard believed that outside invaders do not cause disease. He believed that "the microbe is nothing, the terrain is everything." Others, most notably Antoine Bechamp (1816-1908), a medical doctor, chemist and biochemist, contended that no outside germ is necessary for a healthy person to become sick. Bechamp said, "Disease is born of us and in us."(153)

In the Pottenger's Cats study (see the Ancestry Factor chapter), the healthy cats – fed the healthy diet – were generally kept in close proximity to the sick and diseased cats. The diseased cats had all sorts of diseases that one would normally classify as "contagious." But the healthy cats never got sick – never came down with the "contagious" diseases. Either the healthy cats (who were never immunized) had a strong enough immune system to fend off those nasty germs from the sick cats, or something else was happening.

Dr. Weston Price observed that members of remote tribal villages, who were very healthy before the white man came would start coming down with tuberculosis (among other diseases) after white flour and sugar were introduced into their diets. Tuberculosis is thought to be a contagious disease. However, Dr. Price never got it and the tribes-people who stayed on their original natural diet never got it either, despite constant contact with people (and their germs) who did have it. Price said the reason these people got tuberculosis was because of deficiencies they developed from eating refined sugar and flour, not because of a contagious germ.

Dr. Paul Carton corroborates this with his observations of patients in his clinic in France. He said, "In tuberculosis the soil [our body] is practically everything. One becomes tuberculous by enfeebling one's organism, and the only means of getting rid of the bacillus. . .is the heightening of the spontaneous resisting power. In a word, Koch's bacillus is not much more than a saprophyte, a moss, a parasite which fastens upon failing organisms and seals the fate of those already falling into ruin."(154)

Koch's bacillus is the bacterium that, in 1882, Robert Koch said causes tuberculosis (*Mycobacterium tuberculosis*). Koch developed what is referred to as *Koch's Postulates* (published in 1890), which are used as the guidelines to decide if a germ is the cause of a disease. The First Postulate states that the germ must be found in abundance in all organisms suffering from the disease. This is not always true, however. Walter R. Hadwen, M.D., who was "one of the most experienced men in tuberculosis," said, "Nobody has ever found a tubercle bacillus in the earliest stages of tuberculosis."(155) Even Koch abandoned this postulate when it was shown that people who don't have cholera or typhoid can carry the disease and give it to others (they are termed *asymptomatic carriers,* or *Typhoid Marys*). This, in my opinion, is not even happening, as I'll show in a few minutes.

Another one of Koch's Postulates states that the germ must be capable of producing the original infection. Remember, however, that 90 percent of the people with the polio virus show no signs of the disease, even under epidemic conditions. Koch himself demonstrated that in the cases of cholera and tuberculosis, not everyone exposed to these germs will become infected. Even the website *WebM.D.* says that 15 percent of those with S*treptococcus* in their throats do not have strep throat. So that shoots down Koch's Third Postulate.

There are also major exceptions to the Second Postulate, which has to do with isolating and culturing the microorganism in pure culture, which for some germs, apparently is impossible. Therefore, what do microbiologist do? Make exceptions to the rules, and a lot of them. Some "law" of science, huh? Even so, Koch's Postulates are still taught in medical school as an underpinning to microbiology and the transmission of disease.

Just like any living thing, germs need food, water, and a place to live. When these conditions are present, germs become active. When a lot of food is available, as in undigested food or abundant excretion of waste from the body's cells as they attempt to cleanse themselves from toxicity, these germs will multiply. Herbert M. Shelton, N.D., D.N.Sc. said, "The germs feed on the excretions. They are scavengers. They were never anything else and will never be anything else. They break up and consume the discharge from the tissues. This is the function ascribed to germs everywhere in nature outside the body and is their real and only function in disease. . .The medical profession has cooed itself into hysteria over the germ theory and is using it to exploit an all too credulous public."(156)

Bechamp said that there are, what he called little bodies or microzymas, that exist in all living cells of animal and plant life. They change form depending on the condition of the host organism (this changing form is called *pleomorphism*) and actually help the body get rid of dead and useless matter. If the body is toxic and acidic, the germs turn into certain forms and become active in helping to eliminate excess waste.

Another well-respected German scientist, Guenther Enderlein, also believed in pleomorphism. He contended that bacteria could go through many forms during a life cycle – similar to a caterpillar morphing into a butterfly or a tadpole into a frog. Every living creature I can think of goes through different developmental stages where their appearance changes as they grow. A seed becomes a tree, an egg becomes a fish, an embryo becomes a baby who becomes a girl who becomes a woman. Why would bacteria be any different?

In his book *Bakterien Cyclogenie*, Enderlein explained that when a person is healthy, the bacteria live in a harmonious relationship with it and actually help the immune system. If there are factors such as poor nutrition, dehydration, stress, environmental toxins, alcohol, nicotine or drug use, the internal environment of the body changes and becomes toxic, the pH of the blood becomes imbalanced (it becomes acidic), and then the bacteria change form into disease indicating (not causing) forms.(157) That's why John Tilden, M.D. said, "The disease condition present determines the morphology of the germ and not vice versa."(158)

This also explains why some germs may emit toxins into our bodies, which may have an unhealthy effect on us. But the germs only emit toxic byproducts if the environment they are in is first toxic. It is not the other way around, namely, that the bacteria cause the body's toxicity. Sir Richard Douglas Powell was a leading bacteriologist in the early 20th century. He observed that if tetanus and gas gangrene germs are washed clean and freed from their environment, they are quite harmless. Shelton comments, "It would seem that they [the germs] depend for their toxicity and supposed specificity upon a toxic environment, and if this is so, the chemistry of their environment really determines toxicity."(159)

Other researchers agree. Nancy Appleton, in her book *Rethinking Pasteur's Germ Theory*, recounts the work of Dr. Arthur Kendall, Dean of Northwestern University Research Laboratory in Chicago, Illinois, and Royal Raymond Rife, who said, "The human body is chemical in nature. The bacteria that exist normally in the body feed on these chemicals. If the chemicals change as a result of a toxic environment. . .these same bacteria, or some of them, will also undergo a chemical change. We have often produced all the symptoms of a disease chemically in experimental animals without the inoculation of any virus or bacteria into their tissues."(160)

This is the same reason food poisoning is caused by cooked or partially cooked food that has spoiled. The cooking turns some of the food toxic, and the resulting bacteria who eat it are toxic too. You will never get deadly food poisoning from raw food that has spoiled. You may get an overload of bacteria that may cause diarrhea or other temporary symptoms, but nothing serious and surely nothing deadly. More on bacteria and raw food in a minute.

Florence Nightingale (1820-1910), the famous English nurse, held a similar view. She wrote in her famous book, *Notes on Nursing*, "Is it not living in a continual mistake, to look upon diseases as we do now, as separate entities. . .instead of looking upon them as conditions like a dirty or clean condition, and just as much under our own control; or rather as the reactions. . .against the conditions in which we have placed ourselves? The specific disease doctrine is the grand refuge of weak, uncultured, unstable minds, such as now rule in the medical profession. There are no specific diseases; there are specific disease conditions."(161)

Louis Pasteur contended that *all* diseases are a result of microorganisms invading the body, and that healthy tissues have no microbes present. There are reports that Pasteur, on his death-bed, finally admitted his germ theory was wrong and that the health of the individual is the most important thing in determining the formation and severity of a disease.(162)

Rudolph Virchow, a world famous German pathologist and founder of cellular medicine, stated: "If I could live my life over again, I would devote it to proving that germs seek their natural habitat – 'diseased' tissue – rather than being the cause of the 'diseased' tissue." George White, M.D., states that "If germ theory were founded on facts, there would be no living being to read what's written."(163)

Besides bacteria being abundant in our bodies, they are ubiquitous in the air, and we breathe in an estimated 14,000 germs an hour.(164) You would think that breathing in about 336,000 germs a day, some of them would be the ones that cause disease.

As an environmental engineer, I inspected wastewater treatment plants. Wastewater has a lot of things in it: waste from toilets, sinks, floor drains, hospital bedpans, industrial processes and so on. It's loaded with waste (called the *carbon source*), the exact thing bacteria love to eat. A typical way to treat wastewater involves putting the water into a big lagoon where the bacteria continue to eat the waste. When aerobic bacteria eat, live and grow, they respire (just like humans), taking in oxygen and carbon (from the feces etc.) and giving off carbon dioxide and water. In order to speed up the process and make sure the bacteria don't die, the wastewater in these lagoons is often blown up into the air using a machine called an aerator. This provides more oxygen for the bacteria, so they grow, multiply, and respire even faster, turning more waste into CO_2 and H_2O. This is pure water, which is drawn off a big tank called a clarifier and usually discharged into a river or stream.

The air around the treatment plant is, of course, filled not only with water vapor from the spray produced by the aerators, but bacteria and viruses as well. Therefore, you would think that if there were one place on earth that there are enough bad germs to cause someone to come down with a disease, it would be around a wastewater treatment plant. But I never met a sick wastewater treatment operator, and I never got sick inspecting a plant, even though my system was shocked with a high concentration of germs while being there without having time to build up "immunity." None of my fellow inspectors got sick either. The very things we've been taught to fear, germs, are the main agents used to clean water. Consider water makes up between 60 and 80 percent of the human body.

I've also worked as a county health inspector inspecting restaurants. During our training at the state capital, I asked the head of the certification board just what it was about bacteria that caused illness. He said he didn't know. There isn't a microbiologist alive who can tell you either, because anything they try to pass off as proof is merely anecdotal evidence. There have been no modern scientific studies done to prove germs cause disease. But there *have* been studies to prove that germs do *not* cause disease, as you'll see.

If a doctor took a cell culture of your throat right now, he would likely find *Streptococcus* germs present. But you don't have strep throat do you? Even the textbooks on bacteriology admit that diphtheria, typhoid, tuberculosis, pneumonia, or any other disease germ may be present in an individual without he or she having the disease these germs supposedly cause.

As far as viruses go, as any microbiology textbook will tell you, they are not even alive. They are a dead protein shell with DNA or RNA fragments inside of it. The common belief is that a virus (about 100 times smaller than a bacterium) can inject its DNA into a host cell, take over that cells' metabolism, and force it to reproduce the virus. The science behind this, although very complicated, hi-tech and impressive, is sketchy at best, and some experts are beginning to wonder if viruses actually exist at all. Dr Stefan Lanka and Karl Krafeld, in their book *Vaccination-Genocide in the Third Millennium?* state that there is still no proof of any (medically relevant) virus. Dr. Lanka says that not one virus has ever been isolated and there is no proof of their existence. He points to high-magnification photographs that claim to show the virus particles, but which, in fact, ". . .show cells and typical endogenous particles in them. These structures. . .differ in size and shape and therefore can't be isolated [and can't be viruses because viruses are supposedly the same size and same shape]. . .Nobody claims that they're isolated particles, let alone particles that have been isolated from humans. . .there's not even one publication where the fulfillment of Koch's first postulate is even claimed. . .there is no proof that from humans with certain diseases the viruses have been isolated. Nevertheless, this is precisely what they publicly claim."(165) Dr. Ryke Geerd Hamer, another virus skeptic, prefers to speak of "viruses as 'hypothetical viruses' since lately the existence of viruses has been called into question."(166)

The whole idea behind immunology is to prevent epidemics. Vaccines, the theory goes, protect us from bacteria and viruses that might cause disease in otherwise healthy individuals. These healthy individuals are just that – healthy and strong with no symptoms of the disease (diphtheria, measles, or whatever). Going along with this theory, the germ then has the power to make a healthy person sick. In order to do this, it has to be more powerful in its actions than the defenses and/or biological systems of the healthy and strong individual. Once the person is affected, the person becomes weaker. If the person were now weaker, wouldn't he or she have less power to kill the germ? If a germ can cause disease in a healthy person, then the germ should be able to continue to cause disease in the just-stricken sick person. (And the germ *would be there*. But we've seen that oftentimes the germ is not even present at the very beginnings of a disease it supposedly caused.) The germs would be more powerful and proliferate at a faster and faster rate – with less and less resistance from the body – until they completely overtook the individual and rendered him or her totally powerless – i.e., dead.

According to immunity, it takes about a week for the *adaptive immune system* to mobilize its defenses to combat an infection. But bacteria can multiply fast – doubling as quickly as once every 20 minutes under ideal conditions. After just 12 hours, a single bacterium could multiply to millions. After 7 days? Billions and billions, all the while making the body weaker and less able to combat it. That's why George White, M.D., stated, "If germ theory were founded on facts, there would be no living being to read what's written."

There are two ways to explain sickness if it was a result of germs. One: if the body doesn't have the defenses against that particular germ, then it doesn't have the defenses. So one little germ, one little virus or bacteria, could get into us and take over and make us sick until we were totally overcome and dead. (This is what Pasteur believed.)

Two: let's say that one diphtheria germ won't hurt you. You have enough "immunity" built up to defend against it and render it harmless. But how about a hundred germs or a thousand germs? Still, with just these few, you don't get sick. But let's say that once you get "infected" with one million diphtheria germs, you get sick. Effectively, your defenses and "immunity" are overwhelmed and the germs begin to multiply, and you get even sicker. Diseases just don't start at their peak, they progressively get worse. More and more bacteria mean more and more disease. If your defenses were so overwhelmed at just one million bacteria, which made you weaker and sick, how are they going to defend against a billion at the peak of the disease? The logic of immunity is like saying that some of the enemy made it over the walls of our castle and started killing and maiming us. But somehow, that makes the rest of our army stronger. So now that we're stronger from having some of us killed and maimed, we're better able to defend against the enemy who has breached our walls and is still killing and maiming us and doubling in number every 20 minutes before our very eyes!

If we look at sheer numbers, the germ theory doesn't make sense. The human body consists of about 10 trillion cells. It's estimated that there are many times that number (100 trillion) of microorganisms in the human body, most of which are in the gut. (That's right, folks. You are by number, more bacteria than you are yourself. Your cells are much bigger than the bacteria, though.) Recent research showed that there is an awe-inspiring 5,600 different species of bacteria living in the typical human intestine.(167) Most of these bacteria, or germs, are understood to be beneficial (they help digest carbohydrates, produce hormones and vitamins such as biotin and vitamin K) so much so that the gut bacteria are sometimes termed the "forgotten organ."

There are about 100,000 germs in a sneeze, which sounds like a lot. Let's say you get sneezed on in the face with your mouth wide open and you took in the whole 100,000 germs. You'd be afraid of "catching" that cold, wouldn't you? But consider that there are about 100,000 billion germs in your mouth alone: germs that are, even the doctors admit, doing good things for you – one of which is keeping the "bad" germs in check.(168) So in this scenario, the 100,000 "bad" germs from the sneeze are now in your mouth, which contains 100 billion good germs. Who do you think will win when one side is out-numbered a million to one? That's not to mention all of your own cells (which are much bigger, much more complex, and much smarter than the bacteria in a sneeze) that are there to fight the "bad" germs too. You'd have to be sneezed on directly into your mouth a million times just to get it to the point of it being an even fight of good germs versus bad germs – just in your mouth alone. Add in the good bacteria all over your body, and all the other cells that fight toxicity and disease (which total 110 trillion), and there is no way a sneeze from *Dumbo the Elephant* is going to affect you in any way whatsoever. You cold lick a telephone receiver (25,000 germs per square inch), or toilet seat (49 germs per square inch), or eat a whole kitchen sponge (7.2 billion germs), and still come nowhere near the number of "good" bacteria in your mouth alone.(169)

Let's go further and examine strep throat specifically. The *WebM.D.* says,

"'Strep,' in this case, stands for *Streptococcus pyogenes*, a common strain of bacteria that can live in your throat and nose for months without causing any harm. Tests show that about 15% of healthy people have the strep 'bug' living uneventfully in their mouths or throats, without causing any symptoms. . . Once in a while, though, these bugs can turn on you. Maybe you've been under too much stress or your immune system has been over-taxed. . . whatever the reason, the normally quiet strep organisms can suddenly start spewing out toxins and inflammatory substances to bring on a sore throat and other symptoms."(170)

Sounds plausible, right? Not to me. First, the paragraph says that if your immune system had not been "overtaxed," you would have been able to defend against the germ and no illness would have resulted. This is a caveat that kind of makes the individual responsible (for letting his/her immune system get overtaxed), but kind of blames the germs too. They have to have this caveat because there are so many exceptions to the rules of germs and immunology (in this case, that 15% of healthy people have the strep bug with no sickness), that they know their theories don't hold up most, if not all, of the time. Even in this typical-medical-mentality statement, they are, without realizing it, admitting that the individual's level of health is the determinant of whether or not that person gets sick. (This is the same for any "infectious disease:" You have *Salmonella* germs in you right now, syphilis germs, staph germs, tuberculosis germs – they're all in there as part of the 5,600 species of germs in you. The only thing keeping you from getting any of these diseases is *you* – your level of health.)

Second, the fact that the strep germ is present when the disease itself is not, is in direct contradiction to one of Koch's Postulates, which is what immunology is based on.

Third, why is it that the germ is "spewing out toxins and inflammatory substances?" Where did those harmful substances come from? A smoke stack spews out ash and gases, and these had to be put in the firebox in one form (coal, wood, oil) or another. The "substances" had to have come from somewhere. Even if they do come from the bacteria (which I don't believe they do), where did the bacteria get them? Answer: their environment – the impurities in the blood stream, lymph, or tissues of the body. (I believe the substances for the most part spew not from the bacteria, but from the body's tissues in a cleansing action. The rest come from the bacteria after they have processed this toxic matter.)

During an illness, there are things askew in the body. Perhaps there's an increased temperature, a discharge, or nausea. The whole body (the terrain, the environment) or much of it is usually affected. Although *E. coli.* is a bacterium that is indigenous to humans and, in fact, health enhancing, some scientists believe that a certain strain of it (*E. coli O157:H7*), causes disease. The differences in this strain compared to other strains are small cellular differences, mostly on the surface of the cell membrane. These minor changes on the cell surface can change the environment of the whole body – so the experts say – to the point of causing illness and even death. These bacteria, remember, were vastly outnumbered by healthy bacteria and healthy cells before the "infection," and now they're telling us that just a few little changes on the outer membrane of an otherwise health-producing bacterium can change the whole milieu of the human body? That's like saying my mittens and winter coat caused the snowstorm.

Just as you get normal, fully formed crops when they grow on the proper soil, you get normal, fully formed bacteria when they grow in a healthy environment. Different strains of bacteria manifest when the environment they grow in is not ideal. It's not the kind of bacteria determining the environment; it's the environment determining the kind of bacteria.

The germ theory is crumbling. First, Pasteur said that every illness without exception is caused by bacteria. Now we know that's not true, but the medical community thinks is still is – kind of. Everyone used to think that antibiotics were manna from heaven and could cure everything from allergies to yeast infections, but now many doctors are advising to avoid antibiotics because of their long-term hazards. *Salmonella* (*Salmonella enteritidis*) naturally occurs in the intestines of chickens, dogs, cats, amphibians, and reptiles. It's in chicken poop, dog poop, cat poop, in the carpet, on the lawn. It's even found in the large intestines of humans.(171) Why aren't all the chicken farmers sick and dying? Why doesn't the S*almonella* in Rover's saliva or the litter box kill you or your child? Why does Dr. John Mermen of the CDC say that trying to quash *Salmonella* in an iguana (reptile) "is like trying to do the same with normal levels of *E. coli.* in healthy humans: not a smart thing to do." Everyone used to believe that *Salmonella* in the gut of a reptile indicated disease. Now, they realize it does them no harm, and is even beneficial.(172)

There has been a rash of *Salmonella* scares in the news lately, and many deaths attributed to it. How do I explain that? First, saying *Salmonella* caused a sickness because it's present in the victim, is like saying fingernails caused it. Everyone has fingernails, some longer and slightly different than others, and everyone has *Salmonella*, some at a greater quantity or slightly different than others. If you look hard enough, you'll find *Salmonella* just about anywhere. Same with *E coli*. They are easy things to blame.

Second, if *Salmonella* was, in fact, on the produce or in the peanuts or salsa, it is only there scavenging impurities in or on the product itself. Things like pesticides, herbicides, chemicals, toxic dust of fumigation gasses, incompletely cooked or carelessly preserved food. I'm not saying the food didn't cause a problem, but it wasn't the germ on the food. If the food were pure and properly handled, there'd be no sickness, and no elevated bacteria levels.

In a CDC publication titled "10 Things You Need To Know about Immunizations," the point was made that "Immunizations must begin at birth and most vaccinations completed by age two. . .Children under five are especially susceptible to disease because their immune systems have not built up the necessary defenses to fight infection."(173) My question then is, if the children's systems are not developed enough to fight infection, why are we subjecting them (via vaccines) to the very bacteria and viruses that (supposedly) cause the infection? Not just that, but the vaccines are loaded with impurities and toxins that any healthy body has a difficult time coping with (mercury, formaldehyde, aluminum, etc.). Why would you give an already weak and undeveloped organism – a baby or child – something (bacteria or viruses plus impurities) that is believed to make a healthy child or adult sick?

(Recall the statement by the AAP I referenced earlier where they try to explain why a child can handle vaccines: "At a very young age, children's immune systems are equipped to respond to many antigens at the same time, including those in vaccines." Does that sound consistent with the above statement by the CDC: "Children under five are especially susceptible to disease because their immune systems have not built up the necessary defenses to fight infection"? Another example of them twisting things around to suit whichever agenda they're trying to promote. Are you to trust these people with your child's or your own life?)

"Ah ha!" you may cry, "But you have to build *immunity!* Immunity is the key!" But the theories of immunology are, you are learning, just that – theories – and there are so many exceptions and caveats that the whole science is filled with "maybes", and "we just don't know whys." In my medical school classes, the immunology students were called the "black magicians" because everyone realized they really don't know how immunity works! T-cells, B-cells, phagocytes, lymphocytes, and all those fancy mechanisms that are supposed to somehow remember (if you're lucky) the germ that was injected into you years ago and then come to your rescue when you're exposed to it again. "We don't really know yet how it's remembered, but it is," they say.

They *try* to explain it scientifically (by making it so complicated nobody can see the forest for the trees) and common sense and logic are forgotten. But it's very convenient for the vaccine and drug-makers because if someone gets sick when they weren't supposed to or doesn't get sick when they were, all they have to do is say "Oh, he or she must have a weak/strong immune system." "Ah!!!" you nod your head, "It's their *immune* system! *That* explains it!" You don't want to make trouble or appear stupid, and these people went to school for so long they *have* to know what they're talking about, so you go right along with it. Then if your friend wonders why that person got sick, you can sound so smart saying, "You see, they had a *weak immune system!*"

On one hand, doctors tells us we need antibiotics to kill germs because if germs go unchecked, they will kill us. Immunology, on the other hand, says we need to inject these germs into us, so we can build immunity. Why do the germs in the vaccines not cause the same downward spiral into death that we need to stop with antibiotics? After all, they are the very same germs (or effective facsimiles – if they weren't, they wouldn't use them) in the vaccine as those that also cause a downward spiral into death. Why, when we're exposed to that nasty germ in the atmosphere or by drinking out of the same glass as a sick person (oftentimes having fewer germs than a vaccine does), doesn't our immune system respond in the same way as when we're vaccinated, and just build immunity instead of getting sick? Why is injecting these germs into a child helpful when his or her "immune system" isn't even fully developed yet?

According to immunology, exposure creates immunity; but the only way you can get the disease is by being exposed. Which is it? If the laws of physics, chemistry, biology, and simple logic are followed, it cannot mean both. There is simply no consistency, and too many exceptions, to immunology theories. Apples don't sometimes fall up.

The pharmaceutical companies have the best of both worlds: They have convinced us that we need drugs (antibiotics) to stop germs, so they don't continue to multiply and kill us; and that we need the germs (in vaccines) to start the disease process, so we can build immunity to prevent death later on. The drug companies and most doctors (most of whom are owned by the drug companies) are successful doing this by pointing to a science (immunology) the lay-person doesn't understand and embarrassing them into admitting they don't know enough and the "doctor knows best."

I'm sure you've heard of a "Catch 22." Well, I call this drug/vaccine logic a "Sucker 44." But it doesn't stop there. If you don't make your children get the vaccines, you are endangering their lives and the lives of others and they may try to charge you with child endangerment and arrest you. I call that a "Fascist 66." By the way, Canada does not force schoolchildren to be vaccinated. I wonder why they haven't all died by now. (Check out vaclib.org/exempt/canada.htm)

I've already pointed out how drugs or things manufactured by the drug companies can cause diseases (ADHD, Parkinson's, Alzheimer's, and others), which the drug companies tell us we need other drugs to treat. Autism is no different. First, they make the vaccines that causes autism, then they treat the poor victim with drugs. Pharmacological treatment of autism includes using *Prozac, Dexadrine, Clonidine, Klonpin, Tegriton, Depakote, lamotrigine,* and *Lametol.* As I've said, the drug companies get you coming and going.

In a lot of articles and studies I've read, the point is raised that there is no scientific evidence that proves vaccines cause serious health problems like autism. Just because a high number of children become autistic following vaccines doesn't prove a thing scientifically – it is just anecdotal evidence, not capable of proving a theory.

I would like to extend this argument to germs and how they "cause" disease. I challenge anyone to show me definitive scientific proof using accepted and verified scientific testing protocols that germs do, in fact, cause disease. Just saying, "Oh, everyone knows germs cause disease," doesn't count. (Remember, there were several newspapers that refused to print the story that Orville Wright flew in a self-powdered, heavier than air flying machine because "everyone knows man can't fly." Just saying the incidence of a disease goes down after vaccinations doesn't count either – that's still just anecdotal evidence, which has been disproven anyway and simply is not true.)

Yes, there will be many who think I'm wrong about germs and disease and dismiss what I'm saying here without a second thought. Some will call me a kook or charlatan, or worse. That's OK. That's a natural reaction when a core belief is threatened. But to those people I have just two words: Prove it. If germs really do cause disease and are a fundamental law of science, then proving it shouldn't be difficult. A couple double-blind studies should be enough. Remember, just because germs are present in a sick person isn't proof they caused it. There are typically flies around garbage, but the flies certainly didn't cause the garbage. So until someone proves otherwise, that's my theory, and I'm sticking to it.

Do you think the FDA, CDC, or other agency would commission a study to prove germs cause disease? Of course not. But surprisingly, some people have undertaken the task of showing that exposure to germs does not cause disease. A series of experiments were undertaken between 1914 and 1918 in Toronto, Canada, where numerous volunteers subjected themselves to germs to see if they would become ill. First, they drank water with 50,000 diphtheria germs. No reaction. Then 150,000. Still no reaction. One million, and then literally millions of diphtheria germs were swabbed over the tonsils, under the tongue and in the nostrils. Still no illnesses resulted. They did the same with typhoid germs, meningitis germs, pneumonia germs, and tuberculosis germs, by themselves and in various combinations. The volunteers were observed for several months, and no illnesses were reported. Five years later they were checked on again and not one of the volunteers came down with the diseases these germs were supposed to cause. This study was reported in *Physical Culture* magazine in May 1919. (*Physical Culture* was similar to *Time* or *Life* today) (174)

In the June, 1916 issue of the *London Lancet Medical Journal of Canada*, another similar experiment was documented where a medical doctor and six others were subjected to diphtheria, pneumonia, and typhoid in doses ranging from 50,000 to 1.5 million germs. After two and a half years, no disease.

In 1918 and 1919, about 30 volunteers in the U.S. Navy had blood and secretions from influenza patients' upper respiratory passages sprayed and swabbed in their noses and throats. The Public Health Report summed up the results saying "In no instance was an attack of influenza produced in any one of the subjects."(175) Similar experiments were conducted in San Francisco and Philadelphia resulting in no diseases.(176)

Dr. Thomas Powell challenged his medical colleagues to produce even a single disease in him because of germs. He was subjected to massive numbers of cholera germs, bubonic plague germs, diphtheria germs, and others over the course of many years. His contemporaries did their best to make him sick by inoculating him and having him eat foods laden with these germs. But not once did he become ill.(177) (If you discount these experiments because they took place years ago and science wasn't advanced enough to be reliable back then, may I remind you that the germ theory everyone believes as fact originated in the 1860s.)

These experiments can also be used to illustrate that germs take on the characteristics of the environment, not the other way around. The germs that these people consumed, although considered harmful, did not stay that way. Rather, they reverted into "benign forms" once they were incorporated into the milieu of the healthy person. If you are healthy, any germ you encounter will change into harmless ones once they adapt themselves to your healthy environment. Conversely, if you are laden with toxins and releasing these in a cleansing reaction, any germ you encounter will take on the characteristics of that toxic environment and will change into germs that are considered pathogenic.

You may ask, "What about when my whole family got sick? Isn't that because a contagious germ got passed around?" Sorry, but no. Your family was probably eating a similar diet and leading a similar lifestyle in a similar environment. The residents of whole cities and societies lead similar lifestyles, and thus their bodies react similarly to toxic overload. The bubonic plague first appeared when sugar use sky-rocketed, tribes-people got tuberculosis when they left their natural diet and consumed sugar and flour, and Pottenger's cats succumbed to various "contagious" diseases when fed a deficient diet.

Have you ever noticed the flu season is always after Thanksgiving and Christmas? You would think there would be more bacteria around during the warm summer months than the cold winter months, since they multiply faster in higher temperatures. However, as the days get shorter, so does our exposure to healthy sunlight, we get less exercise, eat fewer fresh foods, and consume more party foods than our system can handle. Our internal environment becomes fouled and overloaded and the body tries to rectify this by accelerating its waste disposal. A runny nose, fever, diarrhea, feeling bad, and so on, arise simply from the body trying to clean itself up, not as a reaction to germs. You'll find that as you clean up your diet and consume more life-giving foods; you won't come down with colds or flus. I haven't had either in over 20 years. Disease is brought on by improper lifestyle and/or toxic contamination and poisoning. The germs only multiply when there is ample food for them to eat.

You see, what most people want is a free pass. They want to be able to stuff themselves with everything from donuts to pizza and then believe getting sick was due to bad luck and they "caught something," and it's someone else's fault or bad luck. Isn't it ironic that with all that hi-tech science behind immunology and the germ theory, getting sick is more a matter of chance than anything else? I'm here to tell you it isn't. Whether you get sick or not can be controlled. That's the good news. The bad news is, it's up to you to control it. But, the more you know, the easier it will be, so let's continue. . .

One of the major byproducts of normal metabolism are acids (uric acid, lactic acid, pyruvic acid), and one of the main jobs of our metabolism to keep our body out of an overly acidic condition. Since many foods and substances, we ingest are either acidic in their own right or create more acid in our body, it's easy for us to slip into an overly acid state. Acids are corrosive, which means they eat away and dissolve things. Too much acid is obviously not a good thing, and the body counters it by mobilizing alkaline (the opposite of acid) minerals out of tissues. Calcium and phosphorus may be taken out of bones and magnesium taken out of the blood and muscle to neutralize the acid, but this can result in the demineralization and weakening of these tissues.

If the acid isn't neutralized fairly quickly, the acidic wastes can accumulate and become stored in a person's tissues, causing them to corrode. This acidic corrosion is essentially a burning (think of what battery acid would do to your skin) – a steady fire that is slowly dissolving the tissues from the inside out.

How do you put out a fire? By dowsing it with water and diluting it until it is no longer raging. The body does this by rushing water with minerals to the site with the acidic build-up, resulting in swelling, inflammation, or edema. These inconveniences are actions the body takes to put out the fire so repairs can get started as soon as possible. They should not be interrupted or suppressed if true healing is to occur. If you take an anti-inflammatory or anti-histamine to stop the swelling, you are stopping the dilution of the acid, and it will continue to eat away at tissue causing more problems later.

An example of why cavities form in teeth illustrates how effects can be mistaken as cause and how the bacteria involved are reactive rather than proactive. We've been told that eating too many sweets will cause cavities. This leads to the misconception that sugar is directly causing holes to develop in our teeth, which is not the primary or even secondary reason cavities are formed. If there is excessive plaque build-up on your teeth, the bacteria that reside among the plaque and the teeth will naturally metabolize their food, which produces very acidic bacterial waste products. These acid waste products demineralize, or corrode, the teeth.(178) These bacteria thrive on carbohydrates (sugar), so they grow and proliferate when it's available. More sugar causes more bacterial growth, which causes more acidic waste, which causes more tooth corrosion.

The sugar didn't cause the corrosion and neither did the bacteria. It's the waste (the acid) from the bacteria that caused it. If you remove the sugar, you eliminate the food for the bacteria and stop the bacterial proliferation, which eliminates the acid wastes and the teeth stay strong and whole.

The bacteria only grow when food – in this case, sugar – is present. They cannot cause harm, unless they can grow, and if there's nothing there for them to eat, they won't. (For completeness, cavities also develop because the teeth are not just demineralized from the outside by the acidic waste from the bacteria, but from the inside due to calcium being extracted from the teeth to keep the blood pH from getting too acidic – similar to when bones get dissolved due to acidic conditions causing osteoporosis.)

This is a perfect illustration of not only how bacteria function in our mouths, but in our whole body as well. They only proliferate when a food source is available (bacteria or viruses cannot eat live human tissue). Think about it – would bacteria, or any other living thing, live and grow where there's no food? Of course not. They are significantly smaller than our cells (if a virus is the size of a baseball, a bacterium would be the size of the pitcher's mound, and a human cell would be the size of the whole baseball stadium), produce waste relative to their size, and are significantly less complex than our cells. They don't have a nervous system or endocrine system. They don't have bones and muscles. They don't communicate with each other. Bacteria don't even have a cell nucleus, which is the part of the cell where the most complicated cellular processes occur (it stores the cell's hereditary material, or DNA, and it coordinates the cell's activities, which include growth, intermediary metabolism, protein synthesis, and reproduction [cell division]).

Bacteria and viruses (which are not even alive) don't have guns, grenades or nuclear weapons, and don't possess magic. We're ascribing all this power to a class of organisms that is nothing special or powerful believing they can bring us to our knees or worse. It's like saying a small band of midget Neanderthals with sticks and rocks can defeat the combined forces of the U.S. military. They can't. You and your intricate matrix of highly evolved, complex cells, are more powerful than microscopic one-celled, primitive, scavengers.

Many cultures all over the world consume bacteria-rich foods on purpose believing they gain health and endurance from them. The Hunzas in Pakistan, Eskimos, Masai, and Samburo tribes of Africa and others regularly consume foods that, according to the germ theory, would be considered pathogenic. In fact, the Hunzas are one of the longest lived people on earth and daily drink raw milk laden with *Salmonella* and *E. coli.* The Eskimos bury their meat in hides for up to six weeks, which increases the bacterial content and when ingested, elevates the mood and increases endurance. This meat is called *high meat* since it makes you feel so good, you feel high. The Chinese emperors used *century eggs* (decomposed eggs aged up to 25 years that have a ton of bacteria) as an aphrodisiac. By modern medicine's standards all these people should have died from pathogenic infections centuries ago.

Nutritionist Dr. Vonderplanitz, reports,

"From desperation, I tried eating raw meats. Thousands of times, I ate raw meats and raw milk that were "microbe-infected" during my 32 years of experimentation and everyday life. According to the assumptions of the medical and scientific communities, I should have suffered bacterial or parasitic food poisoning thousand of times. I did not. Not once. Thousands of other 'at-risk' individuals who switched to eating raw animal products to reverse their diseases and/or to improve their health also did not get sick. I discovered in studies of diarrhea and vomit that more often there were higher concentrations of bacteria in people who ate cooked food than in people who ate raw food. How, then, can the medical and scientific communities adhere to the belief that raw food causes bacterial food poisoning? Their belief is based in fear, with no more rationale than the belief in evil spirits that motivated the witch hunts of medieval times."(179)

Dr. Vonderplanitz has taken a page out of the Eskimo's book and regularly eats, as do many of his clients, his version of high meat: meat that has aged at least a month in the refrigerator in a sealed jar (airing it out every 4 days). During this time, the meat is decomposing due to the active bacteria, which are multiplying and changing form rapidly (going through 17 different stages – the stages Dr. Bechamp talked about with his theory of pleomorphism). He says that eating this meat elevates the mood, reduces pain, reduces waste in the body, and is one of the best things to help cleanse the body.

To some it may sound risky and gross, but hey, I've gotta walk the talk, right? So several years ago I tried it. I put some chunks of beef in a Mason jar, sealed it, and put it in the refrigerator. After about a month, after airing it out a couple of times a week, I took a tentative nibble – and waited for death. But death never came. Since then I've eaten meat aged for over 10 months this way, and find not only does it not bother me in any way (apart from the smell and taste), but clears my sinuses and really does make me happier. Now I eat it several times a week, if not daily. The germs are actually tiny *Pac-men*, who gobble up bodily waste and then are excreted in the feces. (Do NOT do this with cooked meat! Cooked meat contains many toxins, which the bacteria ingest, and will make you sick.)

Consider recent research using microorganisms to treat cancer: *Salmonella* has been used by researchers at Yale University to reverse cancer. Cancer is also being treated with "pathogens" at other notable research facilities: Duke University is using a measles virus; Stanford is using the common cold virus; Harvard is using a herpes virus; and the Mayo Clinic is using a measles virus.[180]

Dr. Henry Heimlich, the originator of the Heimlich Maneuver, has used malaria germs to treat cancer through a process he calls malariotherapy. He contends that introducing the malaria bacteria into the body causes the body to produce heat (fever), which helps eradicate the tumors. He says that his work is based on the work of Julius Wagner-Jauregg, who reported that malariotherapy cured neurosyphilis, and who was awarded the 1918 Nobel Prize in Medicine in 1927 for his work.[181]

Researchers at Johns Hopkins University in Baltimore ". . .have given a new meaning to the term 'friendly bacteria' by discovering a bacterial protein that helps treat cancer," as reported in the journal *Chemistry World* in 2006.[182]

Treating cancer with germs is not something new. A 2003 article in the *Journal of Bacteriology* published by the American Society for Microbiology, reported,

"The use of bacteria or their extracts in the treatment of cancer goes back more than 100 years. . .physician and surgeon William B. Coley of the. . .Memorial Sloan–Kettering Hospital, observed that many of his patients with various forms of cancer had their tumors regress when they were infected with bacterial pathogens. Treatment to eliminate the infections allowed the cancer to come back. . .Several well-coordinated studies have shown a clear relationship between the use of *M. bovis BcG* [a bacterium] immunoprophylaxis after surgical removal of the tumor and the decreased recurrence rate or the delayed period during which recurrence could occur. . .Bacteria such as *Salmonella* are also known to target tumor cells for growth and proliferation and attenuated *Salmonella* mutants, when injected. . .in. . .mice, were reported to allow tumor regression and prolonged survival to the mice. Similar use of *Shigella* and *Clostridia*. . .has been reported."(183)

S.A. Hoption Cann from the Department of Health Care and Epidemiology at the University of British Columbia, Canada sites work by Dr. William Coley that says, "Spontaneous tumor regression has followed bacterial, fungal, viral, and protozoa infections. . .He observed that inducing a fever was crucial for tumor regression. . ."(184)

This leads us into reconsidering the role fever (elevated body temperature) plays in disease. Most people have been led to believe that fever is bad and will cause harm (brain damage) if it isn't suppressed using drugs. However, many doctors used to believe that anytime there's an elevated body temperature (fever or inflammation), the body is in fact in the healing phase, not the disease phase, and this is necessary not just for healing, but sometimes for survival. For thousands of years fever was considered a protective response, and fevers were induced by physicians to combat certain infections. But with the advent of antipyretic drugs, physicians started to reduce fevers, and fever therapy was virtually abandoned. Edda West of the Vaccination Risk Awareness Network, Inc., (VRAN) in Canada, says,

"There is plenty of scientific evidence validating the benefits of fever in fighting viral/bacterial inflammations and its important role in the healing process. Fever increases survival rate during infectious diseases – basic information that has yet to reach the majority of people who remain misinformed and misled by pharmaceutical and medical propaganda which still shamelessly advocates the use of antipyretic [anti-fever] drugs at the first sign of fever. The myth that untreated fevers will lead to seizures and brain damage is perpetuated ad nauseam. Fever is maligned, misunderstood and seen as an enemy to be feared rather than an ally that signals the immune system gearing up for action. Aspirin was once commonly used to suppress fever until it was linked to Reye's syndrome when given to children. . .Reye's syndrome is an often fatal disease affecting the brain and liver, a primary reason doctors switched to acetaminophen, which we now know to be the major cause of liver failure. One disease after another!. . .A recently published article identified acetaminophen overdose as the number one cause of acute liver failure in the U.S. . .Often several preparations of the same brand (*Tylenol Pain*, *Tylenol Sinus*) or several medications for the same symptom (*Tylenol Cold*, *Neo-Citran* and *Sinutab*) are found in the same household and, when used together, can result in an overdose."(185)

Dr. Robert Mendelsohn, a pediatrician and author of *How to Raise a Healthy Child in Spite of Your Doctor* says,

"If your child contracts and infection, the fever that accompanies it is a blessing, not a curse. . .High fevers do not cause convulsions. There is no evidence that those who do have them suffer any serious aftereffects as a result."(186) A study reported in the journal *Pediatrics* said, "Studies. . .have shown that moderate fevers increase survival rate. Many components of the nonspecific host defense response to infection. . .appear to be enhanced by elevations in temperature that simulate moderate fevers."(187)

In a vaccine risk conference in 2000, Dr. Philip Incao cited a study showing this saying,

"The doctors began to think that the higher fevers and rash helped clear the measles virus from the body and enhanced survival. So half-way through this measles epidemic, the doctors revised their treatment and gave no sedatives, no aspirin, or *Tylenol*, nor cough suppressants. . .In this group. . .only 7 percent died compared to 35 percent in the first group [who were given the drugs]. This is a dramatic demonstration, and there are many others, of the vitally important basic principle that it is dangerous to suppress an inflammatory discharge."(188)

It's not just death that can result from suppressing a fever, but long-term chronic health problems too. Some believe that fever suppressant drugs may contribute to the development of autism, allergies, and autoimmune problems. Dr. Incao explains,

"What I read. . .confirmed what I experienced in my own practice, that the children who produced higher fevers and strong rashes, and good discharges of mucous and pus, were healthier and more robust and had stronger immune systems than the children who produced a low intensity of these symptoms. These robust children in my practice. . .had had little or no antibiotics, or antipyretics, or vaccinations in their lives. And the other children who had had all their vaccinations, and lots of antipyretics, and antibiotics – who had had a lot of suppressive, internalizing medical treatments – these children never got high fevers. And these children were the ones who were more likely to have allergies and autoimmune problems."(189)

When we consume toxins, our body tries to eliminate them and it's usually successful using the colon, kidneys, skin, and lungs to do this. But if there are more toxins than these organs of elimination can handle, the body tries to get rid of them in other ways. You may get a runny nose, diarrhea, or a skin eruption. The body may speed up its metabolism to get rid of the toxins faster, raising your temperature and making you feel ill since toxins are now in your bloodstream. Usually, mucus is produced to wrap around toxins and escort them through the lymphatic system and out the body.

This mucus, along with the toxins themselves, is food for the bacteria. Just like the waste in the wastewater is the carbon source for the bacteria, the mucus and toxins within you are too. The bacteria grow, multiply, and may change form. Since their environment is now filled with toxins, they may become toxic themselves, just like we become toxic if we consume toxic things.

If you let go of an apple, it will fall downward every time. If you expose your body to toxins past its ability to handle them, and/or don't nourish your cells correctly, you will become compromised or sick, in one way or another depending on your constitutional weaknesses, every time. There are no exceptions. The reaction by the body may be acute, as with the common cold or the flu, or it may be chronic, as with diabetes, heart disease, arthritis, etc. There's no need for a research grant or an electron microscope. There's no need for complicated theories or the excuse of blaming genetics. There are no "we don't really know whys," and it doesn't take a Ph.D. to understand. It is the real, and only, cause of disease.

Excess Toxins plus Deficient Nutrition equals Disease. Or conversely, No Toxins plus Good Nutrition equals Health: NT + GN = H. This is your simple formula for health. It is true now, and will be true forever, no matter how society changes or technology advances.

Albert Einstein said, "Any intelligent fool can make things bigger, more complex, and more violent. It takes a touch of genius – and a lot of courage – to move in the opposite direction." His formula that changed the world was simple too: $E=mc^2$ (Energy equals mass times the speed of light squared.)

What's the bottom line? Here's the new paradigm for disease: The whole thing – the whole immune system – is nothing but a very intricate, refined, and amazingly efficient waste elimination system. That's all it is. Just like on the macroscopic scale, we eat and we poop – the same thing takes place on the microscopic scale; our cells eat and they poop. In addition, just like our bodies suffer when exposed to poisons, our cells suffer when they're exposed to poisons too. Germs (bacteria and viruses, if they really exist), are nothing but scavengers who multiply and may change form when sufficient waste (from normal cellular processes and toxic overload) is available. When the body has become overly toxic, it may speed up its metabolism (fever, rash) to get rid of the waste quicker. Anytime we interfere with these natural events, we are suppressing the disease and it will just reappear at another time with different symptoms. Note all the degenerative diseases the elderly, and now, not so elderly have. If we allow the scavengers to help us and the fevers to cleanse us, in the long run, we'll be healthier and feel better. Remember, the less bad food (or toxic substances) you put in your body, the less the body will need to cleanse itself, and the fewer fevers and cleansing reactions you will have. The old engineering saying is true – GIGO – which stands for, Garbage In, Garbage Out. If you put garbage into an equation (or the body), you're going to get garbage coming out.

But just calling it a "waste elimination system" isn't very cool or catchy. It's best if we make it sound complicated and sexy, then all the experts

won't be embarrassed to call is something so mundane. So here it is –
drum-roll please. . .The "immune system" is no longer relevant, and we are
replacing it with the term, The Intra and Extra-cellular Debris Elimination
and Acid-Base Maintenance System, or IDEAMS for short. Is that cool
enough? Now when someone gets sick, the doctor can say, "Ah, your
IDEAMS must be stressed." You'll nod your head in acknowledgement,
"Yes! That's it! My IDEAMS has been very stressed! How did you know,
doctor?"

With the IDEAMS you need not be afraid of being sneezed on or
catching syphilis from a toilet seat. You need not be afraid of drinking from
the same cup or getting bodily fluids on you in the wrong places. You need
not be so afraid you sanitize (and poison) just about everything, including
the handle on the buggy in the grocery store. You'll realize you don't need
vaccines, antibiotics, and drugs that curb fever.

You see, bacteria are a necessary thing, and are a big reason humans
exist. Many scientists believe that mitochondria, the bacteria-like looking
organelles inside a cell that produce energy for the cell, are the vestige of
bacteria that adapted to have a symbiotic relationship with the cell. Bacteria
outside the cell also have a symbiotic relationship with us – by consuming
waste and toxicity.

Personally, I am not just unafraid of germs, I appreciate them and the
work they do for me. They help me digest my food, produce vitamins I
need, consume toxins in my body, and help me eliminate them. However,
as much as I like germs, I do not encourage unsanitary conditions.
Cleanliness is good – it is order. Anything in order is in harmony and is
more efficient, and is therefore, healthier.

However, cleanliness is not poisonliness: the use of poisons
(antibiotics, antimicrobial cleansers, sanitizers) that actually create a kind of
disorder by killing off what should naturally be there. Be clean by using
natural things (water, vinegar, lemon, baking soda), keeping your house in
order, and taking out the garbage regularly – just like all those billions of
cells inside you do.

Yes, when you finally know deep in your bones that germs are friends,
not foes, you'll experience a freedom you never knew existed. Remember
how you felt the first time you rode your bike without training wheels? Wow,
what a feeling! "Hey," you said to yourself, "I didn't fall down and get hurt. I
didn't scrape a knee or bang my head or anything! This is fun!" And then it
dawns on you, "Now I can ride my bike all the way down to the end of the
street. Even around the corner and to my friend's house! Then maybe to
the park or school yard. Boy-oh-boy, I can go anywhere I want and not
have to worry about falling and getting hurt!" What a feeling of freedom –
and power! Realizing that germs cannot hurt you will make you feel the
same way. You'll KNOW that you can go anywhere in the world and not

have to worry about catching anything. You'll feel invincible. You'll feel like *Superman* or *Superwoman*. It's freedom. It's a blast. And it's the truth.

Just as there's a price to pay for political and social freedom, there's a price to pay for biological freedom too. You have to be vigilant in order to keep that freedom. That means giving up the sugar, junk foods, and so on and living in harmony with nature. Then nature (and all those germs) will live harmoniously in you.

If you're raised your whole life being told something over and over again, especially by authority figures, it's hard to consider another point of view. Hitler and his goons convinced a whole generation of Germans that Jews were the dregs of the earth and should be exterminated. He said, "If you tell a lie long enough, loud enough, and often enough, people will believe it." It happens.

I realize believing that germs don't cause disease is a stretch for most people – even most natural doctors have never even considered it. But whether germs cause disease or not doesn't really matter because one thing is undeniable: a healthy body does not get sick, even when exposed to germs. That's because either that person has a strong enough "immune system" to fight the germs off, or germs don't cause disease. Take your pick.

If believing that you should get healthy to build up your immune system to fight all those germs who are out to get you is how you want to look at it, that's fine – you'll still have the incentive to improve your health, which is the important thing. If you can understand that germs are not to fear and can actually be helpful, then you also have the incentive to get healthy, because by being so, you won't have to deal with excess waste that causes uncomfortable cleansing reactions and allows germs to multiply.

Whichever is the real truth, your goal is still the same: Do the things in harmony with nature so you can get healthy enough to avoid, and reverse, virtually any disease.

One of the main objectives of this book is to empower you and your family. Knowledge and understanding of our bodies and the environment goes far in this regard. To live in a state of fear and worry does not, especially when it's unwarranted. Remember, many companies make a lot of money from people in fear so they will naturally tend to emphasize the fear factor. The more knowledge and understanding you acquire, the less fear you will have, and the less vulnerable you'll be to deception.

Do me a favor. . .for just a moment or two, imagine that the next time you go to the doctor, he/she greets you with a big smile and handshake, sits you down on the examining table, looks you in the eye, and says, "Boy! Have I got some exciting news! The Harvard School of Medicine, the Mayo Clinic, the American Medical Association, Johns Hopkins Medical School, the FDA and CDC, are all reporting an amazing new scientific discovery and advance in medicine. Here – look at this. . .There's an article in the

Journal of the American Medical Association all about it! The headline reads, 'Germ Theory of Disease Found to be Scientifically Invalid. New Research Proves Bacteria Actually Benefit Mankind!' I knew there was something fishy going on with vaccines and antibiotics and all this fear of germs! But now we have the research to prove it!"

What would you believe then? Really. Think about it. What if since you were a child, you saw ads on TV with smiling, happy people running through fields replete with flowers and butterflies, telling you to take your germs because they're good for you. What do you think you'd believe? Instead of going to the local pharmacist for your dose of toxic drugs, you would go to your local germacist to get your next fresh batch of health-promoting bacteria (or just grow them yourself in your refrigerator)!

Eventually, something similar is going to happen. I predict that in the coming years you're going to hear more and more about "good" bacteria (probiotics) and new ways to use these bacteria to treat diseases. You'll hear about studies like the one published in the journal *Critical Care* reporting that probiotics (germs) are just as effective in preventing pneumonia in critically ill patients as the standard antiseptic treatment currently used – without the nasty side effects and allergic reactions.(190)

Or that researchers at the Albert Einstein College of Medicine said probiotics ". . .may be used to prevent and treat antibiotic-associated diarrhea and acute infectious diarrhea. . .effective in relieving symptoms of irritable bowel syndrome and in treating atopic dermatitis in children. Significant adverse effects are rare, and there are no known interactions with medication."(191)

Other pro-germ things I've read recently include: "The Gut Flora [germs] Plays a Major Role in Metabolizing Dietary Carcinogens," "Bacteria Are Also Implicated in Preventing Allergies," "Some Forms of Bacteria Can Prevent Inflammation." "Certain Bacteria Found in Dirt Can Lift Depression."

The powers-that-be won't admit germs as a whole don't cause disease and are actually good for you – that will come in the next generation (about 30 years from now) – when most of the old-guard doctors and scientists have gone to that great laboratory in the sky. So for now, you'll hear more and more about all the wonderful things probiotics (germs) can do for you as if it's a great new medical advance. Then it will kind of be forgotten or ignored that we once believed germs cause disease. A few years after that, people will look back and shake their heads wondering how we could have believed such nonsense.

Once this drug-chemo-surgery-radiation generation becomes sterile and kills itself off, the only ones left will be a new generation of people who accept not the dogma thrust upon them, but common sense truths. Just as we marvel at the absurdity of drilling a hole in someone's head to relieve evil spirits, the new generation will marvel at the absurdity of injecting poisons into someone's (and especially a child's) arm to prevent disease. If you live long enough to see my prediction come true, just remember, you read it first here.

I'd like to close this section with some notable quotes that echo my thoughts on germs, vaccines, and natural health:

"You cannot have a very severe round of typhoid fever unless you have a 'first-class' physician to give it strength to down you. . .I have not lost a case in 15 years (including typhoid and pneumonia), and I have treated hundreds. Fatality is attributable to the medication." *Dr. John Tilden - a famous natural healer, 1851-1940.* (192)

"Smallpox is considered one of the most virulent of contagious diseases, and it is generally believed that persons exposed are almost invariably attacked, unless protected by vaccination. This is one of the most stupendous exaggerations to be found in medical literature. My experience has been that very few people take it when exposed to it." *Dr. JohnTilden*

"...intelligent people do not have their children vaccinated...The result is not...the extermination of the human race. . . .on the contrary more people are now killed by vaccination. . . " *George Bernard Shaw.*(193)

"Vaccines and serums are employed as substitutes for right living; they are intended to supplant obedience to the laws of life. Such programs are slaps in the face of law and order. Belief in immunizations is a form of delusional insanity." *Herbert Shelton, D.C., famous natural healer* (194)

"I have myself. . .over 16 years, treated all forms and hundreds of cases of typhus and typhoid fevers, pneumonias, measles and dysenteries and have not lost a single patient. The same is true of scarlet and other fevers. No medicine whatever was given." *R.T. Trall, M.D.*

"These diseases (typhoid and pneumonia) are nothing more nor less than a cleansing process – a struggle of the vital powers to relieve the system of its accumulated impurities. The causes of the diseases are constipating foods, contaminated water, atmospheric miasmas, and whatever clogs up the system or befouls the blood. And the day is not far distant when a physician who shall undertake to aid and assist (suppress) nature in her efforts to expel impurities, by the administration of poisons (drugs, medicines, shots, radiation, etc.) will be regarded as an insane idiot. But now this practice is called medical science." *R.T. Trall, M.D.*

"To give drugs is adding to the causes of disease; for drugs always produce disease. Indeed, they cure one disease, when they cure at all, by producing others. Can causes cure causes? Can poisons expel poisons? Can Nature throw off two or more burdens more easily than one? No, never. Poisoning a person because he is impure is like casting out devils through Beelzebub, the prince of devils. It is neither Scriptural nor philosophical. The effect of drug-curing or drug-killing, as the case may be – I mean drug medication – is to lock up, as it were, the causes of the disease within the system, and to induce chronic and worse diseases. The causes should be expelled, not retained. The remedial struggle – the disease – should be aided, regulated, directed, so that it may successfully accomplish its work of purification, not subdued nor thwarted with poisons which create new remedial efforts (drug diseases), and thus embarrass and complicate the vital struggle. To give drugs is to give the living system more work to do. It is aiding and assisting the enemy. It is, in effect, very much like fighting the rebels by firing at our own soldiers in the rear, while they are attacking the enemy in front. Can our army manage two adversaries better than one? It is like tying one hand fast. . .and going at the rebels with the other. Had you not better employ both hands?" *R.T. Trall, M.D.* (195)

I suggest you read this section over and think about it. Put aside popular opinion and even what you think you believe, and consider this from a blank slate. You can go on living in fear, or you can realize that you are the one in control of all aspects of your health. The choice is yours.

Franklin D. Roosevelt said in his presidential inaugural address on March 4, 1933, "The only thing we have to fear, is fear itself." I'd like to make a modern revision to that:

"The only thing to fear, is what we do to ourselves."

Courage, my friend, courage. Because courage is making up your own mind when someone tries to make it up for you. Courage is being healthy when the whole world is sick. Courage is saying no when you have to and yes when you don't. Courage makes you realize you don't need to hurt someone else to help yourself. Courage is the ability to accept the bad times and weather the storms, and the good times and bask in the sunshine. Courage sets you apart, sets you free, and is the first thing you need when you want to change.

Courage is knowing what not to fear.   *Plato*

Courage is being scared to death – and saddling up anyway.
                                                John Wayne

Courage doesn't always roar. Sometimes courage is a little voice at the end of the day that says I'll try again tomorrow.
                                                Mary Anne Radmacher

Have the courage to live. Anyone can die.
                                                Robert Cody

One man with courage makes a majority.
                                                Andrew Jackson

Courage is the power to let go of the familiar.
                                                Raymond Lindquist.

Courage is what it takes to stand up and speak; courage is also what it takes to sit down and listen.   *Winston Churchill*

Courage, my friend, courage.

CHAPTER XVI

The Ancestry Factor

It's highly evident that the health of adults and children is not what it should be. The incidences of degenerative diseases such as cancer and diabetes have increased dramatically over the past 50 years. Disorders such as ADHD that were once rarities are now commonplace. Violent crimes, even by children and adolescents, are happening with greater and greater frequency. It appears that instead of evolving to some higher state of being, we are actually degenerating into a sick, miserable, and highly stressed society. With all our medical knowledge, it seems paradoxical that this is happening. The omnipresent question is, why?

As we have already explored, there are many contributing factors to this dilemma. Pesticides, lead, sugar, water pollution, chemicals, food additives, vaccines, foods lacking in nutrition, TV – the list seems endless. Each one is a straw added onto our backs. As they get piled higher and higher, it gets harder and harder to function normally – physically, mentally, emotionally, and spiritually.

One of the most disturbing trends is that diseases are happening to people at a younger and younger age. First, cancer was rare and only the aged would get it. Now it's commonplace for people to be getting cancer and dying from it in their thirties and younger. Autopsies of teenagers are showing significant amounts of atherosclerosis – their arteries are that of what is expected in an elderly person. One estimate is that by the year 2020, people living in industrialized countries will not be able to successfully reproduce – they will be functionally sterile.(1)

Although the effects of environmental stresses on people are the best evidence we can use, much knowledge is gained by performing experiments on animals. There's been enough scientific evidence to show that experiments on lab animals can be successfully interpreted to be used as guidelines for humans.

An intriguing experiment was conducted on numerous generations of cats between the years of 1932 and 1942. It was not performed under the same scientific protocol as experiments are today, but it was quite advanced for its time. The important thing to realize is that the experiment showed a trend that can be extrapolated to apply to any living system. For example, if I put a cat's paw over a flame, it will get burned. If I put my own hand over the flame, I too will get burned. (Singeing cat's paws was not the experiment – I use this only to illustrate my point.) I know there could be many objections to my thesis in this chapter – from "cats are not people" to highly sophisticated arguments using quantum physics to prove that any experiment is affected by the consciousness of the observer, but let's not throw the baby out with the bathwater. What you are about to learn concerning the cats in this 10-year experiment could be the same thing or at least similar to what's happening to us as a species. All signs point to it as far as I can tell. In fact, it was this evidence and my realization of its profound meaning that led me to write this book. Some people can rationalize anything away. Whether you accept or reject my ideas, here is up to you. But I think that if you observe what is happening in our society, you may agree it's plausible. If you do, you'll see that there is a need to change the direction of our vessel, because right now, it's headed into the perfect storm.

Back to the study: Francis Pottenger Jr., M.D., performed the experiment on more than 900 cats to determine why the cats he was using in some of his other experiments were poor operative risks. Excerpts from the introduction (written by his wife, Elaine Pottenger) of his classic work titled *Pottenger's Cats – A Study In Nutrition,* is fitting. . .

> In his effort to maximize the preoperative health of his laboratory animals, Francis fed them a diet of market grade raw milk, cod liver oil and cooked meat scraps. . . This diet was considered to be rich in all the important nutritive substances by the experts of the day. . . Therefore, Francis was perplexed as to why his cats were poor operative risks. In seeking an explanation, he began noticing that the cats showed signs of deficiency. All showed a decrease in their reproductive capacity and many of the kittens born in the laboratory had skeletal deformities and organ malfunctions.[2]
>
> Pottenger divided the cats into numerous groups and fed them different diets. The result of his study showed that the cats on deficient diets developed: heart problems; nearsightedness and farsightedness; under activity of the thyroid or inflammation of the thyroid gland; infections of the kidney, of the liver, of the testes, of the ovaries and of the bladder; arthritis and inflammation of the joints; inflammation of the nervous system with paralysis and meningitis. . .[The] cats show much more irritability. Some females are even dangerous to handle because of their proclivity for biting and scratching. . .The males, on the other hand, are more docile, often to the point of being nonaggressive and their sex interest is slack or perverted. In essence, there is evidence of a role reversal with the female cats becoming the aggressors and the male cats becoming passive as well as evidence of increasing abnormal activities between the same sexes. Such sexual deviations are not observed among the raw food cats.[3] [Note: the "raw food cats" were fed exclusively raw, uncooked food, which was seen to be sufficient (i.e., not deficient) for these cats.]
>
> The cats fed deficient diets resulted in heterogeneous reproduction and physical degeneration, *increasing with each*

generation. Kittens of third generation cats failed to survive six months. Vermin and parasites abounded. Skin diseases and allergies increased from an incidence of 5 percent in normal cats to over 90 percent in the third-generation. Bones became soft and pliable; calcium and phosphorus content diminished. The cats suffered from adverse personality changes. Females became more aggressive while males became docile. The cats suffered from hypothyroidism and most of the degenerative diseases encountered in human medicine. *They died out completely by the fourth generation. . .*(4) By the time the third deficient generation is born, the cats are so physiologically bankrupt that none survive beyond the sixth month of life, thereby terminating the strain. . .A study of the microscopic sections of the lungs of the second- and third-generation deficient cats show abnormal respiratory tissues. The lungs show hyperemia, some edema and partial atelectasis, (incomplete expansion of the lungs at birth) while the most deficient show bronchitis and pneumonitis. . .At autopsy, cooked meat-fed females frequently present ovarian atrophy and uterine congestion, and the males often show failure in the development of active spermatogenesis. Abortion in pregnant females is common, running about 25 percent in the first deficient generation to about 70 percent in the second generation. Deliveries are generally difficult with many females dying in labor. The mortality rate of the kittens also is high as the kittens are either born dead or are born too frail to nurse. Following delivery, a few mother cats steadily decline in health only to die from some obscure physiological exhaustion in about three months. Other cats show increasing difficulty with their pregnancies and in many instances fail to become pregnant. The mother cats that were fed the deficient diets eventually showed no inclination to care for their offspring. They could not nurse their kittens because their mammary glands were not developed enough for lactation.(5) (Emphasis mine.)

As you can see, there are many similarities to the health of the cats fed deficient diets and the state of our own health:

- *Heart problems, vision problems, kidney, liver, testicle, ovary, bladder problems, arthritis, nervous disorders* – all are reaching epidemic proportions in our society.
- *Irritability* – we and our children are becoming more violent. We are constantly stressed. Violence is in demand in the movies, on TV, and in video games.
- *Sexual deviation* – a deviation from normal biological sexual behavior. Perversion on the Internet and seemingly everywhere else. Role reversal

is occurring where women are more dominant than men. Not just that, but men are becoming women and women are becoming men.

- *Skin diseases and allergies* – who doesn't seem to have allergies these days? Now they are advertising allergy medicine that can be taken by children as young as four years old.

- *Bone became soft and pliable* – soft and pliable bones (osteoporosis) are rampant among the elderly and even teenagers are showing signs of it. Hip replacements are commonplace.

- *Personality changes* – how many times have you seen on TV reports of someone committing a crime no one thought he or she was capable of committing? Adults and children are becoming more distant, reserved, and depressed.

- *Abnormal respiratory tissues* – asthma is increasing at an alarming rate and is at epidemic proportions – especially in our young.

- *Ovarian atrophy and uterine congestion* – blocked fallopian tubes causing infertility.

- *Failure in the development of active spermatogenesis* – male sperm counts are plummeting.

- *Abortion in pregnant females is common* – by this, Dr. Pottenger meant miscarriages. They are increasing in women, especially those who have been exposed to toxic chemicals.

- *No inclination to care for their offspring* – have a baby, put it in day care, and go back to work. Some parents care more about their careers than raising their children. Most have to get a job or a second job to make ends meet. (This itself is a reflection of our stressed society.)

Food for Thought

There are a couple points here I'd like to comment on. The *sexual deviation* definition is by no means a judgment. It is morally neither right nor wrong. However, it is a deviation from the normal biological processes that nature has in place to propagate the species. In that sense, it is a deviation. I'm speaking from a strictly biological point of view. I personally do not care what sexual preference someone has – that's up to them. But there may be biological and physiological causes that manifest psychologically – just as there appeared to be in cases of violence, ADHD, depression, etc.

As for the lack of inclination of diseased cats to care for their off-spring, I see it as a ramification of biological and physiological deficiencies that affect organisms to act in certain ways. If someone is healthy and whole, he or she will likely be loving and caring. If someone is out of sorts and in any kind of diseased or degenerative state, he or she is likely to be more concerned with themselves and less loving and caring towards others. Are you more likely to lose your temper when you're in a good mood and feeling well, or when you're stressed out and feeling poorly? If your body itself is under some sort of physiological stress – from chemicals,

> pesticides, diet, and so on – you'll be more likely to be irritable and selfish. The uncaring atmosphere of our society is, in my opinion, in large part due to subtle biological stresses from environmental stressors that are difficult to avoid and have accumulated in us over the past three generations.

In a way all these aberrations are not our fault. We are victims of our environment (although we as a society created it). It's not a question of willpower to overcome these inadequacies and transgressions. If I'm missing an arm, all the willpower in the world won't give me the power to clap my hands. If my biological system is missing a key nutrient or is hampered by a pollutant that interferes with normal biological function, how can I be at my best? How can I be giving and loving when my own body is crying out in pain and needing attention? How can a child read and write correctly and have a normal attention span if his brain has not developed properly?

What will become of us? In the cat study, the cats on the deficient diet eventually got so diseased and nonfunctional that they could no longer reproduce and went extinct. I call this law of nature "The Ancestry Factor": *An organism under stress or nourished inadequately will pass on its degenerations and weaknesses to its offspring, making that generation weaker and more susceptible to disease earlier in life. This will continue through the generations until reproduction is no longer possible.*

The high infertility rate we are experiencing in our society parallel's those in the cat study. Each generation is becoming less and less efficient at reproducing and carrying on normal reproductive activities. Fertility drugs are prescribed to the tune of a billion dollars a year. *Viagra* and other pharmaceutical solutions to impotency abound. We look to science and think it will solve all our problems. We trust with religious fervor that our intellect and technology will make everything better. But can it? Is it more powerful than nature and the laws of biochemistry and physics themselves?

Throughout this book I have attempted to detail the changes that have occurred in our society over the last century. From the exodus from the small farms to the cities during the industrial revolution to the introduction of pesticides (spawned out of chemical warfare during World War I) to the use of lead and its eventual ban in paint to the escalation in the consumption of sugar, soft drinks, food additives, and nutrient deficient foods, and the use of drugs such as *Ritalin*. All of these things have occurred so quickly that we really haven't taken the time to examine closely enough what their long-term and sometimes even short-term effects might be. We are a proud, sometimes egotistical society that believes that we are not subject to physical law – that even though a pesticide will kill a bug, it won't do us any harm. We myopically believe that food additives are metabolized and have no effect on us or that drinking caffeinated beverages, alcohol, and eating tons of sugar a year are magically rendered harmless.

We are also trusting. We trust that the government will tell us if and when something is bad. The FDA, CDC, EPA, and international organizations such as the WHO, are our watchdogs. If they say something is OK, then it must be so. After all, we have the best universities and research facilities the world has ever seen filled with the brightest minds; they'll tell us when something isn't right. So we go on eating, drinking, consuming harmful foods and beverages, and we continue to subject ourselves to unhealthy environments at work and at home – much out of simple ignorance, some out of egotistical denial, some out of greed, and some out of laziness. The ramifications of this ignorance, denial, greed, and laziness are disastrous. You or someone you love may develop a brain tumor, leukemia, attention deficit disorder, diabetes, cancer, or asthma. He or she may struggle with learning, struggle with others, struggle with their temper, struggle with reality itself. All because he or she has been subjected to agents and conditions not in harmony with the human body.

In the Pottenger's Cats study, the diets that were shown to be deficient were ones that included predominantly cooked meat and cooked milk or condensed milk. The diets shown to be healthy were all raw; no cooked meat and no pasteurized milk. It's easy to come to the conclusion then that a raw-food diet is healthy and a cooked-food diet is deficient. Although an all raw-food diet can be very healthy, it is not the only point of this discussion. There are very few people who will go on an all raw-food diet. And although cooking does destroy many vital nutrients, it also renders some harmful substances in food harmless or makes some foods easier for the human digestive tract to handle.

In exploring the scientific literature further, another reason the cats became sick on the cooked-food diet emerges. It's now known that an essential amino acid of cats is taurine (recall that *essential* means the nutrient must be procured from an outside source – the body cannot manufacture it on its own).[6] Cooking destroys taurine. Since this is now known, cat foods are fortified with taurine. That's why we still have cats around today. Since commercial cat food is cooked and processed, if cooking were the only reason their diets so deficient, then cats would have become sick and died out long ago.

The point here is that the cats' diet was *deficient*. The reason why it was deficient is not as important as the fact that the cats developed diseases and died out on that deficient diet. Even though cats are not people, aren't they subject to the same laws of nature people are?

A typical toxicology study will look at the lethal dose of a substance given to lab animals. In many studies, the LD_{50} is used to set a benchmark for a harmful substance. The LD_{50} is the lethal dose of that substance that causes 50 percent of the test animals to die. As we've seen in exploring numerous studies, many decisions are made on whether a substance can be sold and how much of it can be used based on these kinds of toxicological studies. The point here is that substances like pesticides, heavy metals, food additives and so on do harm similar to the harm that was done to the cats on the deficient diet. A harmful substance in the body is really the same as a deficient diet – it causes stress, does not allow the organism to operate normally, and results in sickness and disease.

In the cat study, the diseases the cats contracted increased with each generation and affected the cats *earlier in their life cycle*. That is, the first generation on the deficient diet developed degenerative diseases late in life. The next generation developed the same degenerative diseases in middle age. The third generation developed these diseases when they were still young so much so that they had trouble reproducing.

The same scenario is happening with us. If we use 1940 as the watershed year when pesticides, food additives, and chemicals became ubiquitous in our environment, then we are now beginning the third generation under these conditions. Each human generation is considered to be 30 years: The first generation under these conditions was from 1940 to 1970; the second, from 1970 to 2000; the third generation will play out around the year 2030. This is not far from the estimate that humans in industrialized nations will be unable to reproduce by the year 2020. The same thing that happened to the cats – extinction after the third generation – could be happening to us.

Not only were numerous manmade substances such as chemicals, pesticides, and fertilizers becoming common around 1940, the soil we grow our crops in had also become deficient, which also leads to disease. In 1936 the U.S. Senate published Document 264, which stated that American soils had become exhausted and were deficient in many minerals. Therefore, the plants grown on these soils and the animals and humans eating these mineral-deficient crops are oftentimes mineral deficient as well. The document states: "Laboratory tests prove that the fruits, the vegetables, the grain, the eggs, and even the milk and meat of today are not what they were a few generations ago – which, undoubtedly explains why our forefathers thrived on a selection of foods that would starve us!" For example, you'd have to eat 60 servings of spinach to get the same amount of iron you would get from just one serving in 1948.[7]

Since minerals are such an important part of our diet – as important as vitamins – these mineral deficiencies can lead to disease. Just as the cats' diet was deficient, the human diet is now deficient as well.

A more recent study (1992) compared the mineral content of today's soils with soils 100 years ago from around the world. The findings showed that today's soils contained far less minerals than those of a century ago. The percentage of fewer minerals were African soils – 74 percent fewer minerals; Asian soils – 76 percent fewer; European soils – 72 percent fewer; South American soils – 76 percent fewer, U.S. And Canadian soils – 85 percent fewer.[8] The World Health Organization reported that in 2000, American soils were 95 percent deficient compared with soils of 100 years ago.[9]

The use of chemical fertilizers does little to replace the minerals lost due to their uptake by plants. As the plants take up the minerals they need to grow, the soil becomes deficient in those minerals. Repeating crops without replenishing those minerals results in deficient soils. A typical fertilizer provides only three minerals (N,P,K). Old-fashioned farming methods used natural fertilizers, which contained most if not all the necessary minerals to support healthy, mineral-rich plants. So the soils were replenished and the plants grew replete with an abundance of minerals. Even then, however, the soils could become deficient. "Bottom land" – land near a river in the flood plain – was prized because when the floods came, minerals were washed down onto the land making the soil mineral-rich again. The progressive depletion of the soils was one of the reasons for western expansion of the U.S. in the 1800s: A farmer would plant for several seasons and deplete the soils; the food would become less nutritious and his family would take ill; they would move to virgin land, grow crops on this new rich soil, and become healthy again.

Food for Thought

I knew a man about ten years ago who was 65 years old. Although he wasn't health-conscious, he was generally healthy and had amazing endurance and stamina. He could work eight hours, go home, eat dinner, and then deliver papers on his paper route until 4 a.m. A few hours of sleep, and then back to work. He could do this for a week or so at a time with no real problem. I use to remarked to him that if I (over 20 years younger) had to do that, I'd probably be dead by the end of the week – even though I'm quite conscious of maintaining a healthy lifestyle. My theory on why he could do it, and I couldn't, is that he has a stronger constitution than I. He grew up on a farm during a time when the soils were richer and they didn't use chemical fertilizers or pesticides. He ate what they grew or slaughtered, had cleaner water and air, and a less stressful lifestyle. Although his grandchildren are having all sorts of health problems, he remains strong and healthy as an ox. He's a first-generation cat. I'm a second-generation cat and am weaker and more prone to breaking down.

Isn't this what we're seeing in our society? Older people, although still susceptible to diseases, get the diseases late in life. Their constitution is stronger than the generations raised on deficient foods and in toxic environments. Now we're seeing middle-aged people – the first generation raised totally on commercially grown food and one that has been exposed to modern toxic chemicals – getting cancer earlier in life; becoming depressed; having difficulty having children; not caring for their young as vigilantly; contracting diabetes, cancer, allergies and so on in epidemic proportions; becoming fatter, lazier, less able to cope with life.

The off-spring of that generation have all sorts of learning disabilities, attention deficit disorders, asthma, allergies, childhood cancers, hyperactivity problems and tendencies towards violence. This generation will – if the trend continues – give rise to a very sick and demented generation. The one after that will not be able to reproduce.

Harold Buttram, M.D., agrees with my assessment. In a personal communication he said, "Yes, many of today's children are in comparable stages of 3rd and even 4th generation Pottenger cats, and the numbers are steadily growing. I believe we will pull through as a society, but I fear our children will pay a fearful price before people come to their senses and the trend begins to reverse itself."[10]

We are coming to a fork in the evolutionary tree. Those who continue to live as is now prevalent in our society will whither in numbers, cease to reproduce and become extinct. Those who heed the warning signs and live within the laws of nature will become stronger with each generation, grow in number and give rise to a new, more enlightened and more harmonious humanity. They will be the beginning of a race of humans that will have everlasting health.

Does it really matter what the soil is like or what kind of farming methods are used? Can we produce more nutritious food? The answer to both is a resounding yes. A study by Firman E. Baer way back in 1949 compared commercially grown produce from different soils around the country. They found that the richer the soil, the more nutrition the crops had. In fact, some crops had from three to 100 times more nutrition as others. Many other essential trace elements are completely absent in some produce whereas trace minerals are abundant in others. Table 6 shows the results of the study.[11]

Table 6
Mineral content of food grown on rich soil vs. poor soil

Vegetable	P	Mg	Na	Mn	Cu	Ca	K	B	Fe	Co
Snap beans										
Rich Soils	0.36	40.5	60	99.7	8.6	73	60	227	69	0.26
Poor Soils	0.22	15.5	14.8	29.1	0.9	10	2	10	3	0
Cabbage										
Rich Soils	0.38	60.0	43.6	148.3	20.4	42	13	94	48	0.15
Poor Soils	0.18	17.5	13.6	33.7	0.8	7	2	20	0.4	0
Lettuce										
Rich Soils	0.43	71.0	49.3	176.5	12.2	37	169	51	660	0.19
Poor Soils	0.16	4.5	4.5	58.8	0	3	1	1	0	0
Spinach										
Rich Soils	0.52	96	203	237	69.5	88	117	158	32	0.25
Poor Soils	0.27	47.5	46.9	84.6	0	12	1	49	0.3	0.2

P, Mg, Na, Ca and K are millequivalents per 100 grams dry weight. Mn, Cu, B, Fe and Co are parts per million dry matter. P = Phosphorus, Mg = Magnesium, Na = Sodium, Ca = Calcium, K = Potassium. Mn = Manganese, Cu = Copper, B = Boron, Fe = Iron, Co = Cobalt

As previously noted, commercial farming methods typically use fertilizers with only three nutrients: nitrogen, phosphorus, and potassium (NPK). Organic farming methods oftentimes use fertilizers that contain many more nutrients, including the trace elements that science is finding are vital to optimal health. Consequently, the organically grown foods will have more nutrients and be better for you, not to mention they are devoid of harmful pesticides.

A more recent study in 1993 compared organically grown food versus commercial supermarket foods for basic element levels. The conclusion was that "...the average elemental concentration in organic foods on a fresh weight basis was found to be about twice that of commercial foods."[12] For example, organically grown sweet corn had 1,000 percent more calcium, 2,200 percent more iodine and 300 percent more magnesium. Organically grown wheat had 360 percent more potassium, 160 percent more copper, and 80 percent more zinc. The 10 percent to 30 percent more you pay for organic food translates to usually more than a 50 percent gain in nutritional value. So, per unit nutrient, you actually pay less for organically raised food than commercially raised food.

It's not just nutritional value that's important with organic food, but the cleanliness of it as well. In a study at the University of Washington, elementary school children tested positive for certain pesticides while eating conventionally grown food. After switching to organically grown food, in just five days, these pesticides (malathion and chlorpyrifos) decreased to nondetectable levels. The authors concluded that "an organic diet provides a dramatic and immediate protective effect against exposures to organophosphorus pesticides that are commonly used in agricultural production."[13]

Is it possible to reverse the trend of degeneration that deficient foods and toxins in our environment cause? Pottenger tried to return some of the degenerating cats back to health. He found that it took four generations on raw meat and milk to bring the kittens of second-degeneration cats back to normal. He wrote, "Improvement in resistance to disease is noted in the second generation regenerating cat, but allergic manifestations persist into the third generation. In the third generation, skeletal and soft tissue changes are still noticeable, but to a lesser degree; and by the fourth generation, most of the severe deficiency signs and symptoms disappear – but seldom completely."[14]

As you can see, the degeneration/regeneration occurs not just in the generation that is fed a certain diet. The deficiencies seem to accumulate through the generations, impacting the next generation more severely. Likewise, it takes several generations for degenerated organisms to return to good health. But it is possible. There is hope.

Food for Thought

An interesting correlation can be made between the state of our health and the actions of our government. As with theater, government is a reflection of society – its wants and needs. A trend in our government over the last 70 years or so is towards more and more programs aimed at helping people. There's welfare, Medicare, Medicaid, Social Security, food stamps, educational programs for the learning impaired, housing assistance programs, handicapped parking and building codes for handicapped accessibility, and so forth. More and more, people are asking for and even demanding that the government step in and help them.

In no way do I denounce these actions. They are – considering the conditions – quite necessary. But *why* are they necessary? Is it because we are just now becoming compassionate toward those less fortunate? Or is it because now there are so many of us in one way or another impaired or needing assistance that it's becoming a driving force in determining government policies?

Since more and more people are getting sicker and less able to care for themselves, you'll see more and more government programs aimed at helping them. The more the government must act to create these programs, the bigger government must become and a more socialistic state will result. As government expands to meet the needs of the many, more money is needed to support this growth, and taxes will inevitably rise. To collect these taxes, even more programs and policies will be needed. "Big Brother" will not arise strictly out of computer technology, but from a simple need – the need for the people to be taken care of.

If we don't reverse the trend of degeneration we see all around us, our health will continue to decline, and so will our society. If the citizens of a country are not independent (i.e. not dependent), how can the country be? For lasting and fundamental change, we must care for our bodies, minds, and spirits in accordance with the laws of nature. Then we will become strong, healthy, and happy, and fewer government programs and laws will be needed. Sound good? Let's take a vote.

All in favor of Everlasting Health say, "Aye."

Those opposed, say, "Nay."

The Ayes have it. Motion is carried.

CHAPTER XVII

Alternative Health Landmines

Throughout this book, I've steered you toward health food stores to obtain many of the items I recommend. But just because you see something in a health food store doesn't automatically mean it's healthy for you or your family. There are many products sold and promoted as being healthy that, in my opinion, are far from good for you. That is especially true now, since many main-stream companies are entering the alternative health industry with the sole intent of exploiting it and making more money. I present this information to give you perspectives that you may not have seen before. I urge you to evaluate it along with any and all other information, and then use your own common sense. Always decide for yourself what's right for you.

The position I take on most issues is, "The closer to nature, the closer to health." All of our knowledge will never compare with the wisdom of nature itself, although our egos like to sometimes think so. The more we tamper with things, the further from nature we get, and the more chances there are for mistakes. If we can consume a food directly from nature – such as a fruit, vegetable, or animal – it will be much better for us than something that can only be consumed after extensive processing (such as soy products) or genetic engineering (such as canola oil). We should remember how humans ate thousands or even millions of years ago. That's closer to the truth of what the body really needs.

Soy

There's no better illustration of something bad turned on its head and made to look good than soy. The contention that soy and soy derived foods are healthy is pure lunacy. To eat a soybean, we must process it extensively with high heat, caustic soda, solvents, and so on. Does that sound to you like something "edible?" Soy isn't just used in foods for adults, but for babies and children as well, which is a crime. To learn how bad soy and soy-based formulas are for babies, please see my book *The Truth about Children's Health*.

I know a lot of people who read this book are already health-conscious, and many of you may think soy is manna from heaven. "Look at all the good things soy has to offer – the phytochemicals (isoflavones), protein, unsaturated fat, and essential fatty acids," you may cry. However, just because something contains a lot of good things doesn't make it good for you. On paper, one of the most nutritious plants in nature is tobacco. It's loaded with vitamins, minerals, and so on. Problem is, it also contains a substance called nicotine, which is deadly.

Should we eat tobacco just because it's a storehouse of nutrients? The overall effect of tobacco in the human body is a negative one. It's the same with soy.

It's my opinion that if we err, we should do so on the side of caution, using nature as the standard. If something is on the borderline and there are questions as to its safety and viability, it's more prudent to exclude it from our experience. Is it possible to achieve superior health without soy? Of course it is. Throughout history, there have been societies, civilizations, and long-lived peoples who have survived and thrived without ever seeing a soybean. Simply use the foods that have nourished mankind for millions of years – before science and agricultural practices started creating new foods to turn a profit.

Do you want to know the real reason soy is touted as a health food and is being embraced by mainstream media and medical doctors? You know what it is: money.

Ask any farmer what he plants on barren land where nothing else will grow. His answer? The soybean plant. It's also easy to cultivate. This gives the farmer and the food processing giants another way to make money from an otherwise unexploited resource. Originally, soy was grown not as a food for human consumption, but as a way to fix nitrogen in the soil. For centuries, soy was only consumed in its nontoxic fermented form (such as soy sauce, tempeh, and miso), even in Asia. It wasn't until recently that processing made soy edible (if you can call it that). To expound on these points, I would like to quote an excellent article by Tim O'Shea, a chiropractor and clinical nutritionist:

> . . .In spite of claims to the contrary, no bean is a complete protein because all beans lack two essential amino acid – cysteine and methionine – which we must get from other sources in our diet. A diet in which soy is the only protein source will cause an abundance of health problems from the ensuing protein deficiency. . .Soy is among the most highly commercially processed of food sources, and after processing it still retains many undesirable substances.[1]

The point is, soybeans are not a healthy food like other vegetables. First of all, soybeans contain high amounts of digestive enzyme inhibitors, blocking the function of the pancreatic enzymes, trypsin in particular. These enzyme inhibitors are not removed by cooking. They interfere not only with the digestion of the soy-beans, but also with the digestion of other foods that happen to be present in the tract.

The second main antinutrient soybeans contain is phytic acid. Present to some degree in all types of beans, phytic acid blocks the uptake of important minerals, such as iron, magnesium, calcium, and especially zinc. Soybeans have the highest phytic acid levels of any legume, and as such have an extraordinary ability to cause mineral deficiencies. Third World countries with diets high in grains and soy have the most profound deficiencies of these minerals.

This is especially bad for infants. The soy in infant formulas robs zinc from the baby's system. Since zinc controls iron uptake, abnormally high iron levels may occur if zinc is not present and liver damage can result. Zinc is crucial for growth and brain and nervous system development (remember, it's sometimes called the *intelligence mineral*), as well as protein digestion. It is also necessary for immune system development and normal insulin function.

Another component of soy that is problematic is hemagglutinin – an agent that causes red blood cells to clot. When red cells clump together, the oxygen supply to the entire body is diminished. Those who already have a history of heart problems should be especially wary of soy.

Aluminum, another toxin found in some processed soy products, is said to be 10 times higher in infant soy formulas than in milk-based formulas – and 100 times higher than in unprocessed milk. Aluminum can damage the newly forming kidneys of an infant who drinks soy formula. Worse yet, it directly damages the infant brain because the blood-brain barrier has not yet formed. – Soy products may also be a causative factor in cancer. O'Shea states:

> Processed soy can also contain a known carcinogen called lysinoalanine. It is a by-product of a processing step called alkaline soaking, which is done to attempt to eliminate enzyme inhibitors. Even though the beans are thoroughly rinsed, the lysinoalanine by-product can remain from the interaction of the soybeans with the alkaline solution.

It's ironic that the same manufacturing processes used to render soy edible from a marketing perspective are the very processes that renders soy inedible from a health perspective. The beneficial soy enzymes, minerals, fiber, vitamins and nutrients are lost, rendering the end products – soybean oil and soy protein isolate and concentrate – totally devitalized commercial foods.[2]

If wholesomeness is what you're looking for, don't turn to soy. Producing it sounds like some kind of chemical manufacturing process. The first step in soy processing is high-temperature cooking to try and get rid of the phytic acid. High temperatures denature the natural enzymes of the soybean. Without enzymes, any plant becomes a devitalized food, very difficult to digest in the human digestive tract. Consider that enzymes, vitamins, and minerals are three legs of the tripod of metabolic activity. Take away any one and the other two cannot function properly.

After cooking, soy oil is removed by one of two paths: pressing, or solvent extraction. Soybean oil is rarely cold-pressed, as many claim, but is usually subjected to heat, which produces destructive free radicals. The easier method of oil extraction is by the use of solvents. Several are used in soybean oil processing. Hexane, a petroleum distillate and known carcinogen, is the standard chemical used. Traces of this toxic solvent may be left behind in the finished products, both in the oil and in the protein isolate.

The next step in the refining process is degumming, the removal of residual fiber, or gum, from the oil. The problem is that valuable trace minerals like calcium, copper, magnesium, and iron, as well as chlorophyll, are removed as well.

Next, the refined oil is mixed with sodium hydroxide (which is what drain cleaners are made of) at a temperature of 167° F. The purpose of this step is to remove any remaining free fatty acids. To remove extra pigments and make the oil completely clear, bleaching is done by using more high heat followed by filtering. Other free radicals called peroxides are thus introduced.

Deodorizing is then thought to be necessary to destroy any natural aromatics. This process uses extreme heat, up to 518° F, which destroys whatever vitality and antioxidants the oils might have left. The oil is rendered absolutely tasteless, colorless, and odorless and devoid of any useful vitamins, minerals, enzymes or nutrients whatsoever. Even though it has undergone extreme high temperatures at several steps, as long as no external heat was added during the actual pressing step, the oil can still be sold as "cold-pressed."

As if no further biological indignity could have been levied against the life-less processed oil, researchers in the 1930s at DuPont figured out a way to harden the oil into a perfectly engineered non-food: margarine. They found out that if they subjected the refined oil to yet another round of high temperatures – up to 410° F – and also forced hydrogen gas in the presence of an aluminum catalyst through the oil, they could produce a substance with the desired spread-ability and shelf-life. That's what hydrogenated margarine means. At least 80 percent of the margarine made in the U.S. comes from refined soybean oil.(3)

Most soybeans on the market these days have been genetically modified and have had a gene inserted that makes them resistant to herbicides. Then the soybeans can withstand more herbicides being sprayed near them to kill weeds. Less weeding equals more profit. But what about the buildup of herbicides within the soybean plant itself? Won't the plants exposed to all these herbicides become unsafe for human consumption? No one knows because no one has ever tested them.

To underscore how much the role of money plays into the contention that soy is healthy, O'Shea tells us more unsettling facts:

> The soy protein fad also has an uneasy background – it stems from the soy oil manufacturing process. With six million tons of soybeans being made into oil every year, there was a lot of product waste. After the oil was removed, what was left? Soy protein – the perfect remedy for the American obsession with obesity and cholesterol. Suddenly everyone was dining on soy burgers to meet their protein requirements. They are unaware that they are eating the residue of the oil-refining process. Soy protein isolate is just as toxic and foreign to the human body as processed soybean oil.

Soy protein isolate is big business. We must appreciate the brilliance of taking a waste product from an already extremely processed food source and getting the majority of the population to think of it as a natural food.(4)

Soy is supposedly great for women approaching menopause, so the advertisers claim, because it supplies a "natural" estrogen, or phytoestrogen, which may prevent osteoporosis and other problems. These estrogen-like compounds come from the isoflavones in soy.

Most isoflavones come from genetically modified soy and are definitely not natural. The amount that soy isoflavones increase estrogen levels in the body may well be pathological (but it's never been studied). But it *is* known that high levels of estrogen compounds may cause sex organ malformation, tumors and menstrual disruption. So do you think it's good for infants who eat soy to have phytoestrogen blood levels from 13,000 to 22,000 times higher than normal? I don't.

The soybean is America's third largest crop and supplies more than 60 percent of the world's soybean demand – that's a crop value of close to $20 billion per year. If we take into account the retail market value of the dozens of *finished* soy food products sold in supermarkets, the total value approaches $100 billion per year.

Yes, you can find soy in burgers, margarine, cooking oil, and soy milk. But soy is hidden in a lot of other foods where it's not even listed on the label. Soy can be in items like chocolate, soup, French fries, and potato chips. Other names used to disguise soy are "vegetable flavoring," "natural flavoring," "vegetable shortening," " hydrolyzed protein," and "textured vegetable protein." These disclosures, which are all the FDA requires, are terms that indicate that the product contains hydrogenated soybean oil or protein isolate (probably from genetically modified plants). Yet you might never know it.

Soy products are not adequate for human protein requirements. They are devitalized, nonfoods with many toxic substances and little to no nutrient content. The only soy product that is not detrimental to your health is traditional soy sauce that's been naturally brewed. Modern processing methods produce large amounts of the kind of unnatural glutamic acid that is found in MSG. Buy only the kind of soy sauce that says *Naturally Brewed* on the label.

Vegetarianism

Over the past 40 years or so it's been more and more popular to be a vegetarian. Proponents cite moral as well as health reasons. Vegetarians must very careful and vigilant to ensure adequate nutrition. In his article *Vegetarianism: An Anthropological/Nutritional Evaluation*, H. Leon Abrams, a noted anthropologist, says, "No culture in the history of mankind has been based on a 100 percent vegetarian diet, and although one can theoretically, in the light of contemporary nutritional scientific knowledge, obtain all the nutrients needed to provide good health, the technology to ensure such has not been developed and such a vegetarian diet is extremely risky."(5)

That is especially true for children. As already discussed, children need a high fat diet or else their nervous system and brain will not develop normally. They need iron in adequate amounts and vitamin B_{12}, which is absent or lacking in non-animal foods. Children need to eat meat or animal products every day once they stop breast feeding and start eating solid food. For more on the diet of infants, see my book *The Truth About Children's Health*.

Abrams goes on to talk about the *macrobiotic diet*, which primarily consists of cooked grains and no animal products:

> Research and clinical observation found that babies who eat no animal protein fail to grow at a normal rate; this study found that infants on 'vegan' diets, except for early breast feeding, did not grow nor develop as normally as babies on diets containing animal products or vegetarian diets supplemented with cow's milk. . .The results of such diet can be scurvy, anemia, hypoproteinemia, hypocalcemia, emaciation and even death.(6)

He also reported that the Hindus of India, although not 100 percent vegetarian, come the closest of any culture. He said that ". . .the greater percentage of the population, who subsist almost entirely on vegetable foods, suffer from kwashiorkor, other forms of malnutrition, and have the shortest life span in the world." (Kwashiorkor is a severe protein deficiency that is marked by severe tissue wasting and retarded growth.)

Food for Thought

Some of you reading this may be hard-core vegetarians. I was a vegetarian (vegan, and even a fruitarian for a while) for about 10 years, but started eating animal products again about 15 years ago. I changed because of scientific evidence, personal observation, and the fact that my health wasn't improving.

The findings of researchers examining the diets of primitive cultures and long-lived and healthy peoples were very instrumental in changing my mind. Consider that for the 3 million to 4 million years mankind has been on this planet (if carbon dating is correct), 99 percent of the time mankind was a hunter/gatherer. That means mankind ate large amounts of animal food. It wasn't until 10,000 years ago that people finally started cultivating plants – only because they had in large part exhausted the supply of wild game.

Interestingly, this stationary agricultural activity spawned political organizations (societies) and religions. Some religions imposed dietary restrictions – such as not eating meat – out of population growth pressures and for other pragmatic reasons. The Hindus, for example, once consumed beef. But because of the increased population and the fact that cows were valuable for their milk, dung (as fuel for cooking), and as draft animals, they were banned as food and became religious icons.(7)

Clearly, mankind has been, and should now be, an omnivore, consuming a wide variety of foods, including meat. (For a more detailed discussion on this, see *The Cambridge World History of Food, Volume Two*, Cambridge University Press, 2000.)

My personal observation also showed that the vegetarian people I knew were frankly, not very healthy and always struggling with one problem or another. I think part of the problem with most vegetarians is that they eat a high percentage of cooked foods – rice, especially. Cooking robs the foods of vital nutrients. Rice, unless soaked overnight, contains enzyme and growth inhibitors, which interfere with digestion and normal metabolism.

When I was a vegetarian, I ate a lot of uncooked foods, mostly pre-soaked nuts and seeds, and not too many cooked grains. I didn't get sick, but I wasn't healing either. Now that I eat animal foods, I consume virtually all of them in their uncooked form. I eat only organic raw milk cheese, take unheated glandular supplements (liver, kidney, heart), and have been eating raw meat for about 10 years (and haven't gotten ill once because of it). Every long-lived culture consumed unheated animal products to some degree – cultured milk, organ meats, eggs, butter, and so on. It's a stretch for us to think of eating meat raw, but I now believe eating some animal products in their natural state is vital to optimal health.

If we examine the history of primitive man, Dr. Abrams tells us,

"Ancient cave-man was a flesh eating animal. Perhaps he ate a few wild fruits and plants which he found in the area, but for the most part he preferred meat. . .Man depended almost entirely, if not completely, on meat for his subsistence. . .He probably ate most of his meat raw, and that which was cooked was most likely rare."(8) If you think that that might be fine for a cave-man, but not for us, consider that "man hasn't changed physiologically from ancient cave-man, and not at all from the men of 10,000 or more years ago."(9)

Did this diet of mostly raw animal food suit early man? "...the skeletal remains which we have, show that he was very healthy. He had to be in order to survive..."(10) (If you counter that man's lifespan was significantly shorter then than now, consider my comments about electricity in the first chapter.)

Sally Fallon clues us in on more of the history and culture behind raw food:

"Almost all traditional societies incorporate raw, enzyme-rich foods into their cuisines – not only vegetable foods but also raw animal proteins and fats in the form or raw dairy foods, raw muscle and organ meats, and raw fish. These diets also traditionally include a certain amount of cultured or fermented foods, which have an enzyme content that is actually enhanced by the fermenting and culturing process. The Eskimo diet, for example, is composed in large portion of raw fish that has been allowed to autolate or predigest, that is, become putrefied or semi-rancid; to this predigested food they ascribe their stamina."(11)

This shows that the germs in their semi-rancid food did nothing to harm them, and in fact made them stronger – more evidence that germs do us no harm and even good.

One more point worth noting is that pre-industrial cultures that consumed cooked meat usually included fermented vegetables such as sauerkraut, pickled cucumbers, beets or carrots, with their meals. This increases the enzyme content of the meal making it easier to digest. So if you eat a steak, chop or hot dog, don't hold the 'kraut!

Aajonus Vonderplanitz, Ph.D., is a nutritionist who has been eating a diet of predominately raw meat and animal products for over 20 years. (Check out his book *The Recipe for Living Without Disease* for raw meat recipes.) He claims to have healed himself of numerous ailments, including cancer, and has reported success within three months time with 236 out of 240 cancer cases (the cancer was checked) that he put on his diet.(12) His findings are further validation that raw animal products are necessary for good health. In fact, he says that "experience has shown me that over time raw animal products produce the calmest, most balanced human nature with excellent mental clarity."(13) Vonderplanitz also cites the Eskimo, saying,

"By several accounts of world travelers and explorers they considered the Eskimo the happiest of all races. . .the Eskimo ate 99% raw animal products and lived free of degenerative disease before white men introduced cooking cauldrons, breads, and refined sugar to them. . .Their first case of dental decay was 50 years after [these] were introduced. The dental caries only existed among those who ate some or all of white man's food. Cancer never occurred among primitive Eskimo."(14)

Some vegetarians will cite physiological reasons for their choice, saying that the human body is not equipped to handle animal foods. Science disagrees. Again I quote Dr. Abrams:

> Actually, the digestive mechanism of man is adapted to a mixed meat and vegetable diet. Human teeth consist of three types: canines or piercing teeth of the meat-eating animals, and the molars or grinders of grain-and-nut-eating animals. With respect to structure, human teeth are conclusive proof that the human body is adapted to a mixed animal and plant diet. Man has specific digestive ferments for meat proteins and other special digestive juices for carbohydrates. His stomach and intestinal tract are equipped to handle both.(15)

Speaking of teeth, how strong and resistant to decay they are is a measure of how strong your bones are and how healthy you are in general. Healthy people (and animals) will simply not have cavities. Although tooth decay has been known throughout human history, it was extremely rare through the Paleolithic period, which spanned some 3 to 4 million years. It wasn't until mankind started agriculture (abandoning hunting because of lack of game) and consumed a diet high in unhealthy carbohydrates (i.e., grains), did tooth decay become a major problem. Skeletal remains of ancient societies showed increases in tooth decay between 75 percent and 85 percent around the time agriculture became predominant and the diets became largely vegetarian.[16] Weston Price also found a dramatic increase in tooth decay of people of primitive cultures who abandoned their traditional diets and started consuming more agricultural products such as white flour.

Of particular concern for vegetarians is obtaining adequate amounts of vitamin B_{12}. Cyanocobalamin is critical for healthy blood and a properly functioning nervous system. Since vegetarian sources cannot supply adequate amounts of B_{12}, deficiencies in vegetarians are the rule instead of exception. Once one becomes a vegetarian, this deficiency may not become apparent for a while since the body stores a supply of B_{12} that can last from two to five years.

Deficiencies can cause pernicious anemia, panic attacks, impaired eyesight, schizophrenia, hallucinations, weakness, loss of balance, numbness in the hands and feet, and irregular menstruation including sparse flow or no flow.[17,18] An article in the *British Medical Journal* reported that a deficiency of vitamin B_{12} brought on devastating mental and emotional symptoms such as difficulty in thinking and remembering, mood disorders, confusion, agitated depression, paranoia, delusions, visual and auditory hallucinations, maniacal behavior, and epilepsy.[19] Another study found that an extremely high percentage of inmates in psychiatric wards suffer from low blood levels of B_{12}.[20]

Vegetarian women are not only making themselves vulnerable to a vitamin B_{12} deficiency, but their children as well. Many may eat sea vegetables, tempeh, miso, and tamari that theoretically contain adequate amounts of vitamin B_{12}, thinking they are supplying the body's vitamin B_{12} requirement. However, tests reveal that individuals who ingested such products showed no increase in vitamin B_{12} blood levels leading to a B_{12} deficiency in their baby. Dutch bio-chemists demonstrated that ingested seaweed products did not correct vitamin B_{12} deficiencies in infants. Neither did spirulina, a microalgae. Why? Vitamin B_{12} is only well absorbed from animal sources. The Dutch searchers reported that infants of many vegetarian women have abnormal red blood cells, delayed motor skills, and slow growth, compared with control group babies.

What are the best sources of vitamin B_{12}? You won't find them growing on trees. They're liver, sardines, mackerel, herring, salmon, lamb, Swiss cheese, eggs, haddock, beef, blue cheese, halibut, scallops, cottage cheese, chicken, and milk.

As you can see, children and infants are especially vulnerable to the inadequacies of a strictly vegetarian diet. A research team made up of scientist from the University of Cincinnati, Harvard School of Public Health, Vanderbilt and Brandies Universities reported that strict vegetarian women who breastfeed their infants may be subjecting them to possible long-term brain damage.[21]

As I mentioned before, examining the diets of primitive cultures and our ancestors is interesting and enlightening. Native Americans were healthy and robust (before the white man came). They were not vegetarians. Recalls John Lame Deer, a full-blooded Sioux born 90 years ago on the Rosebud Reservation in South Dakota,

> We always had plenty of food for everybody, squaw bread, beef, the kind of dried meat we called *papa*, and *wasna*, or pemmican, which was meat pounded together with berries and kidney fat. . . *wasna* kept a man going for a whole day. . .In the old days we used to eat the guts of the buffalo, making a contest of it, two fellows getting hold of a long piece of intestines from opposite ends, starting chewing toward the middle, seeing who can get there first; that's eating. Those buffalo guts, full of half-fermented, half-digested grass and herbs, you didn't need any pills and vitamins when you swallowed those.[22]

Vegetarian men have a slightly higher annual all-cause-death rate than nonvegetarian men (0.93 percent vs. 0.89 percent), and vegetarian women have a significantly higher annual all-cause-death rate than nonvegetarian women (0.86 percent vs. 0.54 percent). Vegetarianism is not better for your heart, either. The International Atherosclerosis Project found that vegetarians had just as much atherosclerosis as meat eaters.[23]

As far as children are concerned, I believe they are headed for trouble if some high-fat animal food is not included in their diets. If you're worried about cholesterol, remember that it is vital to the proper functioning and development of the brain (see detailed discussion in the chapter on cardiovascular problems). Low cholesterol levels are believed to contribute to aggressive and violent behavior, depression, and suicidal tendencies. Cholesterol is needed for the proper functioning of serotonin (the feel-good neurotransmitter) receptors in the brain; is a precursor to hormones; is an antioxidant; is necessary for healthy cell membranes and is a precursor to vitamin D (needed for healthy bones and nervous system, insulin production, immune system function, proper growth, and mineral metabolism). Nature knows best, so it's no surprise that mother's milk is very high in cholesterol, and 50 percent of its calories come from fat (much of it saturated fat). That should be evidence enough that growing infants and children need a high-fat diet.

A popular item vegetarians consume is alfalfa sprouts. Although other kinds of sprouts are generally nutritious, alfalfa sprouts contain a substance called cadaverine that can be toxic. Tests indicate that alfalfa sprouts can inhibit the immune system and can contribute to inflammatory arthritis and lupus.(24)

My advice? Eat animal products. And above all, have your kids eat them regularly. There's a reason why they love hot dogs so much. (But please get them the best at the health food store.)

Canola Oil

In recent years many nutritionists have claimed that canola oil is a good, healthy oil, especially for the heart. They make these claims based on the accepted medical dogma, which says that polyunsaturated and unsaturated fats and oils are healthy, and saturated fats like those found in animal products are unhealthy and lead to cardiovascular and heart problems as well as cancer.

At the turn of the 20th century, most fat in the diet was either in the saturated or monounsaturated form, coming primarily from lard, butter, coconut oil, and olive oil. Heart disease was rare, as was cancer. Today, heart disease is the leading killer and cancer is an epidemic – and as much as 30 percent of the calories in our diet comes from polyunsaturated oils. This is in large part due to the abundance of margarine in our diets along with vegetable oils derived from soy, corn, safflower, and rape seeds (canola oil).

Primitive, healthy populations in temperate and tropical regions consume about 4 percent of their calories in the polyunsaturated form – far less than the 30 percent in Western diets. (These come from legumes, grains, nuts, green vegetables, fish, olive oil, and animal fats.) Studies have shown that polyunsaturated oils actually increase cancer and heart disease, damage the liver, reproductive organs and lungs, cause digestive disorders, depress learning ability, and impair growth and weight gain.(25) Why? Polyunsaturated oils become rancid easily when subjected to heat, oxygen, and moisture (when cooking or processing). When oil is rancid, it has many free radicals that attack cell membranes and red blood cells, damage DNA/RNA and cause mutations in tissues, blood vessels, and skin.

Free radicals cause skin to wrinkle, organs to develop tumors, and blood vessels to develop plaque. Not only have numerous studies shown that high consumption of polyunsaturated oils causes heart disease and cancer, but also contribute to premature aging, arthritis, Parkinson's disease, Lou Gehrig's disease, Alzheimer's, cataracts, and autoimmune disorders.

Most of the polyunsaturates in commercial vegetable oils are in the form of omega-6 linoleic acid. Too much omega-6 in the diet can cause blood clots to form, high blood pressure, depressed immune function, sterility, cancer, weight gain, inflammation, and irritation of the digestive tract. Too little omega-3 linolenic acid in the diet can cause asthma, heart disease, and learning problems. The healthy ratio of omega-6 to omega-3 fatty acids in the diet is about one to one. However, our modern diet contains far too much omega-6 and not enough omega-3, due largely to the prevalent use of polyunsaturated vegetable oils.

Canola oil has twice as much omega-6 as omega-3, making it unbalanced oil. Even worse, during the processing of canola oil, much of the omega-3 fatty acids are transformed into *trans*-fatty acids, similar to those found in margarine and known to be dangerous.(26)

Mold develops very quickly in baked goods made with canola oil. Canola oil also contains a very long-chain fatty acid called erucic acid, which is associated with fibrotic heart lesions. Even though canola oil is bred to contain little erucic acid, it is likely still present. Even though canola oil is touted as being good for the heart, a recent study has shown that it may actually cause a deficiency in vitamin E, which is needed for a healthy cardiovascular system.(27)

While we're on the topic of fats and oils, it's important to realize that hydrogenated fats (like margarine – made from rancid vegetable oils) and partially hydrogenated vegetable oils have a very deleterious effect on the human body. They have been associated with cancer, diabetes, obesity, low-birth-weight babies, birth defects, sterility, atherosclerosis, immune system dysfunction, lactation difficulties, sexual dysfunction, and increased blood cholesterol. The next time you pick up a product in the supermarket, read the label. Many foods contain partially hydrogenated vegetable oil. It's a testimony to the advertisers that they could brainwash generations of people into thinking that natural fats, such as those in animal products, are bad and manmade products from rancid and over-processed oils are good.

On the other hand, good old-fashioned butter contains short- and medium-chain fatty acids that are easily metabolized by the body and have antimicrobial and antitumor qualities. Butter also contains virtually the only dietary source of butyric acid, which has antitumor as well as antifungal properties.

CHAPTER XVIII

How to Avoid and Reverse Disease

Disclaimer: The ideas and strategies contained in this book are not intended as a substitute for the appropriate care of a licensed health care practitioner. Qualified medical assistance should always be sought before beginning any treatments. The following is intended for educational purposes only. Suggestions are not made to treat a specific condition. The following has not been evaluated by the FDA.

The following are ideas and strategies for you to consider to help you and your family deal with many of the health problems discussed this book. An important thing to keep in mind is that you don't need to be perfect in your implementation of these strategies. The human body is designed to take a fair amount of abuse and thrive in less than ideal conditions. The anguish and frustration that may result from trying to do everything and do it perfectly in some cases would be worse than not doing anything at all. Your mental health and peace of mind are just as important as eliminating the problem. Do the best you can, and realize that it's going to take some time. But a change here, a change there, and in time, you'll be surprised at how far you've come. You may eliminate a specific problem in a few hours or a day, or it may take years. Realize that you are doing something great and something of true value. Not just for you and your children, but for society and future generations.

The dietary guidelines presented below are simply the basic fundamentals we've lost sight of that have nourished and healed the body for millions of years. Changes to our foods were initially made during the industrial revolution to preserve those foods to get them to market. With such changes, we discovered these foods didn't taste or look that good. So we added flavor enhancers, artificial flavors, preservatives, dyes, and colorings. All to make us think we were getting the real thing. The problem is, altered foods are not just deficient in their nutrient content, but also polluted by the additives.

In our quest to produce more food with less labor, we developed pesticides, herbicides, and chemical fertilizers. They further degraded the food supply and added to air and water pollution. We want to avoid foods with any of these in them as much as possible. They interfere with normal cellular processes and are also less nutritious. Anything not found in nature is suspect. The closer to nature, the closer to health.

- **Buy and eat as much organically raised food as possible.**

Not only is it cleaner, it's more nutritious. Nutrient for nutrient, it is actually less expensive than conventionally grown foods. You won't need to eat as much (since your body will be satisfied sooner), and you'll be saving untold medical bills down the road. If you must buy nonorganic produce, soak it in a sink full of water with one-teaspoon hydrogen peroxide or apple cider vinegar added. Soak about 10 minutes and then rinse well. That will help remove pesticides and other impurities. Most people believe that fruits and vegetables are the main sources of pesticide contamination. This is not the case, since these impurities bioaccumulate up the food chain and animal foods have higher concentrations of pesticides than produce, so it's very important to obtain organically raised meat, poultry, eggs, and dairy products.

- **Eat as much whole, natural, unprocessed food as possible.**

Scientists believe that there is less than 1/100,000th of a difference between the metabolism of modern man and that of people 10,000 years ago.[1] But our diets would be unrecognizable to those ancestors. Our digestive system is just not made for and has not adapted to the 50,000 synthetic chemicals in our food supply and all the modern processing we do to our food. Think of it this way: If our ancestors of 500 years ago didn't eat it, we shouldn't eat it either. That means no soft drinks, no *Doritos*, no white bread, pasteurized milk, and so on. We should consume animal products regularly. The important thing here is to be sure the meat, dairy, and eggs are clean, organically raised and prepared properly (and oftentimes raw). You can still have hot dogs, but buy them from a health food store. Serve them on whole wheat buns or Ezekiel bread (a special kid of "sprouted grain" bread at health food stores). Buy organic mustard, ketchup, relish, sauerkraut, and so on.

- **Eat a lot of raw food.**

You should make it a goal to consume at least 50 percent to 70 percent of your food in an uncooked state. Cooking destroys many nutrients and changes many others to unusable and sometimes harmful forms. Remember Pottenger's cats? The cats fed only cooked food degenerated and died out in just a few generations. Life begets life. Everyone needs some uncooked food every day.

- **Eat at least one raw egg a day.**

Eggs are rich in many nutrients you need. Your child needs these nutrients for proper development and growth. Include a raw egg yolk in your family's diet every day, preferably from fertile eggs from organically raised chickens. Eggs contain sulfur, which binds with mercury, helping to eliminate it from the body. If you must cook, poach or soft-boil eggs rather than frying or scrambling them.

Here's a simple, nutritious, fast, and delicious recipe to start your off right. It's loaded with enzymes, protein, good fatty acids, vitamins, and minerals. One great thing about this meal is that it sticks to your ribs. Since your body is getting a lot of wholesome nutrients, it realizes it's being well fed and doesn't get hungry. Since the ingredients are raw, you won't gain weight on this meal, and in fact, you may lose weight if you have to since it's so nutrient dense without empty calories. Take 3-6 raw eggs, 1 banana, ½ teaspoon unheated honey, 2-3 ounces raw cream or 1-2 teaspoons raw, unsalted butter. Add to blender and blend on medium for several seconds. You can put this in a coffee mug and eat it on the run. You can use other fruits besides bananas or a mixture.

• Avoid canned vegetables, frozen dinners, and commercial fruit juices.

Canned vegetables are overcooked and usually contain salt or sugar. Frozen dinners are usually filled with preservatives, dyes, and other chemicals (including MSG), and are usually packaged in aluminum. Commercial fruit juices have too much sugar and fluoride and have been shown to be harmful for kids. Make your own dinner, and make your own juice. Please note that even freshly prepared fruit juices are high in sugar and may disrupt blood sugar levels, so go easy on these. Avoid are candy, pastry, jam, jelly, ice cream, crackers, cereals, catsup, soft drinks, coffee, tea (herbal is OK), and processed, canned, preserved or packaged foods.

• Cook in the right cookware, store food in glass containers.

Cook only in glass, unchipped enamel, Corning, or stainless steel cookware. Do not use aluminum or nonstick cookware. The wrong cookware can introduce toxic chemicals into your food. Store your food in glass as much as possible. Instead of plastic-ware, get some Mason jars with lids. They're inexpensive and can be found at most grocery stores. Freezing in plastic is all right.

• Cook properly to preserve nutrients

Cook food as little as possible to preserve nutrients. Light steaming is the most preferable way of cooking vegetables, followed by boiling, baking, and then quick frying. Meat and fowl are best slow-roasted or broiled. Poach, broil, or bake seafood.

• Avoid irradiated foods.

Many fruits and produce now are irradiated in order to preserve the food and increase shelf life (and profits). However, it's been shown that irradiation of our food can cause kidney damage, chromosomal damage, mutations, and heart damage. Extending shelf life is not a good trade-off for shortening human life. More on this subject can be found in the book *The Food That Would Last Forever: Understanding the Dangers of Food Irradiation* by Gary Gibbs, M.D. Shopping at health food stores and buying organically raised products will help you avoid buying this kind of food. Avoid genetically engineered (GE) foods (also known as genetically modified organisms or GMOs).

- **Do not microwave your food or your baby's food.**

Microwaving your food distorts the electrical integrity of the food. It's believed to alter fats, proteins and vitamins, making them more difficult to digest and assimilate. Eating microwaved food results in abnormal blood profiles, which are very similar to those found in the early stages of cancer. Please don't use a microwave to heat your baby's bottle since microwaved milk can be toxic to the liver and nervous system, especially for infants.(2) It also presents a burn risk since microwaving heats unevenly, potentially leaving pockets of heat you can't detect with a test drop on your wrist.

Yes, microwaved food is bad news. In fact, mcirowaves are so potentially harmful the Soviet Union banned their use in 1976. Consistently eating microwaved food shorts out electrical impulses in the brain, causing permanent brain damage, loss of memory, concentration, and emotional stability. It can shut down or alter hormone production, cause immune system deficiencies, decrease intelligence, and cause intestinal cancerous growths. Minerals, vitamins, and other nutrients of all microwaved food are reduced and altered so the body gets little or no benefit or also absorbs altered compounds that it cannot break down.(3)

- **Use only butter and extra virgin olive oil or virgin coconut oil.**

Avoid margarine and all commercial vegetable oils, including canola oil and corn oil and any products made with these in them. They're abundant in the wrong kinds of fats – *trans*-fatty acids – and contribute to weight gain, depression, cardiovascular disease, and other health problems. Eat butter, preferably raw (not pasteurized), unsalted and organic from grass fed cows. It has a valuable fatty acid (butyric acid) that is difficult to obtain from any other source. Butyric acid has antifungal and antitumor properties.

- **Eliminate ALL soy foods** (unless it's naturally fermented)

Soy upsets hormonal balances and tofu is loaded with aluminum.

- **Eliminate ALL SUGAR.**

Sugar in every way, shape, and form must be removed from the diet. No high-fructose corn syrup, added sucrose or fructose, or any other form of added sugar. Now they try to hide the added sugar by calling it "carbohydrates." Yes, sugar is a carbohydrate, so they're not lying, just being deceptive. The only way is to make sure the product says *No Sugar Added* on the label. That's supposed to ensure that no sugar was added. (In this day and age though, who knows.) If you follow just one dietary guideline, this would be it since sugar is so bad. Use raw, unheated honey instead. It's loaded with enzymes and minerals. See my discussion on the evils of sugar in the chapter on diabetes.

For many of you new to the health food arena, this may seem like quite a stretch. Do the best you can. Some go all out and just throw away everything in their cupboards with sugar and start over from scratch. Others go gradually, using up what they have and replacing it with more wholesome products. Usually, gradual dietary changes are best since the enzyme systems in your body take a little time to adjust to a new diet. In extremely critical situations, more drastic changes may be warranted.

- **Eliminate all products that contain aspartame or other artificial sweeteners.**

This includes the brand names of *Equal* and *Sweet 'n Low*, *Splenda*, among others. Avoid any other kind of artificial sweetener. Again, unheated honey is best sweetener. Others, in order of whole-food goodness, are *Stevia*, powdered dates, Grade A or B dark amber maple syrup, blackstrap molasses, and succanate (unprocessed cane sugar).

A great-tasting, very nutritious and refreshing drink that will replace *Kool-Aid* and sodas in your child's diet is to squeeze a lemon or lime into a couple of glasses of water add a tablespoon or two of the dark amber maple syrup or unheated honey, and blend. Adjust ingredients to suit your taste. Also try the Total Health Drink (see Obesity chapter) with orange juice or a little lemon juice added.

- **Avoid white flour products.**

White flour products are not only nutrient-deficient, but are poisoned from bleaching agents including cadmium and aluminum. They also, more often than not, contain some amount of sugar and bromine. That includes bagels, any pastries, pizza, spaghetti, most brown-looking bread at the regular grocery store (coloring the bread is another trick to make you think it's healthy), and so on.

Remember, white flour products have had the germ removed, which is the source of B vitamins in the wheat. Lack of B vitamins creates stress in the body. The best bread to buy is called *Ezekiel*. You'll only find it at the health food stores. There are other whole-grain or sprouted grain products at the health food stores too. Once you eat them for a while, and then you taste regular bread again you'll see that regular white-flour products taste and feel like paste. You'll find that many whole grain and sprouted grain products are kept refrigerated. They have to be or they'll soon go rancid, since they don't have preservatives and are real food.

The best pasta to buy is called *Vita-Spelt*. It has significantly more protein and nutrients than other brands. Eating brown-looking spaghetti may seem weird at first, but you'll get used to it. Pasta made from kamut is good too. Whole-wheat pastas are OK, but not as good as spelt or kamut since the spelt and kamut grains have more nutrients in them to begin with. (Most regular wheat on the market is from hybridized plants that are not that nutrient dense.)

One of the biggest problems with wheat products is that many people are allergic to them. That's because of the high amount of gluten (the sticky stuff) in these products. Not so with the whole-grain and sprouted grain products. You may find a lot of your and your child's allergies diminishing when you switch to these more nutritious, less allergic foods.

- **Avoid cereal products.**

Especially those found in regular supermarkets. If you do use cereals, make sure they're whole-grain with no added sugar and add your own sweetener (if you must). Use good old fashioned raw whole milk. Above all, stay away from the common supermarket milk. Soy-milk and soy products are bad – no matter how much they advertise to the contrary.

- **Eliminate all pasteurized milk and pasteurized milk based products, but use plenty of raw dairy.**

If milk is raw and from cows fed organically, cow's milk is a great food for babies, children, and adults. Cow's milk also contains lactose, which most people cannot metabolize if the milk is pasteurized. However, in its raw state, the milk contains lactase, the enzyme necessary to digest this sugar. Therefore, those with lactose intolerance will not experience problems with raw dairy products. Most cows raised at conventional dairies are injected with hormones to make them produce more milk faster (to make more money, of course). A century ago, a cow that produced 600 pounds of milk a year was considered a high producer. In 1972, an American cow named Hattie produced 44,019 pounds of milk in one year! This is very unnatural. Chickens are similarly treated so they will produce more and more eggs and farmers are now experimenting with new and different lighting systems to increase egg production to 400 or 500 eggs a year – up from the current (and forced) one egg a day.(4)

Many healthy populations throughout history have relied on unpasteurized dairy products as a major part of their diet; The Swiss, Greeks and other inhabitants of the Mediterranean; Africans; Tibetans; the long-lived citizens of Soviet Georgia; the hearty Mongols of Northern China; Americans up to the first World War; and the long-lived people of Austria and Switzerland.(5) These cultures consumed dairy products primarily in the cultured or fermented form. In Europe before industrialization, people consumed raw milk as yogurt, cheese, clabber or curds and whey. Fermentation, due to the lactic-acid-producing bacteria, preserves the milk for days or weeks, and in the case of cheese, for several years. Y*ogurt* comes from Bulgaria. The beverages *kefir* and *Koumiss* come from Russia, Scandinavians drink a cultured milk product called *longfil Dahi*, a soured milk product is consumed in India with almost every meal.

Fermenting milk results in beneficial changes. For one, milk protein (casein) is broken down and essentially predigested. If you are troubled by allergies, switching from regular dairy products to raw, cultured dairy products will really help. Culturing increases the lactase content, which helps digest lactose (milk sugar). Many traditional societies give fermented milk products to the sick, aged, and nursing mothers because they value their health-promoting properties. Vitamins B and C increase when milk is fermented (due to the benefitial activity of bacteria), and cultured dairy provides beneficial bacteria and lactic acid to the digestive tract.

Can you get enough calcium without drinking raw milk? Some researchers think not. Sally Fallon, in a personal communication, says, "Children cannot get adequate calcium from green vegetables (and adults can't either). The only two good sources of calcium in human diets are milk products and bone broths. In cultures where milk products are not used, bone broths are an essential part of the diet. Parents who cannot find decent milk products need to make bone broth and serve it at almost every meal. By the way, when children get plentiful calcium and fat-soluble activators in the diet they are well protected against many of the toxins in our food, including the toxic metals."

Don't turn to calcium pills to get your calcium. Most calcium supplements on the market have the wrong kind of calcium because it's the cheapest kind. Squeeze some fresh oranges or invest in a juicer and make vegetable juices (carrots, celery, cucumber, parsley, tomato, etc.) and drink an 8-oz. glass a day with some cream, butter, or milk (the fat in these help with vitamin and mineral absorption.) There's plenty of calcium in that one little glass of fresh, unpasteurized orange juice or vegetable juice with raw milk added. You can get a little hand-squeezer – the kind you twist an orange half on – for a couple of dollars. Decent juicers can be found at most department stores.

• Don't drink much water.

Chemists consider water to be the universal solvent. It dissolves just about anything, including bones and tissue. The more pure the water is, the more it will dissolve. Distilled water, being devoid of all minerals, is very hungry, aggressive water that should not be drunk. If you are distilling water that has been treated with chlorine, a toxic byproduct of the distillation process called trihalomethanes will end up in the distilled water. If you do distill water, be sure there's a carbon filter attachment on the distiller to get rid of the trihalomethanes. Distilled water is bad enough for adults, but is catastrophic for kids. They don't need minerals leached out of their growing bodies.

The only water that is tolerated by the body is mineral water from pure sources. The Hunzas, one of the longest lived people on earth, drink mineral-dense water from melting glaciers called glacial milk. Water from natural springs, like *Perrier* water from France, is fine. Ideally, you and your child should get most of the water your body needs from the food you eat, raw milk, and vegetable juices. Drinking large quantities of raw milk is fine and even healthful. Fruit juices tend to dissolve and leach minerals out of the body too. Eating food in its raw state will also help you stay hydrated since the water in this live food is very bioavailable and beneficial.

If you're craving a soft drink or glass of iced tea, have a glass of milk, juice or mineral water with some lemon first or the Total Health Drink. Drink juice, milk, or mineral water whenever you like, and you don't have to drown yourself with the prescribed eight glasses a day. Drink when you're thirsty – don't force yourself. The less cooked food you eat, the less water you'll need to drink.

- **Avoid salt.**

If you must use salt, use only *Celtic Sea Salt* since it is unheated and has a good mineral balance. I discussed salt in detail in the Cardiovascular Disease chapter.

- **Get enough and the correct kind of fat.**

Without the correct fats, your nervous system and brain cannot function properly and children's minds can't develop. Do not put your child on a low-fat diet, even if he or she is over-weight. A child can always slim down, but the window of nervous system development is short, and you may be doing him or her irreversible harm in restricting fats in their diets. A better alternative is to limit sugar and other high-carbohydrate foods (like pizza and pasta), since the excess sugar gets stored as unhealthy fat. Fat is so important for growing children, that they actually benefit from a diet that contains more calories as fat than as protein.

Fat is also important to maintain everybody's brain and nervous system. I discussed that at length in the chapter on cardiovascular disease. Again, a good practice is to eat at least a raw egg a day. Egg yolks are a good source of eicosapentaenoic acid (EPA) and docasahexaenoic acid (DHA), which are not essential, but are oftentimes difficult to manufacture by the body. Consuming eggs, liver, and other organ meats, fish oils, and organically raised chickens will supply EPA and DHA. GLA can be found in borage oil and evening primrose oil, and AA is found in butter and organ meats. If you want a good supplement with DHA in it, try Neuromins. Neuromins is a purified form of DHA and has been clinically shown to be safe for infants, children, and pregnant and lactating women. There are other DHA products on the market made from fish oils that can be used also, but Neuromins is DHA from a plant source, which has been shown to have less contamination (especially mercury) than fish oil DHA. Arachidonic acid (AA) and gamma-linolenic acid (GLA) are two other fatty acids that are difficult for the body to manufacture, so these must be obtained from the diet as well.

- **Get enough vitamin A**

Dr. Weston Price considered Vitamin A to be the catalyst on which all other biological processes depend, so it's important to get enough of it daily. An egg a day will help, but you need more vitamin A than that. Some say that carotenes are metabolized into vitamin A, but please realize that carotenes can only be converted to vitamin A under optimal conditions. Cod liver oil, liver, butter, egg yolks, fresh cream, and shellfish are good sources of vitamin A. I also recommend getting a good supply of essential fatty acids – especially the omega 3s. You should look for ones that are cold-pressed from organic sources and kept in the refrigerator section. These oils can go rancid easily so you need to keep them refrigerated.

- **Soak all nuts, seeds, and grains overnight. Avoid roasted nuts and seeds.**

All seeds and grains have substances called phytates, which block absorption of iron, calcium, magnesium, copper, and zinc. Nuts, seeds, and grain also contain enzyme inhibitors that interfere with digestion. Both phytates and these enzyme inhibitors are inactivated by water. If you've had trouble digesting nuts or seeds, this is probably the reason. If you soak them overnight, they'll be easy to digest. Even rice and wheat should be soaked at least overnight and as long as a couple of days. Only whole grain, brown rice should be consumed. Most vegetarians eat a lot of rice, yet I haven't met many that know this about phytates and rice. I think that this, along with the fact that many vegetarians eat a lot of soy products, is the reason you hardly ever meet a healthy vegetarian. Roasting nuts and seeds turns their fats rancid and alters their proteins and carbohydrates. It's best to buy your nuts and seeds raw (organic), and sprinkle some soy sauce over them. They are best stored in the refrigerator or freezer.

- **Avoid most nutritional supplements.**

Over the years, I have researched and experimented with a variety of health supplements such as vitamin and mineral supplements. What I've discovered is a vast majority of them are bad. Nor can we be sure whether we really need all or any of the ingredients. For one thing, most vitamin or mineral pills contain a host of impurities that cannot only make their ingredients unusable by the body, but are themselves health hazards. (See Chapter II) The human body is designed to acquire its nutrition from foods, not from pills made in some laboratory. The vitamins, minerals, fatty acids, proteins, and carbohydrates in whole foods are in the right forms for your body to use as nourishment. If we ate nothing but wholesome, clean, and nutritious food, we wouldn't need supplements of any kind.

There are, however, a few things I recommend, and I've discussed these at length: The right kinds of cod liver oil, iodine, and magnesium will help overcome critical deficiencies and allow other nutrients to be used by the body easier. Bee pollen contains everything the body needs (it's a food, not a supplement), and should be your new "multivitamin."

- **Get your blood levels checked for iodine, magnesium, and vitamin D, and supplement if necessary.**

These are the three things most people are deficient in, and they are each vital for optimum health. It's best to test to see if you are, in fact deficient, and below are the places you can contact to do this. I strongly recommend you play it safe and get the tests and take the supplements under medical supervision, especially if you're presently taking any medication. If you choose to go it alone, start slowly with conservative dosages and pay attention. If you start feeling worse, stop, and seek professional help.

- **Eliminate as many toxins from your environment as possible.**

Avoid using dishwasher powder you buy at the supermarket since it is extremely poisonous – there are more pure dishwasher powders available at health food stores. Avoid fluoridated toothpastes, tablets, gels, and all other fluoridated products. Fluoride is basically a pesticide since it works by poisoning the bacteria and plaque in your mouth. It is particularly unsafe for children, since they tend to swallow much of the toothpaste they use. Avoid drinking fluoridated water. Do not drink water from municipal water supplies since it contains chlorine and oftentimes fluoride, and drink only pure spring water. Eliminate using pesticides and herbicides in and around the house. Clean the toxins that tend to settle on floors, toys, and surfaces children play on and put in their mouths. Reduce or eliminate deodorants, cosmetics, and nail polish, since they are all laden with poisons and can get into the air you breathe.

- **Eliminate all drugs.**

All drugs are toxic – I've shown that time and again throughout this book. Decrease and eliminate all drugs under the supervision of a qualified health care professional. The healthier you become by making positive changes to your lifestyle, the less you will think you need them.

- **Avoid EMF pollution — sleep grounded.**

Do not sleep with electric blankets, or with a waterbed heater on. These disturb the electromagnetic fields of the body. In fact, electromagnetic pollution is becoming quite a problem in our highly technological society. EMFs (electromagnetic fields) have been implicated in a wide variety of illnesses such as sleep disorders, stress-related and autoimmune diseases including arthritis, asthma, fibromyalgia, lupus, cardiovascular disease, and many more. Our bodies take on some of the electromagnetic charges around us, and we actually act like a battery and store some of these charges. Our electrical system (our nervous system) operates on very low voltage. When we take on too much voltage from the environment, we get overcharged, which leads to stress and overproduction of adrenaline and other stress hormones. One solution is to be grounded, and I discussed this in the chapter on sleep disorders. It's good to walk barefoot on the bare earth often to discharge the EMFs. See the Insomnia chapter for more.

- **Get plenty of rest and sleep.**

Allow yourself and child and yourself to sleep as much you like. Sleep is the time when the body makes repairs, and processes new information, and it knows just how much time it needs make them. Adequate sleep is essential for learning. "A full night's sleep is one of the most important factors for learning and absorbing information," says Mark DiDea, M.D. Bruce D. Perry, M.D., agrees, "Sleep is probably the most important period of the day for processing new information. Children have many new concepts to learn in school. A good night's sleep not only lets them process what they learned but also helps them be alert in class."[7]

It's not just kids who learn, but adults are learning every day too. It's best for children to go to bed early, say around 7:00 p.m. And 8:00 p.m. At the latest, and adults to go to bed before 11:00 pm. This keeps the body in tune to the natural nocturnal rhythms of humans in general. Benjamin Franklin's advice "Early to bed and early to rise makes a man (and woman) healthy, wealthy, and wise" is true, and especially important for youngsters. Oftentimes when the body starts healing, it will require more sleep. If you make some positive changes to your diet and lifestyle this may be the reason.

• Don't smoke.

That means both tobacco and marijuana. Marijuana smoke contains nine times the amount of the toxic heavy metal cadmium as tobacco smoke.

• Exercise.

We all know that exercise is important. It increases circulation and improves overall cardiovascular health. It burns fat and increases your metabolism so you will burn fat even when you're not exercising. It's very helpful and sometimes great cure for depression because when you exercise, serotonin and endorphins are produced, which make you feel good. I discuss the best kind of exercise in the cardiovascular chapter.

• Do the special breathing exercise to get an extra shot of oxygen.

I described a special kind of breathing (not deep breathing) in the chapter on asthma. It delivers a big dose of oxygen to all the cells and tissues in your body. Do it at least once a day (10-30 minutes) or more, especially if you're not feeling your best.

• Love your family and friends.

The emphasis of this book has been on the physical, chemical, and physiological aspects health. My belief is that if we are physically and mentally sound, we will naturally be loving and caring. As your health improves your life will become easier. However, as physically and mentally healthy as we may become, we still need love.

Love makes things grow and bring joy into our lives. We need that warm and fuzzy feeling, and kids need it more than anyone. Give your kids and your spouse a hug every day. Tell them you love them. Hold them close and whisper sweet nothings in their ears. For some, this may sound corny. To a child, it's the breath of life. Don't be ashamed to verbalize and demonstrate your love and make a habit of it. If you're afraid or ashamed to, it probably means you weren't raised in a loving atmosphere yourself, so break that chain and be brave.

The Reverend Wayne Muller, author of *Sabbath: Finding Rest, Renewal and Delight in Our Busy Lives*, said, "We can tell children we love them and we can mean it. However, the only way the kids are ever going to know what we mean by 'love' is the time we spend playing with them on the carpet." Remember when you were a kid? You know that's true.

Show your child you care by laying down the law when needed and making sure they understand you're doing it for their betterment. You don't need to be your child's best friend, but you do need to be a loving and caring steward, directing them with gentle firmness toward the truly good things in life.

If you're having trouble in your marriage, it's best to try and work it out. But you don't want to live in an untenable situation either. I am definitely not a marriage counselor but here's my advice anyway:

You as a family can take this book and make it a project. Husband and wife reading it and then working on it together as a team to improve your family's life. If your child is old enough, have him or her read it too. Analyze it and discuss it – maybe even do some research on your own. Try putting some of the recommendations in this book to work and watch things change. Read some of the books in the Recommended Reading section.

You'll see that as you get healthier and closer to the real you, personality conflicts will dissolve by themselves without any effort. You and your spouse will remember why you fell in love with each other, and you'll start feeling that magic feeling again. Not just emotionally, but physically as well. I guarantee that if you follow my recommendations, your sex life will improve dramatically.

Tell your spouse "I love you," even if you have to fake it to start. Remember, "In the beginning was The Word. . ." Have some fun along the way. Get some joke books out of the library and make it a family tradition to have someone tell a joke every evening before dinner. Laughter lifts the mood and helps digestion. To get you started, here are two pretty bad golf jokes:

1. Husband and wife sitting at the breakfast table eating toast and eggs – he reading a golf magazine as usual. She says, "Harry, all you think about is golf, golf, golf! You haven't even noticed this fine Sunday breakfast you're eating." "Sure I have dear," he replies. "Oh, and would you please pass the putter."

2. "Darling, remember the day we got married?" she asks. "Sure do," he replies with a smile, "Sank a 45-foot putt the day before!"

Don't make getting healthy a bore or a chore, but try to make it fun and an exploration. I know it's a complicated world, and sometimes it seems overwhelming. Take one little step at a time and try not to worry. Take a break now and then. Go and treat yourself and your kids for a job well done, even if it means going out for pizza or ice cream every now and then. The healthier you and your kids become, the less you'll be attracted to junky foods. Once you start reversing the downward spiral and see some positive things happen, you'll be able to do more and more with less and less effort. Give it some time, be patient, and don't give up.

- **Get some sunshine every day.**

That means real sun without any sunscreen or sun block, without getting burned. Sunlight is needed for proper vitamin D production and thus calcium absorption and hormonal regulation. Too much of anything is harmful. Be sensible and cautious, but get some sun and use full spectrum lighting.

- **Watch less TV, or none at all.**

- **Avoid Heavy Metals**

Mercury is very toxic to life and can create all sorts of problems in the human body and mind. The best thing to do is to avoid mercury exposure as much as possible. There are hundreds if not thousands of products in today's society that contain mercury. A complete list of everyday items with heavy metal can be found in the book, *It's All In Your Head* by Hal A. Huggins, D.D.S.

I cannot emphasize enough that many vaccines contain thimerosal and other trace amounts of mercury (as well as aluminum). As Congressman Dan Burton said, "How is it that mercury is not safe for food additives and OTC drugs, but is safe in vaccines and dental amalgams?"[10]

I recently talked with a mother of four who got the necessary exemptions and not one of her children received even one vaccine. They are all alive and well, and she says they hardly ever get as much as a sniffle. She also feeds them well and keeps them off junk foods as much as possible. I asked her how she got the exemptions, and she said she simply wrote letters saying she didn't believe in them. I don't know if this approach will work in every case, but it may be worth a try. You may consider home-schooling your kids to avoid the requirements for vaccines. Call the National Vaccine Information Center (NVIC) at (800) 909-SHOT for more information or for help in getting your child out of getting vaccinated. I also included a letter in the vaccine chapter that might help.

I have a friend who has her own dog-training business. She mentioned that a friend of hers who breeds dogs professionally had stopped giving the dogs shots because he noticed that the dogs themselves are not only healthier in the long run, but they give birth to healthier and heartier puppies. Since the unvaccinated dogs were not sickened on purpose by vaccines, which weaken their cellular constitution, that strength is passed on to the next generation. Likewise, cellular weakness is passed on too.

Do not get silver-mercury amalgams dental fillings. Not only does the mercury leech into the bloodstream, but it also out-gasses from the filling. As it interacts with the saliva, it creates significant electrical charges in the mouth that may interfere with the functioning of the nervous system.

If you already have amalgams in your teeth, it's wise to get them removed as soon as possible. Your dentist will probably tell you there's no problem, and that you're crazy for wanting to remove them. Don't listen. The state of California actually requires dentist to post a health warning about amalgam fillings. There are plenty of dentists who understand that mercury is a problem and will be happy to remove the fillings. The fillings need to be removed in a certain order, depending on their respective electrical discharges. You need to find a dentist who has the appropriate testing equipment and knows what he's doing. See the Resource Guide. There are plenty of other kinds of materials (called composites) to fill cavities with. Dentistry has come a long way in just the last couple decades. Most of the newer materials are non-toxic. However, they all may not be suited to your specific body chemistry. It's a good idea to get a Compatibility Test, where a sample of blood is analyzed for allergic-type reactions to the various dental materials on the market. If your dentist does not know about this or says it's unnecessary, you need to get another dentist.

Another thing to consider is the effect of braces. The metal itself not only corrodes to some degree in the acidic environment of the mouth, but the interaction of this metal and any other metals in the mouth (i.e., in fillings) sets up an electrical storm in the mouth. This can cause severe personality shifts and problems in the adolescent during a time when their hormones are giving them enough trouble as it is. For a detailed discussion on these effects, read the book *Uninformed Consent* by Dr. Hal Huggins.

- **Getting the Heavy Metals Out**
   Although heavy metals have and tend to stay in the body a long time and, as you now know, can cause many problems, it *is* possible to eliminate them from your body using the right foods and juices. I do not recommend you use chelating agents or supplements claiming they will remove heavy metals. Most of them are toxic in their own right and will, over the long haul, cause problems. It's important to realize that heavy metals and other toxins in the body are eliminated by binding to fats in the diet. Butter, coconut oils and meat, olive oil, eggs, cream, and milk fats are excellent for this. In order to mobilize the toxins out of the tissues, certain vegetable juices can be consumed. Juicing fresh cilantro, parsley, celery, and zucchini, with some carrots mobilizes the toxins and nourishes the tissues as well. Be sure to consume some fat with the juice. Putting a couple of ounces of raw cream in the juice will do nicely or taking a tablespoon of coconut oil or cod liver oil works too.

Some foods are believed to help with eliminating mercury from the body. These are foods high in sulfur, which is believed to bind with mercury. You may consider adding these foods to your diet on a regular basis: eggs, garlic, onions, cilantro, parsley, cabbage, and broccoli. Try the *Chelation Pesto* I discussed in the ADHD chapter.

Epilogue

We live in a complicated world. Society, science, and technology are moving so fast it can make your head spin. However, as complicated as things might get, there are some simple truths we as living organisms must adhere to in order to survive and thrive. These truths will never change for they are universal laws of chemistry, physics, and biology that all matter and every organism is subject to.

The objective of this book has been to show you things that may be affecting your and your loved ones' health in unnatural and therefore, unhealthy ways. Science, technology, and greed have produced many things that cause biological malfunctions. The malfunctions can be immediate, like a drug overdose, or take years and even generations to manifest, like the rising infertility rate.

Getting treatments without knowing the true cause of the problem will only cause more havoc. If we know the real cause, then taking the proper corrective actions will be simple. Oftentimes it's a case of eliminating an offending substance from our environment or diet. Sometimes it's making sure we have the correct nutrition. Merely treating the symptom, as with drugs, in the short run may provide some comfort, but it will do nothing to stop the symptom or other symptoms from eventually reappearing.

We like to think humanity is advancing toward some higher good and getting stronger, healthier, and more enlightened. But if you look around, is that really what you see? Why have heart disease, diabetes, asthma, ADHD, and autism become epidemics? Why are children shooting each other? Is it because we're rising to a higher state of being?

Society is made up of individuals, and individuals are made up of living cells. How can we expect society to function well when its individuals are sick and impaired? How can we expect an individual to function well when his or her cells are toxic and malnourished?

The next 30 years will be very interesting. Will we wise up and make wholesale changes to our environment, eliminating toxic substances and cleaning up our food, water, and air? Or will we continue to stick our heads in the sand and deny that unnatural things beget unhealthy beings? Will science and politics, influenced by corporate profits, keep hiding behind sayings such as: "there is no observable effect" or "there is no real scientific evidence" when simple common sense tells us otherwise?

Will we see the continual decline in people's and children's health, with each generation getting sicker and weaker at younger and younger ages? Will aggression, violence, stupidity, perversity, and immorality keep rising? Or will we realize that the body and mind need to be treated in certain ways for harmony to exist? The saying "you are what you eat" has become "you are what you consume." If we continue to consume and subject ourselves to substances that cause biological discord (mercury, chlorine, fluoride, sugar, aspartame, *Ritalin*, vaccines), we will continue to see discord and disease in our lives and our society. If we continue to consume with our mind television, video and movie violence, we will continue to be influenced by it.

Throughout this book, I debunked and criticized government agencies such as the FDA and CDC and certain government policies. I have admittedly been harsh, to the point that you may have gotten the impression that I am un-American. Nothing could be further from the truth. I believe, even with all the problems we have, the U.S. of A. is the greatest country in recorded history, and mankind took a quantum leap away from injustice, malice, greed, and slavery when it was born.

However, there are some among us who place money and power above all else. They prey on the weak and innocent, yes, but as is the case with America, the prosperous and trusting. You see, a pirate doesn't plunder a barren ship. He finds the grandest, richest ship afloat, attacks it, weakens it, boards it, and seizes its gold. Such is what is happening to America.

These modern-day pirates, who only care about how much gold they have in their coffers and how much power they have over others, haven't used swords and cannon to weaken us, but psychology, inculcation, and fear. They have brainwashed us into believing their products and services are better than what God and nature provide and are necessary not just for a more comfortable life, but for survival itself. They are enslaving us, not with shackles, but with sickness and infirmity. They have infiltrated the government and schools and have even changed history so their stranglehold and pilfering can continue.

Sadly, I have little hope for the masses. Most people do not have the courage to question authority and think for themselves. Furthermore, since drugs and our toxic environment are affecting people's intellect and reasoning powers, they will be less and less able to separate truth from dogma. They will listen and follow until they can literally no longer hear, walk, or reproduce. Along the way, people and our society will get more violent, barbaric, immature, and immoral. Then, when the pirates have taken everything there is to take, they will turn their backs on the huddled, suffering masses, and, without blinking an eye, find someone else to plunder. Such is the heart of darkness.

However, some will recognize cause and effect, truth and dogma, right and wrong, nature and Godliness, and have the courage and energy to take a different path. A path that may be hard in some ways, but immensely fulfilling in others. A path that is cooperative instead of antagonistic, enlightening instead of confusing, harmonious instead of discordant. A path you won't be able to resist, because when you are of the light, you gravitate towards the light. There is a reason you are reading this.

Then there will arise out of this country of twisted bones, twisted minds, and twisted values, a new nation. Not a nation necessarily bound by rivers or mountains or geographical lines on a map – but a nation of people bound together by knowledge and truth. A truth that will enable them to overcome their confusion, greed, and malice, and develop into the species they were meant to be – one of compassion, courage, and grace. A group of individuals devoted to becoming more and more and reaching higher and higher, not just for themselves, but for their progeny. For each generation will become greater and greater, stronger and stronger, more and more compassionate, until compassion is rarely needed. They will build on the strength of those enlightened ones before them so that they too may become more enlightened. And the earth will become the paradise it once was, and even more.

You are the first of this small but powerful wave and your struggle against the lies and misinformation is greater due to the momentum it has gathered over the centuries. But stem that tide you must – *as best you can*. For we are not supermen, superwomen, and superkids. . .yet.

Future generations will look back and call you their forefathers and heroes. Forefathers of the people we were meant to be. Heroes because of your courage, initiative, wisdom, resilience, and nobility. In time, there will be another declaration of independence – not just for a nation of healthy and sovereign individuals, but for humanity itself. A humanity that can, and will, have Everlasting Health.

Recognizing the truth and acting on it: That is your greatness and your genius. Good luck, and Godspeed.

> . . .*Stood alone on a mountain top, staring out at the Great Divide.*
> *I could go east, I could go west, it was all up to me to decide.*
> *Just then I saw a young hawk flying and my soul began to rise*
> *And pretty soon, my heart was singing. . .*
> *Roll, roll me away, I'm gonna roll me away tonight.*
> *Gotta keep rolling, gotta keep riding,*
> *Keep searching 'till I find what's right.*
> *And as the sunset faded I spoke to the faintest first starlight,*
> *And I said,*
> *Next time. . .*
> *Next time. . .*
> *We'll get it right.*
> *Bob Seger*

Resource Guide

It's important that only the brands listed be used for each product. Others may not be effective, and may even be harmful. Many products can be found in most health food stores, but other sources are also listed.

Everlasting Health Newsletter
A bimonthly publication that continues to explore, expose, educate, and enlighten. To request your copy, send an email to proreach@aol.com. In the subject line, put *ELH Newsletter* and your name and address in the body of the email. To request by mail, write *ELH Newsletter* on a postcard or in a letter, along with your name and address, and mail to: PRI Publishing, 1130 E. Main Street, Suite 183, Ashland, OH 44805.

Bee Pollen
www.ccpollen.com (800) 875-0096
www.ysorganic.com (800) 654-4593

Unheated Honey
Beware brands that say they are raw but are still heated somewhat. The only two brands I am sure are unheated are below, and are in most health food stores.
www.reallyrawhoney.com (800) REAL-RAW
www.ysorganic.com (800) 654-4593

Cod Liver Oil
Blue Ice High Vitamin Cod Liver Oil: (402) 858-4818
Radiant Live Premier High Vitamin Cold Liver Oil: (888) 593-8333

Vitamin D Testing
www.zrtlab.com (866) 600-1636
www.directlabs.com (800) 908-0000

Zinc Test
Oral Zinc Tally test: www.thewayup.com (800) 289-8487

Iron and Red Blood Cell, or Complete Blood Count (CBC) Tests
www.healthcheckusa.com (800) 929-2044
www.directlabs.com (800) 908-0000

Hair Analysis or Heavy Metal Fecal Test
www.genovadiagnostics.com (800) 522-4762
www.directlabs.com (800) 908-0000

Mercury Free Dentists
www.mercuryfreedentists.com

Vaccine Information
National Vaccine Information Center (NVIC) (800) 909-SHOT
Vaccine Liberation: www.vaclib.org

Magnesium Oil
www.magneticclay.com (800) 257-3315

RBC Magnesium Test
www.directlabs.com (800) 908-0000

Nascent Iodine
www.magneticclay.com (800) 257-3315

Iodine Testing
www.ffplab.org (877) 900-5556
www.labrix.com (877) 656-9596

Alternatives to mammograms and prostate exams
   Power Color Doppler Sonography
      www.cancerscan.com (212) 355-7017
      www.4wecare.com (602) 493-2159
   Thermography
      www.breastthermography.com (650) 361-8908

Grounding Products
www.barefoothealth.com (800) 620-9912

Juicers
www.omegajuicers.com (717) 561-1105
www.greenstar.com (888) 254-7336

Apple Cider Vinegar
www.bragg.com (Braggs)
www.spectrumorganics.com (Spectrum Naturals)

Neuromins
www.mmspro.net, www.emersonecologics.com

Oils and **Essential Fatty Acid Products**
These oils are pressed below 96° F, which preserves their nutrients. They can usually be found at health food stores, but if not, here's contact info You can get extra virgin olive oil, coconut oil, coconut butter, flax seek oil etc.
www.florahealth.com, (800) 446-2110
www.omeganutrition.com (800) 661-3529
www.spectrumnorganics.com (800) 434-4246

Organic Food

You can find organically raised foods at most health food stores or national chains like Whole Foods and Wild Oats. Some mail order sources:

Jaffe Brothers
(877) 975-2333
www.organicfruitsandnuts.com

Boxed Greens
Boxedgreens.com

Diamond Organics
(888) ORGANIC
www.diamondorganics.com

D'Artagnan
(800) 327-8246
www.dartagnag.com

Raw Milk and Dairy Products

You can check with local dairy farmers to see if they sell raw dairy products. Finding one may be difficult, so I suggest you contact The Weston A. Price Foundation who publishes listings of providers of unpasteurized dairy products.
www.westonaprice.org (202) 333-HEAL.
www.realmilk.com.

Eggs

To obtain raw, fertile eggs from free range hens, check at your health food store or find a local farmer.

Salt

Salt should be avoided. But, if you are going to eat it, eat only Celtic Sea Salt. You can find it at most health food stores or at
www.celticseasalt.com (800) 867-7258

Water

Use *Perrier* water or other good mineral water bottled at the source with natural, not added carbonation.

Personalized Nutritional Counseling

David Getoff, CCN, CNC, FAAIM
www.naturopath4you.com (831) 423-7554

Nontoxic Household Products

www.seventhgeneration.com (800) 456-1191
www.solutions-4-you.com (800) 301-9111
Two good books are:
Nontoxic, Natural, & Earthwise by Debra Lynn Dadd
Better Basics for the Home: Simple Solutions for Less Toxic Living
by Annie Berthold-Bond

Recommended Reading

The Truth about Children's Health by Robert Bernardini. Hailed as "One of the most important books of our time." Complete natural health for your child.

PRI Publishing at (419) 869-7901, proreach@aol.com

The Complete Children's Safety and Protection Kit, with 14 Days to a Safer Child Lesson Plan, by PRI Publishing. www.supersafechild.com, (419) 869-7901.

Iodine: Why You Need it, Why You Can't Live Without It by David Brownstein, M.D.   3rd Edition. Medial Alternatives Press, 4173 Fieldbrook, W. Bloomfield, MI 48323.(888) 647-5616.

Transdermal Magnesium Therapy by Mark Sircus, Phaelos Books, 860 N McQueen Rd, #1171, Chandler, AZ 85225.(480) 275-4925.

We Want to Live by Aajonus Vonderplanitz. Published by Carnelian Bay Castle Press, P.O. Box 66663, Los Angeles, CA 90066.(800) 247-6553.

The Recipe for Living Without Disease, by AajonusVonderplanitz, Carnelian Bay Castle Press, P.O. Box 66663, Los Angeles, CA 90066.(800) 247-6553.

Health & Healing Wisdom Journal. Published by the Price-Pottenger Nutrition Foundation, P.O. Box 2614, La Mesa, Ca 91943.(800) 366-3748.

The Crazy Makers by Carol Simontacchi. Published by Penguin Putnam, Inc., 375 Hudson St., New York, NY, 10014. Available through the Price-Pottenger Nutrition Foundation, (800) 366-3748.

Vaccination, Social Violence, and Criminality by Harris L. Coulter, North Atlantic Books, Berkeley California.

A Shot in the Dark by Harris L. Coulter and Barbara Loe Fisher. Avery Publishing, NY, NY. www.909shot.com

The Consumer's Guide to Childhood Vaccines by Barbara Loe Fisher. Published by the National Vaccine Information Center, 512 W. Maple Ave., Suite 206, Vienna, VA, 22180.(800) 909-SHOT.

For Tomorrow's Children – A Manual for Future Parents. Published by Preconception Care, Inc., P.O. Box 357, Blooming Glen, PA 18911. Price-Pottenger Nutrition Foundation (800) 366-3748.

The Curse of Louis Pasteur – Why Medicine is Not Healing a Diseased World by Nancy Appleton. Published by Choice Publishing, P.O. Box Santa Monica, CA 90403 & Price-Pottenger Nutrition Foundation (800) 366-3748.

Sugar Blues by William Dufty. Published by Warner Books, Inc., 1271 Avenue of the Americas, New York, NY 10020. Available at most book stores or Amazon.com.

Uninformed Consent – The Hidden Dangers in Dental Care by Hal A. Huggins and Thomas E Levy. Published by Hampton Roads Publishing Company, Inc, 1125 Stoney Ridge Road, Charlottesville, VA 22902.(800) 766-8009.

It's All in Your Head – The Link Between Mercury Amalgams and Illness by Hal A. Huggins. Published by Avery Publishing Group, Inc., Garden City Park, NY.

Nourishing Traditions by Sally Fallon. New Trends Publishing, Inc., Washington, D.C.(877) 707-1776.

Wise Traditions Newsletter. Published quarterly by The Weston A. Price Foundation, PMB (202) 333-HEAL.

Training the Brain to Pay Attention the Write Way by Jeanette Farmer, www.retrainthebrain.com. (303) 740-6161

Braingym   www.braingym.com. (888) 388-9898

Bibliography

Introduction
1. Bromfield, L. *Pleasant Valley.* The Wooster Book Company, Wooster, OH. 1977.
2. Buttram, Harold, Richard Piccola. *Who is Looking After Our Kids? A Guide for Parent's to Protect Their Children From Environmental Hazards.* Foresight America Foundation, Quakertown, PA . December 1997; www.healing.org/Child-intro.html.
3. Fallon, Sally, and Mary G. Enig, Ph.D. *Nourishing Traditions,* Washington, DC: New Trends Publishing, Inc. 1999.

Chapter I—People of the USA
1. U.S Census Bureau, www. census.gov.
2. CDC/NCHS National Vital Statistics System & www.cia.gov/cia/publications/factbook/rankorder/2102rank.html.
3. *JAMA,* July 26, 2000;284(4):483-5.
4. Douglass WC. "Dial –a-side-effect Hotline." Daily Dose Newsletter, June 2, 2008.
5. Landrigan, Philip J., et al. *Pesticides in the Diets of Infants and Children.* National Research Council. National Academy Press: Washington, DC, 1993, p. 61.
6. Wiles, Richard, et al. "Pesticides in Children's Food." Washington, DC: Environmental Working Group, June 1993. www.ewg.org.
7. Landrigan, et al. Op cit. p. 43.
8. Carlson, Elisabeth, et al. "Evidence for Decreasing Quality of Semen During Past 50 Years." *British Medical Journal* 305: 609-613 (1992).
9. Gray, J.R., and Leon Earl. "Chemical-Induced Alterations of Sexual Differentiation: A Review of Effects in Humans and Rodents." In *Advances in Modern Environmental Toxicology,* edited by M.A. Mehlman. Princeton, NJ: Princeton Scientific Publishing Co. Inc., 1992, pp. 203-230.
10. *Infant Risks From Pesticides,* Washington, DC: Environmental Working Group, 2001. www.ewg.org.
11. Peto, R., et al. "Effects on 4080 Rats of Chronic Ingestion of N-Nitrosodiethylamine or N-Nitrosodimethylamine: A Detailed Dose-Response Study." *Cancer Research* 51 (1991): 6415-51.
12. McConnell, Ernest. *Comparative Responses in Carcinogenesis Bioassays as a Function of Age at First Exposure. Similarities & Differences Between Children and Adults.* Washington, DC: ILSI Press, 1992, pp. 66-78.
13. Snodgrass, Wayne R. "Physiological and Biochemical Difference Between Children and Adults As Determinants of Toxic Response to Environmental Pollutants." In *Similarities and Differences between Children and Adults: Implications for Risk Assessment,* edited by Philip S. Guzelian, Carol J. Henry, and Stephen S. Olin. Washington, DC: International Life Sciences Institute, 1992, pp. 35-42.
14. Landrigan, Philip J., et al. Op cit.
15. Ibid.
16. Ibid
17. Ries, L., et al. *Cancer in Children, SEER Cancer Statistics Review, 1973-1990.* Washington, D.C.: U.S. Department of Health and Human Services, 1993.
18. Masters, Roger D., Brian Hone, and Anil Doshi. "Environmental Pollution, Neurotoxicity and Criminal Violence." In *Environmental Toxicology,* edited by J. Rose. New York: Gordon and Breach Publishers, 1997.
19. Executive Order. *Protection of Children From Environmental Health Risks and Safety Risks.* The White House, Office of the Press Secretary. April 21, 1997.
20. *Preventing Child Exposures to Environmental Hazards: Research and Policy Issues.* Children's Environmental Health Network/California Public Health Foundation. 1994.

Chapter II – Obesity
1. Heart Disease and Stroke Statistics - 2005 Update, American Heart Association
2. *Annals of Internal Medicine.* June 18, 2002; 136:857-864, 923-925
3. Horlick, Mary. Endocrine Society's 2000 annual conference, 2000.
4. Olshansky, SJ et al. "A Potential Decline in Life Expectancy in the U.S. in the 21st Century." *New England Journal of Medicine,* March 17, 2005, Vol. 352, no.11:1138-1145.
5. Yahoo! News January 6, 2004.
6. "More in U.S. Obese Than Just Overweight." Reuters. Dec. 9 2008.
7. Yahoo! News January 6, 2004.
8. *USA Today,* June 27, 2005.
9. cdc/gov/nccdphp/dnpa
10. Yahoo! News January 29, 2004.
11. Ibid.
12. Hale, Ellen. "Youths Untouched by Health Trends: Obese Young People Invite Heart Disease with Unhealthy Diets." *Iowa Press-Citizen.* December 18, 1986.
13. Ibid.
14. Yahoo! News April 28, 2004.
15. "Vegetable without Vitamins." *Life Extension Magazine* March 2001.
16. www.en.allexperts.com.
17. U.S. National - Reuters. CDC Says Carbs to Blame for Rising Calorie Intake. February 5, 2004.
18. Berkey, CS. "Milk, Dairy fat, Dietary Calcium, and Weight Gain: a Longitudinal Study of Adolescents," *Archives of Pediatrics & Adolescent Medicine,* June 2005: 159(6): 543-550.
19. Biser S. *The Last Chance Health Report.* University of Natural Healing. Charlottesville, VA 1994,4:9
20. National Academy of Sciences. *Regulating Pesticides: The Delaney Paradox.* 1987.
21. Lowengart, R et al. "Childhood Leukemia and Parents' Occupational and Home Exposures." *Journal of National Cancer Resources Institute.* 79:39-46 1987
22. Tebbey PW, Buttke TM. "Molecular Basis for the Immunosuppressive Action fo Stearic Acid on T-cells." *Immunology,* 1990 July;379-80
23. Ulloth JE, Casiano CA, DeLeon M. Department of Microbiology and Immunology, East Carlina University School of Medicne. PMID:112562519 (PubMed
24. Sparaga GC, Hickson-Bick, DL. *American Journal of Medical Science.* 318(1):15, July 1999.
25. Healy M. "With Vitamin-enriched foods, More Isn't Always Better." LA times, May 22,2008
26. "Fast Food 'As Addictive As Heroin." BBC News Jan. 30, 2003
27. arthritistrust.org
28. garynull.com
29. Robinson W, "Delay in the Appearance of Palpable Mammary Tumors in C3H Mice Following the Ingestion of Pollenized Food." *Journal of the National Cancer Institute,* Oct. 1948:9 119-123
30. Wojcicki J, et al. "Effect of Pollen Extract on the Development of Experimental Atherosclerosis in Rabbits." *Atherosclerosis.* 1986 Oct:62(1) 39-45
31. Chen J, Chu L, Aerospace Medicine & Life Sciences.
32. *BBC News,* "Honey Could help Fight Cancer," December 5, 2004. www.bbc.co.uk.
33. www.garynull.com.
34. Johnston CS, Kim CM, Buller AJ. "Vinegar Improves Insulin Sensitivity to a High-carbohydrate Meal in Subjects withb Insulin Resistance or Type 2 Diabetes." Diabetes Care 27:281-282.
35. Jushimi, T, et al. "Acetic Acid Feeding Enhances Glycogen Repletion in Liver and Skeletal Muscle of Rats." *Journal of Nutrition,* 2001;131:1973-1977.
36. Kishi M, et al. "Enhanding Effect of Dietary Vinegar on the Intestinal Absorption of Calcium in Ovariectomized Rats." Biosci Biotechnol Bochem. 1999;63:905-910.
37. Honsho S., "A Red Wine Vinegar Beverage Can Inhibit the Rennin-angiotensin System: Experimental Evidence in Vivo. Biol Pharm Bull. 2005:28:1208-1210.
38. Kondo, S. "Antihypertensive Effects of Acetic Acid and Vinegar on Spontaneously Hypertensive Rats." Biosci Biotechnol Biochem. 2001;65:2690-2694.
39. Aminifarshidmehr N. "The Management of Chronic Suppurative Otitis Media with Acid Media Solution" Am J Otol. 1996:17:24-25.
40. Shaw T. "Peru Tries Vinegar Against Cervical Cancer." Bull World Health Org. 2003;81:73-74
41. Abraham, GE, Flechas, JD, "Management of Fibromyalgia: Rationale for the Use of Magnesium and Malic Acid." *Journal of Nutritional Medicine* (1992) 3, 49-59.
42. Jarvis, DC. *Folk Medicine.* Fawcet. 1985.
43. Puotinen, J. *Encyclopedia of Natural Pet Care.* Keats Publishing. 2000.

44. Hale, Ellen. Op cit.
45. "Media Education," *Pediatrics.* 104, no. 2, August 1999.
46. Robinson, Thomas N. "Reducing Children's Television Viewing to Prevent Obesity; A Randomized Controlled Trial," *Journal of the American Medical Association* 282, no. 6. October 1999.
47. American Heart Association website 2003 study, Mark Periera and www.turnoffyoutv.com
48. "Media Education." Op cit.
49. Ibid.
50. "Children, Adolescents and Advertising." *Pediatrics* 95, no. 2 (February 1995).
51. "Violence on Television" (brochure). American Psychological Association, 2001.
52. National Coalition on Television Violence.
53. "Violence on Television," Op cit.
54. Marks, Alexandra. "What Children See and Do: Studies on Violence on TV." *Christian Science Monitor,* April 17, 1998.
55. "Violence on Television." Op cit.
56. Ibid.
57. Krugman, H.D. "Brain Wave Measurements of Media Involvement," *Journal of Advertising Research.* 11:1, Feb. 1971.
58. Setzer, Valdemar. "TV and Violence: A Perfect Marriage." 2001. www.ime.usp.br/~vwsetzer.
59. Ott, John N. *Health and Light.* New York: Pocket Books, 1973.
60. 21CFR1030.10. (Code of Federal Regulations, Title 21, Volume 8, Part 1030. "Performance Standards for Microwave and Radio Frequency Emitting Products." Section .10, Revised as of April 1, 2001)
61. Naisbitt, John. *High Tech, High Touch: Technology and Our Search for Meaning.* London: Nicholas Breadley. 2000.
62. Setzer, Valdemar, W. "The Risks to Children Using Electronic Games." 2001. www.ime.usp.br/~vwsetzer.

Chapter III – Cancer
1. www.breastcancer.org
2. *Dorland's Pocket Medical Dictionary.* W.B. Saunders Company, Philadelphia: Harcourt Brace Jovanovich, Inc., 1989.
3. U.S. Bureau of the Census, *Statistical Abstract of the United States: 1955.* (Seventy-sixth edition.) Washington, D.C., 1955.
4. Landrigan, Philip J. "Commentary: Environmental Disease—A Preventable Epidemic." *American Journal of Public Health* 82 (July 1992): 941-943.
5. American Cancer Society Cancer Facts and Figures, 2004. www.cancer.org
6. *USA Today.* January 20, 2005
7. Ries, L.A.G., et al., eds. *Cancer Incidence and Survival among Children and Adolescents: United States SEER Program 1975-1995,* National Cancer Institute, SEER Program. NIH Pub. No.99-4649 (1999): 1.
8. Schmidt, Charles W. "Childhood Cancer: A Growing Problem." *Environmental Health Perspectives* 106, no. 1 (1998): A18-A23.
9. Ries, L.A.G., et al. eds. *SEER Cancer Statistics Review, 1973-1995.* National Cancer Institute, http://www.seer.ims.nci.nih.gov (1998).
10. Kosary, C.L., et al. eds. *SEER Cancer Statistics Review, 1973-1992: Tables and Graphs,* National Cancer Institute. NIH Pub. no. 96-2789 (1995): 455.
11.   Miller, B.A., et al. eds. *SEER Cancer Statistics Review 1973-1990.* NIH Publ. no. 93-2789 (1993).
12.   Ries, L.A.G. Op cit. p. 5.
13. Schmidt, Charles W. Op cit.
14. Montague, Peter. "Children's Cancer and Pesticides." Environmental Research Foundation. *Rachel's Environment & Health Weekly,* no. 588: 1 (March 5, 1998).
15.   Lichtenstein, P., et al. "Environmental and Heritable Factors in the Causation of Cancer— Analyses of Cohorts of Twins from Sweden, Denmark, and Finland." *New England Journal of Medicine* 343, no. 2: 28-85 (2000).
16. Davis, Robert, Cancer Stats Cite New Danger, *USA Today,* Jan 14, 2004
17. *Preventing Child Exposures to Environmental Hazards: Research and Policy Issues.* Children's Environmental Health Network/California Public Health Foundation. Emeryville, CA. 1994,1995. www.cehn.org.
18. Barich, Bob. "Hedging Your Bets." Greatlife. January, 2001, p10.
19. Li, Frederick P., et al. "Cancer Mortality Among Chemists." *Journal of the National Cancer Institute* 43: 1159-1164 (1969).
20. Walrath, Judy, et al. "Causes of Death Among Female Chemists." *American Journal of Public Health* (August 1985): 883-885.
21. Thomas, Terry L., and Pierce Decoufle. "Mortality Among Workers Employed in the Pharmaceutical Industry: A Preliminary Investigation." *Journal of Occupational Medicine* 21: 619-623 (September 1979).
22. Arnetz, Bengt B. "Mortality Among Petrochemical Science and Engineering Employees." *Archives of Environmental Health* 46: 237-248 (July/August 1991).
23. Sinclair, Wayne. "Chemicals and Pesticides. Environmental Causes of Child Cancers and Remission Information." 2000. www.chemtox.com./cancerchildren/default/htm.
24. Mercola.com. How to Avoid the Top 10 Most Common Toxins
25. "A Short History of Pesticides." *Simplelife.* 1995/96. www.simplelife.com.
26. Needham, Larry L., et al. "The Priority Toxicant Reference Range Study: Interim Report." *Environmental Health Perspectives* 103, supplement 3 (April 1995).
27. Landrigan, Philip J. "Commentary: Environmental Disease—A Preventable Epidemic." *American Journal of Public Health* 82 (July 1992): 941-943.
28. "Pesticide Exposure During Pregnancy." www.chem-Tox.com/pregnancy/pregpest.htm.
29. "Pesticide Statistics." *Simplelife.* 1995/96. www.simplelife.com
30. Pearce, Fred, and Debora Mackenzie. "It's Raining Pesticides: The Water Falling From Our Skies is Unfit to Drink." *New Scientist:* 23 (April 3, 1999). www.newscientist.com.
31. Montague, Peter, "Pesticides in the News." *Rachel's Environmental & Health Weekly.* Environmental Research Foundation. July 22, 1999.
32. Schmidt, Charles W. "Childhood Cancer: A Growing Problem." *Environmental Health Perspectives* 106, no. 1 (1998): A18-A23.
33. Burros, Marian. "High Pesticide Levels Seen in U.S. Food." *New York Times,* February 19,1999. (http://-archives.nytimes.com.)
34. Pogoda, Janice M., and Susan Prestonu-Martin. "Household Pesticides and Risk of Pediatric Brain Tumors." *Environmental Health Perspectives* 105, no. 11 (1997): 1214-1220.
35. Montague, Peter. "Children's Cancer and Pesticides," *Rachel's Environmental & Health Weekly.* Environmental Research Foundation. March 5, 1998.
36. Lewis, R.G., et al. "Measuring Transport of Lawn-Applied Herbicide Acids from Turf to Home: Correlation of Dislodgeable 2,4-D Turf Residues with Carpet Dust and Carpet Surface Residues." *Environmental Science and Technology* 30, no. 11 (2000): 3313-3320.
37. Fenske, Richard A., Kathleen Black, and Kenneth P. Elkmer. "Home Pesticide Flea Treatments Cause Illegally High Air Levels." *American Journal Public Health* 80, no. 6 (1990): 689-693.
38. Hayes, Howard M., et al. "Case-Control Study of Canine Malignant Lymphoma: Positive Association with Dog Owner's Use of 2,4-Dichlorophenoxyacetic Acid Herbicides. *Journal of the National Cancer Institute* 83 (September 4, 1991): 1226-31.
39. Landrigan, Philip J., et al. National Research Council. *Pesticides in the Diets of Infants and Children.* National Academy Press: Washington, D.C., 1993.
40. Montague, Peter. "Pet Dogs Get Cancer From Week Killers." *Rachel's Environmental & Health Weekly.* Environmental Research Foundation. September 11, 1991.
41. Aschengrau, Ann, and Richard R. Monson. "Paternal Military Service in Vietnam and the Risk of Late Adverse Pregnancy Outcomes." *American Journal of Public Health* 80 (October 1990): 1218-24.
42. Fenske, Richard and Todd Sternbach. "Indoor Air Levels of Chlordane in Residences in New Jersey." *Bulletin Environmental Contamination Toxicology* 39 (1987): 903-910.
43. Ozonoff, David, et al. "Leukemias and Blood Dyscrasias Following Exposure to Chlordane and Heptachlor." *Teratogenesis, Carcinogenesis and Mutagenesis* 7 (1987): 527-540.
44. Kliburn, Kaye H. and John C. Thornton. "Chlordane Causes Neurological Disorders ADD Symptoms in 216 Adults Tested." *Environmental Health Perspectives* 103 (1995) 690-694.
45. Montague, Peter. "Children's Cancer and Pesticides." *Rachel's Environmental & Health Weekly.* Environmental Research Foundation. March 5, 1998.
46. Barich, Bob. "Hedging Your Bets." Greatlife. January, 2001, p10.
47. Nordstrom, M., et al. "Occupational Exposures, Animal Exposure and Smoking as risk Factors for Hairy Cell Leukaemia Evaluated in a Case-Control Study." *British Journal of Cancer* 77 (1998): 2048-2052.
48. Hardell, Lennart, and Mikael Eriksson. "A Case-Control Study of Non-Hodgkin Lymphoma and Exposure to Pesticides." *Cancer.* 85, no. 6 (1999): 1353-60.
49. Buckley, J.D., et al. "Pesticide Exposure in Children with Non-Hodgkin Lymphoma." *Cancer* 89, no.11 (2000).
50. Montague, Peter. "Pesticides and Aggression." *Rachel's Environmental & Health Weekly.* Environmental Research Foundation. April 29, 1999.

51. Guillette, Elizabeth A., et al. "An Anthropological Approach to the Evaluation of Preschool Children Exposed to Pesticides in Mexico." *Environmental Health Perspectives* 106, no. 6 (1998): 347-353.
52. Koop, C.E., and G.D. Lundberg. "Violence in America: A Public Health Emergency." *Journal of the American Medical Association* 267, no. 22 (1992): 3075-3076.
53. Cummins, Ronnie, Being Aware of Gene-Altered Foods. *Well Being Journal* 10, no. 3 (Summer 2001): 26.
54. Ibid.
55. Montague, P. "Pet Dogs Get Cancer From Week Killers." Op cit.
56. Montague, P. "Hazardous Waste is Legally 'Recycled' into Pesticides and Labeled 'Inert.'" *Rachel's Environmental & Health Weekly*. Environmental Research Foundation. November 6, 1991.
57. You, L., et al. "Impaired Male Sexual Development in Perinatal Sprague-Dawley and Long-Evans Hooded Rats Exposed in Utero and Lactationally to p,p'-DDE." *Toxicological Sciences* 43, no. 2 (1998): 162-173.
58. Loeffler, I.K., and R.E. Peterson. "Interactive Effects of TCDD and p,p'-DDE on Male Reproductive Tract Development in Utero and Lactationally Exposed Rats." *Toxicology and Applied Pharmacology* 154, no. 1 (1999): 28-39.
58. Mitchell, J.A., and S.F. Long. "The Behavioral Effects of Pesticides in Male Mice." *Neurotoxicology and Teratology* 11 (1989): 45-50.
60. Landrigan, Philip J. "Commentary: Environmental Disease—A Preventable Epidemic." Op cit., pp. 941-943.
61. Davis, Geoff. "Household Cleaners: Part 2-Dirty Little Secrets." Natural Home. www.gaiam.com.
62. www.epa.gov.
63. SafeScience. "The Need for Chemically Safe Cleaners." 2000. www.safescience.com.
64. Davis, Op cit.
65. Ibid.
66. Prochko, Judy. "The Air You Breathe-Part 2." The League of Women Voters of the Fairfax Area. www.lwv-fairfax.org.
67. Ruder, AM, et al. "Mortality in Dry-Cleaning Workers: An Update." *American Journal of Industrial Medicine*. Vol. 39. Feb. 2001: 121-132.
68. www.hopeforcancer.com, www.stopcancer.com
69. Higginbotham, S. et al. "Dietary Glycemic Load and Risk of Colorectal Cancer in the Women's Health Study." *Journal of the National Cancer Institute*, February 4, 2004;96(3):229-233.
70. Larsson, SC, Bergkvist, L., Wolk, A. "Consumption of Sugar and Sugar-sweetened Foods and the Risk of Pancreatic Cancer in a Prospective Study." *American Journal of Clinical Nutrition*, November 2006; 84(5): 1171-1176
71. Vonderplanitz, Aajonus, *We Want to Live*, Carnelian Bay Castle Press, Santa Monica, 1997
72. U.S. Food and Drug Administration. "Food Additives" (brochure). FDA/IFIC. January 1992.
73. U.S. Food and Drug Administration, Center for Food Safety & Applied Nutrition. "'Everything' Added to Food in the United States (EAFUS)." Office of Premarket Approval. June 8, 2001.
74. "Adverse Effects of 'Inactive' Ingredients." www.feingold.org/effects.html (Sources: The American Academy of Pediatrics Committee on Drugs in Pediatrics in October 1985 "E is for Additives"; *Health Letter* by Public Citizen Health Research Group, March/April 1985)
75. U.S. Food and Drug Administration. January 1992.
76. Strubbe, B. "Killing Me Sweetly." ECHO Magazine 4, no. 10 (November 2000).
77. Gold, M.D. "The Bitter Truth About Artificial Sweeteners," *Nexus Magazine* 2, no. 28 (October-November 1995); 3, no.1 (December 1995-January 1996).
78. Ibid.
79. "Cover Story Interview with Mary Nash Stoddard," *Nutrition & Healing* 2, issue 11 (November 1995).
80. Ibid.
81. Blaylock, R.L., M.D. *Excitotoxins: The Taste That Kills*. Santa Fe, NM: Health Press, 1997.
82. Ibid.
83. Gold. M.D., 1996. Op cit.
84. Blaylock, R.L., 1997. Op cit.
85. Mullarkey, Barbara. "How Safe Is Your Artificial Sweetener?" *Informed Consent Magazine*, September/October 1994.
86. "Cover Story Interview with Mary Nash Stoddard." Op cit.
87. Walton, R.G., M.D. "Analysis Shows Nearly 100% of Independent Research Finds Problems With Aspartame." www.holisticmed.com/aspartame/100.html. October 17, 1996.
88. Schiffman, S.S., et al. "Aspartame and Susceptibility to Headache." *New England Journal of Medicine* 317, no. 19: 1181-1185.
89. Camfield, P.R., et al. "Aspartame Exacerbates EEG Spike-Wave Discharge in Children with Generalized Absence Epilepsy: A Double-Blind Controlled Study." *Neurology* 42, issue 5: 1000-1003 (1992).
90. Rowen, J.A., et al. "Aspartame and Seizure Susceptibility: Results of a Clinical Study in Reportedly Sensitive Individuals." *Epilepsia* 26, no. 3:270-275 (1995).
91. Woodrow, M.C. "Aspartame: Methanol and the Public Health." *Journal of Applied Nutrition* 36, no. 1: 42-53.
92. Gold, Mark D. "Scientific Abuse in Methanol/Formaldehyde Research Related to Aspartame." Aspartame Toxicity Information Center. 2000. www.holisticmed.com/aspartame/abuse/seizures.html.
93. Gold, Mark D. "Aspartame is Dangerous For Everyone." Aspartame Toxicity Information Center. 2000. www.holisticmed.com/aspartame/abuse/seizures.html.
94. Congressional Record SID 835:131 (August 1, 1985)
95. National Cancer Institute SEER Program Data.
96. Olney, J.W., et al. "Diet Drinks Suspected for Increasing Brain Cancer Risks." *Journal of Neuropathology & Experimental Neurology* 55, no. 11: 1115-1123 (1996).
97. Roberts, H.J. *Aspartame (NutraSweet), Is it Safe?* City: The Charles Press, Publishers, 1992.
98. Ibid.
99. Walton, R.G., Robert Hudak, Ruth Green-Waite. "Adverse Reactions to Aspartame: Double Blind Challenge in Patients from a Vulnerable Population." *Biological Psychiatry* 34: 13-17 (1993).
100. Mullarkey, Barbara. Op cit.
101. Gold, M.D. "Aspartame (NutraSweet)." Aspartame Toxicity Information Center. 1996. www.holisticmed.com/aspartame/aspart2.txt.
102. Ibid.
103. Mullarkey, B., ed. "Bittersweet Aspartame—A Diet Delusion." *Health Watch Book*, April 1992.
104. Gold, MD. "Aspartame is Dangerous For Everyone." Aspartame Toxicity Information Center. 2000. www.holisticmed.com/aspartame/abuse/seizures.html.
105. www.mercola.com/2000dec/3/sucralose_dangers.htm
106. www.americancancersociety.com
107. RxPG News. April 3, 2006
108. www.dailymail.co.uk
109. superfoodsnews.com
110. Olesen, PT. et al. "Epidemiology: Acryamide Exposure and Incidence of Breast Cancer Among Menopausal Women in the Danish Diet, Cancer and Health Study." *International Journal of Cancer*. January 8, 2008
111. Michaud, DS, et al. "Meat Intake and Bladder Cancer Risk in 2 Prospective Cohort Studies." *American Journal of Clinical Nutrition*. November 2006;84(5)1177-1183
112. Honolulu Star Bulletin, http://starbulletin.com/2005/04/21/news/story1.html
113. Douglass WC. *Big Secrets Behind Junk Medicine*
114. "Honey Could Help Fight Cancer." *BBC News*, December 5, 2004. www.bbc.co.uk

Skin Cancer
115. Journal of the National Cancer Institute
116. Hughes, JR, et al. "Increase in Non-melanoma Skin Cancer - the King's College Hospital Experience (1970-92)." Blackwell Science Limited, 1995
117. Christenson, LJ. et al. "Incidence of Nonmelanoma Skin Cancer in a Population Younger than 40Years. *Journal of the American Medical Association*. Vo. 294, no. 6:681-690, Aug 9, 2005.
118. McCormac, Patricia. "Role of Light In Health." *Los Angeles Times*, February 17, 1980, p. 9,10.
119. Ott, John N. *Light, Radiation, & You*, New York: Devin-Adair Publishers, 1985.
120. Hollwich, F., and B. Dieckhues. "The Effect of Natural and Artificial Light Via the Eye on the Hormonal and Metabolic Balance of Animal and Man," *Opthalmologica* 180, no. 4 (1980).

121. Mughal, Zulf, M.D. "Air Pollution May Cause Vitamin D Deficiency," *Proceedings, 22nd Meeting of the American Society for Bone and Mineral Research,* 2001.
122. Ibid.
123. Waldie, K.E., et al. "The Effects of Pre-and Post-natal Sunlight Exposure on Human Growth: Evidence from the Southern Hemisphere." *Early Human Development* 60: 35-42. (November 1, 2000).
124. Helland, IB, et al., "Maternal Supplementation with Very-long-chain n-3 Fatty Acids During Pregnancy and Lactation Augments Children's IQ at 4 Year of Age." Pediatrics Online, Jan 2003; 111:e39-e44.
125. McGrath, J., "Low Maternal Vitamin D as a Risk Factor for Schizophrenia: A Pilot Study Using Banked Sera." Schizophrenia Research Vol. 63, Issue 2, (2003) 73-78.
126. Cannell, J. "Even Nature's Most Perfect Food Deficient in This Crucial Vitamin," Press Release The Vitamin D Council. www.mercola.com/2004/feb/7/vitamin_d.htm
127. Holick, Michael, *The UV Advantage,* 1 Books, 2004.
128. Kime, Zane R. M.D., M.S. *Sunlight,* Penryn, CA: World Health Publications, 1980.
129. Grant WB. "An Estimate of Premature Cancer Mortality in the United States Due to Inadequate Doses of Solar Ultraviolet-B Radiation Cancer," March 2002; 94:1867-75
130. Nelemans PJ et al. "Effect of Intermittent Exposure to Sunlight on Melanoma Risk Among Indoor Workers and Sun Sensitive Individuals." *Environmental Health Perspectives* 1993; 101(3): 252-55
131. The Healing Power of Sunlight, www.mercola.com
132. *Archives Environmental Health.* 1990;45:261-267
133. Ott, John N. *Health and Light.* Op cit.
134. "Sunblock can Actually Increase Your Cancer Risk." http://articles.mercola.com/sites/articles/archive/2003/07/02/sunblock-cancer-part-one.aspx
135. Raloff, Janet. "Understanding Vitamin D Deficiency." *Science News.* 2005;167(18).
136. Holick MF. "Sunlight and Vitamin D for Bone Health and Prevention of Autoimmune Diseases, Cancers and Cardiovascular Disease." *American Journal of Clinical Nutrition* 2004; 80(6): 1678S-88S
137. Garland CF et al. "The Role of Vitamin D in Cancer Prevention." *AJPH* 2005; 12/27/2005.
138. *American Journal of Clinical Nutrition.* Dec, 2007;86(6):1657-1662
139. Vieth R. "Vitamin D Supplementation, 25-hydroxyvitamin D Concentrations, and Safety." *American Journal of Clinical Nutrition* 1999;69:842-856
140. "Update on Cod Liver Oil, December 2008." www.westonaprice.org.
141. Blum, H.F. *Carcinogenesis by Ultraviolet Light.* Princeton NJ: Princeton University Press, 1959.
142. Sissonn, Thomas R., M.D., et al. "Retinal Changes Produced by Phototherapy," *Journal of Pediatrics* 77, no. 2: 221-227
143. Ott, John N. *Health and Light,* op cit.
144. *BBC News,* "Denmark World's Happiest Nation." Friday, July 28, 2006
145. "Fatty Diet Does Not Increase Risk of Skin Cancer. Science Daily. May 30, 2006.
146. Miller, DW Jr. "Vitamin D in a New Light." Lewrockwell.com/miller/miller25.htm
147. Kassandra L, et al. "Serum 25-hydroxyvitamin D Levels and Risk of Multiple Sclerosis."*JAMA.* 2006;296:2832-2828
148. Ponsonby AL, McMichael A, van der Mei I. "Ultraviolet Radiation and Autoimmune Disease: Insights From Epidemiological Research "*Toxicology.* 2002;181-182:71-78.

Lung Cancer
149. SEER Stat Fact Sheet.
150. *USA Today.* August 9, 2005.
151. Marcus, PM, et al. "Lung Cancer Mortality in the May Lung Project: Impact of Exxtended Follow-up." *Journal of the National Cancer Institute,* Vol 92 No. 16. 1308-1316, August 16, 2000.
152. "Sunshine, Vitamin D Improve Lung Cancer Survival." HealthDay News, April 18, 2005. www.lifeclinic.com
153. Slatore CG, Littman AJ, Au DH, Satia JA, White E. "Long-term Use of Supplemental Multivitamins, Vitamin C, Vitamin E, and Folate Does Not Reduce the Risk of Lung Cancer." *Am J Respir Crit Care Med.* 2008 Mar 1;177(5):524-30.
154. 219th National Meeting of the American Chemical Society. San Diego, March 19, 2000
155. Clark LC et al. "Effects of Selenium Supplementation for Cancer Prevention in Patients with Carcinoma of the Skin. *JAMA.* 1996;276:1957-1963.
156. Knekt, P et al. "Is Low Selenium status a Risk Factor for Lung Cancer?" *AM J Epidemiol.* 1998;148:975-82
157. Press Release, Garlic: Slows Growth of Lung Cancer Cells. April 16, 1996. www.gourmetgarlicgardens.com
158. Fleischauer, AT, et al. Garlic Consumption and Cancer Prevention: Meta-analyses of Colorectal and Stomach Cancers. *American Journal of Clinical Nutrition* October 2000 Vol. 72, No. 4, 1047-1052.
159. Challier B, Perarnau JM, Viel JF. Garlic, onion and cereal fiber as protective factors for breast cancer: A French case-control study. *European Journal of Epidemiology* 1998; 14(8):737–747.
160. Chan JM, Wang F, Holly EA. Vegetable and fruit intake and pancreatic cancer in a population-based case-control study in the San Francisco bay area. *Cancer Epidemiology Biomarkers & Prevention* 2005; 14(9):2093–2097.
161. Bongiorno PB et al. Potential Health Benefits of Garlic: A Narrative Review. *Journal of Complementary and Integrative Medicine,* Vol 5, Issue 1, 2008.
162. Tilli CM, Stavast-Kooy AJ, Vuerstaek JD, et al. "The Garlic-derived Organosulfur Component Ajoene Decreases Basal Cell Carcinoma Tumor Size by Inducing Apoptosis." *Archives of Dermatological Research* 2003; 295(3):117–123.
163. Mimura A et al. "Induction of Apoptosis in Human Leukemia Cells by Naturally Fermented Sugar Cane Vinegar (Kibizu) of Amami Ohshima Island." Biofactors. 2004;22:93-97.
164. Nanda K, et al. "Extractof Vinegar Kurosu from Unpolished Rice Inhibits the Proliferation of Human Cancer Cells." J Exp Clin Cancer Res. 2004;23:69-75.
165. Shimoji Y et al. "Extract of Kurosu, a Vinegar from Unpolished Rice, Inhibits Azoxymethane-induced Colon Carcinogenesis in Male F344 Rats." Nutr Cancer. 2004;49:170-173.
166. Seki T, et al. "Antitumor Activity of Rice-shochu Post-Distillation Slurry and Vinegar Produced from the Post-distillation Slurry via Oral Administration in a Mouse model." Biofactors. 2004;22:103-105.
167. Hong FU et al. "Effect of Short-chain Fatty Acids on the Proliferation and Differentiation of the human Colonic Adenocarcinoma Cell Line Caco-2." Chin J Dig Dis. 2004;5:115-117.
168. Augenlicht LH et al. "Short Chain Fatty Acids and Colon Cancer." J Nutr 2002;132:3804S-3808S.
169. Nishino H, et al. Cancer Prevention by Phytochemicals. Oncology. 2005;69 (Suppl 1):38-40.
170. Nishidain S, et al. "Kurosu, A Traditional Vinegar Produced from Unpolished Rice, Suppresses Lipid Peroxidation in Vitro and in Mouse Skin. Biosci Biotechnol Biochemn. 2000;64:1909-1914.
171. SEER Stat Fact Sheet
172. *Targeting Tobacco Use: The Nation's Leading Cause of Death, At-A-Glance.* Atlanta, GA: Centers for Disease Control and Prevention. November 2, 2000. www.cdc.gov/tobacco.
173. American Heart Association. "Cigarette Smoking and Cardiovascular Diseases." 2000. www.americanheart.org.
174. *USA Today,* January 19, 2005
175. "Targeting Tobacco Use: The Nation's Leading Cause of Death, At-A-Glance." Op cit.
176. *American Heart Association.* "Cigarette Smoking Statistics." 2000. www.americanheart.org.
177. *American Heart Association.* "Cigarette Smoking and Children." 2000. www.americanheart.org.
178. Gidding, Samuel S., et al. "Active and Passive Tobacco Exposure: A Serious Pediatric Health Problem." *American Heart Association:* AHA Medical/Scientific Statement." June 16, 1994.
179. *American Heart Association.* "Clean Indoor Air Laws." 2000. www.americanheart.org.
180. diFranza, J, Lew, R. "Morbidity and Mortality in Children Associated with the Use of Tobacco Products by Other People." *Paediatrics* 97 (1996): 560-568.
181. DeNoon, Daniel J. "Parents' Smoking Gives Children Asthma, Wheezing." *WebM.D. Medical News.* Healtheon/WebM.D. Corporation. December 2, 1999.
182. "Smoking Around Children." Michigan Department of Public Health. Lansing, MI. 2000.
183. Action on Smoking and Health. "Parents Are Deliberately Making Their Kids Sick: At What Point Does It Become Child Abuse or Endangerment?" 2001. http://ash.org.
184. Tobacco Free Kansas Coalition. "Impact of Smoking: Children's Health." 1999. www.tobac-cofreekansas.org.
185. Gilliland, Frank. "Smoking During Pregnancy Impairs Child's Future Lung Function." *Thorax* 55, no. 4 (2000): 271-276.
186. Frost, Pam. "Environmental Tobacco Smoke Harms Non-Smoking Children for Years." *Environment News Service* (ENS). 1999.
187. "Smoking During Pregnancy Damages Children's Lungs." 2000. www.antenna.nl/nietrokers/e/n/14030.html.
188. National Clearinghouse on Tobacco and Health. "Youth and Tobacco: Smoking Around Children and During Pregnancy." 2001. www.cctc.ca.

189. Gidding, Samuel S., et al. "Active and Passive Tobacco Exposure: A Serious Pediatric Health Problem." American Heart Association: AHA Medical/Scientific Statement. June 16, 1994.
190. Ibid.
191. *The Health Consequences of Smoking for Women: A Report of the Surgeon General.* Rockville, M.D.:U.S. Department of Health and Human Services, 1981.
192. Stathis, Stephen L., et al., "Study Links Maternal Smoking During Pregnancy to Children's Ear Troubles." American Academy of Pediatrics electronic pages. 104 (2):e16, August, 1999.
193. Kleinman, J.C., et al. "The Association of Maternal Smoking With Age and Cause of Infant Death." *American Journal of Epidemiology* 128 (1988): 46-55.
194. Centers for Disease Control and Prevention. "Ingestion of Cigarettes and Cigarette Butts by Children—Rhode Island, January 1994-July 1996." *Morbidity and Mortality Weekly Report* 46, no. 6 (1997): 125-128.
195.Gidding, Samuel S., et al. "Active and Passive Tobacco Exposure: A Serious Pediatric Health Problem." American Heart Association: AHA Medical/Scientific Statement. June 16, 1994.
196. Tobacco Free Kansas Coalition. Op cit.
197. Milberger, S., et al. "Is Maternal Smoking During Pregnancy a Risk Factor for Attention Deficit Hyperactivity Disorder in Children?" *The American Journal of Psychiatry* 153 (1996): 1138-1142.
198. Brennan, Patricia, et al. "Study Shows Smoking During Pregnancy Can Affect Behavior of Children." *Archives of General Psychiatry.* March 1999.
199. Marcus, Adam. "In Teens, Smoking and Sleep Don't Mix." *HealthScout.* August 7, 2000. www.healthscout.com.
200. Henningfield, J.E., R. Clayton, and W. Pollin. "Involvement of Tobacco in Alcoholism and Illicit Drug Use." *Br. J. Addit* 85 (1990): 279-291.
201. Food and Drug Administration. "President's Plan to Reduce Children's Use of Tobacco." Press release. January 5, 2001. www.wellweb.com.
202. American Heart Association. "Tobacco Industry's Targeting of Youth, Minorities and Women." www.americanheart.org.
203. American Heart Association. "Smoking Cessation." 2000. www.americanheart.org.
204. epa.gov
205. *Natur.* May 10, 2004

Prostate Cancer, BPH & Male Virility
206. Federal Citizen Information Center, The Prostate, www.pueblo.gsa.gov
207. Douglass WC. "Prostate Problems: Safe, Simple, Effective Relief." Rhino Publishing, S.A., 2003. www.rhinopublish.com
208. Ibid.
209. Ibid.
210. www.proscar.com, www.nlm.nih.gov/medlineplus/print/druginfo/uspdi/202649.
211. Douglass, W.C. Op cit.
212. http://w.anniesremedy.com/herb_detail255.php
213. What is the Prostate Gland, www.pueblo.gsa.gov
214. Douglass, WC. Op cit.
215. "Considering Your Chances of Survival." www.pueblo.gsa.gov.
216. http://articles.mercola.com/sites/articles/archive/2001/11/10/prostate-cancer-part-two.aspx
217. Annual Meeting of the American Society of Clinical Oncology, Orlando, FL, May 20, 2002, mercola.com
218. Douglass, W.C. Op cit.
219. Okihara K et al. "Transrectal Power Doppler Imaging in the Detection of Prostate Cancer." *British Journal of Urology.* June 2000
220. ACRIN 2008 Multicenter Trial and personal communication with Robert L. Bard, M.D.
221. National Prostatic Cancer Project.
222. Douglass, WC. Op cit.
223. Douglass, WC. Op cit.
224. http://articles.mercola.com/sites/articles/archive/2001/11/10/prostate-cancer-part-two.aspx
225. "Testosterone Deprivation Makes Men Forget." *Science Daily,* October 22, 2004
226. Shahinian, VB, et al. "Risk of Fracture after Androgen Deprivation for Prostate Cancer." *New England Journal of Medicine,* Vol. 352:154-164 No. 2. Jan. 13, 2005.
227. Sears, Al, 12 Secrets to Virility, Welllness Research & Consulting, Inc., 2006.
228. Shike, M, et al. "Lack of Effect of a Low-fat, High-fruit, Vegetable, and Fiber Diet on Serum Prostate-specific Antigen of Men without Prostate Cancer: Results fro a Randomized Trial." *Journal of Clinical Oncology* 2002:20:3570-3571, 3592-3598.
229. Giovannucci, E. et al. "Prospective Study of Predictors of Vitamin D Status and Cancer Incidence and Mortality." *Journal of the National Cancer Institute,* April 5, 2006 98: 451-459.
230. Annual Meeting of the American Association for Cancer Research, April 3, 2000, San Francisco, CA.
231. www.cancer.org.
232. Reuter's Health, May 1, 2003.
233. Sears, A. Doctor's House Call Newsletter, November 13, 2006
234. Giovannucci, E et al. "A Prospective Study of Tomato Products, Lycopene, and Prostate Cancer Risk." Journal of the National Cancer Institute, March 6, 2002 94:391-398.
235. Cohen, JH. et al. "Fruit and Vegetable Intakes and Prostate Cancer Risk. *Journal of the National Cancer Institute,* January 5, 2000;92:61-68.
236. Le H., et al. "Plant-derived 3,3 Diindolylmethane is a Strong Androgen Antagonist in Human Prostate Cancer Cells." J. Biol Chem, 2003 Jun 6; 278(23): 21136-21145.
237. *BBC News,* Healthy Combos Ward off Cancer. Friday, 16 July, 2004.
238. Le H., et al. Op cit.
239. USAWeekend.com, Food, EatSmart by Jean Carper, CookSmart by Pam Anderson.
240. Clark L.C. et al. "Decreased Incidence of Prostate Cancer with Selenium Supplementation: Results of a Double-blind Cancer Prevention Trial." *British Journal of Urology* 1998;81:730-734.
241. Clark L. et al. "Effects of Selenium Supplementation for Cancer Prevention in Patients with Carcinoma of the Skin. *Journal of the American Medical Association* 1996;276:1957-1963.
242. Zhang Z-F, Winton MI, Rainey C. "Boron is Associated with Decreased Risk of Human Prostate Cancer." FASEB J, 15:A1089,2001.
243. Gallardo-Williams MT, Maronpot RR, King PE. "Effects of Boron Supplementation on Morphology, PSA Levels, and Proliferate Activity of LNCaP Tumors in Nude Mice." *Proc Amer Assoc Cancer Res* 43:77, 2002.
244. Kurahashi, N. et al. "Association of Body Mass Index and Height with Risk of Prostate Cancer Among Middle-aged Japanese Men." *Br J Cancer.* March 7, 2006 94: 740-742.
245. Leitzmann, MF, et al. Dietary Intake of n-3 and n-6 Fatty Acids and the Risk of Prostate Cancer." *American Journal of Clinical Nutrition,* July 2004 80(1);204-216
246. 2005 Multidisciplinary Prostate Cancer Symposium, Orlando, Fl, Feb 17-19, 2005. News Release, Brigham and Women's Hospital and Harvard University School of Public Health.
247. *Annals of Internal Medicine,* October 2004
248. Heinonen, OP, Albanes, D. "The Effect of Vitamin E and Beta Carotene on the Incidence of Lung Cancer and Other Cancers in Male Smokers." *New England Journal of Medicine,* Vol. 330:1029-35. April 14, 1994, No. 15.
249. Vonderplanitz, Aajonus, The Recipe for Living Without Disease, Carnelian Bay Castle Press, 2002.
250. Lopez-Bote et al. "Effect of Free-range Feeding on Omega-3 Fatty Acids and Alpha-tocopherol Content and Oxidative Stability of Eggs. *Animal Feed Science and Technology,* 1998. 72:33-40
251. Wu X, Radcliffe J. "Papers on Alpha-tocopherol Intake and Bladder Cancer Risk." Presented at the Annual Meeting of the American Association of Cancer Research, Orlando, FL May 23, 2004
252. Ho, E., Yan, M., *Zinc and Prostate Cancer,* Linus Pauling Institute Spring/Summer 2005 Research Report.
253. UC Berkeley. *Wellness Guide to Dietary Supplements,* www.wellnessletter.com
254. Ho, E., op cit
255. Hyun T, Barrett-Connor E, Milne D. "Zinc Intakes and Plasma Concentrations in Men with Osteoporosis: the Rancho Bernardo Study." *Am J Clin Nutr,* Sept. 2004:80(3): 715-721
256. Smith, Matthew R., et al. "Low Bone Mineral Density in Hormone-naive Men with Prostate Carcinoma." *Cancer,* Vol. 91, June 15, 2001, pp. 2238-45
257. prevention.com

258. Jayaprakasam B, Seeram NP, Nair MG. "Anticancer and Anti-inflammatory Activities of Cucurbitacins from Cucurbita Andreana." *Cancer Letters.* 2003 Jan 10; 189(1):11-6 2003
259. Carani C, et al. "Urological and Sexual Evaluation of BPH and Pygeum." *Arch Ital Urol Nefrol Androl.* 1991, 63(3):341-5
260. Schiebel-Schlosser G, et al. "Phytotherapy of BPH with Pumpkin Seeds." *Zeitschrift fur Phytotherapie* (Germany), 1998, 19/2 (71-76)
261. Sears, Al, 12 Secrets to Virility, Wellness Research & Consulting, Inc., 2006
262. Ibid
263. Sears, Op cit.
264. Hamalainen E, Adlercruetz H, Puska P, Pietinen P. "Diet and Serum Sex Hormones in Healthy Men." *J Steroid Biochem.* 1984;20(1):459-64
265. Sears, Op Cit.
266. Ibid.
267. Boyd IW. "HMG-CoA Reductase Inhibitor-induced Impotence (letter)." *Ann Pharac.* 1996: 30(10): 1,199.
268. Mirkin, G, M.D., "Smoking Causes Impotence," www.drmirkin.com.
269. Feldman HA, Goldstein I, et al. "Impotence and its Medical Correlates: Results of the Massachusetts Male Aging Study." *J Urol.* 1994: 151(1):54-61.
270. Tengs, TO, Osgood, ND, *Preventive Medicine,* 2001 Vol. 32, Iss. 6, pp 447-452.
271. Rosen RC, Fisher W, et al. "The Multinational Men's Attitudes to Life Events and Sexuality (MALES) Study." *Curr Med Res Opin* 2004;20(5):607-617.
272. Cooper M.D. MPH, Kenneth H, *Advanced Nutritional Therapies,* Thomas Nelson, Inc. Publishers, Nashville, 1996, Pp 87-88, 93, 94.
273. Lamm, M.D., Steven and Couzens, Gerald Secor, *Younger at Last: The New World of Vitality Medicine,* Simon & Schuster, 1997, Pp 62-64.
274. Klatz, DO, Ronald , Kahn, C. *Grow Young with HGH,* Harper Collins Publishers, New York, 1997
275. Hendler, M.D., Ph.D., Sheldon Saul, *The Doctor's Vitamin and Mineral Encyclopedia,* Fireside, New York, 1990, Pp 209-215.

Breast Cancer
276. www.breastcancer.org.
277. www.cancer.org.
278. Sherman, Janette D, *Life's Delicate Balance; The Causes and Prevention of Breast Cancer,* New York and London: Taylor and Francis, 2000.
279. American Cancer Society.
280. Hanse NM, et al. "Manipulation fo the Primary Breast Tumor and the Incidence of Sentinel Node Metastases from Invasive Breast Cancer." Arch Surg. 2004;139:634-640.
281. www.cancer.org.
282. Douglass, WC, Real Health Breakthroughs, Vol 5 No. 10, March 2006.
283. Cancer statistics, 2004. *Cancer. Clin.* 2004;54:8-29.
284. www.alternativemedicine.com.
285. Miller AB, Baines CJ, Wall C. "Canadian National Breast Screening Study-2: 13-year Results of a Randomized Trial in Women Aged 50-59 Years." *J Natl Cancer Inst,* 2000 Sep 20;92(18):1490-9.
286. Miller AB, Baines CJ, Wall C, "Mammograms in Women Age 40 to 49: Results of the Canadian Breast Cancer Screening Study." *Annals of Internal Medicine.* 3 Sept 2002 Vol 137, Issue 5, Part 1, Page 1-28.
287. Miller, AB et al. "Canadian National Breast Screening Study-2: 13-Year Results of a Randomized Trial in Women Aged 50-59 Year." *Journal of the National Cancer Institute.* September 20, 2000; 92:1490-1499.
288. www.mercola.com.
289. Northstar Nutritionals newsletter, 12/11/2008.
290. Zahl et al. "The Natural History of Invasive Breast Cancers Detected by Screening Mammography." Arch Intern Med. 2008;168(21):2302-2303
291. *The Lancet,* July 11, 1992.
292. www.nci.gov.
293. www.nih.gov.
294. NewsTarget.com, August 15, 2005.
295. *The Daily Dose,* Douglass, WC, Feb 17, 2004.
296. Ibid.
297. Personal Communication, Tracy Cousins, M.D., Wausau, WI
298. *The Lancet,* July 11, 1992, p. 122
299. Douglass, Op cit.
300. Gofman, JohnW, Preventing Breast Cancer, Committee for Nuclear Responsibility; 2nd edition, Feb. 1996.
301. Cochrane Database Syst Rev. 2001:(4):CD001877, Cochrane Database Syst Rev. 2006:(4):CD001877.
302. Wright CJ, Mueller CB, "Screening Mammography and Public Health Policy." *The Lancet,* July 1995.
303. Caplan A. "Breast Cancer Tests – Not Worth the Price" MSNBC Oct. 8, 2008.
304. Parikh YR et al. "Efficacy of Computerized Infrared Imaging Analysis to Evaluate Mammographyically Suspicious Lesions." *American J Roentgenolgy.* 180 (2003):263-269.
305. Gamagami P. "Indirect Signs of Breast Cancer: Angiogenesis Study." *Atlas of Mammography,* Cambridge, MA, Blackwell Science pp 231-26, 1996.
306. Okihara K et al. "Transrectal Power Doppler Imaging in the Detection of Prostate Cancer." British Journal of Urology. June 2000
307. www.cancerscan.com and*AmericanJournalofRadiology.*January, 2000
308. "What Causes Breast Cancer?" *Rachel's Environment & Health News,* #723 - April 26, 2001.
309. Westin, Jerome B., and Elihu Richter. "The Israeli Breast-Cancer Anomaly." In *Trends in Cancer Mortality in Industrial Countries,* edited by Devra L. Davis and David Hoel. New York: Academy of Sciences, 1990, pp 259-268.
310. Montague, Peter. "Breast Cancer Epidemic Continues; Prevention Philosophy is Ignored," *Rachel's Environmental & Health Weekly.* Environmental Research Foundation. December 25, 1991.
311. Montague, Peter. "Human Breast Milk is Contaminated," *Rachel's Environmental & Health Weekly.* Environmental Research Foundation. August 8, 1990.
312. Foster, Warren, et. al. "In Utero Exposure of the Human Fetus to Xenobiotic Endocrine Disrupting Chemicals." Presented at the Endocrine Society's 81st Annual Meeting in San Diego, CA, June 14, 1999.
313. Davis, Devra L., et al. "Medical Hypothesis: Xenoestrogens as Preventable Causes of Breast Cancer." *Environmental Health Perspectives* 101 (October 1993):372-377.
314. Montague, Peter. "Chemicals and Health – Part I." Rachel's Environmental & Health Weekly. Environmental Research Foundation. December 23, 1993.
315. National Institutes of Health - National Heart, Lung and Blood Institute Press Release, "NHLB Stops Trial of Estrogen Plus Progestin Due to Increased Breast Cancer Risk, Lack of Overall Benefit." July 9, 2002.
316. www.nlm.nih.gov/medlineplus/print/ency/article/007111.htm.
317. www.equineadvocates.com.
318. www.mercola.com.
319. Writing Group for the Women's Health Initiative Investigators. "Risk and Benefits of Estrogen Plus Progestin in Healthy Postmenopausal Women: Principal Results from the Women's Health Initiative Randomized Controlled Trial. *JAMA.* 2002; 288:321-333.
320. "Breast Cancer Drop Tied to Less Hormone Therapy." *MSNBC News Services,* Dec 14, 2006.
321. Sherman Janett D. *Life's Delicate Balance; The Causes and Prevention of Breast Cancer.* New York and London: Taylor and Francis, 2000
322. Cone, M., "Banned Elsewhere, Compounds Still Used in U.S." *LA Times,* October 8, 2006
323. Sherman JD. Op cit.
324. Eliassen AH, et al. "Adult Weight Change and Risk of Post-menopausal Breast Cancer." *JAMA.* 2006;296:193-201.
325. Darbre, PD. "Underarm Cosmetics and Breast Cancer." *Journal of Applied Toxicology,* 2003. Mar-Apr;23(2):89-05.
326. McGrath, K. "An Earlier Age of Breast Cancer Diagnosis Related to More Frequent Use of Antiperspirants/deodorants and Underarm Shaving. *European Journal of Cancer Prevention,* Vol. 12, p. 479.
327. www. breastcancerfund.com.
327a. Velicer CM, et al. "Antibiotic use in Relation to the Risk of Breast Cancer." *JAMA,* Feb. 18, 2004;291(7):827-35.
328. Marshall, SF, et al. "Nonsteroidal Anti-Inflammatory Drug Use and Breast Cancer Risk by Stage and Hormone Receptor Status." *Journal of the National Cancer Institute.* June 1, 2005, Vol. 97, No.11:805-812.
329. Cotterchio, M. et al. "Antidepressant Medication Use and Breast Cancer Risk." *American Journal of Epidemiology,* May 2000 151:951-957.
330. 35th Annual Meeting of the Society for Epidemiologic Research, Seattle, June 2000.
331. *BBC News,* Jan. 7, 2004.
332. www.breakthechain.org.
333. Ibid.

334. Bromfield, L. *Pleasant Valley*. Wooster Book Company, 1997.
335. Grant WB. "An Estimate of Premature Cancer Mortality in the U.S. due to Inadequate Doses of Solar Ultraviolet-B Radiation." Cancer. 2002;94:1867-1875.
336. Garland, et al. *Prev Med.* 1990;19:614-622.
337. Laino, C. "Suggestions that Vitamin D May Protect against Breast Cancer (AACR Annual Meeting). " *Oncology Times.* Vol 28(12)25 June 2006 p 50-51.338. American Association of Cancer Research Annual Meeting, Washington, DC, April 1-6, 2006.
339. Lowe LC, et al. "Plasma 25-hydroxy Vitamin D Concentrations, Vit D Receptof Genotype and Breast Cancer Risk in a UK Caucasian Population." *Eur J Cancer.* 2005;41:1164-1169
340. Bertone-Johnson ER, et al. "Plasma 25-Hydroxyvitamin D and 1,25-Dihydroxyvitamin D and Risk of Breast Cancer" Cancer Epidemiol Biomarkers. Prev. 2005;14:1991-1997.
341. Laino, Charlene. Vitamin D may protect against cancer. WebM.D. April 4, 2006.
342. Sircus, M. *Transdermal Magnesium Therapy.* 2007. Phaelos Books, Chandler AZ.
343. Werbach, M. M.D., *J Alt & Comp Med.* Feb. 1994;12(2)
344. Sircus, M., Op cit.
345. Eskin, BA. "Iodine and Mammary Cancer." Tanscript, NY Acadamy of Sciences. 1970
346. Drouse, T. Age-related changes in iodine-blocked. Proc. Amer. Ass. Cancer Research. 18. 1977
347. Brownstein, D. *Iodine, Why you need it why you can't live without it.* Medical Alternatives Press, W. Bloomfield, MI. 2008.
348. Eskin, BA. "Mammary gland dysplasia in iodine deficiency." *JAMA.* May 22, 1967.
349. Brownstein, D., Op Cit.
350. Finley, JW et al. "Breast Cancer and Thyroid Disease." *Quart. Rev. Surg. Obstet. and Gyn.* 1960 17:139
351. Miller, Jr., DW. "Extrathyroidal Benefits of Iodine," *Journal of American Physicians and Surgeons.* Vol. 11, No. 4, Winter 2006.
352. Cann SA, van Netten JP, van Netten C. "Hypothesis: Iodine, Selenium and the Development of Breast Cancer." *Cancer Causes Control.* 2000;11:121-127.
353. Eskin BA, et al. "Identification of Breast Cancer by Differences in Urinary Iodine." *Proc Am Assoc Cancer Res.* 2005;46:504.
354. Bogardus, AG. *Surgery.* 1960, 49, 461. and Finley, J. rev. *Obstet. Gynec.* 1960, 49, 17.
355. Beaston, G. "Adjunvant Use of Thyroid Extract in Breast Cancer." *Lancet.* 104:no.2,pg.162,1896.
356. Vishniakova YY, Murav'eva NI. "On the Treatment of Dyshormonal Hyperplasia of Mammary Glands." *Vestn Akad Med Nauk* (USSR) Russian, 1966;21(9);19-22.
357. Ghent WR, Eskin BA, Low DA, Hill LP. "Iodine Replacement in Fibrocystic Disease of the Breast." *Can. J. Surg.* 1993;36-453-460.
358. Kessler JH. "The Effect of Supraphysiologic Levels of Iodine on Patients with Cyclic Mastalgia." *Breast J.* 2004;10:328-336.
359. Brownstein, D., Op cit.
360. Miller, Jr. Op cit.
361. www.helpmythyroid.com .
362. Ibid.
363. Horowitz, B. "Bromism from Excessive Cola Consumption." *Clinical Toxicology*, 35(3(315-320. 1997.
364. 35th Annual Meeting of the Society for Epidemiologic Research, Seattle, WA June, 2000.
365. Cantor KP, Hildesheim ME, Lynch CF, et al. "Drinking Water Source and Chlorination Byproducts: Risk of Bladder Cancer." *Epidemiology.* 1998;9(part 1):21-28. and; Hildesheim ME, Cantor KP, Lynch CF, et al. "Drinking Water Source and Chlorination Byproducts: Risk of Colon and Rectal Cancers." Epidemiology 1998;9(part 2):29-35. *Epidemiology.* May 1999. 10:233-237.
366. Brownstein, op cit.
367. Miller, DW Jr., *Iodine for Health.* Lewrockwell.com
368. Journal of Biological Chemistry. June 6, 2003.
369. "Organically Grown Foods Higher in Cancer-fighting Chemicals than Conventionally Grown Foods." *ScienceDaily*, Mar. 4, 2003. and Asami DK, et al. "Comparison of the Total Phenolic and Ascorbic Acid Content of Freeae-dried and Air-dried Marionberry, Strawberry, and Corn Grown using Conventional Organic, and Sustainable Agricultural Practices." *Journal of Agricultural and Food Chemistry.* Feb. 26 2003 51(5);1237-41.
370. Challier B, Perarnau JM, Viel JF. "Garlic, Onion and Cereal Fibre as Protective Factors for Breast Cancer: A French case-control study. *European Journal of Epidemiology* 1998; 14(8):737-747.
371. Maskarinec G et al. "A 2-year Soy Intervention in Premenopausal Women Does Not Change Mammographic Densities. *Journal of Nutrition*, Nov. 2004; 134:3089-3094.
372. Annual Meeting of the American Association for Cancer Research. April 3, 2000
373. Macrae, Fiona, "Frying Can Increase Cancer Risk." Mail Online, www.dailymail.co.uk. April 10, 2006.
374. Arbanas, C. "Girls, Young Women Can Cut Risk of Early Breast Cancer Through Regular Exercise," Washington University School of Medicine, Press Release, May 13, 2008
375. Holmes, M.D., et al., "Physical Activity and Survival after Breast Cancer Diagnosis." *JAMA.* May 25, 2005:293:2479-2486.
376. www.cancer.org.
377. *Newsinferno.com.* "FDA Lifts 14-Year Ban on Silicone Breast Implants," November 20, 2006.
378. Brinton LA, et al. "Breast Cancer Following Augmentation Mammoplasty,(U.S.)" *Cancer Causes & Control* 2000;11(9):819-827.
379. Brinton LA et al. "Cancer Risk at Sites other than Breast Following Augmentation Mammoplasty." *Annals of Epidemiology.* May 2001;11(4):248-256.
380. Brinton, LA, et al. "Mortality among Augmentation Mammoplasty Patients." *Epidemiology.* May 2001;12(3):321-326.
381. Villeneuve, PJ, et al. "Mortality among Canadian Women with Cosmetic Breast Implants." *American Journal of Epidemiology.* 2006. 164(4):334-341, August 15, 2006.

Chapter IV - Cardiovascular Diseases

1. www.americanheart.org, Heart Disease and Stroke Statistics - 2005 Update, American Heart Association.
2. www.americanheart.org, Heart Disease and Stroke Statistics - 2005 Update, American.
3. Schlesinger K, "Knoublach (allium sativum) als Helimittel bei Artiosklerose Wein Ned Wochenschr. 1926;76:1076-77.
4. Taubman G. "Therapie Mit Drogen." *Med Klin* 1934;32:1067-1069.
5. Rahman K. "Historical Perspective of Garlic and Cardiovascular Diseases." *American Society for Nutritional Sciences.* 2001; 977-979.
6. Bongiorno PB, et al., "Potential health Benefits of Garlic (Allium Sativum): A Narrative Review." *Journal of Complementary and Integrative Medicine*, Vol 5, Issue 1, 2008.
7. Ackermann RT, et al. "Garlic Shows Promise for Improving Some Cardiovascular Risk Factors." *Arch Intern Med.* 2001;161:813-24.
8. "Honey and nuts fight cholesterol." *BBC News*, August 19, 2002.
9. Kondo S, et al. "Antihypertensive Effects of Acetic Acid and Vinegar on Spontaneously Hypertensive Rats." *Biosci Biotechnol Biochem* 2001;65:2690-2694.
10. Hu FB, et al. "Dietary intake of Alpha-linolenic acid and risk of Fatal Ischemic Heart Disease Among Women." *Am J Clin Nutr.* 1999;69:890-897.
11. Johnston CS, et al. "Vinegar: Medicinal Uses and Antiglycemic Effect" *MedGenMed.* 2006;8(2):61.
12. Murshed R. "The Sweet Solution -2." *The Daily Star*, May 24, 2008. www.thedailystar.net.
13. McMurray JJ, Pfeffer MA. Heart failure. *Lancet.* 2005;365:1887-1889.
14. Frustaci, A, et al. "Marked Elevation of Myocardial Trace Elements in Idiopathic Dilated Cardiomyopathy Compared with Secondary Dysfunction." Department of Cardiology, Catholic University, Rome Italy. Journal of the American College of Cardiology. Vol. 33, No. 6, 1999, pp. 1578-1583
15. Byrnes, Stephen, Ph.D. "Are Saturated Fats Really Dangerous For You?" www.mercola.com/2002/feb/23/vegetarianism_myths_06.htm
16. Debakey, M, et al. "Serum Cholesterol Values in Patients Treated Surgically for Atherosclerosis." *JAMA*, 1964, 189:655-59.
17. Howard BU, Van Horn L, Hsia J. "Low-fat Dietary Pattern and Risk of Cardiovascular Disease: Women's Health Initiative Randomized Controlled Dietary Modification Trial." JAMA, 2006;295:655-666.
18. Wolf, RL, et al. "Factors Associated with Calcium Absorption Efficiency in Pre- and Perimenopausal Women." *American Journal of Clinical Nutrition,* Aug. 2000; 72: 466-471.
19. Knopp, RH et al. "Long-term Cholesterol-lowering Effects of 4 fat-restricted Diets in Hypercholesterolemic and Combined Hyperlipidemic Men. The Dietary Alternatives Study." *JAMA.* 1997; 278(18); 1509-1515. and . *Medicine Science of Sports Exercise.* July 2000; 32(7); 389-95.
20. Fallon, S, Enig, ME. Ph.D. *Nourishing Traditions.* New Trends Publishing, 1999.
21. Ibid.
22. Mercola, J. "Trans-fat: What exactly is it and why is it so dangerous?" www.mercola.com/2003/jul/19/trans_fat.htm.
23. Ibid.
24. Vonk, Brian, M.D. "How to Determine Your cardiovascular Health." www.mercola.com/2003/jan/4/cardiovascular_health.htm.
25. MSNBC, September 29, 2005.
26. Peat, R. *Coconut Oil*, www.coconutoil.com.

27. Fried, Susan K., and Salome P Rao, "Sugars, Hypertriglyceridemia and Cardiovascular Disease." *American Journal of Clinical Nutrition*, Vol 78, No. 4, 873S-880S, October, 2003.
28. Fallon S, Enig MG., *Dangers of Statin Drugs: Wat you Haven't Been Told About Popular Cholesterol-Lowering Medicines.* www.westonaprice.org/moderndiseases/statin.html.
29. Laise E. "The Lipitor Dilemma". *Smart Money: The Wall Street Journal Magazine of Personal Business.* Nov 2003.
30. Gaist D et al. *Neurology.* 2002 May 14;58(9):1321-2.
31. Langsjoen PH. "The clinical use of HMG Co-A reductase inhibitors (statins) and trhe associated depletion fo the essential co-factor coenzyme Q10: a review of pertinent human and animal data". www.fda.gov/ohrms/dockets/dailys/02/May02/052902/02p-0244-cp00001-02-Exhibit A-vol1.pdf.
32. Clark AL et al. *J Am Coll Cardiol.* 2003;42:1933-1943.
33. Fallon S, Op cit.

34. Zipes DP, Wellens HJ. "Sudden Cardiac Death." *Circulation.* 1998;98:2334-2351.
35. Burr ML, Fehily AM, Gilbert JF, et al. "Effects of Changes in Fat, Fish and Fiber Intakes on Death and Myocardial Reinfarction: Diet and Reinfarction Trial (DART)." *Lancet.* 1989;2:757-761.
36. Gruppo Italiano per lo studio della Sopravvivenza nell'infarto Miocardico. "Dietary Supplementation with n-3 Polyunsaturated Fatty Acids and Vitamin E after Myocardial Enfarction: Results of the GISSI-Prevenzione Trial." *Lancet.* 1999; 354:447-455.
37. Fife, B. The Healing Miracles of Coconut Oil, Healthwise Publications, 2001.
38. Price, W.S., Nutrition and Physical Degeneration, 1939, Keats Publishing, 1998.
39. Genco RJ, et al. "Periodontal microflora related to the risk of myocardial infarction: a case-control study (abstract 2811). *J Dent Res* 1999;78(special issue):457.
40. DeStefano F, et al. "Dental Disease and Risk of Coronary Heart Disease and Mortality." *British Medical Journal* 306:688-691, 1993.
41. Campbell, W.C. Second Opinion Newsletter.
42. Fife, B. The Healing Miracles of Coconut Oil. Healthwise Publications, 2001
43. Ibid.
44. *Journal of the American College of Nutrition*, October, 2000(Supplement)
45. International Journal of Cardiology March 10, 2005; Volume 99, Issue 1, 65-70
46. www.alsearsmd.com
47. *Journal of the American College of Nutrition*, October, 2000 (Supplement) from mercola, www.mercola.com/2000/nov/12/eggs.htm
48. "Where Would We Be Without The Egg? A Conference About Nature's Original Functional Food." Journal of the American College of Nutrition, October, 2000 (Supplement). Vol 19.
49. Fallon, S. Op cit, p. 45.
50. "An Overview of the Salmonella Enteritidis Risk Assessment for Shell Eggs and Egg Products." US. Department of Agriculture. Risk Analysis, April, 2002 22(2) 203-18.
51. Fallon, S, Enig, ME. Ph.D. *Nourishing Traditions*. New Trends Publishing, 1999. pp. 6,7.
52. Weil, J., Colin-Jones D., et al., "Prophylactic Aspirin and Risk of Peptic Ulcer Bleeding." *British Medical Journal* , April 1, 1995, Vol. 310, pp 827-829.
53. Otsuka H, et al. "Studies on anti-inflammatory Agents. VI. Anti-inflammatory Constituents of Cinnamon sieboldii Meissn (author's transl)." Yakugaku Zassh 1982 Jan;102(2):162-72. PNMID:12260.
54. Page I. MBBS, and Henry D. MBchB, "Consumption of NSAIDs and the Development of Congestive Heart Failure in Elderly Patients." *Archives of Internal Medicine*, March 27, 2000, Vol. 160, pp. 777-784.
55. Larsen, HR., "Parkinson's disease: Is Victory in Sight?" *International Journal of Alternative and Complementary Medicine*. Vol. 15, No. 10, October 1997, pp. 22-24.
56. Janet E. Joy, Stanley J. Watson, Jr., and John A Benson, Jr., "Marijuana and Medicine: Assessing the Science Base," Division of Neuroscience and Behavioral Research, Institute of Medicine, Wash DC. National Academy Press, 1999. www.samhsa.gov.
57. "Estrogen Replacement and Coronary-Artery Atherosclerosis Trends in the Incidence of Coronary Disease and Changes in Diet and Lifestyle in Women." *New England Journal of Medicine*, August 24, 2000; 343: 522-529, 530-537.
58. Bath, PMW, Bray, LJ. "Association Between Hormone Replacement Therapy and Subsequent Stroke. A Meta-analysis." Division of Stroke Medicine, Institute of Neuroscience, Queen's Medical Centre, University of Nottingham, Nottingham NG7 2UH. http://bmj.bmjjournals.com/cgi/content/abstract/bmj.38331.655347.8Fv1?maxtoshow=&H
59. Wassertheil-Smoller, S, et al. "Association Between Cardiovascular Outcomes and Antihypertensive Drug Treatment in Older Women." *JAMA*, December 15, 2004; 292:2849-2859.
60. Carolyn, D, Op cit.
61. Teo KK. et al. "Effects of Intravenous Magnesium in Suspected Acute Myocardial Infarction: Overview of Randomized Trals." Grit Med J, Vol. 303, pp 1499-1503, 1991.
62. Teo KK, Yusuf S. "Role of Magnesium in Reducing Mortality in Acute Myocardial Infarction. A Review of the Evidence." *Drugs*, Vol 46, pp 247-259, 1993.
63. Woods KL, Fletcher S, Roffe C, Haider Y. "Intravenous Magnesium Sulphate in Suspected Acute Myocardial Infarction: Results of the Second Leicester Intravenous Magnesium Intervention Trial (LIMIT-2)." *Lancet* 1992;339:1553-8.
64. Dean. Op cit.
65. Wassertheil-Smoller, Sylvia et al., "Association Between Cardiovascular Outcomes and Antihypertensive Drug Treatment in Older Women." *JAMA*, Dec 15, 2004;292:2849-2859.
66. Furberg, CD. "Calcium Channel Blocker Meta-Analysis." 22nd Congress of the European Society of Cardiology." August 26-30, 2000. Amsterdam, the Netherlands. and, http://circ.ahajournals.org/cgi/content/full/103/8/e41 and http://heartdisease.about.com/library/weekly/aa0092000b.htm)
67. Press Release - University of Maryland Medical News, December 3, 2002, Study Suggests Possibility of New Heart and High Blood Pressure Medications
68. Devine A et al. "A Longitudinal Study of the Effect of Sodium and Calcium Intakes on Regional Bone Density in Postmenopausal Women." *Am J Clin Nutr.* 1995;62:740-745.
69. Nordin BEC et al. "Metabolic Consequences of the Mebnopause: A Cross-sectional and Longitudinal Intervention Study on 557 Normal Postmenopausal Women. *Calcif Tiss Int.* 1987;41:S1-S59.
70. Matkovic V et al. "Urinary Calcium, Sodium and bone mass of young females." *Am J Clin Nutr.* 1995;62:417-425.
71. Cappucci FP. "Dietary Prevention of Osteoporosis: Are We Ignoring the Evidence?" *Am J Clin Nutr* 63, 787-788.
72. Nordin BEC et al. "The Nature and Significance of the Relationships Between Urinary Sodium and Urinary Calcium in Women." *J Nutr.* 1993;123:1615-1622.
73. Vonderplanitz, A., *We Want to Live*, Op cit., p 278.
74. Bragg P "How to Keep Your Heart Healthy and Fit. The Truth About Salt." www.living-foods.com.
75. www.living-foods.com
76. Shelton HM. "Salt Eating Pernicious." Hygienic Review Vol 34 No 7, 1973
77. Brody, JE. "A New Look at an Ancient Remedy: Celery." *NY Times*, June 9, 1992.
78. Le QT and Elliott WJ. "Hypotensive and Hypocholesterolemic Effects of Celery Oil May be due to BuPh." *Clin Res* 1991; 39:173A.
79. Yu Sr, et al.: The Protective Effect of 3-n-butyl phthalide on Rat Brain Cells." *Yao Hsueh Hsueh Pao* 1988;23:656-61.
80. Chong ZZ and Feng YP. "dl-3-n-butyl phthalide Improves Regional Cerebral Blood Flow after Experimental Subarachnoid Hemorrhage in Rats." *Chung Kuo Yao Li Hsueh Pao* 1999; 20:509-12.
81. Chong ZZ and Feng PY. "dl-3-n-butyl phthalide Attenuates Reperfusion-induced Blood-brain Barrier Damage after Focal Cerebral Ischemia in Rats." *Chung Kuo Yao Li Hsueh Pao.* 1999;20:696-700.
82. Yan CH, Feng YP and Zhang JT.: "Effects of dl-3-n-butyl phthalide on Regional Cerebral Blood Flow in Right Middle Cerebral Artery Occlusion in Rats." *Chung Kuo Yao Li Hsueh Pao.* 1998;19:117-20
83. Lin JF and Feng YP. "Effect of dl-3-n-butyl phthalide on Delayed Neuronal Damage after Local Cerebral Ischemia and Intrasynaptosome Calcium in Rats." *Yao Hsueh Hsueh Pao.* 1996;31:166-7.
84. Liu XG and Feng YP. "Protective Effect of dl-3-n-butyl phthalide on Ischemic Neurological Damage and Abnormal Behavior in Rats Subjected to Focal Ischemia." *Yao Hsueh Hsueh Pao.* 1995;30:896-903.
85. Zhang LY and Feng YP. "Effect of dl-3-n-butyl phthalide (NBP) on Life Span and Neurological Deficit in SHRsp Rats." *Yao Hsueh Hsueh Pao.* 1006;31:18-23
86. Kurl S, Tuominanen TP, Laukkanen JA et al. "Plasma Vitamin C Modifies the Association between Hypertension and Risk of Stroke." *Stroke* Jun:33(6):1568-73 2002.

87. Venkat S, Soundararajan S, Daunter B and Madhusudhan S. "Use of Ayurvedic medicine in the treatment of rheumatic illness. Department of Orthopaedics, Kovai Medical Center and Hospitals, Coimbatore, India, 1995.
88. HuD, Huang XX and Feng YP: Effect of dl-3-n-butyl phthalide (NBP) on Purine Metabolite in Striatum Extracellular Fluid in Four-vessel Occlusion Rats. *Yao Hsueh Hsueh Pao*. 1996;31:13-7.
89. Sarwat Sultana, et al. "Inhibitory Effect of Celery Seeds Extract on Chemically Induced Hepatocarcinogenesis: Modulation of Cell Proliferation, Metabolism and Altered Hepatic Foci Development." *Cancer* Letters Volume 221, Issue 1, 18 April 2005, Pp. 11-20.
90. www.nutrasanus.com
91. Sesso, HD. et al. "Physical Activity and Coronary Heart Disease in Men : The Harvard Alumni Health Study." *Circulation*. 2000;102:975-980.
92. Manson JE et al. "A Prospective Study of Walking as Compared with Vigorous Exercise in the Prevention of Coronary Heart Disease in Women." *New England Journal of Medicine* 1999;341:650-658.
93. LeMura, LM and Maziekas, MT "Factors that Alter Body Fat, Body Mass and Fat-free Mass in Pediatric Obesity." *Med Sci Sports Exerc* 2002;34:487-496.
94. Foster, T, McKnight, EF. Society for Neuroscience 35th Annual Meeting. Washington DC, November 12, 2005. and EurekAlert November 12, 2005.
95. Carlson, JF, et al. "Disability in Older Adults, Physical Activity as Prevention. *Journal of Behavioral Medicine*, 1999; 24:157-168.
96. Whang W et al. "Physical Exertion, Exercise and Sudden Cardiac Death in Women." *JAMA*, March 22/29, 2006;295:1399-1403.
97. Miller JC, et al. "A Meta-analysis of the Past 25 Years of Weight Loss Research using Diet, Exercise, and Diet plus Exercise Intervention." *Int. J. Obes Relat Metab Disord*, 1997; 21(10) 941-7.
98. "Impact of Exercise Intensity on Body Fatness and Skeletal Muscle Metabolism." *Metabolism* 1994; 43(7): 814-18.
99. Fallon, S. *Nourishing Traditions*. Op cit.
100. American Heart Association, Stroke Risk Factors, www.americanheart.org.
101. "Stroke Statistics" www.theuniversityhospital.com.
102. "Western Diets may be Linked to Greater Stroke Risk." Stampfer, Meir, J., et al., Stroke: Journal of the American Heart Association, Stroke Journal Report, 7-1-2004
103. Nagano, Jun, et al. Fruits and Vegetables May Protect Against Major Types of Stroke. Stroke: Journal of the American Heart Association. Stroke Journal Report, 9-19-2003
104. He, Jiang, et al., Foods Rich in Folate May Reduce Risk of Stroke, Stroke: Journal of the American Heart Association. *Stroke News*, 5-3-2002
105. Carolyn Dean, Op cit.
106. Ibid.
107. "MIT: Magnesium May Reverse Middle-Age Memory Loss." *Medical News Today*, 12-1-04, medicalnewstoday.com
108. Davalos, A., et al. "Body Iron Stores and Early Neurologic Deterioration in Acute Cerebral Infaction." *Neurology*, April 25, 2000; 54:1568-1574.
109. American Journal of Clinical Nutrition March, 2004;79(3);437-43
110. "Vitamin D Deficit: Women's Silent Bone Threat." webM.D. Medical News www.webmd.com 5-20-05.
111. He, K, et al. "Fish Consumption and Risk of Stroke in Men." *JAMA* December 25, 2002;288(24);3130-6.

Chapter V – Diabetes

1. National Institute of Diabetes and Digestive and Kidney Diseases, "Diabetes Statistics." National Diabetes Information Clearinghouse, National Institutes of Health. 2000. www.niddk.nih.gov.
2. National Institutes of Health. *Conquering Diabetes: A Strategic Plan for the 21st Century, A Report of the Congressionally Established Diabetes Research Working Group*. NIH Publication no. 99-4398. 1999.
3. National Diabetes Fact Sheet, www.diabetes.org.
4. Montague, Peter. "Diabetes is Increasing," *Rachel's Environmental & Health Weekly*. Environmental Research Foundation. August 7, 1997.
5. Christian, Henry A. *The Principles and Practice of Medicine*, 16th Edition, p. 582. New York: D. Appleton-Century, 1947.
6. Coulter, Harris. "Childhood Vaccinations and Juvenile-Onset (Type 1) Diabetes." Testimony before the Congress of the United States, House of Representatives, Committee on Appropriations, Subcommittee on Labor, Health and Human Services, Education, and Related Agencies. April 16, 1997. (Available from the National Vaccine Information Center, www.909shot.com.)
7. Centers for Disease Control and Prevention. CDC's Diabetes Program, 1990-1998. 2000. www.cdc.gov.
8. Pinhas-Harniel, Orit, et al. "Increased Incidence of Non-Insulin-Dependent Diabetes Mellitus Among Adolescents, Part I." *The Journal of Pediatrics* 128, no. 5: 608-615. May 1996.
9. National Institutes of Health. "Conquering Diabetes, A Strategic Plan for the 21st Century: A Report of the Congressionally Established Diabetes Research Working Group." NIH Publication no. 99-4398. 1999.
10. Ibid.
11. Ibid.
12. LaPorte, RE., Matsushima, M. and Chang, Y. *Diabetes in America, 2nd Edition*, National Diabetes Data Group, NIH Publication No. 95-1468. 1995.
13. Pinhas-Harniel, Orit, et al. Op cit.
14. Langer, Stephen E. and James F. Scheer. *Solved: The Riddle of Illness*. New Canaan, CT: Keats Publishing, Inc. 1984, p. 92.
15. Ibid.
16. Ibid, p. 94.
17. Ibid, p. 96.
18. Notkins, Abner L. "Environmental Etiology of Type 1 Diabetes: Viruses and Other Factors. Environmental Etiology Workshop Final Report," NIDDK, National Institutes of Health. September 1998.
19. Henriksen, Gary L., et al. "Serum Dioxin and Diabetes Mellitus in Veterans of Operation Ranch Hand." *Epidemiology* 8, no. 3: 252-258 (May 1997).
20. Kohlmeier, Lenore, and Martin Kohlmeier, "Adipose Tissues as a Medium for Epidemiologic Exposure Assessment." *Environmental Health Perspectives Supplements* 103, Supplement 3: 99-106 (April 1995).
21. Dean, Carolyn, M.D., N.D., *The Miracle of Magnesium*, Random House Publishing, New York, NY, 2003.
22. Ibid.
23. Galland L, *Superimmunity for Kids*, Bantam Doubleday Dell, New York, 1988.
24. Ibid.
25. Wyshak, G., and R.E. Frisch, "Carbonated Beverages, Dietary Calcium, the Dietary Calcium/Phosphorus Ration, and Bone Fractures in Girls and Boys." *Journal of Adolescent Health* 15, no. 3: 210-215 (1994).
26. Center for Science in the Public Interest. Op cit.
27. Hitti, M. "Soft Drink Consumption Soars." WebM.D. Medical News, Sept 17, 2004. www.webmd.com.
28. Valentine, J., "Soft Drinks – America's Other Drinking Problem." Wise Traditions in Food, Farming, and the Healing Arts. Summer 2001.
29. Ibid.
30. National Soft Drink Association. "Soft Drinks and Nutrition." Washington, DC. Undated.
31. Associated Press. "Consumer Group Attacks Artificial Sweetener." August 1, 1996.
32. Jacobson, Michael F. "Liquid Candy—How Soft Drinks are Harming Americans' Health." Center for Science in the Public Interest. October 1998.
33.   Center for Science in the Public Interest. "Soft Drinks Undermining Americans' –Teens Consuming Twice as Much 'Liquid Candy' as Milk." CSPI News Release, October 1998.
34. Valentine, J. Op cit.
35. Nakamura, David. *The Washington Post*. "Schools Hooked on Junk Food." February 27, 2001, p. A1, A8.
36. Center for Science in the Public Interest. Op cit.
37. Jacobson, MF. Op cit.
38. Federal Register. 44:37212-37221. 1979.
39. Baldwin, J.L., A.H. Chou, and W.R. Solomon. "Popsicle-induces Anaphylaxis Due to Carmine Dye Allergy." *Allergy Asthma Immunology* 79 (1997): 415-419.
40. Analyses by Environment Inc. based on USDA CSFII 1994-1996 two-day data. September 1998.
41. Wyshak, Grace. "Teenaged Girls, Carbonated Beverage Consumption, and Bone Fractures." *Pediatrics & Adolescent Medicine* 154, no. 6 (June 2000).
42. Wyshak, G., and R.E. Frisch, "Carbonated Beverages, Dietary Calcium, the Dietary Calcium/Phosphorus Ration, and Bone Fractures in Girls and Boys." *Journal of Adolescent Health* 15, no. 3: 210-215 (1994).
43. Center for Science in the Public Interest. Op cit.
44. "Caffeine: The Inside Scoop—Osteoporosis." *Nutrition Action Healthletter*. December 1996. Center for Science in the Public Interest. www.cspinet.org.
45. Barger-Lux, M.J., and R.P. Heaney. "Caffeine and the Calcium Economy Revisited." *Osteoporosis Intern* 5, no. 2: 97-102 (March 1995).
46. Ismail, A.I, et al. "The Cariogenicity of Soft Drinks in the United States." *Journal of the American Dental Association* 109, no. 2: 241-245 (1984).

47. Valentine, Judith. Op cit.
48. Ibid.
49. Freedman, David S., et al. "The Relationship or Overweight to Cardiovascular Risk Factors Among Children and Adolescents: The Bogalusa Heart Study." *Pediatrics* 103: 1175-1182 (1999).
50. National Institute of Diabetes and Digestive and Kidney Diseases. www.niddk.nih.gov.
51. Shuster, J., et al. "Soft Drink Consumption and Urinary Stone Recurrence: A Randomized Prevention Trial." *Journal of Clinical Epidemiology* 45, no. 8: 911-916 (1992).
52. Jacobson, MF. Op cit.
53. Center for Science in the Public Interest. "Label Caffeine Content of Foods, Scientists Tell FDA." Press Release. July 31, 1997. www.cspinet.org.
54. "Caffeine: The Inside Scoop—Birth Defects & Miscarriages." *Nutrition Action Healthletter*. December 1996. Center for Science in the Public Interest. www.cspinet.org.
55. Ibid.
56. Nehlig, Astrid, "Consequences on the Newborn of Chronic Maternal Consumption of Coffee During Gestation and Lactation: A Review." *Neurotoxicology and Teratology* 6: 531-43 (1994).
57. *Nutrition Action Healthletter*. Op cit.
58. Nehlig, Astrid. Op cit.
59. Gordon, Serena. "One in Five Kids May Have Mental Problem. Psychological Disorders in Kids Almost Tripled in Last 20 Years." *HealthScout Newsletter*, 2000. www.healthscout.com
60. 40CFR 261.22 (Code of Federal Regulations, Title 40, Volume 22, Part 261 – "Identification and Listing of Hazardous Waste." Revised as of July 1, 2001.)
61. Dufty, William. *Sugar Blues*. New York: Warner Books, Inc., 1975.
62. Martin, W.C., "When is a Food a Food—and When a Poison?" *Michigan Organic News*, March 1957, p. 3.
63. Dufty, William. Op cit.
64. Ibid.
65. Ibid.
66. Pauling, Linus. "Orthomolecular Psychiatry." *Science* 160: 265-271 (April 19, 1968).
67. Hoffer, Abram. "Orthomolecular Approach to the Treatment of Learning Disabilities." Synopsis of reprint article issued by the Huxley Institute for Biosocial Research, New York.
68. Tintera, John W. *Hypoadrenocorticism*. Mt. Vernon, NY: Adrenal Metabolic Research Society of the Hypoglycemia Foundation, Inc., 1969.
69. Fallon, Sally, and Mary G. Enig, Ph.D. *Nourishing Traditions*, 2nd ed. Washington, DC: New Trends Publishing Inc. 1999.
70. Dufty, William. Op cit.
71. Ibid.
72. Ibid.
73. Ibid.
74. Center for Science in the Public Interest. "America: Drowning in Sugar." Press release. www.cspinet.org. August 3, 1999.
75. Center for Science in the Public Interest. "FDA Weighing Sugar Labeling." Press release. www.cspinet.org. June 26, 2000.
76. Johnston, CS et al. "Vinegar Improves Insulin Sensitivity to a High-Carbohydrate Meal in Subjects with Insulin Resistance or Type 2 Diabetes." *Diabetes Care* 27:281-282 2004.
77. Telephone interview with Carol Johnston, April 25, 2008 by Jack Challem of www.dLife.com. "A Spoonful of Vinegar Makes the Blood Sugar Go Down."
78. Ostman, E, et al. "Vinegar Supplementation Lowers Glucose and Insulin Reponses and Increases Satiety after a Bread Meal in Healthy Subjects." *Eur J Clin Nutr* 2005;59,983-988.
79. Banerjee SK, Maulik SK. "Effect of Garlic on Cardiovascular Disorders: A Review." Nutr J. 2002;1:4
80. Eide A, et al., "Antidiabetic Effect of Garlic "Allium sativum L>) in normal and Streptozotocn-induced Diabetic Rats. *Phytomedicine*. 2006;13(9-100:624-9.
81. Bongiorno PB, et al. "Potential Health Benefits of Garlic (Allium sativum): A Narrative Review." *Journal of Complementary and Integrative Medicine*, Vol 5, Is 1. 2008
82. Khan, A, et al. "Cinnamon Improves Glucose and Lipids of People with Type 2 Diabetes." *Diabetes Care* 26:3215-32:8, 2003.
83. Broadhurst CL et al. "Insulin-like Biological Activity of Culinary and Medicinal Plant Aqueous Extracts In Vitro." *J Agric Food Chem* 2000 Mar;48(3):849-52 2000
84. Hlebowicz J et al. "Effect of Cinnamon on Postprandia Blood Glucose, Gastric Emptying, and Satiety in Healthy Subjects." *Am J Clin Nutr*. 2007 Jun;85(6):1552-6. PMID:17556692.
85. Quin B et al. "Cinnamon Extract Prevents the Insulin Resistance Induced by a High-fructose Dies." *Horm Metab Res*. 2004 Feb;36(2):119-25. PMID:15002064.
86. Mucia MA et al. "Antioxidant Evaluation in Dessert Spices Compared with Coommon Food Additives. Influence of Irradiation Procedure." *J Agric Food Chem*. 2004 Apr 7;52(7):1872-81. PMID:15053523

Chapter VI -Asthma
1. Sheffer, A.L., and V.S. Taggart. "The National Asthma Education Program: Expert Panel Report Guidelines for the Diagnosis and Management of Asthma. *Med Care* 31(suppl) (1993): MS20-MS28.
2. www.cdc.gov
3. HSI e-alert, Dec 16, 2008. hsibaltimore.com, LLC
4. "New Survey Suggests Growing Awareness of COPD, Nation's Fourth Leading Killer." NIH News Nov 13, 2008.
5. Drummond BM, et al. "Inhaled Corticosteroids in Patients with Stable Chronic Obstructive Pulmonary Disease." JAMA, Vol 300, No. 20, Nov 26, 2008
6. "Steroid inhalers Raise Pneumonia Risk for Lung Disease Patients." HealthDay News, Nov 25, 2008, nlm.nih.gov.
7. Fulwood, R., et al. "Asthma-United States, 1980-1987." *Morbidity and Mortality Weekly Report* 39, no. 29 (1990): 493-497.
8. Sly, Michael R. "Mortality From Asthma, 1979-1984." *Journal of Allergy and Clinical Immunology* 82, no. 5 (1988): 705-717.
9. American Lung Association, Epidemiology & Statistics Unit, Research and Program Services, *Trends in Asthma Morbidity and Mortality*, May 2005.
10. National Library of Medicine. *Understanding Allergy and Asthma*. National Institutes of Health
11. Centers for Disease Control. Surveillance for Asthma – U.S., 1960-1995, MMWR. 1998;47 (SS-1)
12. CDC Fast Facts A-Z. Vital Health Statistics, 2003.
13. Mannino, David M., et al. "Surveillance for Asthma—United States, 1960-1995." *Morbidity and Mortality Weekly Report* 47(SS-1) (April 24, 1998): 1-28.
14. U.S. Department of Health and Human Services. "Action Against Asthma—A Strategic Plan for the Department of Health and Human Services." May 2000. http://aspe.hhs.gov/sp/asthma/
15. American Lung Association, Op cit.
16. Montague, Peter. "Asthma is Increasing Among U.S. Children," *Rachel's Environmental & Health Weekly*. Environmental Research Foundation. January 30, 1991.
17. U.S. Department of Health and Human Services. "Action Against Asthma—A Strategic Plan for the Department of Health and Human Services." May 2000. http://aspe.hhs.gov/sp/asthma/
18. Gardiner H. "Warning Given on Use of 4 Popular Asthma Drugs, but Debate Remains." NY Times, Dec. 6, 2008.
19. Dominguez LJ et al. "Bronchial Reactivity and Intracellular Magnesium: a Possible Mechanism for the Broncho Dilating Effects of Magnesium in Asthma." Clin Sci (Colch), vol 95, no. 2, pp 137-142, 1998.
20. Britton J. "Dietary Magnesium, Lung Function, Wheezing and Airway Hyperactivity in a Random Population Sample." *Lancet*, Vol. 344, pp 357-362, 1994.
21. Dean, C. *The Miracle of Magnesium*, p186.
22. Stark J, Stark R., *The Carbon Dioxide Syndrome*, Buteyko On Line Ltd, 2002.
23. Hickling KG, et al., Low Mortality Rate in Adult Respiratory Distress Syndrome Using Low-volume, Pressure-limited Ventilation with Permissive Hypercapnia: a Prospective Study." *Critical Care Medicine*, 1994, 22 pp 1568-1578.
24. Laffey JG, Kavanagh BP. "Carbon Dioxide and the Critically Ill - Too Little of a Good Thing?" *Lancet*. 1999. 354(9186). pp 1283-1286.
25. Lumb. AB. *Nunn's Applied Respiratory Physiology*. Reed. London. 2000 pp 3-12, 237,2676,321,362.
26. Stark J, Stark R. Op Cit. p. 69.
27. Buteyko, "Escape from Asthma" pamphlet. www.wt.com.au.
28. Wenger W, Poe R *The Einstein Factor*. Prima Publishing. 1996.
29. Brody, J, A Breathing Technique Offers Help for People with Asthma. NY Times. Nov 3, 2009
30. Dr. Julian Whitaker's Health & Healing, November 2006, Vol 16, No. 11.
31. Sprott, TJ. *The Cot Death Cover-Up?* Auckland, New Zealand: Penguin Books., 1996. Also see www.healthychild.com.
32. *USA Today*, Oct. 6, 2008. Fan in Baby's Room May Help Prevent SIDS.

33. Carbon Dioxide handout. The Buteyko Method workshop by Carol Baglia.

Chapter VI -ADHD
1. Montague, Peter. "ADHD and Children's Environment," *Rachel's Environment & Health Weekly*, no. 678 (December 2, 1999): 2. Environmental Research Foundation.
2. "CHADD Facts." Children and Adults with Attention-Deficit/Hyperactivity Disorders (CHADD). 1996. www.chadd.com.
3. Ibid.
4. "Focus: Reading, Writing, 'Rithmetic, and Ritalin." *Education Reporter*. July 1996. www.eagleforum.org.
5. Montague, Peter. Op cit., p. 1.
6. "CHADD Facts." Op cit.
7. LeFever, G.B, K.V. Dawson, and A.L. Morrow. "The Extent of Drug Therapy for Attention Deficit-Hyperactivity Disorder Among Children in Public Schools." *American Journal of Public Health* 89 (1999): 1359-1364.
8. *Medical News Today*, Survey of adults reveals life-long consequences of ADHD, May 7, 2004. www.medicalnewtoday.com
9. Montague, Peter. Op cit., p. 1.
10. Elias KM,*USA Today*, "Number of Adults on ADHD Drugs Doubles." September 14, 2005.
11. Bellanti, Joseph A., Crook, WG, Layton, RE, eds. *ADHD Attention Deficit Hyperactivity Disorder, Causes and Possible Solutions: Conference Syllabus of Presentation Papers, November 4-7, 1999, Arlington, VA*. Alexandria, VA: International Research Consultants. November 1999.
12. *American Academy of Neurology*. "Brain Abnormalities Found in Children with ADHD." Press Release. April 19,1999. (This can be found at the CHADD website www.chadd.com.)
13.Montague, Peter. Op cit.
14. Loporto, Gaarret, *The DaVinci Method*, 2005, Preview Edition, www.DaVinciMethod.com.
15. Montague, Peter. Op cit.
16. Ibid.
17. Jacobson, Michael F., and David Schardt. *Diet, ADHD & Behavior; A Quarter-Century Review*. Washington, DC: Center for Science in the Public Interest. November 1999. www.cspinet.org. (Also see: "Food Additives," brochure. U.S. Food and Drug Administration [FDA/IFIC], January 1992.)
18. Shaywitz, Bennett A. "Food Colorings Given Following Birth Generate Attention Deficit Disorder Symptoms." *Neurobehavioral Toxicology* 1, no. X (year): 41-47.
19. Reif-Lehrer, Liane. "Infant Seizures Improve After MSG Removal." *Federation Proceedings* 1, no. 11 (1976): 2205-2212.
20. Pressinger, Richard W. "MSG & Aspartame During Pregnancy." www.chem-tox.com.
21. Olney, John W. "MSG & Aspartate Cause Brain Damage Following A Single Low Level Dose." *Nature* 227 (August 8, 1970).
22. Olney, John W. "Obesity-Shorter Growth-and-Reproduction Problems from MSG Intake." *Science* 164 (1969): 719-721.
23. Ibid.
24. Reif-Lehrer, Liane, Op cit.
25. Schettler, Ted, M.D., M.P.H., and Jill Stein, M.D. *In Harm's Way: Toxic Threats to Child Development*. Boston: Greater Boston Physicians for Social Responsibility, 2000.
26. Ibid.
27. Ibid.
28. Landrigan, Philip J. "Commentary: Environmental Disease – A Preventable Epidemic." *American Journal of Public Health* 82 (July 1992): 941-943.
29. Environmental Protection Agency. "Lead in Your Home: A Parent's Reference Guide." EPA 747-B-99-003. May 1999.
30. Committee on Environmental Health, American Academy of Pediatrics. "Lead Poisoning: From Screening to Primary Prevention." *Pediatrics* 92 (July 1993): 176-183.
31. Montague, Peter. "Dumbing Down the Children—Part 3," *Rachel's Environmental & Health Weekly*. Environmental Research Foundation. March 2, 2000.
32. Landrigan, Philip J. Op cit.
33. Committee on Environmental Health, American Academy of Pediatrics. Op cit.
34. Rubin, Rita." ADHD Focuses on Adults." *USA Today*, December 2, 2003.
35. CDC. "The Adult Blood Lead Epidemiology and Surveillance Program (ABLES)" www.cdc.gov/niosh/ables.html
36. Agency for Toxic Substances and Disease Registry. "Toxicological Profile for Lead." July 1999, pp. 26-29.
37. Lanphear, Bruce P. "The Paradox of Lead Poisoning Prevention." *Science* 281 (September 11, 1998): 1617-18.
38. Montague, Peter. Op cit.
39. Environmental Protection Agency. Drinking Water Standards Program. "Lead & Copper." Office of Water, Ground Water and Drinking Water. www.epa.gov/safewater/leadcop.html.
40. Needleman, Herbert L., et al. "Bone Lead Levels and Delinquent Behavior." *Journal of the American Medical Association* 275, no. 5 (1996): 363-369.
41. de la Burde, Brigitte, and McLin S. Choate. "Early Asymptomatic Lead Exposure and Development at School Age." *Journal of Pediatrics* 87, no. 4 (1975): 638-642.
42. Bellinger, David, et al. "Pre-and Postnatal Lead Exposure and Behavior Problems in School-Aged Children." *Environmental Research* 66 (1994): 12-30.
43. Marlowe, Mike, and John Errera. "Low Lead Levels and Behavior Problems in Children." *Behavioral Disorders* 7 (1982): 163-172.
44. Montague, Peter. "Toxins Affect Behavior." *Rachel's Environmental & Health Weekly*. Environmental Research Foundation. January 16, 1997.
45. Byers, Randolph K. and Elizabeth E. Lord. "Late Effects of Lead Poisoning on Mental Development." *American Journal of Diseases of Children* 66, no. 5 (November 1943): 471-494
46. Masters, Roger D., Brian Hone, and Anil Doshi. "Environmental Pollution, Neurotoxicity, and Criminal Violence." In *Environmental Toxicology*, edited by J. Rose. New York: Gordon and Breach Publishers, 1997.
47. Environmental Protection Agency. *Lead in Your Home: A Parent's Reference Guide*. EPA 747-B-99-003. May 1999.
48. National Research Council. *Measuring Lead Exposure in Infants, Children, and Other Sensitive Populations*. Washington, DC: National Academy Press, 1993.
49. Flegal, Russell A., and Donald R. Smith. "Lead Levels in Preindustrial Humans." *New England Journal of Medicine* 326 (1992): 1293-1294.
50. Masters, Roger D., Brian Hone, and Anil Doshi. Op cit.
51. Motluck, Alison. "Pollution May Lead to a Life of Crime." *New Scientist* 154, no. 2084 (1997): 4. and Masters, RD., "Silicofluorides and Higher Blood Lead: A National Problem that Particularly Harms Blacks." Videoconference - Appalachian Environmental Lab, Frostburg State University, Frostburg, M.D. November 15, 2001.
52. Montague, Peter. "Dumbing Down the Children—Part 3," Op cit.
53. Pear, R. "States Called Lax on Tests for Lead in Poor Children." *New York Times*, August 22, 1999, p. A-1.
54. Montague, P. Op cit.
55. Lanphear, Bruce P. "Racial Differences in Urban Children's Environmental Exposures to Lead." *American Journal of Public Health* 86, no. 10 (1996): 1460-1463.
56. Schulte, A., et al. "Urinary Mercury Concentrations in Children With and Without Amalgam Restorations." *Journal of Dental Restoration* 73, no. 4 (1994): A-334.
57. Abraham, J.E., C.W. Svare, and C.W. Frank. "The Effect of Dental Amalgam Restorations on Blood Mercury Levels." *Journal of Dental Restoration* 663, no. 1 (1984): 71-73.
58. Five Common Toxic Metals to Avoid, and Where You'll Find Them. www.mercola.com. 12, 27, 2003
59. Associated Press. "Mercury Poses Health Risk." November 8, 1990.
60. Schettler, Ted, M.D., M.P.H., and Jill Stein, M.D. *In Harm's Way: Toxic Threats to Child Development*. Boston: Greater Boston Physicians for Social Responsibility. 2000.
61. Spyker, Joan, Sheldon B. Sparber, and Alan M. Goldberg. "Low Level Mercury Causes Behavior Problems During Pregnancy." *Science* (August 1972): 621-623.
62. Huggins, Hal A. *It's All in Your Head: The Link Between Mercury Amalgams and Illness*. Garden City Park, NY: Avery Publishing Group, Inc. 1993.
63. Bartolome, George, and Patricia Trepanier. "Dopamine Uptake in Brain Cells Changed by Methyl mercury." *Toxicology and Applied Pharmacology* 65 (1982): pp. 92-99.
64. Pressinger, Richard W. "Mercury Exposure During Pregnancy—Links to Learning Disabilities, ADD, and Behavior Disorders." 2000. www.chemtox.com.
65. Siblerad, Robert L., John Moti, and Eldon Kienholz. "Psychometric Evidence That Mercury From Silver Dental Fillings May be an Etiological Factor in Depression, Excessive Anger, and Anxiety." *Psychological Reports* 74 (1994).
66. "Mercury Amalgam & Mental Illness." www.whale.to
67. Lichtenberg, H.J. "Elimination of Symptoms by Removal of Dental Amalgam From Mercury Poisoned Patients, as Compared With a Control Group of Average Patients." *Journal of Orthomolecular Medicine* 8 (1993) 145-148.

68. Huggins, Hal A. Op cit., pp. 32-33.
69. Huggins, Hal A. "Birth Defects." 2000. www.whale.to or www.hugnet.com.
70. Huggins, Hal A. *It's All in Your Head, The Link Between Mercury Amalgams and Illness.* Op cit.
71. DAMS, Inc. www.dams.cc or www.amalgam.org. or (800) 311-6265.
72. Huggins, Hal A. Op cit., pp. 35, 54,150.
73. Huggins, Hal A. "Politics of Medicine—The Struggle for Freedom of Medical Choice. California Dentists Forced Out of State of Denial." *Alternative Medicine* 41 (May 2001): 114-117.
74. "Mercury Inducing Disease in Animal Experiments." 2000. www.whale.to.
75. Weintraub, Skye. Natural Treatments for ADD and Hyperactivity. P. 187. Pleasant Grove, UT: Woodland Publishing, Inc. 1997.
76. Wilson, Lawrence. "Evidence for Traditional Diets From Hair Mineral Analysis." *Health & Healing Wisdom, the Journal of the Price-Pottenger Nutrition Foundation* 23, no. 31 (Spring 1999): 9
77. Weintraub, Skye. *Natural Treatments for ADD and Hyperactivity.* Pleasant Grove, UT: Woodland Publishing, Inc., 1997, p. 187.
78. Ibid.
79. Wilson, L. Op cit.
80. Jacobson, MF, and Schardt, D. Op cit.
81. Rudlin, Donald. *The Omega-3 Phenomenon, The Nutrition Breakthrough of the 80s.* New York: Rawson Associates, 1989.
82. Evans, Lara, "Life in the Fat Lane." *Delicious Living,* December 2000, p. 28.
83. Weintraub, S. Op cit.
84. Ibid.
85. Wilson, L. Op cit.
86. Weintraub, S. Op cit.
87. Ibid.
88. Evans, L. Op cit.
89. Enig, Mary G., *Know Your Fats. The Complete Primer for Understanding the Nutrition of Fats, Oils & Cholesterol.* Bethesda, M.D.: Bethesda Press, 2000.
90. Kane, PC. "Lifting Depression." *Alternative Medicine Digest,* issue 22: 64-70.
91. Weintraub, S. Op cit.
92. Evans, L. Op cit.
93. www.allergyconnection.com.
94. Weintraub, S. Op cit.
95. Ibid.
96. *For Tomorrow's Children.* Blooming Glen, PA: Preconception Care, Inc. 1990.
97. Whitaker, J. "Nature's Perfect Food? A Second Opinion!" *Health & Healing, Tomorrow's Medicine Today* 8, no. 10 (October 1998).
98. Vonderplanitz, Aajonus. "What Started Pasteurization?" *Right to Choose Healthy Food.* Right to Choose Healthy Food. 1999. ww.odomnet.com/rawmilk.
99. Vonderplanitz, A, "Micro-Phobia Destroys the Nutrients in our Food and, in Turn, Destroys our Health." *Right to Choose Healthy Food.* 1999. ww.odomnet.com/rawmilk
100. "Milk: Why is the Quality so Low?" *Consumer Reports,* January 1974, pp. 70-76.
101. Vonderplanitz, Aajonus, Micro-Phobia Destroys the Nutrients in our Food and, in Turn, Destroys our Health." Op cit.
102. Cousens, Gabriel, *Conscious Eating.* Patagonia, AZ: Essene Vision Books, 1992.
103. Ibid.
104. Pouls, Maile. Personal communication.
105. Fallon, S, Enig, M. *Nourishing Traditions,* Washington, DC: New Trends Publishing, Inc. 1999, p. 35.
106. Weintraub, S. Op cit.
107. Ibid.
108. Ibid.
109. Ibid.
110. Tucker, P. "More Kids Are Hyper and Sad Inside." *HealthScout.* 2000. www.healthscout.com.
111. Gordon, S. "One in Five Kids May Have Mental Problem." *HealthScout.* 2000. www.health-scout.com.
112. Ibid.
113. National Institute of Mental Health, "Depression in Children and Adolescents, A Fact Sheet for Physicians." NIH Publication no. 00-4744. 2000. www.nimh.nih.gov.
114. Ibid.
115. Ibid.
116. Ibid.
117. Weintraub, S. Op cit.
118. Science ,1997;277:1859-1861
119. Eberstadt, Mary. "Why Ritalin Rules." Policy Review, The Heritage Foundation, April & May 1999, no. 94.
120. Diller, Lawrence H. *Running on Ritalin: A Physician Reflects on Children, Society, and Performance in a Pill.* Bantam Books, 1998.
121. Hollowell, Edward M., Ratey, J. *Driven to Distraction, Recognizing and Coping with Attention Deficit Disorder from Childhood Through Adulthood.* New York: Pantheon Books, 1994.
122. Eberstadt, Mary. Op cit.
123. Breggin, PR., Breggin, GR. "The Hazards of Treating 'Attention-Deficit/Hyperactivity Disorder' with Methylphenidate (Ritalin)." *The Journal of College Student Psychotherapy* 10, no. 2 (1995): 55-72.
124. Ibid.
125. Eberstadt, M. Op cit.
126. Golden, G.S. "Role of Attention Deficit Hyperactivity Disorder in Learning Disabilities." *Seminars in Neurology* 11, no. 1 (1991): 3541.
127. Children and Adults with Attention-Deficit/Hyperactivity Disorders (CHADD) "CHADD Facts." 1996. www.chadd.com.
128. Langer, Stephen E., and James F. Scheer. *Solved: The Riddle of Illness.* New Canaan, CT: Keats Publishing, Inc., 1984.
129. Mason, N, *The New Psychiatry.* New York: Philosophical Library, Inc., 1959, p. 21.
130. Elwood, C. *Feel Like a Million.* New York: Devin-Adair Co., 1956, p. 235.
131. Holmes, J.M. "Cerebral Manifestations of Vitamin B12 Deficiency." *British Medical Journal* (1956) 2:1394-1398.
132. Langer, SE., and Scheer JF. Op cit.
133. Breggin, PR. and Breggin GR. Op cit.
134. Ibid.
135. Chira, Susan. "Is Small Better? Educators Now Say Yes for High School." *New York Times,* July 14, 1993, Section A, Page 1.
136. Breggin, PR. and Breggin GR. Op cit.
137. Montague, P. Op cit.
138. "Focus: Reading, Writing, 'Rithmetic, and Ritalin." *Education Reporter.* July 1996. www.eaglefo-rum.org.
139. Eberstadt, M. Op cit.
140. Ibid.
141. Montague, P. Op cit.
142. Gibbs, N, "The Age of Ritalin." *Time,* November 30, 1998, p. 94.
143. Ibid, p. 96.
144. Ibid, p. 90.
145. Ibid, p. 92.
146. Weintraub, S. Op cit.
147. Ibid.
148. Eberstadt, M. Op cit.
149. Ibid.
150. American Psychiatric Association, *Treatments of Psychiatric Disorders – A Task Force Report of the American Psychiatric Association, Volume 2.* Washington, DC, American Psychiatric Association, (1989, p. 1221.)
151. Goodman, A.G., et al. *The Pharmacological Basis of Therapeutics,* 8th Edition. New York: Pergamon Press. 1991.
152. Spotts, J.V., Spotus, C.A. (eds.), *Use and Abuse of Amphetamine and its Substitutes.* Rockville, M.D.: National Institute on Drug Abuse. DHEW Publication no. (ADM) 80-941. 1980.

153. "Focus: Reading, Writing, 'Rithmetic, and Ritalin." Op cit.
154. Eberstadt, M. Op cit.
155. Ibid.
156. Hollowell, EM., Ratey, J. Op cit.
157. Gibbs, N. Op cit.
158. Breggin, PR. and Breggin GR. Op cit.
159. Ibid.
160. Jacobson, MF, Schardt, D. Op cit.
161. Eberstadt, M. Op cit.
162. Gibbs, N. Op cit., p. 94.
163. Eberstadt, M. Op cit.
164. *USA Today*, June 30, 2005, Mercola 7-26-05
165. Ibid.
166. Medical News Today, 4-8-06, Get Your ADHD Drug From a Patch.mercola.com
167. Eberstadt, M. Op cit.
168. Diller, LH. Op cit.
169. Shalin, L. *The Alphabet versus the Goddess*. New York: Penguin/Compass, 1999.
170. Barkley, Russell, *ADHD and the Nature of Self-Control*. New York: Guilford Press, 1997.
171. Farmer, Jeanette. *Training the Brain to Pay Attention the Write Way*. Denver, CO: WriteBrain Press. 1995.
172. Ibid.
173. Ibid.
174. Hannafore, Carla. *Smart Moves: Why Learning is Not All In Your Head*. Arlington, VA: Great Ocean Publishers, Inc. 1995.
175. *Source: National Right to Read Foundation. www.nrrf.org.*
176. Farmer, Jeanette. Op cit.
177. Hedges C. "America the Illiterate." Nov. 10, 2008. truthdig.com.
178. McGinness, Diane. *Why Our Children Can't Read and What We Can Do About It*. New York: Simon & Schuster. 1997.
179. Joseph, R. *The Right-brain and the Unconscious, Discovering the Stranger Within*. New York: Plenum Press, 1992.
180. Farmer, Jeanette. Op cit.
181. Ibid.
182. Beckett, Cheryl. *Growing Up Inside Out*. Fort Collins, CO: Higher States Publishing. 1994.

Chapter VIII - Depression
1. NIMH fact sheet, The Numbers Count, www.nimh.gov.
2. Ibid.
3. mercola.com/2002/dec/11/depression.htm. and mercola The Ultimate Drug for Treating Depression.
4. NIH Publication No. 03-5299, March 2003.
5. mercola.com/2002/dec/11/depression.htm.
6. mercola.com/2002/dec/11/depression.
7. Freeman EW, Sammnel M.D., Lin H, et al. "Association of Hormones and Menopausal Status with Depressed Mood in Women with No History of Depression." *Archives of General Psychiatry*. 2006;63:375-382.
8. Lehrer JA, et al. "Depression Symptomatology as a Predictor of Exposure to Intimate Partner Violence among U.S. Female Adolescents and Young Adults." *Archives of Pediatrics and Adolescent Medicine*. 2006;160:270-276.
9. Klerman GL. "The Current Age of Youthful Melancholia. Evidence for Increase in Depression among Adolescents and Young Adults." *Br J Psychiatry* 1998; 152:4-14
10. Klerman GL, Weissman MM. "Increasing Rates of Depression." *JAMA* 1989: 261: 2229-35
11. Depression Statistics Information, Attention Deficit Disorder Help Center, info@add-adhd-help-center.com - get permission.
12. Facts about Depression in Older Adults, 2005 American Psychological Association, Public Policy Office, 750 First St. NE, Washington DC 20002.
13. Depression: Depression Caused by Chronic Illness, WebM.D. Medical Reference in collaboration with The Cleveland Clinic.
14. NIH Publication No. 01-4591.
15. mercola.com/2002/dec/11/depression.
16. mercola What do Prozac and NSAIDs have in common? You don't want to know. MSNBC May 16, 2005, www.mercola.com/2005/may/31/prozac_nsaids.htm.
17. Ibid.
18. O'Meara, Kelly P, Special Report Prescription Drugs May Trigger Killing, Insight on the News magazine, Sept 2, 2002.
19. Drug Report Barred by FDA - Scientist Links Antidepressants to Suicide in Kids, San Francisco Chronicle, Feb 1, 2004.
20. Pringle, Evelyn J. Bush-backed Drug Marketing Schemes www.dissidentvoice.org, April 26, 2005.
21. Ziot, JM, et al. "Trends in the Prescribing of Psychotropic Medications to Preschoolers." *JAMA* February 23, 2000;283:1025-1030, 1059-1060.
22. Drug Report Barred by FDA - Scientist Links Antidepressants to Suicide in Kids, *San Francisco Chronicle*, Feb 1, 2004.
23. Hawkins, Beth, *A Pill is Not Enough*, Citypages.com. Vol. 25, # 1225, May 26, 2004
24. mercola.com/2004/feb/21/antidepressant_suicides.htm.
25. Pringle, Evelyn J. Bush-backed Drug Marketing Schemes www.dissidentvoice.org, April 26, 2005.
26. Keating, Gina, War in Courtroom over Paxil Drug TV Ads, Yahoonews. Aug. 22, 2002.
27. Ibid.
28. Hawkins, Beth, *Paxil is Forever*, Citypages.com. Vol. 23, # 1141, Oct. 16, 2002.
29. *BBC News*, June 10, 2003
30. Blood, April 1, 2002, Vol. 99. No. 7. pp. 2545-2553
31. CNN April 28, 2004. Mercola.com/2004/may/15/pregnancy_prozac.htm
32. StarNewsOnline.com Has the Romance Gone? Was it the Drug? May 4, 2004.
33. Ibid.
34. Adams, Mike. "President's Bogus Mental health Screening Initiative is a Thinly Veiled Scam to Boost Pharmaceutical Profits." August 7, 2004, NewsTarget.com/z001688.html.
35. Pringle, Evelyn, "Big Pharma Bankrupting U.S. Health Care System." Scoop., Sept. 1, 2006
36. Ibid.
37. Ibid.
38. Robinson, Bryan. "Pills vs. Talking, When it Comes to Mental Illness, Parents Face Dilemmas Over Medication, Talk Therapy." ABCnew.com. Jun 7, 2004.
39. Hawkins, Beth, *Paxil is Forever*, Citypages.com. Vol. 23, # 1141, Oct. 16, 2002.
40. "Getting Off Antidepressants, Antidepressant Discontinuation Syndrome." HealthyPlace.com.
41. Homeland Stupidity, Homelandstupidity.us. March 24, 2006.
42. Kirsch, I, et al. "The Emperor's New Drugs: An Analysis of Antidepressant Mediation Data Submitted to the U.S. Fod and Drug Administration." Prevention & Treatment, Vol. 5, Article 23, July 15, 2002.
43. Hawkins, Beth, *A Pill is Not Enough*, Citypages.com. Vol. 25, # 1225, May 26, 2004
44. Connor, Steve, Glaxo Chief: Our Drugs Do Not Work on Most Patients, Independent News/UK, Dec 8, 2003.
45. Keating, Gina, War in Courtroom over Paxil Drug TV Ads, Yahoonews. Aug. 22, 2002
46. Sears, Al, M.D., Doctor's House Call Newsletter, October 30, 2006.
47. Ibid.
48. "Getting Off Antidepressants, Antidepressant Discontinuation Syndrome." HealthyPlace.com.
49. Rider, Dawn. "Judge Orders Pharmaceutical Giant GlaxoSmithKline to Pull TV Commercials that Claim the Antidepressant Drug *Paxil* is Non Habit-forming." Baum, Hedlund, Aristei, Guilford & Schiavo. Press Release. Los Angeles, CA, Aug. 19, 2002. and, http://www.namiscc.org/News/2002/Fall/PaxilAds.htm.
50. Attachment to FDA Approval Letter NDA 20-031/S-029.
51. Gardiner Harris, "Device Won Approval Though FDA Staff Objected." *New York Times*, 17 February 2006.
52. Loudon, M. "The FDA Exposed: An Interview with Dr. David Graham, the Vioxx Whistleblower." August 30, 2005. www.naturalnews.com.
53. Sears, Al, M.D., *Doctor's House Call Newsletter*, October 30, 2006

54. Borkin, Joseph. *The Crime and Punishment of I.G. Farbin*. FreePress. June, 1978.
55. Waknine, Yael. "FDA Safety Changes Paxil, Paxil CR, Cardura, Zyprexa, Zyprexa Zydis, CME/CD." May 31, 2006. www.medscape.com.
56. Rayburn WF, et al. "Effect of Antenatal Exposure to Paroxetine (*Paxil*) on Growth and Physical Maturation of Mice Offspring. *J Maternal Fetal Med* 9(2): 136-14 (2000).
57. Chambers CD, et al., "Weight Gain in Infants Breastfed by Mothers who Take Fluoxetine." *Pediatrics* 104 (5):e61 (1999).
58. "Thyroid." www.health911.com/remedies/rem_thyr.htm.
59. Shomon, Mary J. *Living Well with Hypothyroidism: Second Edition*/2005. HarperCollins/Harper Resource.
60. Dranov, Paula. *Tired? Depressed? Check Your Thyroid*, Condensed from American Health (May '94) www.mentalhealth.com/mag1/p51-thyr.html.
61. Key Thought of Joseph Mercola, D.O. From Mary Shomon.
62. Shomon, Mary, Op.cit.
63. Benevicius, R, Et Al. "Effects of Thyroxine asCompared with Thyroxine plus Triiodothyronine in Patients with Hypothyridism." *New Eng J Med.* 340 (1999):424-429,469-70.
64. Wright, Jonathan V., M.D., One Mineral Can Help a Myriad of Conditions From Atherosclerosis to COPD to Zits. Reprinted from *Nutrition and Healing*. www.tahoma-clinic.com/iodide.shtml
65. Conklin, Sarah, Ph.D., et. al. "Omega 3 Fatty Acids Influence Mood, Impulsivity and Personality." University of Pittsburgh Medical Center, March 3, 2006.
66. Adams PB, Lawson S, Sanigorski A, Sinclair AJ. "Arachidonic Acid to Eicosapentaenoic Acid Ratio in Blood Correlates Positively with Clinical Symptoms of Depression." *Lipids* 1996: 31: S157-S-161.
67. Peet M, Murphy B, Shay J, Horrobin D. "Depletion of Omega-3 Fatty Acid Levels in Red Blood Cell Membranes of Depressive Patients." *Biol Psychiatry* 1998;43: 315-319.
68. Maes M, et al. "Lowered n-3 Polyunsaturated Fatty Acids in the Serum Phyospholipids and Cholesterol Esters of Depressed Patients." *Psychiatry Res* 1999; 85:275-291.
69. Tiemeier H, van Tuijl HR, Hofman A, et al. "Plasma Fatty Acid Composition and Depression are Associated in the Elderly: the Rotterdam Study." *Am J Clin Nutr* 2003; 78:40-46.
70. Peet, M., Horrobin, DF. "A Dose-ranging Study of the Effects of Ethyl-eicosapentaenoatein Patients with Ongoing Depression Despite Apparently Adequate Treatment with Standard Drugs." *Arch Gen Psychiatry* 2002: 59: 913-919.
71. Stol, AL, Severus, WE, Freeman,MP, et al. "Omega 3 Fatty Acids in Bipolar Disorder; a Preliminary Double-blind, Placebo-controlled Trial." *Arch Gen Psychiatry* 1999: 407-412.
72. Sampalis, F, Bunea R, Pelland MF, et al. "Evaluation of the Effects of Neptune Krill Oil on the Management of Premenstrual Syndrome and Dysmenorrhea." *Altern Med Rev* 2003; 8: 171-179.
73. Hibbeln JR, et al., Fish consumption and major depression (letter). *Lancet* 1998: 351: 1213.
74. Hibbeln JR. "Seafood Consumption, the DHA Content of Mothers' Milk and Prevalence Rates of Postpartum Depression: A cross-national, Ecological Analysis." *Journal of Affective Disorders*. 2002 may;69(1-3):15-29.
75 Holub BJ. "Clinical Nutrition: 4. Omega-3 Fatty Acids in Cardiovascular Care." *CMAJ* 2002, 166;608-615.
76. Kimbrell TA, Ketter TA, George MS, Little JT, et al. "Regional Cerebral Glucose Utilization in Patients with a Range of Severities in Unipolar Depression." *Biol Psychiatry* 2002; 51: 237-52.
77. Logan, Alan C, "Omega-3 Fatty Acids and Major Depression: A Primer for the Mental Health Professional. Integrative Care Centre of Toronto." *Lipids in Health and Disease* 2004, 3:25.
78. Seaton, R.B., et al. "Thermic Effect of Medium-chain and Long-chain Triglycerides in Man." *American Journal of Clinical Nutrition* 1986 44:620-629.
79. Bray, GA et al. "Weight Gain of Rats Fed Medium-chain Triglycerides is Less than Rats Fed Long-chain Triglycerides." *Int. J. Obes*, 1980, 4:27-32.
80. Geliebter, A. "Overfeeding with Medium-chain Triglycerides Diet Results in Diminished Deposition of Fat." *American Journal of Clinical Nutrition*, 1983, 37:1-4.
81. Dean, C. Op cit., *Miracle of Magnesium*, p 45.
82. Rimonen, M, et al. "Insuln Resistance and Depression: Cross Sectional Study." *British Medical Journal* January 1, 2005;330:17-18.
83. Dunn, AL et al. "Exercise Treatment for Depression: Efficacy and Dose Response." *American Journal of Preventive Medicine* January 2005;28(1):1-8.
84. Dimeo, et al. "Benefits from Aerobic Exercise in Patients with Major Depression: A Pilot Study." *British Journal of Sports Medicine* April 2001;35:114-117.
85. More, Lee Krens, "It's Wintertime: Lighten up!" Gannett News Service, December 26, 1994.
86. Lambert, CW. et al. "Effect of Sunlight and Season on Serotonin Turnover in the Brain." *Lancet* December 7, 2002:360:1840-1842.
87. Rosenthal, NE, *Winter Blues*, Giliford Press, New York, NY. 2006.
88. More, LK. Op cit.

Chapter IX – Alzheimer's disease
1. Alzheimer's Foundation. www.alzfdn.org.
2. Ibid.
3. Ibid.
4. American Health Assistance Foundation website. www.ahaf.org.
5. www.alzfdn.org.
6. Butler, Robert. "Early Determinants of Disease in the Elderly." International Longevity Center.
7. "Alzheimer drugs don't work." www.mercola.com/2004/apr/24/alzheimer_drugs.htm.
8. Terry, RD., et al., editors, *Alzheimer Disease*. Raven Press, New York, NY 1994.
9. The Burton Goldberg Group. *Alternative Medicine - The Definitive Guide*. Future Medicine Publishing Inc., Puyallup, WA 1993.
10. Bolla, DL, et al. "Neurocognitive Effects of Aluminum." *Archives of Neurology*, Vol. 49, Octover 1992, pp. 1021-26.
11. Terry, RD. Op cit.
12. The Facts about Human Health and Alluminum in Drinking Water, ES&E, Jan 1997. www.esemag.com.
13. Is aluminum a dementing ion? The *Lancet* Vol 339, March 21, 1992, pp. 713-14.
14. McLachlan C, Donald R. "Would Decreased Aluminum Ingestion Reduce the Incidence of Alzheimer's disease?" *Canadian Medical Association Journal*, Vol. 147, No 6, September 15, 1992, pp. 846-47.
15. Campbell, WCD, Real Health Daily Dose, 5-27-03 www.realhealthnews.com.
16. Zoladz P et al. "Cinnamon Perks Perfomance." Paper Presented at the annual meeting of the Association for Chemoreceptin Sciences held in Sarasota, FL, April 21-25. 2004
17. Conquer, JA. "Fatty Acid Analysis of Blood Plasma of Patients with Alzheimer's disease, other Types of Dementia, and Cognitive Impairment." *Lipids*, Vol 35 No. 12, 2000, pp. 1305-1312.
18. Kalmijn, S., et al. "Dietary Fat Intake and the Risk of Incident Dementia in the Rotterdam Study." *Ann Neurol*, Vol 42, No. 5, 1997, pp. 776-782
19. Fallon, Sally, and Mary G. Enig, Ph.D. *Nourishing Traditions*, 2nd ed. Washington, DC: New Trends Publishing, Inc., 1999, p. 237.
20. Douglas, WC. "A Substance Found in Breast Milk Helps Depression, Alzheimer's." *Second Opinion* XI, No. 3. March 20010.
21. Stehlin, IB. "Infant Formula: Second Best but Good Enough." U.S. Food and Drug Administration. www.fda.gov.
22. Sears, B, *The Omega Rx Zone*, 2002 New York, Harper-Collins.
23. Yehuda, S et al. "The Role of Polyunsaturated Fatty Acids in Restoring the Aging Neuronal Membrane." *Neurobiology of Aging*, Vol, 23, No 5, 2002, pp. 843-853.
24. Yehuda, S., et al. "Essential Fatty Acids Preparation (SR-3) Improves Alzheimer's Patients Quality of Life." *Int. J. Neuroscience*, Vol. 87, No 3-4, 1996, pp. 141-149.
25. *American Journal of Clinical Nutrition*, Sept. 2006: 84(3):616-622
26. Whyte, EM, et al. "Cognitive and Behavioral Correlates of Low Vitamin B12 Levels in Elderly Patients with Progressive Dementia." *Am J Geriatr Psychiatry*, Vol. 10, No. 3, 2002, pp. 321-327.
27. Wang, HX, et al. "Vitamin B(12) and Folate in Relation to the Development of Alzheimer's disease." *Neurology*, Vol. 56, No. 9, 2001, pp. 1188-1194.
28. Clarke, R., et al. "Folate, Vitamin B12 and Serum Total Homocysteine Levels in Confirmed Alzheimer Disease." *Arch. Neurolo.*, Vol. 55, No. 11, 1998, pp. 1449-1455.
29. Snowdon, DA, et al. "Serum Folate and the Severity of Atrophy of the Neocortex in Alzheimer Disease: Findings from the Nun Study." *American Journal of Clinical Nutrition*, Vol. 71. No. 4, 2000, pp 993-998.
30. Yoon et al. "Changes in Folate, Vitamin B12, and Homocysteine Associated with Incidnet Dementia." *Journal of Neurology, Neurosurgery, and Psychiatry* 2008 Aug;79(8):864-8.
31. Bonaa KH. "NORVIT: Randomized Trial of Homocysteine-lowering with B-vitamins for Secondary Prevention of Cardiovascular Disease after Myocardial Infarction. Program and Abstracts from the European Society of Cardiology Congress 2005:Sept 3-7, 2005 Stockholm, Sweden.

32. Quinlivan EP, Gregory JF. "Effect of Food Fortification on Folic Acid Intake in the United States." *American Journal of Clinical Nutrition.* 2003 Jan;77(1):221-5
33. Ann Pharmacother, 1999, May: 33:641-3
34. White LR, Petrovitch H, Ross GW, et al. "Brain aging and midlife tofu consumption." *J Am Coll Nutr* 2000;19:242–55.
35. Journal of the American College of Nutrition, April 2000; 19-207-209, 242-255.
36. Tyas SL, et al. "Midlife Smoking and late-life Dementia: the Honolulu-Asia Aging Study." *Neurobiol. Aging* 2003;24:589-96.
37. Luchsinger JA, et al., "Alcohol Intake and Risk of Dementia." *J Am Geriatr Soc.* 2004:52:540-6.
38. Larrier S, et al. "Nutritional Factors and Risk of Incident Dementia in the PAQUID Longitudinal Cohort." *J Nutr Health Aging* 2004,:8:150-4.
39. Neurology, October 24, 2006; 67(8): 1370-1376.
40. "Research Indicates Mental Activity Prevents Alzheimer's disease - Brief Article." *Better Nutrition,* June 2002, Primedia Intertech.
41. Byrd, JB., Sr. "High Mental Activity Protects Against Alzheimer's disease in Mice." Alzheimer's Center & Research Institute, June 13, 2006
42. Larson, EB, Cole, GM. Alzheimer's disease Research Center, University of California, Los Angeles; Jan. 17, 2006 Annals of Internal Medicine.
43. Mozes, A. "Regular Exercise May Delay Alzheimer's." *HealthDay Reporter,* Jan 16, 2006.
44. Proceedings of the National Academy of Sciences Early Edition, February 16, 2004.
45. "Studies Reinforce Links Between Cognitive Function and Cardiovascular Health. Alzheimer Risk Factors Linked to Physical Activity and Diet." 10th International Conference on Alzheimer's disease and Related Disorder (ICAD), presented by the Alzheimer's Association, Madrid, July 18, 2006.
46. BBC News June 23, 2003, mercola.com/2003/jul/9/power_naps.htm.
47. EurekaAlert! March 15, 2003, mercola.com/2004/mar/31/alzheimers_symptoms.htm

Chapter X – Parkinson's disease
1. www.parkinsonsdisease-guidebook.com.
2. Larsen, HR. "Parkinson's disease: Is Victory in Sight?" *International Journal of Alternative and Complementary Medicine*, Vol. 15, No. 10, October 1997, pp. 22-24.
3. Parkinson's disease Foundation, www.pdf.org.
4. Fahn, Stanley. Parkinson disease, the effect of levodopa, and the ELLDOPA trial. Archives of Neurology, Vol. 56, May 1999, pp. 529-35
5. www.brainandspine.org.uk
6. Chabolla, David R., et al. Drug-induced parkinsonism as a risk factor for Parkinson's disease: a historical cohort study in Olmsted County, Minnesota. May Clinic Proceedings, Vol. 73, August 1998, pp. 724-27.
7. Bower, James H. et al. Incidence and distribution of parkinsonism in Olmsted County, Minnesota, 1976-1990. Neurology, Vol. 52, April 12, 1999, pp. 1214-20
8. Muller, Thomas, et al. Nigral endothelial dysfunction, homocystene, and Parkinson's disease. The Lancet, Vol. 354, July 10, 1999
9. Lang, Anthony E. Surgery for Parkinson disease: a critical evaluation of the state of the art. Archives of Neurology, Vol. 57, August 2000, PP. 1118-25
10. Meara, Jolyon, et al. Accuracy of diagnosis in patients with presumed Parkinson's disease. Age and Ageing, Vol. 28, March 1999, pp. 99-102
11. Bhatt, Mohit H., et al. Acute and reversible parkinsonism due to organophosphate pesticide intoxication. Neurology, Vol. 52, April 22, 1999, pp. 1467-71
12. New Scientist, November 11, 2000, p. 16
13. New Scientist, May 25, 2006
14. Larsen, Hans, R., Parkinson's disease: Is Victory in Sight? International Journal of Alternative and Complementary Medicine, Vol. 15, No. 10, October 1997, pp. 22-24
15. Dean, Carolyn, Op cit.
16. Powers, K.M. et al. Parkinson's disease risks associated with dietary iron, manganese and other nutrient intakes, Neurology 2003;60:1761-1766
17. Hellenbrand, W., et al. Diet and Parkinson's disease II: a possible role for the past intake of specific nutrients. Neurology, Vol. 47, September 1996, pp. 644-50
18. Vonderplanitz, Aajonus. We Want to Live, Carnelian Bay Castle Press, LLC, Santa Monica, CA, 1997
19. *USA Today,* May 15, 2006
20. MSNBC, September 29, 2005
21. *Neurology,* March 22, 2005;64(6):1047-1051
22. Journal of Korean Medical Science, June 2005;20(3):495-98. mercola.com/2005/jul/14/vitamin_d.htm. full text available link
23. Larsen, Hans, R., Op cit.
24. Neurology, February 22, 2005; 64(4):664-9

Chapter XI – Arthritis, Osteoporosis & Cavities
1. CDC. Prevalence of disabilities and associated health conditions among adults. U.S., 1999.
2. MMWR. 2001;50:120-125.
3. Hootman JM, Helmick CG. "Projections of U.S. Prevalence of Arthritis and Associated Activity Limitations." *Arthritis Rheum.* 2006;54:226-229.
4. www.Arthritis.org.
5. Medizine's Healthy Living, Second quarter 2007.
6. Bystrianyk, R., "Toxic and Deadly NSAIDS, An Investigative Report." www.healthsentinel.com, August 19, 2001.
7. Singh G. "Recent Considerations in Nonsteroidal Anti-Inflammatory Drug Gastropathy," *The American Journal of Medicine,* July 27, 1998, P. 315.
8. Wolfe M, Lichtenstein D, Singh. "Gastrointestinal Toxicity of Nonsteroidal Anti-inflammatory Drugs." *The New England Journal of Medicine,* June 17,1999, Vol 340, No 24, pp. 1888-1889.
9. "Arthritis Drug may Lead to Heart Risks, Study Says." *Toronto Star* July 12, 2004.
10. Douglass, WC. *The Daily Dose,* November 29, 2004.
11. Ibid.
12. "Courts Reject Two Major *Vioxx* Verdicts." *New York Times* May 30, 2008.
13. Summey BT, Yosipovitch G. "Glucocorticoid-induced Bone Loss in Dermatologi Patients: An Update." *Arch. Dermatol.* 2006;142:82-90.
14. *JAMA,* March 15, 2006. Vol. 295, No 11.
15. "High Doses of Tylenol May Hurt Liver." *Akron Beacon Journal* March 5, 2006.
16. Watkins PB et al. "Aminotransferase Elevations in Healthy Adults Receiving 4 Grams of Acetaminophen Daily." *JAMA* 2006;296:87-93.
17. Murshed, R. "The Sweet Solution – 2" The Daily Star Dec 8, 2008 www.thedailystar.net
18. Garlic & Vinegar How to use Them for Fold Remdies, Recipes, health & Beauty Tips. American Media Mini Mags, Inc. 2006.
19. www.nof.org.
20. Summey BT, Op cit.
21. *New York Times,* June 2, 2006.
22. Heckbert et al. "Use of Alendronate and Risk of Incident Atrial Fibrillation in Women" *Archives of Internal Medicine,* April 28, 2008;168(8):826-31.
23. Ibid.
24. Tylavsky FA et al. "Fruit and Vegetable Intakes are an Independent Predictorof Bone Size in Early Pubertal Children." *American Journal of Clinical Nutrition.* February 2004;79(2) 311-317.
25. *American Journal Clinical* Nutrition. February, 2003;77:495-503
26. Belch, PA *Prescription for Nutritional Healing, 4th Edition.* Avery Publishers. 2006
27. Ibid.
28. *Journal of the American Geriatrics Society.* Vol 51, p 1533.
29. Sigurdsson G, et al. "The Association Between Parathyroid Hormone, Vitamin D and Bone Mineral Density in 70-year-old Icelandic Women." *Osteoporosis. Int.* 2000;11:1031-5.
30. *American Journal Clinical Nutrition.* December 2002. 76:1446-1453.
31. Eriksen W, Sandvik L, Bruusgaard D. "Does Dietary Supplementation of Cod Liver Oil Mitigate Musculoskeletal Pain?" *Eur. J Clin Nutr* 1996;50:689-93.
32. Lips P. "Vitamin D Deficiency in a Multicultural Setting." *Ned. Tijdschr. Geneeskd.* 2001;145:2060-2.
33. Rowen, RJ. *Second Opinion Newsletter.* October 2001. Vol XI, No. 10.
34. Mancino M, Ohia E, Kulkarni P. "A Comparative Study Between Cod Liver Oil and Liquid Lard Intake on Intraocular Pressure on Rabbits." *Prostaglandins Leukot. Essent. Fatty Acids.* 1992;45:239-43.
35. Vilaseca J, et al. "Dietary Fish Oil Reduces Progression of Chronic Inflammatory Lesions in a Rat Model of Granulomatous Colitis." *Gut.* 1990;31:539-44.
36. Guarner F, Vilaseca J, Malagelada JR. "Dietary Manipulation in Experimental Inflammatory Bowel Disease." *Agents Actions.* 1992;Spec No:C10-C14.
37. Shu XO, et al. "A Population-based Case-control Study of Childhood Leukemia in Shanghai." *Cancer* 1988. Aug 1;62(3):635-44.

38. Terkelsen LH, et al. "Topical Application of Cod Liver Oil Ointment Accelerates Wound Healing: an Experimental Study in Wounds in the Ears of Hairless Mice." *Scand. J Plast. Reconstr. Surg. Hand Surg.* 2000;34:15-20.
39. Blunt K, Cowan R. *Ultraviolet Light and Vitamin D in Nutrition.* University of Chicago Press, Chicago, May 1931.
40. "Cod liver Oil Number One Super Food." www.newmediaexplorer.com.
41. "Did Government Approve Citizens as Toxic Waste Sites? Are We Being Poisoned?" *The Winds.* 1998, p. 12. www.thewinds.org.
42. Schuld, Andreas. "Fluoride—Worse Than We Thought." *Wise Traditions* 1, no. 3 (Fall 2000). Weston A. Price Foundation.
43. "The Effect of Fluorine on Dental Caries." *Journal of the American Dental 8ssociation* 31 (1944): 1360.
44. "Did Government Approve Citizens as Toxic Waste Sites? Are We Being Poisoned?" Op cit.
45. Schuld, A. Op cit.
46. "Achievements in Public Health, 1900-1999— Fluoridation of Drinking Water to Prevent Dental Caries." *CDC Morbidity and Mortality Weekly Report* 48(41) (1999): 933-940.
47. Green, Jeff. "Just What is Fluoride?" *Health & Healing Wisdom, the Journal of the Price-Pottenger Nutrition Foundation* 23, no. 1 (Spring 1999):
48. Borne, Gregory. "Phosphoric Acid Waste Dialogue, Report on Phosphoric Wastes Dialogue Committee, Activities and Recommendations; Southeast Negotiation Network." *EPA Stakeholders Review.* September 1995.
49. "Did Government Approve Citizens as Toxic Waste Sites? Are We Being Poisoned?" Op cit., p.11.
50. National Research Council, Committee on Toxicology, Board on Environmental Studies and Toxicology, Commission on Life Sciences, Subcommittee on Health Effects of Ingested Fluoride. *Health Effects of Ingested Fluoride.* August 1993, p. 59.
51. *Fluorides and Human Health.* World Health Organization. 1970, p. 239.
52. Carton, R.J., and J.W. Hirzy. "Applying the NAEP Code of Ethics to the Environmental Protection Agency and the Fluoride in Drinking Water Standard." *Proceedings of the 23rd Annual Conference of the National Association of Environmental Professionals.* GEN 51-61 (June 1998): pp. 20-24.
53. Carton, Robert J. "Corruption and Fraud at the EPA." *The Winds.* July 28, 1995. www.thewinds.org.
54. Mullenix, Phyllis. "Neurotoxicity of Sodium Fluoride in Rats." *Journal of Neurotoxicology and Teratology* 17, no. 2 (1995).
55. Ibid. See also, Joel Griffiths and Chris Bryson's "Fluoride Teeth and the Atomic Bomb," 1997, an article originally commissioned by the *Christian Science Monitor* but never published in it. You can find it at www.winds.org.
56. "Did Government Approve Citizens as Toxic Waste Sites? Are We Being Poisoned?" Op cit.,p.10.
57. Masters, Roger D., "Silicofluorides and Higher Blood Lead: A National Problem that Particularly Harms Blacks." Videoconference - Appalachian Environmental Lab, Frostburg State University, Frostburg, M.D. November 15, 2001.

Chapter XII – Sleep Disorders, Migraine Headaches

1. Ancoli-Israel S. "The Impact and Prevalence of Chronic Insomnia and other Sleep Disturbances Associated with Chronic Illness." *The American Journal of Managed Care.* Vol 12, No 8 Sup.
2. www.merck.com.
3. "The Role of the Pharmacist in Treating Insomnia." medscape.com.
4. www.mercola.com/2000/7/cure_insomnia.htm.
5. Ancoli-Israel S. Op cit.
6. *BBC News.* May 27,2005.
7. Douglass WC. *Daily Dose Newsletter*, July 20, 2004.
8. *LA Times*, October 9, 2006.
9. Ibid.
10. Gottlieb DJ, et al. "Association of Usual Sleep Duration with Hypertension: The Sleep Heart Health Study." *Sleep* 2006; 29:1009-1014.
11. JAMA, June 28, 2006, Vol 295, No 24, P2851-2858.
12. "NIH State of the Science Statement on Manifestations and Management of Chronic Insomnia in Adults." National Institute of Health June 13-15, 2005.
13. Sleep. 2005: 28:1049-1057
14. Medizine's Healthy Living, Second quarter 2007, p85.
15. Stoschitzky K, et al. "Influence of Beta-blockers on Melatonin Release." *European Journal of Clinical Pharmacology* 1999;55(2):111-5.
16. Maas, J. *Power Sleep* Collins Living; 1st edition, December 9, 1998.
17. NIH Press Release, Dec. 19, 2005. www.nih.gov.
18. Medizine, Op cit.
19. Borge S, et al. "Cognitive Behavioral Therapy vs. Zopiclone for Treatment of Chronic Pulmonary Insomnia in Older Adults." *JAMA.* 2006;295:2851-2858.
20. Morin CM et al. "Behavioral and Pharmacological Therapies for Late-life Insomnia: a Randomized Controlled Trial." *JAMA.* 1999;281:991-999.
21. Wenger W, Poe R. *The Einstein Factor.* Prima Publishing. 1996
22. "Sharing Bed Drains Men's Brains." *BBC News* July 20, 2006.
23. www.mercola.com/2000/7/cure_insomnia.htm
24. Gomez RL et al. "Naps Promote Abstraction in Language-Learning Infants." Psychological Science. August 2006;17(8):670.
25. www.barefoothealth.com.
26. Thomas J, Thomas E, Tomb E. "Serum and Erythrocyte Magnesium Concentrations and Migraine." *Magnes Res.* 1992 Jun;5(2):127-30.
27. Dean C, *The Miracle of Magnesium.* Ballantine Books, 2003
28. Mauskop A, Altura BT, Cracco RQ, Altura BM. "Intravenous Magnesium Sulfate Rapidly Alleviates Headaches of Various Types." *Headache.* 1996 Mar;36(3):154-60.
29. Dean C, Op cit.
30. Peikert A, Wilimzig C, Kohne-Volland R. "Prophylaxis of Migraine with Oral Magnesium: Results from a Prospective, Multi-center, Placebo-controlled and Double-blind Randomized Study." *Cephalalgia.* 1996 Jun:16(4):257-63.
31. Weaver K. "Magnesium and Migraine." *Headache*, Vol 32, p 168, 1990.
32. Facchinetti F, et al. "Oral Magnesium Successfully Relieves Premenstrual Mood Changes." *Obstet Gynecol.* 1991 Aug;78(2):177-81.
33. Guillem E, Pelissolo A, Lepine JP. "Mental Disorders and Migrane: Epidemiologic Studies." *Enciphale.* 1999 Sep-Oct;25(5):436-42.
34. Sircus M. *Transdermal Magnesium Therapy.* Phaelos Books. 2007.
35. Tobias K et al. "Migraine and Risk of Cardiovascular Disease in Women." *JAMA.* Vol 296 No 3, July 19, 2006.
36. "Migraine Sufferers have Increased Risk of Heart Attacks and Strokes." Telegraph.co.uk, Apr 2008.

Chapter XIII – Birth Defects

1. March of Dimes, Birth Defects Information, 1999. www.modimes.org.
2. Centers for Disease Control and Prevention, "Birth Defects and Pediatric Genetics." CDC, 2000. www.cdc.gov.
3. "Major Advances in Biology should be Used to Assess Birth Defects From Toxic Chemicals." National Research Council of the National Academies Press Release. June 1, 2000. www.books.nap.edu/catalog/9871.
4. U.S. Bureau of the Census, *Statistical Abstract of the United States, 1955* (76th edition.), Washington, DC, 1955, p. 71; and 83rd edition, 1962, p. 66; and 101st edition, p. 90, 1980; and 121st edition, 2000.
5. *National Vital Statistics Reports.* Table 30, 47, no. 19. June 30, 1999.
6. Edmonds, Larry D. "Temporal Trends in the Prevalence of Congenital Malformations at Birth Based on the Birth Defects Monitoring Program, United States, 1979-1987." *Morbidity and Mortality Weekly Report, CDC Surveillance Summaries* 39, no. SS-4 (December 1990): 19-23.
7. Skjaerven, Rolv, et al. "A Population-Based Study of Survival and Childbearing among Female Subjects with Birth Defects and the Risk of Recurrence in Their Children." *The New England Journal of Medicine* 340, no. 14 (1999): 1057-1062.
8. Lie, RT, Wilcox AJ, Skjaerven R. "Survival and Reproduction Among Males With Birth Defects and Risk of Recurrence in Their Children." *JAMA* 285, No. 6 2001.
9. "Alarming Rise in Birth Defects." *BeijingReview.com* No. 49 Dec. 6, 2007.
10. Montague, Peter. "Birth Defects—Part 2: Why Birth Defects Will Continue To Rise," Environmental Research Foundation. *Rachel's Environment & Health Weekly*, no. 411 (October 13, 1994).
11. Bennett, J.V., et al. "Infectious and Parasitic Diseases." In *Closing the Gap: The Burden of Unnecessary Illness*, edited by R. Amler and H.B. Dull. Oxford, England: Oxford University Press. 1987. (The figure cited is not an official CDC estimate, though it was informally developed by CDC scientists.)
12. Morris R., Levin, R. "Estimating the Incidence of Waterborne Infectious Disease Related to Drinking Water in the United States." In *Assessing and Managing the Health Risks From Drinking Water Contamination*, edited by E. Richard. London: International Association of Hydrological Sciences, 1996.
13. "40 CFR Parts 9,141,132." *Federal Register* 63, no. 241 (December 16, 1998).
14. Thornton, J. "Chlorinated Tap Water Linked to Birth Defects." *The Electronic Telegraph*, February 20, 2000.

15. Klotz, JB., Pyrch, LA. *Case-Control Study of Neural Tube Defects and Drinking Water Contaminants.* Atlanta, GA: Agency for Toxic Substances and Disease Registry. January 1998.
16. Cantor, KP. "Drinking Water and Cancer—Epidemiologic Research on Cancer Risk and Chlorination By-Products in Drinking Water." *Cancer Causes and Control* 8 (1997).
17. Waller, K, et al. "Trihomethanes in Drinking Water and Spontaneous Abortion." *Epidemiology* 9, no. 2 (March 1998): 134-140.
18. Cantor, Kenneth P. Op cit.
19. Betts, Kellyn S. "Miscarriages Associated With Drinking Water Disinfection Byproducts, Study Says." *Environmental Science & Technology* (April 1, 1998): 169A-170O.
20. Zaslow, Sandra A., and Glenda M. Herman. "Health Effects of Drinking Water Contaminants." North Carolina Cooperative Extension Service, publication he-393 (May 1992).
21. Durant, John L., et al. "Elevated Incidence of Childhood Leukemia in Woburn, Massachusetts: NIEHS Superfund Basic Research Program Searches of Causes." *Environmental Health Perspectives* 103: Supplement 6 (September 1995).
22. Physicians for Social Responsibility. "Physicians Give Failing Grade to Congress on Child Health Issues." August 26, 1998. www.psr.org/reportcard.htm.
23. Physicians for Social Responsibility. www.atsdr.cdc.gov/toxhazsf.html.
24. Zaslow, Sandra A., and Glenda M. Herman. Op cit.
25. Natural Resources Defense Council. "Clean Water and Oceans: Drinking Water: In Brief: FAQs. Arsenic in Drinking Water." June 30, 2000. www.nrdc.org/water/drinking/quarsenic.asp
26. WatersafeTM. "Pocket Guide—Have You Tested Your Drinking Water Lately?" Silver Lake Research, Monrovia, CA.
27. Self, James R., and Reagan M. Waskom. "Nitrates in Drinking Water." Colorado State University Cooperative Extension Service. June 1992.
28. Natural Resources Defense Council. "Clean Water and Oceans: Drinking Water: In Brief: FAQs. Bottled Water: Pure Drink or Pure Hype?" April 29, 1999. www.nrdc.org/water/drinking/nbw.asp.
29. March of Dimes. "Birth Defect Information, Thalidomide." www.modimes.org.
30. March of Dimes. "Folic Acid Fact Sheet." www.modimes.org.
31. Centers for Disease Control and Prevention. "Folic Acid Now." CDC, 2000. www.cdc.gov.

Chapter XIV- Infertility

1. National Women's Health Information Center. "Infertility." Office on Women's Health, Department of Health and Human Services. 2000. www.4woman.gov.
2. Wright, Lawrence. "Silent Sperm." *New Yorker.* January 15, 1996.
3. Pinchbeck, Daniel. "Downward Motility." *Esquire.* January 1996.
4. Montague, Peter. "Sperm in the News," Environmental Research Foundation. *Rachel's Environment & Health Weekly,* no, 477, January 18, 1996.
5. Herman-Giddens, Marcia E. "Secondary Sexual Characteristics and Menses in Young Girls Seen in Office Practice: A Study from the Pediatric Research in Office Settings Network." *Pediatrics,* 99 no. 4 (1997): 505-512.
6. Sinclair, Wayne, and Richard W. Pressinger. "Environmental Causes of Infertility." 2000. www.chem-tox.com.
7. Wright, Lawrence. Op cit.
8. Giwercman, Aleksander, et al. "Sperm Counts Decline Since 1940s, Testicle Abnormalities Increase." *Environmental Health Perspectives* 101, no. 2 (1993): 65-71.
9. CDC.gov.
10. The Ottawa Citizen, January 21, 2007
11. Sherman, J.K. "Lower Sperm Count Increases Risk of Miscarriage, University of Arkansas Study." *Washington Star,* January 7, 1979.
12. Furuhjelm, Mirjam, Birgit Jonson, and C.G. Lagergren. "Miscarriages Linked to Men With Low Sperm Counts." *International Journal of Fertility* 7, no. 1: 17-21.
13. Giwercman, Aleksander, et al. Op cit.
14. Carlson, Elisabeth, et al. "Evidence for Decreasing Quality of Semen During Past 50 Years." *British Medical Journal* 305: 609-613 (1992).
15. Wright, Lawrence. Op cit.
16. Ibid.
17. Pressinger, Richard. "Damaged Sperm & Common Chemical Exposure." 2000. www.chem-tox.com.
18. Ibid.
19. Little, Ruth and Charles Sing. "Father's Drinking Lowers Birth Weight of Babies." *Miami Herald,* June 19, 1986, p. 24A.
20. Strohmer, H., Andrea Boldizsar, and Barbara Plockinger. "Low Sperm Counts and Infertility More Common in Agricultural Workers." *American Journal of Industrial Medicine* 24 (1993): 587-592.
21. Omura, M., M. Hirata, and M. Ahao. "Pesticide Causes Testicle Damage, Reduces Sperm Counts." *Bulletin of Environmental Contamination Toxicology* 55 (1995): pp. 1-7.
22. Scott, Patricia P. J.P. Greaves, and M.G. Scott. "Surprising Testicle/Sperm Abnormalities Appear After Consumption of Chemically Grown Foods." *Journal of Reproductive Fertility* 1 (1960): 130-138.
23. Vine, Marilyn. "Smokers Have Lower Sperm Counts." *Fertility Sterility Journal* 6 no. 1 (1994): 35-43.
24. Joffee, Michael, and Zhimin Li. "Male and Female Factors in Fertility." *American Journal of Epidemiology* 140, no. 10 (1994): 921-928.
25. "Tolerance Develops to the Disruptive Effects of Delta-9 Tetrahydrocannabinol on Primate Menstrual Cycle." *Science* 219, no. 4591 (March 25, 1983).
26. Pressinger, Richard. "Environmental Causes of Infertility." 2000. www.chem-tox.com.
27. Ibid.
28. National Women's Health Information Center. "Infertility." Office on Women's Health in the Department of Health and Human Services. 2000. www.4woman.gov.
29. Pressinger, Richard. Op cit.
30. Ibid.
31. Ibid.
32. Center For Science in the Public Interest. "Caffeine: The Inside Scoop, Infertility." *Nutrition Action Newsletter,* December 1996. www.cspinet.org.
33. Ibid.
34. Pressinger, Richard. Op cit.
35. Baird, Donna D., and Allen J. Wilcox. "Cigarette Smoking Associated with Delayed Conception." *Journal of American Medical Association* 253, no. 20 (1985): 2979-2983.
36. Pizzi, William J., et al. "Reproductive Dysfunction in Male Rats Following Neonatal Administration of Monosodium L-Glutamate." *Neurobehavioral Toxicology* 1(1) (Spring 1979): 1-4.
37. *Fertility and Sterility.* August 2008.
38. *Harvard Health Letter.* October 1992.
39. Pressinger, Richard. Op cit.
40. "Chemical Caution: Miscarriages Are Linked to Two Solvents Used on Microchips." *Time.* October 26, 1992, p. 27.
41. Baranski, Boguslaw. "Conference of the Impact of the Environment and Reproductive Health Held in Denmark September 4, 1991." *Environmental Health Perspectives* 101 (suppl 2) (1993): 85.
42. Ibid.
43. Montague, Peter. "Warning on Male Reproductive Health." *Rachel's Environmental & Health Weekly,* Environmental Research Foundation. April 20, 1995.
44. Pressinger, Richard. Op cit.

Chapter XV - Vaccines

1. Talkaboutcuringautism.org.
2. "Vaccine case draws new attention to autism debate" CNN.com, March 7, 2008.
3. www.909shot.com – website of the National Vaccine Information Center. and, Coulter, HL, Fisher, BL. *A Shot in the Dark: Why the P in DPT Vaccination May be Hazardous to Your Child's Health.* Garden City, Park, NY: Avery Publishing Group, 1991.
4. Coulter, Harris L. and Barbara Loe Fisher. *A Shot in the Dark: Why the P in DPT Vaccination May be Hazardous to Your Child's Health.* Garden City Park, NY. Avery Publishing Group, 1991.
5. McBean, Eleanor. *Poisoned Needle.* Mokelumne Hill, CA. Health Research.
6. Fisher, Barbara Loe. Shots in the dark, Discussion group on…Attempts at Eradicating Infectious Diseases are Putting Our Children at Risk. www.nextcity.com. and
7. www.whale/to/a/edward_jenner.html.
8. World Health Organization, Parents' Forum. Op cit.

9. Douglass, WC. *Lethal Injections: Why Immunizations Don't Work and the Damage They Cause.* Atlanta: Second Opinion Publishing, Inc., 2000.
10. World Health Organization, Parents' Forum. Op cit.
11. "Vaccine Facts." www.access1.net.
12. "Vaccines: The Truth Revealed." www.odomnet.com. and www.vaers.hhs.gov.
13. Office of Special Programs. "National Vaccine Injury Compensation Program Monthly Statistics Report," U.S. Department of Health and Human Services, Health Resources and Services Administration, January 31, 2002. www.hrsa.gov/osp/vicp.
14. Cassel, Ingri. "Vaccinations - Do They Even Work and At What Price?" Vaccination Liberation Conference, Coeur d'Alana, ID. February 8, 2000. www.whale.to/vaccines/cassel.
15. Ostrom, Neenyah. "First Do No Harm, Barbara Loe Fisher and the National Vaccine Information Center Work to Prevent Vaccine-Related Injuries and Deaths by Educating the Public About Rights and Responsibilities." 2000. www.shronicillnet.org.
16. "Vaccine Facts." Op cit.
17. www.909shot.com.
18. Balkan, Michael. "Shoot First and Ask Questions Later." Presented at the 2nd International Public Conference on Vaccination 2000. Arlington, Virginia. October 22, 2000. www.mercola.com.
19. Schlafly, Phyllis. "Congressional Hearing Exposes Conflicts of Interest." June 28, 2000. www.chem-tox.com.
20. Ibid.
21. Balkan, Michael. Op cit.
22. "Vaccine Facts." Op cit.
23. Coulter, Harris, L. *Vaccination, Social Violence, and Criminality: The Medical Assault on the American Brain.* Berkeley, CA: North Atlantic Books, 1990.
24. Ibid.
25. Ibid.
26. Cowart, V.S. "Attention-Deficit Hyperactivity Disorder: Physicians Helping Parents Pay More Heed." *Journal of American Medical Association* 259, no. 18 (May 13, 1988): pp. 2647-2652.
27. Coulter, Harris, L. Op cit.
28. Coulter, Harris L. and Barbara Loe Fisher. Op Cit.
29. Coulter, Harris, L. Op cit.
30. Cowart, V.S. Op cit.
31. Coulter, Harris, L. Op cit.
32. Ibid.
33. Ibid.
34. Workman-Daniels, K.L., et al. "Childhood Problem Behavior and Neuropsychological Functioning in Persons at Risk for Alcoholism." *Journal of Studies on Alcoholism* 43, no. 3 (1987): 187-193.
35. "1 in 150 Children in U.S. Has Autism, New Survey Finds." washingtonpost.com, Feb 9, 2007.
36. Yazbak, Edward F. Autism in the United States: a Perspective. *Journal of American Physicians and Surgeons.* Vol. 8, No. 4. Winter 2003.
37. Ibid. and www.peninsulautism.org/factsheet.htm
38. Schettler, Ted, M.D., M.P.H. and Jill Stein, M.D. *In Harm's Way: Toxic Threats to Child Development.* Boston: Greater Boston Physicians for Social Responsibility, 2000.
39. Autism At a Glance, *USA Today*, Nov. 3, 2008, and Yazbak, Edward F. "Autism 99, A National Emergency." 1999.www.garynull.com.
40. Balkan, Michael. Op cit.
41. Mendelsohn, Robert. *How To Raise A Healthy Child.In Spite of Your Doctor.* Chicago: Contemporary Books, 1984.
42. Keusch, Gerald T. "Vitamin A Supplements—Too Good Not to Be True." *New England Journal of Medicine.* 323, no. 14 (October 4, 1990): 985-987.
43. Coulter, Harris. "Childhood Vaccinations and Juvenile-Onset (Type-1) Diabetes." Testimony before the Congress of the United States, House of Representatives, Committee on Appropriations, Subcommittee on Labor, Health and Human Services, Education, and Related Agencies. April 16, 1997.
44. "Juvenile Diabetes and Vaccination: New Evidence for a Connection." National Vaccine Information Center. 1996. www.909shot.com.
45. Coulter, Harris L. Op cit.
46. Yazbak, Edward F. Autism in the United States: a Perspective. *Journal of American Physicians and Surgeons.* Vol. 8, No. 4. Winter 2003.
47. Ibid.
48. Coulter, Harris, L. Op cit.
49. Ibid.
50. Ibid.
51. Yazbak., Edward F. Autism in the United States: a Perspective. Op cit.
52. www.fda.gov/cber/vaccine/Thimerosal.htm
53. Sircus, MA, "Mercury, Vaccines and Medicine." http://articles.mercola.com/sites/articles/archive/2004/10/30/mercury-vaccines-medicine-part-one.aspx
54. Halsey, Neal A. "Limiting Infant Exposure to Thimerosal in Vaccines and Other Sources of Mercury [Editorial]." *Journal of the American Medical Association* 282, no. 18 (1999):1763-1765.
55. www.fda.gov.
56. Groves, Bob. Op cit.
57. Groves, Bob. "CDC Says Vaccine to be Mercury-Free." The Record Online. Bergen Record Corp. June 16, 2000. www.bergen.com.
58. "Thimerosal." www.whale.to/vaccines/thimerosal.htm.
59. Ibid.
60. Sircus, op Cit.
61. Ibid.
62. Ibid.
63. Sears, A. Doctor's House Call, Feb. 18, 2008
64. "Thimerosal." Op cit.
65. Halsey, Neal A. Op cit.
66. Gibbwake, "Thimerosal in Vaccnes Doesn't Lead to Autism? Black Listed News, January 10, 2008
67. Ibid.
68. "AAP Addresses FDA Review of Vaccines." American Academy of Pediatrics Press Release, July 14, 1999. www.aap.org.
69. Burbacher T, et al., "Comparison of Blood and Brain Mercury Levels in Infant Monkeys Exposed to Methyl mercury or Vaccines Containing Thimerosal. Environmental Health Perspectives. 113:1015-1021. 2005.
70. Harry, GJ et al. "Mercury Concentrations in Brain and Kidney Following Ethyl mercury, Methyl mercury and Thimerosal Administration to Neonatal Mice." Toxicology Letter, Vol. 152, No. 3, Pp. 183-189. 2004.
71. www.whale.to/vaccine/olmsted_h.html and www.ageofautism.com
72. www.aap.org.
73. "No Autism for Unvaccinated Amish? The age of Autism: 'A Pretty big secret'." UPI. December 7, 2005.
74. Madsen KM et al. "*A Population-Based Study of Measles, Mumps, and Rubella Vaccination and Autism.*" New England Journal of Medicine November 7, 2002 (Vol. 347 No. 19
75. www.vaclib.org/news/table1.htm
76. Merck Misled on Vaccines. *LA Times*, March 7, 2005
77. Kasemodel, T. Rebuttal of Misleading Statements. www.ageofautism.com/2008/06/thimerosal-and.html
78. "Study: Counties with more rainfall have higher autism rates." *USA Today*, Nov. 3, 2008
79. Prate, D, The Great Thimerosal cover-up: Mercury, vaccines, autism and your child's health. NaturalNews.com
80. Sircus, op Cit.
81. Ibid.
82. Ibid.
83. Ibid.
84. Prate, D, op Cit.
85. Ibid.
86. www.CDC.gov.
87. Halsey, NA. Op cit.
88. www.CDC.gov.
89. Sircus, op Cit.

90. www.fda.gov/cber/vaccine/thimfaq.htm#q4
91. Gibbwake, op Cit.
92. Kasemodel, T, op cit.
93. "Calculation of Mercury Content in Thimerosal-Containing Vaccines." October 26, 2001. www.whale.to/vaccines/thimerosal3.html.
94. Halsey, NA. Op cit.
95. Sircus, op Cit.
96. www.whale.to/whaley.htms.
97. Ibid.
98. Burton, Dan. "Autism: Present Challenge, Future Needs—Why the Increased Rates?" Opening Statement, Government Reform Committee, U.S. House of Representatives. April 6, 2000.
99. Sircus, op Cit.
100. Ibid.
101. Schettler, Ted, M.D. M.P.H. and Jill Stein, M.D. In Harm's Way: Toxic Threats to Child Development. Boston: Greater Boston Physicians for Social Responsibility, 2000.
102. Healy, Jane M. Endangered Minds: Why Our Children Don't Think. New York: Simon & Schuster, Inc. 1990.
103. Yazbak, F. Edward, and Kathy L. Lang-Radosh. "Adverse Outcomes Associated with Postpartum Rubella or MMR Vaccine." Medical Sentinel 6, no. 3 (2001): 95-99, 108.
104. Yazbak, F. Edward. Personal communication.
105. Yazbak, F. Edward, and Kathy L. Lang-Radosh. Op cit.
106. Yazbak, F. Edward. "Autism 99, A National Emergency." Op cit.
107. Harkins, Don. "Comprehensive, Independent Study Proves MMR Vaccine Link to Nation's Autism Epidemic." Idaho Observer. 4(3) (June 2000), p. 11.
108. Mendelsohn, Robert S. How to Raise a Healthy Child... In Spite of Your Doctor. Contemporary Books, Inc, Chicago, Illinois, 1984.
109. Coulter, Harris L. "Childhood Vaccinations and Juvenile-Onset (Type-1) Diabetes." Testimony before the Congress of the United States, House of Representatives, Committee on Appropriations, subcommittee on Labor, Health and Human Services, Education, and Related Agencies. April 16, 1997.
110. Ibid.
111. Juvenile Diabetes and Vaccination: New Evidence for a Connection. Op cit.
112. Ibid.
113. Ibid.
114. Coulter, Harris L. and Barbara Loe Fisher. Op cit.
115. Ibid.
116. Appleton, Nancy. Rethinking Pasteur's Germ Theory. Frog, Ltd., Berkely, CA. 2002.
117. Coulter, Harris L. and Barbara Loe Fisher. Op cit.
118. Mendelsohn, Robert S. Immunizations: The Terrible Risks Your Children Face That Your Doctor Won't Reveal. Atlanta: Second Opinion Publishing,1993.
119. Mendelsohn, Robert, "The Medical Time Bomb of Immunization Against Disease." East West Journal. November 1984. www.whale.to/vaccines/mendelsohnlhtm.
120. Coulter, Harris L. and Barbara Loe Fisher. Op cit.
121. Mendelsohn, Robert S. How to Raise a Healthy Child... In Spite of Your Doctor. Contemporary Books, Inc, Chicago, Illinois, 1984, p228. Also, Baraff, Larry, Pediatric Infectious Disease, January, 1983.
122. Torch, W.C., American Academy of Neurology 34th Annual Meeting: Diphtheria-pertussis-tetanus (DPT) Immunization: A Potential Cause of the Sudden Infant Death Syndrome (SIDS). Neurology, Vol. 32, No. 4. Pt. 2.
123. "Vaccine Facts." Op cit.
124. Ostrom, Neenyah. Op cit.
125. Coulter, Harris L. and Barbara Loe Fisher. Op cit.
126. "Vaccine Facts." Op cit.
127. Mendelsohn, RS Op cit.
128. Funk & Wagonells New Encyclopedia., 1971. Funk & Wagonells, Inc. N.Y., Vol 19, pp 228-229.
129. Ibid.
130. Mendelsohn, RS. Op cit.
131. Ibid.
132. www.whale.to/v/sandler.html, and, Sandler, Benjamin P. "Diet Prevents Polio." The Lee Foundation for Nutritional Research. 1951.
133. McBean, Eleanor. Poisoned Needle. Op cit.
134. Intensive Immunization Programs, Hearings before the Committee on Interstate & Foreign Commerce, House of Representatives, 87th Congress, 2nd Session on H.R. 10541, Washington, DC, May 1962, Pp 96-97.
135. Los Angeles County Health Index Morbidity & Mortality, Reportable Disease. and; Kent, C, Gentempo P. Immunization: Fact, Myth, and Speculation. International Review of Chiropractic, Nov/Dec 1990.
136. Ibid.
137. Bayly, M. Beddow. The Case Against Vaccination. London: William H. Taylor & Sons, Ltd., June, 1936.
138. "Vaccine Law." www.whale.to vaccines/law.html (click on Barbara Loe Fisher).
139. www.whale.to/vaccines/marchini.html
140. www.whale.to/v/shawl.htm.
141. Nathan Seppa. "The Dark Side of Immunizations? A Controversial Hypothesis Suggests That Vaccines May Abet Diabetes, Asthma." Science News 152, no. 21 (November 22, 1997): 332. November 22, 1997.
142. "Plagued by Cures." The Economist 344, no. 8044 (1997), p. 95.
143. Prevots, Rebecca D., et al. "Outbreaks in Highly Vaccinated Populations: Implications for Studies of Vaccine Performance." American Journal of Epidemiology 146, no. 10 (1997): 881.
144. Tomaselli, KP. "More Parents Refusing to Get Kids Vaccinated." American Medical News, Vol. 7, No. 6., Feb 9, 2004.
145. Schultze, Richard. "Cold and Flu Special Report: Influenza Facts." Get Well Newsletter. November 2000.
146. Mendelsohn, Robert, "The Medical Time Bomb of Immunization Against Disease." East West Journal. November 1984. www.whale.to/vaccines/mendelsohnlhtm.
147. www.909shot.com.
148. National Vaccine Information Center, Opening Statement by Barbara Loe Fisher, Workshop on Risk Communication and Vaccination, May 13, 1996.
149. National Vaccine Information Center, "Statement on Vaccine Safety Research Needs— Perspective From Parents," April 1, 1996. National Vaccine Information Center. 1996.
150. Verner, J.R., et al. Rational Bacteriology, 2nd ed. New York: H. Wolff, 1953. 151. Lavelle, P. Modern Bug Battlegrounds.www.abc.net
152. Vonderplanitz, Aajonus. "What Started Pasteurization?" Right to Choose Healthy Food, 1999. www.odomnet.com/rawmilk.
153. Appleton, Nancy. The Curse of Louis Pasteur—Why Medicine is Not Healing A Diseased World. Santa Monica, CA: Choice Publishing, 1999.
154. Shelton, Herbert M. Human Life, Its Philosophy and Laws, An Exposition of the Principles and Practices of Orthopathy, Mokelumne Hill, CA: Health Research, 1979, p. 194.
155. Ibid, p. 193
156. Ibid, p. 189.
157. Appleton, Nancy. Rethinking Pasteur's Germ Theory. Frog, Ltd., Berkely, CA. 2002.
158. Shelton, HM. Op cit. p. 194.
159. Shelton, HM. Op cit, p. 188.
160. Appleton, N. Op cit.
161. Nightingale, Florence. Notes on Nursing (1859). Reprint. Philadelphia: J.B. Libbincott Company, 1946.
162. Hume, DE. Bechamp or Pasteur: A Lost Chapter in the History of Biology. Kessinger Publishing.
163. Appleton, N. Op cit.
164. Shelton, HM. Op cit., p. 188.
165. "Dr. Stefan Lanka Exposes the 'Viral Fraud,' Pictures of 'Isolated Viruses' Debunked. www.neue-medizin.con/lanka2.
166. Dr;. Med. Ryke Geerd Hamer, German New Medicine.ca.
167. "Human Gut Loaded with More Bacteria than Thought." LiveScience Staff. Nov 18, 2008.
168. www.bio-medicine.org.
169. The Germ Freak's Guide to Outwitting Colds and Flu

170. www.webM.D.com
171. www.textbookofbacteriology.net.
172. www.anapsid.org.
173. "Ten Things You Need to Know About Immunizations." National Immunization Program. Centers for Disease Control and Prevention. March 28, 2000. www.cdc.gov.
174. Shelton, Herbert M. Op cit., p. 191.
175. Ibid, p. 192.
176. Ibid, p. 193.
177. Ibid.
178. Oral Bacteria and Dental Caries, Bacteriology.suite101.com. June 23, 2008
179. Vonderplanitz, Aajonus.*The Recipe for Living Without Disease.* Carnelian Bay Castle Press, LLC, 2002.
180. Ibid.
181. Anglen, R."Scientist Linked to Heimlich Investigated." *Cincinnati Enquirer.* Feb. 16, 2003.
182. "Bacteria that Help Fight Cancer." *Chemistry World,* Nov. 23, 2006
183. Chakrabarty, AM. "Microorganisms and Cancer: Quest for a Therapy." *J Bacteriol.* 2003 May; 185(9):2683-2686
184. *Postgraduate Medical Journal* 2003;79:672-680.
185. West, E. "Is Fear of Fever Hurting Our Children?" VRAN Newssletter, Jan-Mar, 2003. www.whale.to/a/west8.html and Health Canada Advisory, Feb 13, 2003. www.hc-sc.gc.ca/english/iyh/.
186. Mendelsohn, RS. Op cit.
187. Kluger, MJ. "Fever." *Pediatrics.* 1980 Nov;66(5):720-4.
188. Incao, P. National Vaccine Information Center (NVIC) Conference, Alexandria, VA, April, 2000.
189. Ibid.
190. Klarin B, et al. "Use of the Probiotic Lactobacillus planarum 299 to Reduce Pathogenic Bacteria in the Oropharynx of Intubated Patients: a Randomised Controlled Open Pilot Study." Critical Care 12(6), R136, Nov 6, 2008
191. Kligler B, Cohrssen A, "Probiotics." American Family Physician Nov 1 2008 Vol.78 No.9, 1073-1078) and ("Findings May Help Patients Better Tolerate Antibiotcs: Albert Einstein College of Medicine, Dec 17, 2008
192. http://www.whale.to/vaccines/tilden.html.
193. www.whale.to/v/shawl.htm.
194. www.whale.to/vaccines.
195. Trall, RT., "The True Healing Art: Or, Hygienic vs. Drug Medication. An Address Delivered at the Smithsonion Institute," Washington, D.C. New York, Fowler & Wells, Reprinted 1880. http://www.whale.to/v/trall.htm and Soil and Health Library, www.soilandhealth.org.

Chapter XII -The Ancestry Factor
1. Montague, Peter. "Chemicals and Health—Part 1," *Rachel's Environmental & Health Weekly,* Environmental Research Foundation. December 23, 1993.
2. Pottenger, Francis M. *Pottenger's Cats: A Study in Nutrition.* La Mesa, CA: Price-Pottenger Nutrition Foundation, Inc. 1983, p. 10.
3. Ibid, p. 11.
4. Price-Pottenger Nutrition Foundation, Resource Catalog, Spring/Summer 1999.
5. Pottenger, Francis M. Op cit., p. 11.
6. www.beyondveg.com.
7. Sears, B. *Doctor's House Call Newsletter,* November 27, 2006.
8. Redmon, George S. "Minding the Minerals." *Healthy & Natural,* October 2000, p. 92.
9. Ibid.
10. Buttram, Harold. Personal communication.
11. Baer, Firman, Stephen J. Toth, and Arthur L. Prince. "Variation in Mineral Composition of Vegetables." *Soil Science Society of America* 13, 1949.
12. Smith, Bob L. "Organic Foods vs. Supermarket Foods: Element Levels." *Journal of Applied Nutrition* 45, no. 1 (1993).
13. Chengsheng L, et al. "Organic Diets Significantly Lower Children's Dietary Exposure to Organophosphorus Pesticides." Envir Health Perspectives. Vol 114, No. 2,Feb 2006.
14. Pottenger, Francis M. Op cit. p. 13.

Chapter XIII—Alternative Health Land Mines
1. O'Shea, Tim. "Soy Con: Soy is Not a Health Food." *Alternative Medicine,* no. 41 (May 2001): 51-65.
2. Ibid.
3. Ibid.
4. Ibid.
5.Abrams, Leon H. "Vegetarianism: An Anthropological/Nutritional Evaluation." *Journal of Applied Nutrition* 32, no. 2 (1980).
6. Ibid.
7. Kiple, Kenneth F, and Krienhild Conee Ornelas, eds. *Vegetarianism: Another View. Cambridge World History of Food, vol. 2.* Cambridge: Cambridge University Press, 2000, pp. 1564-1571.
8. Page, Melvin E., and H.Leon Abrams, Jr. *Your Body is Your Best Doctor!* New Canaan, CT: Keats Publishing, Inc., 1972, p. 215.
9. Ibid, p. 216.
10. Ibid, p.215.
11. Fallon, Sally, and Mary G. Enig, Ph.D. *Nourishing Traditions,* Washington, DC: New Trends Publishing, Inc. 1999, p. 47.
12. Bass, Stanley S., "Interview with Aajonus Voderplanitz." *Super Nutrition & Superior Health.* Jan, 2000. www.drbass.com.
13. Ibid.
14. Ibid.
15. Kiple, Kenneth F. and Krienhild Conee Ornelas, eds. Op cit., pp.1564-1571.
16. Ibid.
17. Fallon, Sally, and Mary G. Enig, Ph.D. Op cit. p. 28.
18. Langer, Stephen E. and James F. Scheer. *Solved: The Riddle of Illness.* New Canaan, CT: Keats Publishing, Inc. 1984, p. 52.
19. Ibid, p. 77.
20.Fallon, Sally and Mary G. Enig, Ph.D. Op cit., p. 28.
21. Ibid, p. 250.
22. Ibid, p. 245.
23. Ibid, pp. 253, 288.
24. Ibid, p. 113.
25. Ibid, p. 10.
26. Ibid, pp. 11,19.
27. Ibid, p. 20.

Chapter XIV—How to Prevent and Reverse Disease
1. *The H.O.P.E. Report.* p. 1-b-11. Health Excel, Inc.
2. Fallon, Sally and Mary G. Enig, Ph.D. *Nourishing Traditions.* 2nd ed. Washington, DC: New Trends Publishing, Inc. 1999, p. 68.
3. Wayne, Anthony, and Lawrence Newell. The Christian Law Institute. http://lawgiver.org.
4. PPNF News, "Food for Thought, But Not for Humans." *Health & Healing Wisdom, Journal of the Price-Pott Nut Fnd.* 22, no. 4 (Winter 1998): 17
5. Ibid, p. 19.
6. Fallon, Sally and Mary G. Enig, Ph.D. Op cit., p. 80.
7. Owens, Darryl. "Lack of Sleep Hurts Child's Grades." *Orlando Sentinel.* As quoted in *Caring for Your School-Age Child: Ages 5 to 12, Rev. Ed.* edited by Edward L. Schor, M.D. New York: Broadway Books, 1999.
8. EPA, *Lead In Your Home: A Parent's Reference Guide. EPA 747-B-99-003, May 1999.*
9. Brewitt, Barbara, and H. Hynn Amsbury, "MMR Vaccine and Autism." *Well Being Journal* 10, no. 3 (Summer 2000): 1.
10. Upledger, John E. *An Etiologic Model for Autism.* Committee on Government Reform, Rep. Dan Burton Chairman. www.house.gov/reform/hearings/healthcare/00.06.04/upledger.htm.

Index

2

2,4,5-T, 41
2,4-D, 40, 44

A

acetylcholine, 247, 317, 324, 325, 337
acid reflux, 17, 18, 225, 362
acne, 15, 140, 213, 256, 313, 352
AD. *See* Alzheimer's disease
ADD, 226, 230, 270, 276, 277, 284, 329
ADHD, i, v, 15, 86, 226, 227, 228, 229, 230,
    231, 234, 236, 237, 238, 245, 252, 253,
    254, 255, 256, 257, 262, 263, 264, 266,
    267, 269, 270-89, 291, 294, 308, 326,
    329, 355, 419, 420, 497
adolescence, vi, 87, 133, 142, 183, 267, 272,
    350
Adverse Reaction Monitoring System, 53
Advisory Committee on Immunization
    Practices (ACIP), 397
Agency for Toxic Substances and Disease
    Registry, 238, 249, 355, 375, 376, 415
Agent Orange, 41, 187
aggressive behavior, 22, 23, 24, 42, 76, 153,
    188, 234, 239, 240, 243, 289
agnosia, 323
agoraphobia, 291
AIDS, 58, 115, 185, 345
air fresheners, 47, 88
air pollutants, 212
air pollution, 6, 47, 210, 225, 326, 375
alcohol, 59, 61, 78, 87, 90, 97, 106, 110,
    112, 127, 134, 147, 150, 154, 176, 189,
    202, 204, 215, 229, 241, 243, 244, 249,
    257, 333, 334, 347, 350, 361, 369, 370,
    374, 382, 384, 385, 388, 400, 438, 465
allergens, 212, 262
allergies, 15, 41, 54, 123, 131, 159, 200,
    202, 209, 210, 215, 216, 252, 256, 257,
    258, 259, 261, 262, 263, 367, 374, 394,
    396, 404, 424, 444, 454, 463, 464, 468,
    489
alpha-1 blockers, 90
Aluminum, 251, 326, 474
Alzheimer's disease, 47, 58, 95, 99, 100,
    128, 158, 177, 251, 291, **322-36**, 337,
    338, 340
amalgam fillings, 245, 246, 247, 248, 249,
    326, 405

amalgams, 245, 247, 249, 250, 496
Ambies, 360
American Academy of Child and
    Adolescent Psychiatry, 279
American Academy of Pediatrics, 21, 22,
    237, 238, 258, 279, 391, 403, 406, 420,
    424
American Chemical Society (ACS), 35, 141
American Dental Association, 247, 250,
    354, 405
American Diabetes Association, 57, 62, 183
American Medical Association (AMA), 2,
    21, 95, 117, 128, 149, 209, 239, 346, 353,
    373, 400, 420, 457
American Psychological Association, 23,
    24, 279
amnesia, 188, 294, 322
amphetamines, 273, 275, 277
anemia, 176, 177, 179, 180, 238, 241, 258,
    332, 341, 477, 480
anencephaly, 380
anger, 41, 247, 249, 317
angina pectoris, 144
animal food, 477, 478, 481
animal products, 160, 251, 332, 334, 451,
    477, 478, 479, 482, 483, 485
anorexia nervosa, 291
antacids, 17, 326, 340, 362
antibiotics, v, 128, 129, 253, 260, 389, 396,
    444, 454, 456
antidepressants, 63, 128, 129, 139, 277, 293,
    294, 295, 298, 299, 300, 301, 302, 310,
    361
Anti-Malignant Antibody Screen (AMAS),
    120
aphasia, 323
aphrodisiacs, 109, 170, 451
apple cider vinegar, 17, 18, 19, 20, 49, 80,
    104, 146, 207, 327, 347, 485
arachidonic acid, 161, 255
arginine, 80, 110, 111
arsenic, 49, 52, 65, 78, 83, 137, 222, 376,
    377
arteriolosclerosis, 55
arteriosclerosis, 108, 164
arthritis, v, 8, 12, 15, 16, 18, 20, 55, 72, 100,
    104, 164, 168, 170, 213, 218, 219, 259,
    294, 303, 320, 332, 338, 344, 345, 346,
    347, 348, **344–49**, 351, 358, 364, 366,
    368, 462, 463, 482, 493
artificial colors, 231
artificial insemination, 385
aseptic meningitis, 401, 428

Great Publications from PRI Publishing

To Order, Call 24 hours: **(419) 869-7901** or Fax (419) 869-7935
Email: proreach@aol.com
MasterCard, Visa Accepted

PRI Publishing
Suite 183
1130 E. Main Street,
Ashland, OH 44805

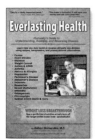
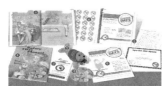
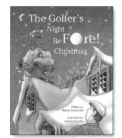
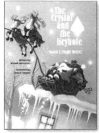